AF326903

IADVL Textbook of Pemphigus and other Autoimmune Bullous Diseases

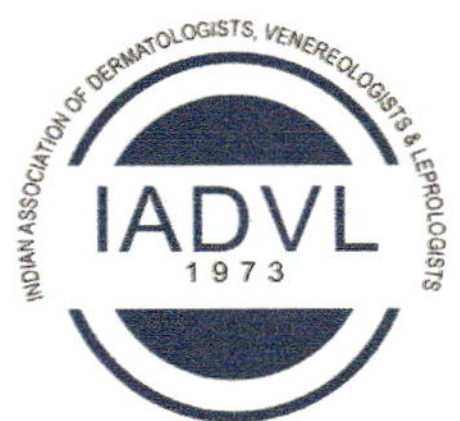

Indian Association of Dermatologists, Venereologists and Leprologists

IADVL Textbook of Pemphigus and other Autoimmune Bullous Diseases

Editor-in-Chief

Sujay Khandpur MD DNB MNAMS
Professor
Department of Dermatology and Venereology
All India Institute of Medical Sciences
New Delhi, India

Associate Editors

Raghavendra Rao MD DNB
Professor and Head
Department of Dermatology, Venereology and Leprosy
Kasturba Medical College
Manipal Academy of Higher Education (MAHE)
Manipal, Karnataka, India

Vinay Keshavamurthy MD DNB MNAMS MRCP FRCP (London)
Associate Professor
Department of Dermatology, Venereology and Leprology
Postgraduate Institute of Medical Education and Research
Chandigarh, India

Assistant Editors

Atiya Yaseen MD DVD
Medical Officer, Dermatologist
Department of Health and Medical Education
Sub District Hospital Pampore
Jammu & Kashmir, India

Saritha Mohanan MD DNB
Associate Professor
Department of Dermatology, Venereology and Leprosy
Indira Gandhi Medical College and Research Institute
Kathirkamam, Puducherry, India

Foreword

Takashi Hashimoto

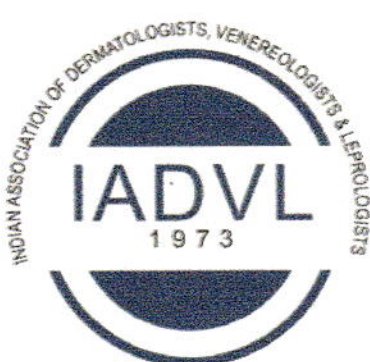

Under the Aegis of IADVL Academy

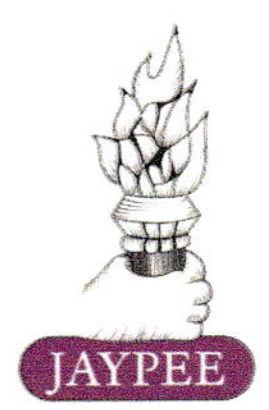

JAYPEE BROTHERS MEDICAL PUBLISHERS
The Health Sciences Publisher
New Delhi | London

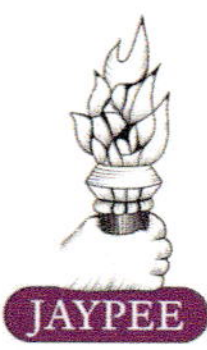

Jaypee Brothers Medical Publishers (P) Ltd

Headquarters

EMCA House
23/23-B, Ansari Road, Daryaganj
New Delhi 110 002, India
Landline: +91-11-23272143, +91-11-23272703
+91-11-23282021, +91-11-23245672
E-mail: jaypee@jaypeebrothers.com

Corporate Office

Jaypee Brothers Medical Publishers (P) Ltd.
4838/24, Ansari Road, Daryaganj
New Delhi 110 002, India
Phone: +91-11-43574357
Fax: +91-11-43574314
E-mail: jaypee@jaypeebrothers.com

Overseas Office

JP Medical Ltd.
83, Victoria Street, London
SW1H 0HW (UK)
Phone: +44-20 3170 8910
Fax: +44(0)20 3008 6180
E-mail: info@jpmedpub.com

Website: www.jaypeebrothers.com
Website: www.jaypeedigital.com

© 2024, IADVL - Indian Association of Dermatologists, Venereologists and Leprologists

The views and opinions expressed in this book are solely those of the original contributor(s)/author(s) and do not necessarily represent those of editor(s) or publisher of the book.

All rights reserved. No part of this publication may be reproduced, stored or transmitted in any form or by any means, electronic, mechanical, photocopying, recording or otherwise, without the prior permission in writing of the publishers.

All brand names and product names used in this book are trade names, service marks, trademarks or registered trademarks of their respective owners. The publisher is not associated with any product or vendor mentioned in this book.

Medical knowledge and practice change constantly. This book is designed to provide accurate, authoritative information about the subject matter in question. However, readers are advised to check the most current information available on procedures included and check information from the manufacturer of each product to be administered, to verify the recommended dose, formula, method and duration of administration, adverse effects and contraindications. It is the responsibility of the practitioner to take all appropriate safety precautions. Neither the publisher nor the author(s)/editor(s) assume any liability for any injury and/or damage to persons or property arising from or related to use of material in this book.

This book is sold on the understanding that the publisher is not engaged in providing professional medical services. If such advice or services are required, the services of a competent medical professional should be sought.

Every effort has been made where necessary to contact holders of copyright to obtain permission to reproduce copyright material. If any have been inadvertently overlooked, the publisher will be pleased to make the necessary arrangements at the first opportunity.

Inquiries for bulk sales may be solicited at: jaypee@jaypeebrothers.com

IADVL Textbook of Pemphigus and other Autoimmune Bullous Diseases / *Sujay Khandpur*

First Edition: **2024**

ISBN: 978-93-5696-144-9

Printed in India

Dedication

*To my late parents Jayanti and Subhash, my teachers, my wife Shaifali,
and children Saanchi and Shaurya.*
—Sujay Khandpur

*To my late father Haridas Rao and my dear mother Mohini Rao,
my wife Dr Chythra, and our children Pranav and Prateeksha.*
—Raghavendra Rao

To my loving wife Ashwini and daughters Aarya and Ahana.
—Vinay Keshavamurthy

*To my late mother who instilled in me that I can do anything I set my mind to
and that could only be accomplished if I work hard.*
—Atiya Yaseen

To our patients whose suffering teaches us many things.
—Saritha Mohanan

Contributors

EDITOR-IN-CHIEF

Sujay Khandpur MD DNB MNAMS
Professor
Department of Dermatology and Venereology
All India Institute of Medical Sciences
New Delhi, India

ASSOCIATE EDITORS

Raghavendra Rao MD DNB
Professor and Head
Department of Dermatology, Venereology and Leprosy
Kasturba Medical College
Manipal Academy of Higher Education (MAHE)
Manipal, Karnataka, India

Vinay Keshavamurthy MD DNB MNAMS MRCP FRCP (London)
Associate Professor
Department of Dermatology, Venereology and Leprology
Postgraduate Institute of Medical Education and Research
Chandigarh, India

ASSISTANT EDITORS

Atiya Yaseen MD DVD
Medical Officer, Dermatologist
Department of Health and Medical Education
Sub District Hospital Pampore
Jammu & Kashmir, India

Saritha Mohanan MD DNB
Associate Professor
Department of Dermatology, Venereology and Leprosy
Indira Gandhi Medical College and Research Institute
Kathirkamam, Puducherry, India

CONTRIBUTING AUTHORS

Abir Saraswat MD DNB MNAMS
Consultant Dermatologist
Department of Dermatology
Indushree Skin Clinic
Lucknow, Uttar Pradesh, India

Ajithkumar Kidangazhiathmana MD DD FRCP (London) FRCP (Edinburgh)
Professor
Department of Dermatology, Venereology and Leprosy
Government Medical College
Kottayam, Kerala, India

Alpana Sharma PhD FAMS FIABS
Professor
Department of Biochemistry
All India Institute of Medical Sciences
New Delhi, India

Amitha Ramesh MDS
Professor and Head
Department of Periodontics
AB Shetty Memorial Institute of Dental Sciences
NITTE Deemed-to be-University
Deralakatte, Mangaluru, Karnataka, India

Ananya Sharma MD DNB MRCP (SCE)
Senior Resident
Department of Dermatology and Venereology
All India Institute of Medical Sciences
New Delhi, India

Anuradha Bishnoi MD FRCP
Assistant Professor
Department of Dermatology, Venereology and Leprology
Postgraduate Institute of Medical Education and Research
Chandigarh, India

Contributors

Atiya Yaseen MD DVD
Medical Officer, Dermatologist
Department of Health and Medical
Education
Sub District Hospital Pampore
Jammu & Kashmir, India

Bhavya Swarnkar MD DNB
Former Senior Resident
Department of Dermatology and
Venereology
All India Institute of Medical Sciences
New Delhi, India

Binod K Khaitan MD FAMS
Professor
Department of Dermatology and
Venereology
All India Institute of Medical Sciences
New Delhi, India

C Udayashankar MD MBA
Professor and Head
Department of Dermatology,
Venereology and Leprosy
Indira Gandhi Medical College and
Research Institute
Kathirkamam, Puducherry, India

Chandana Shajil MD DNB
Assistant Professor
Department of Dermatology,
Venereology and Leprosy
Sri Venkateswaraa Medical College
Hospital and Research Institute
Nallur, Chennai, Tamil Nadu, India

Chitra Shivanand Nayak MD DDV
DHA AFIH
Professor and Head
Department of Dermatology
Topiwala National Medical College and
BYL Nair Charitable Hospital
Mumbai, Maharashtra, India

Debajyoti Chatterjee MD DM
Assistant Professor
Department of Histopathology
Postgraduate Institute of Medical
Education and Research
Chandigarh, India

Deepika Pandhi MD FAMS
Director Professor
Department of Dermatology and STD
University College of Medical Sciences
and Guru Teg Bahadur Hospital
Delhi, India

Dharshini Sathishkumar MD DDVL
Fellowship in Pediatric Dermatology
(Birmingham, UK)
Professor
Department of Dermatology
Christian Medical College and Hospital
Vellore, Tamil Nadu, India

Dipankar De MD
Professor
Department of Dermatology,
Venereology and Leprology
Postgraduate Institute of Medical
Education and Research
Chandigarh, India

Gayatri Vitthal Gund MD
Senior Resident
Department of Dermatology
Topiwala National Medical College and
BYL Nair Charitable Hospital
Mumbai, Maharashtra, India

Geethanjali S MD DNB PDCC (Pediatric
Dermatology) MRCP (SCE)
Assistant Professor
Department of Dermatology,
Venereology and Leprosy
Government Medical College
Kottayam, Kerala, India

Geeti Khullar MD DNB
Assistant Professor
Department of Dermatology and STD
Lady Hardinge Medical College and
Associated Hospitals
New Delhi, India

Hitaishi Mehta MD DNB MRCP (SCE)
Senior Resident
Department of Dermatology,
Venereology and Leprology
Postgraduate Institute of Medical
Education and Research
Chandigarh, India

Krina Bharat Patel MD DVD
Professor and Head
Department of Dermatology
GMERS Medical College, Sola
Ahmedabad, Gujarat, India

Kyle T Amber MD FAAD
Assistant Professor and Director of the
Dermatology Infusion Center
Department of Dermatology and
Internal Medicine
Rush University Medical Center
Chicago, Illinois, USA

Laxmisha Chandrashekar MD DNB
Professor
Department of Dermatology and
Venereology
Jawaharlal Institute of Postgraduate
Medical Education and Research
Puducherry, India

Luca Borradori MD
Chairman and Professor
Department of Dermatology
University Hospital of Bern
Bern, Switzerland

Minu Jose Chiramel MD DNB PDF
(Pediatric Dermatology)
Assistant Professor
Department of Dermatology
Christian Medical College and Hospital
Vellore, Tamil Nadu, India

M Ramam MD
Professor
Department of Dermatology and
Venereology
All India Institute of Medical Sciences
New Delhi, India

Neha Taneja MD DNB MRCP (SCE)
Assistant Professor
Department of Dermatology and
Venereology
All India Institute of Medical Sciences
New Delhi, India

Neirita Hazarika MD
Additional Professor and Head
Department of Dermatology,
Venereology and Leprosy
All India Institute of Medical Sciences
Rishikesh, Uttarakhand, India

Pallavi Hegde MD
Senior Resident
Department of Dermatology
Kasturba Medical College, Manipal
Manipal Academy of Higher Education
Manipal, Karnataka, India

Pooja Desai MD
Senior Resident
Department of Dermatology
GMERS Medical College, Sola
Ahmedabad, Gujarat, India

Raghavendra Rao MD DNB
Professor and Head
Department of Dermatology
Kasturba Medical College
Manipal Academy of Higher Education
(MAHE)
Manipal, Karnataka, India

Rahul Mahajan MD FRCP (Edinburgh)
Associate Professor
Department of Dermatology,
Venereology and Leprology
Postgraduate Institute of Medical
Education and Research
Chandigarh, India

Rajat Choudhary MD
Senior Resident
Department of Dermatology and
Venereology
All India Institute of Medical Sciences
New Delhi, India

Ramesh Bhat M MD DVD DNB MNAMS
Professor and Vice Dean
Father Muller Medical College
Mangaluru, Karnataka, India

Rashmi Sarkar MD FAMS
Director Professor
Department of Dermatology,
Venereology and Leprosy,
Lady Hardinge Medical College and
associated Hospitals
New Delhi, India

Rhea Ahuja MD DNB
Senior Resident
Department of Dermatology and
Venereology
All India Institute of Medical Sciences
New Delhi, India

Riti Bhatia MD
Assistant Professor
Department of Dermatology,
Venereology and Leprosy
All India Institute of Medical Sciences
Rishikesh, Uttarakhand, India

Rochelle C Monteiro MD
Associate Professor
Department of Dermatology
Father Muller Medical College
Mangaluru, Karnataka, India

Sanjeev Handa MD FAMS FAAD
FRCP (Edinburgh)
Professor (HAG) and Head
Department of Dermatology,
Venereology and Leprology
Postgraduate Institute of Medical
Education and Research
Chandigarh, India

Saritha Mohanan MD DNB
Associate Professor
Department of Dermatology,
Venereology and Leprosy
Indira Gandhi Medical College and
Research Institute
Kathirkamam, Puducherry, India

Shikha Shah MD DNB
Senior Resident
Department of Dermatology,
Venereology and Leprology
Postgraduate Institute of Medical
Education and Research
Chandigarh, India

Sonal Sachan MD
Assistant Professor
Department of Dermatology,
Venereology and Leprosy
Hind Institute of Medical Sciences
Barabanki, Uttar Pradesh, India

Sujay Khandpur MD DNB MNAMS
Professor
Department of Dermatology and
Venereology
All India Institute of Medical Sciences
New Delhi, India

Sunil Dogra MD DNB FAMS FAAD Dip
Dermatology (Glasgow) FRCP (London)
FRCP (Edinburgh)
Professor
Department of Dermatology,
Venereology and Leprology
Postgraduate Institute of Medical
Education and Research
Chandigarh, India

Swastika Suvirya MD
Additional Professor and Head
Department of Dermatology,
Venereology and Leprosy
King George's Medical University
Lucknow, Uttar Pradesh, India

Takashi Hashimoto MD
Specially Appointed Professor
Department of Dermatology
Osaka Metropolitan University
Graduate School of Medicine
Abeno, Osaka, Japan

Vignesh Narayan R MD
Senior Resident
Department of Dermatology,
Venereology and Leprosy,
MS Ramaiah Institute of Medical
Sciences
Bengaluru, Karnataka, India

Vinay Keshavamurthy MD DNB MNAMS
MRCP FRCP (London)
Associate Professor
Department of Dermatology,
Venereology and Leprology
Postgraduate Institute of Medical
Education and Research
Chandigarh, India

Vishakha Hooda MSc
PhD Student
Department of Biochemistry
All India Institute of Medical Sciences
New Delhi, India

Vishal Gaurav MD DNB
Senior Resident
Department of Dermatology and
Venereology
All India Institute of Medical Sciences
New Delhi, India

Vishal Gupta MD
Assistant Professor
Department of Dermatology and
Venereology
All India Institute of Medical Sciences
New Delhi, India

Xiaoguang Li MD
Associate Professor
Department of Laboratory Medicine
Chronic Disease Research Center,
Medical College, Dalian University
Dalian, Liaoning, China

Message from the President, IADVL 2022

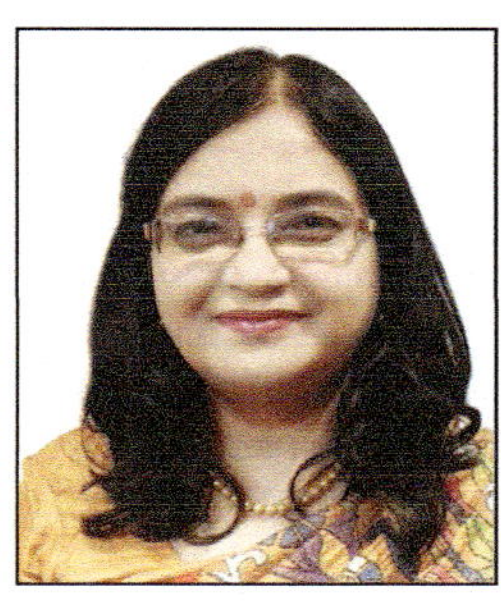

Dr Rashmi Sarkar MD FAMS
President, IADVL 2022
LM/ND/1543

Dear IADVL members,

The year 2022 was special since it marked 50 years of the Indian Association of Dermatologists, Venereologists and Leprologists (IADVL) or Golden Jubilee Year of IADVL. Out of all the Presidential projects, I felt that in India, we still face a challenge treating pemphigus and other immunobullous diseases. We do have a rich knowledge of this disease, but do not have a textbook to do justice to the topic. Hence, it was decided to take up this project on *"IADVL Textbook of Pemphigus and other Autoimmune Bullous Diseases"*. I am very glad it has Dr Sujay Khandpur as the eminent editor, who has worked extensively on this topic with Dr Raghavendra Rao and Dr Vinay Keshavamurthy as the Associate Editors and Dr Atiya Yaseen and Dr Saritha Mohanan as the Assistant Editors. The book is divided into several sections and chapters written by both national and international experts. We hope this book is able to fill the gaps in the subject and satisfy institutional colleagues, private practitioners, and postgraduates in the subject. I wish you all have happy reading and congratulate the editorial board for their hard work.

Long live IADVL!

Message from the IADVL Academy

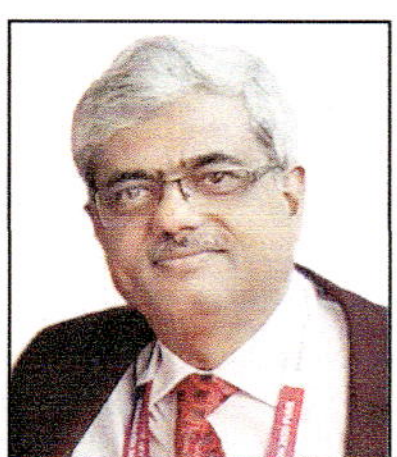

Lalit Kumar Gupta MD FAAD
Chairperson, IADVL Academy 2022–2023
Senior Professor
Department of Dermatology
RNT Medical College
Udaipur, Rajasthan, India

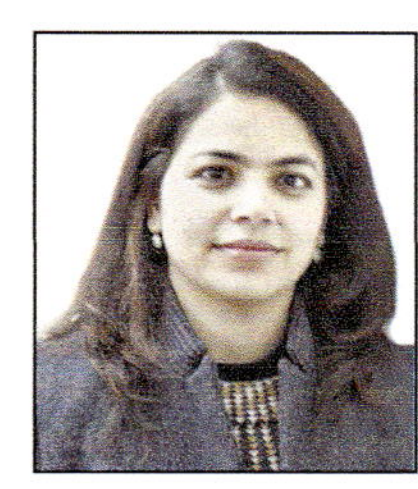

Rashmi Jindal MD
Convener, IADVL Academy 2022–2023
Professor
Department of Dermatology, Venereology
and Leprosy
Himalayan Institute of Medical Sciences
Dehradun, Uttarakhand, India

We are happy to learn that the much awaited, first edition of *"IADVL Textbook of Pemphigus and other Autoimmune Bullous Diseases"* is being released.

The autoimmune bullous diseases (AIBD) are common in India as well as globally and pose a huge diagnostic and therapeutic challenge. A comprehensive textbook on this subject, particularly in the Indian population was a long felt need and this master piece written by eminent experts in the field of autoimmune bullous diseases will certainly fill this void and help clinicians in managing these diseases better.

We recognize and deeply appreciate the hard work of the editorial team led by Professor Sujay Khandpur (Editor-in-Chief), Dr Raghavendra Rao, Dr Vinay Keshavamurthy (Associate Editors) and Dr Atiya Yaseen, Dr Saritha Mohanan (Assistant Editors) in meticulously designing the contents and systematically compiling and editing the book well in time. We also sincerely thank and acknowledge the contribution of all the erudite authors who spared their time in sharing their wisdom and expertise with the readers.

The book covers all the aspects of AIBDs, from basics, clinical, diagnostic, and therapeutic aspects in a very practical and easy to understand manner using high quality clinical images, tables, and flowcharts.

We are sure the book will serve as a reference book and a "must have resource" on the desk of every dermatologist and clinician caring for the patients with AIBDs. We wish the book *"IADVL Textbook of Pemphigus and other Autoimmune Bullous Diseases"* a great success.

Happy reading!!

Foreword

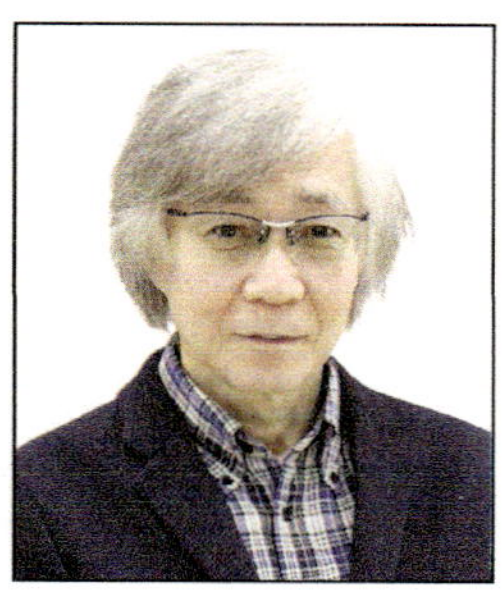

Takashi Hashimoto MD
Specially Appointed Professor
Department of Dermatology
Osaka Metropolitan University
Graduate School of Medicine
Abeno, Osaka, Japan
E-mail: *hashyt@gmail.com*

Pemphigus and other autoimmune bullous diseases (AIBDs) are intractable and potentially fatal tissue-specific autoimmune diseases of the skin, which are characterized clinically by mucocutaneous blistering lesions. This group of diseases is classified into two subgroups, i.e., intraepidermal immunobullous diseases (pemphigus diseases) and subepidermal immunobullous diseases (pemphigoid diseases), which show IgG and/or IgA autoantibodies against keratinocyte cell surfaces and epidermal basement membrane zone, respectively. Various biochemical studies have identified a number of different autoantigens of the skin, leading to the development of distinct diagnostic methods. Various in vitro and in vivo experimental models have clarified the pathogenic mechanisms in these diseases, leading to the development of novel therapies.

Pemphigus and AIBDs are first suspected by clinical and histopathological features, and then various immunological examinations make the final diagnosis. The accurate diagnoses are essential for the best treatments for the patients of this group of diseases.

The *"IADVL Textbook of Pemphigus and other Autoimmune Bullous Diseases"*, edited by Professor Sujay Khandpur and other associate and assistant editors, has been written by both Indian and international experts in the field of immunobullous diseases. This textbook is aimed to be a comprehensive textbook mainly for dermatology postgraduates and dermatologists, who are in-charge of clinical practice of these diseases.

This textbook combines all the topics on scientific advances, clinical presentations, diagnostic methods, and managements of this group of diseases. The textbook is prepared very systematically, utilizing many figures, tables, flowcharts, and therapeutic algorithms, which makes it very easy to read. Although this textbook has been originally prepared for the Indian readers, I am convinced that it will be extremely useful as a reference book for the clinical practice of pemphigus and other AIBDs, not only for Indian dermatological practitioners but also for all dermatologists in the world. I wish the editors and authors great success.

Osaka, Japan, February 2023

Preface

Sitting in a busy dermatology OPD, we see a plethora of cases of pemphigus and other autoimmune bullous diseases. Though some come to us at early stages with only occasional blisters or mucosal ulcers, the majority present with extensive denudation associated with pain, itching, and secondary infection. These patients are sick and sometimes present as a dermatological emergency that requires prompt intervention to avoid serious consequences. They form a significant proportion of our inpatients. We also encounter patients with mucocutaneous blistering due to other causes, being inadvertently treated as pemphigus and vice versa, both situations being deleterious to them. To add to the burden, in India unlike the west, this group of diseases affects a relatively younger population causing misery among the working community. Justifiably, significant emphasis is given to this subject during postgraduate training. In fact, no residency exit examination is complete without these diseases being extensively discussed as either a long case, a spotter, slide examination for histopathological features, medical management, or nursing care. To cater to the needs of this group of patients, the tertiary centers of our country that see the bulk of these patients, have tried to equip themselves with the requisite facilities, with access to good nursing care and sophisticated medications, and some departments have devised innovative treatment regimens. Many centers run special clinics and laboratories to prioritize management of these diseases. Significant research on different aspects is being undertaken. Treatment guidelines have also been formulated.

Remarkable work on this subject has been done globally, and extensive literature is available. However, it mostly caters to the needs of specific demographic regions which may not be relevant to our population or situations. Hence, IADVL felt the need to bring out comprehensive literature on this subject in the form of a book that encompasses all aspects, in an easy-to-read format. This book has brought together specialists in the field of autoimmune bullous diseases from all over our country to document their experiences, along with experiences shared by international experts. Clinical images of our own patients supplemented with tables, flowcharts, and line diagrams have been incorporated for better understanding.

This work is a culmination of the experience gathered from our seniors and teachers who have done exhaustive work in the field, long hours of deliberations and discussions with our colleagues and students, information assimilated from world authorities, and most of all, through our stories of success and failures in treating our patients. We hope that this book finds a place of pride on your table.

Sujay Khandpur
Raghavendra Rao
Vinay Keshavamurthy
Atiya Yaseen
Saritha Mohanan

Acknowledgments

I am very fortunate to have received guidance from wonderful teachers like Professor BSN Reddy, Professor JS Pasricha, Professor Vinod K Sharma and Professor M Ramam who inculcated my interest and gave me several opportunities in the field of immunobullous diseases. I have always admired their passion, dedication, and knowledge. I feel blessed to have had parents who were my ideals and who provided me a very loving and conducive environment to fulfil my dreams and passions. My gratitude to my wife Dr Shaifali and children Saanchi and Shaurya for their immense love and selfless support.

Sujay Khandpur

I would like to acknowledge my colleagues in the department and all my teachers. I also would like to remember (Late) Balbir S Bhogal (former scientist, Immunodermatology Laboratory, St John's Institute of Dermatology, Guys and St Thomas Hospital, London, UK) for teaching me the finer aspect of immunological diagnosis of AIBDs. A gem of a person he was!

Raghavendra Rao

I would like to acknowledge Professor Amrinder J Kanwar for mentoring during the early days of my career.

Vinay Keshavamurthy

The *IADVL Textbook of Pemphigus and other Autoimmune Bullous Diseases* is very close to my heart as it is the first book for which I am the one of the editorial board members. I am optimistic that it will serve the purpose of catering dermatology postgraduates and practicing dermatologists. I would like to express my special appreciation to the Editor-in-Chief, Professor Sujay Khandpur whose able guidance was pivotal for editing this book. My special thanks goes to all other members of the editorial team for their efforts. I especially like to thank my family—my beloved husband and my kids who have encouraged me throughout this experience. Their prayers and love for me is what sustained me thus far. I thank God for letting me through all difficulties.

Atiya Yaseen

I am grateful to my teachers, who were inspiring and encouraging. I am grateful to my parents who always supported me. I will not be able to do much, if not for the kindness showed to me by my husband and children. I am obliged to my colleagues, who work with me in cooperation. I am grateful to God who blessed me with all these people in my life.

Saritha Mohanan

Contents

Section 5: Other Therapeutic Interventions for Pemphigus
and other Autoimmune Bullous Diseases

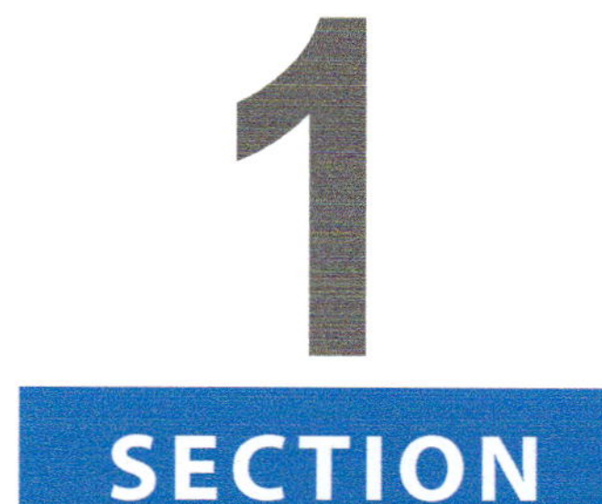

Basic Science in Pemphigus and other Autoimmune Bullous Diseases

Ultrastructure of the Skin in Relation to Pemphigus and other Autoimmune Bullous Diseases

Rajat Choudhary, Neha Taneja

- Molecular structure of the skin
- Adhesion between keratinocytes
- Adhesion of basal keratinocytes with underlying dermis
- Autoimmune bullous diseases occurring due to defects in adhesion molecules of skin

INTRODUCTION

Adhesion between the keratinocytes and adhesion of basal keratinocytes with the underlying dermis is required for maintaining the integrity of skin. The major structures required for cell-to-cell (keratinocyte) adhesion are desmosomes, while for adhesion between the epidermis and dermis, hemidesmosome-basement membrane complex plays a key role. Although ultrastructurally hemidesmosomes appear as half of the desmosomes, but at a molecular level they are markedly different.

Recent advances in genetics and proteomics have allowed us to understand the structure of desmosomes and basement membrane zone (BMZ), their functions and role in various human diseases. Apart from being autoantigens in various autoimmune bullous diseases (AIBDs), more than 25 genetic mutations in these proteins have been linked to inheritable genetic diseases. In this chapter, we will discuss their structure and role in AIBDs along with a brief enumeration of the associated genetic diseases.

We will be discussing under two headings:
1. Adhesion between keratinocytes (cell-to-cell adhesion)
2. Adhesion of basal keratinocytes with underlying dermis

ADHESION BETWEEN KERATINOCYTES (CELL-TO-CELL ADHESION)

Adhesion between keratinocytes is maintained by four mechanisms—(1) desmosomes (2) adherens junction (3) tight junction and (4) gap junction. Among these,

desmosomes are the major adhesion complex in keratinocytes and the only one affected in intraepidermal AIBDs.

Desmosomes—The Major Adhesion Complex in Epidermis

Desmosomes, also known as macula adherens, are transmembrane molecular complexes which anchor keratin intermediate filaments (KIFs) to the cell membrane, bridge the keratinocytes, and provide strength against trauma. Besides skin epithelium, desmosomes are also found in the myocardium, meninges, and lymph nodes. However, the other organs are not targeted in AIBDs due to structural differences among the various isoforms of proteins in different organs.

Although desmosomes were described on light microscopy as intercellular bridges in a spongiotic epidermis, their ultrastructure can only be appreciated on electron microscopy (EM). On EM, the cell membrane of adjacent keratinocytes creates a junction with the intercellular electron-lucent space. Desmosomes appear as transcellular electron dense plaques running parallel to the cell membrane at junctional regions. Within this electron dense region of the desmosome, three bands can be seen as moving away from the cell membrane—an electron dense region near the cell membrane followed by a relatively less dense zone, and then a fibrillar area.

Desmosome can be structurally divided into the desmosomal plaque and a transcellular portion-desmosomal cadherins.

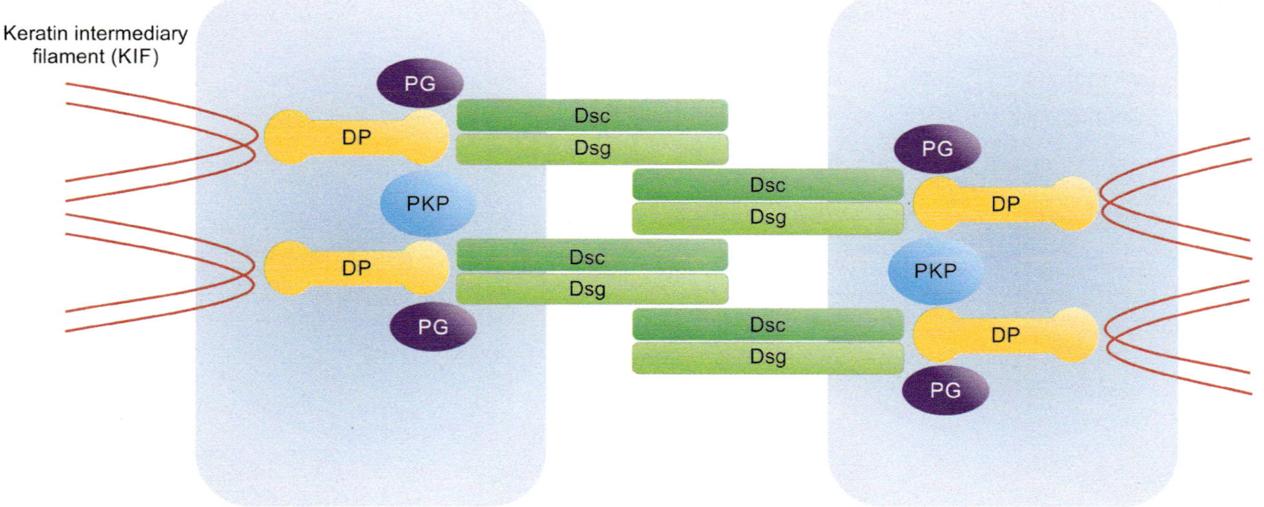

Fig. 1: Schematic overview of the desmosome structure (not to scale).
(DP: desmoplakin; Dsc: desmocollin; Dsg: desmoglein; PG: plakoglobin; PKP: plakophilin)

Desmosomal Plaque

The major components of the desmosomal plaque are plakins [e.g., desmoplakin (DP)], which bind to the KIFs at one end and to plakoglobin (PG) and plakophilin (PKP) at the other end. Finally, PG and PKP get attached to the intracellular portion of the cadherins **(Fig. 1)**.

Desmosomal Cadherins

Desmocollins (Dsc) and desmogleins (Dsg) are calcium-dependent E cadherins that form the transmembrane part of desmosomes. Like other proteins, they are synthesized as prepro-proteins in the endoplasmic reticulum (ER) and get converted to pro-proteins in late Golgi complex.

The cadherins, Dsg and Dsc, are made up of extracellular and intracellular domains. The extracellular domain consists of four cadherin repeats and an anchor domain, all of which are separated by calcium binding motifs. The cytoplasmic domain of cadherins have a and b isoforms, which bind to PG, PKP, DP, envoplakin, and periplakin, while the extracellular domains undergo both heterophilic (i.e. Dsg-Dsc) and homophilic (i.e. Dsg-Dsg and Dsc-Dsc) interactions to provide adhesion to cells. However, heterophilic interactions are more likely to contribute the major part in epidermal adhesion. Recent research has shown that apart from cell binding, these molecules are also involved in regulation of cell signaling and transcription.

Desmosomes are not only physically and functionally coupled to the cytoskeleton and other cell junctions, but also to cell organelles. It has been recently demonstrated using volume EM approaches that a close spatial proximity exists between the desmosomal plaque, KIFs, and ER. Genetic perturbations and live-cell optical imaging experiments suggest that desmosomes are required for dynamics and positioning of the ER complex, and likewise, ER appears to contribute to keratin organization and desmosome assembly at nascent sites of cell contact formation. Although the precise functional consequences are not fully resolved yet, these results might have implications for conditions like *Darier's disease*, in which loss-of-function mutations of ATP2A2 (encoding Ca^{2+}-ATPase SERCA2) leads to impaired desmosome function.

In humans, four isoforms of Dsg and three of Dsc have been identified in epidermal cells and other organs. The expression of each isoform varies within and among different epithelia, e.g., the upper layers of human epidermis express predominantly Dsgs1 and 4 and Dsc1 isoforms, whereas basal layers predominantly express Dsg3 and Dsc2. Similarly, among the various epithelial tissues, types 1 and 3 of Dsg and Dsc are expressed predominately in the stratified squamous epithelium of skin and oropharynx, Dsg2 is found in most of the simple and transitional epithelia of the body and heart, while Dsg4 is found in hair, testes, and prostrate **(Table 1)**. This differential expression explains involvement of only the skin and oropharynx in pemphigus [except in paraneoplastic pemphigus (PNP)].

Autoantibodies against the various desmosomal antigens are found in pemphigus group of disorders **(Table 1)**, e.g., pemphigus vulgaris (PV) has antibodies against Dsg3 and 1, pemphigus foliaceus (PF) against Dsg1, while in PNP, autoantibodies against multiple antigens such as Dsg1 and 3, DP 1 and 2, envoplakin, periplakin, plectin, and hemidesmosome BP230 are found. Due to many target antigens in PNP, almost all mucosae can be involved and multiple morphologies of cutaneous lesions can be seen. While Dsg3 (90% of patients) and Dsg1 (50–60% of patients) are the major autoantigens in PV, additional structural and metabolic autoantigens have been identified including Dsc1 and 3, muscarinic and nicotinic acetylcholine receptors, mitochondrial antigens, thyroid peroxidase, hSPCA1, PKP 3, and PG. Studies have shown that autoantibodies against these additional targets may complement the effects of anti-Dsg autoantibodies and explain individual variations in pemphigus disease severity. Dsc1 has been identified as

TABLE 1: Desmosomal components: Distribution and association with various diseases.

	Desmosomal component	Distribution	Autoimmune diseases	Genetic diseases
Desmosomal cadherins	Desmoglein 1	Differentiated cells of superficial epidermis	Pemphigus foliaceus, pemphigus vulgaris, IgA pemphigus (intraepidermal neutrophilic type), pemphigus herpetiformis, paraneoplastic pemphigus	Striate PPK (AD)
	Desmoglein 2	Most of the simple and transitional epithelia of the body and heart		ARVC (AD)
	Desmoglein 3	Basal and/or supra-basal layer of epidermis of skin, epithelium of oral cavity and oropharynx, thymic epithelial cells	Pemphigus vulgaris, paraneoplastic pemphigus, IgA pemphigus (intra-epidermal neutrophilic type), pemphigus herpetiformis (less common)	
	Desmoglein 4	Differentiated cells of superficial epidermis, hair, testes and prostrate		Hypotrichosis (AR), monilethrix (AR)
	Desmocollin 1	Differentiated cells of superficial epidermis	IgA pemphigus (subcorneal pustular dermatosis type), pemphigus herpetiformis, pemphigus vegetans	
	Desmocollin 2	Basal and/or supra-basal layers of epidermis	IgA pemphigus (intra-epidermal neutrophilic type), pemphigus herpetiformis, pemphigus vulgaris	ARVC (AR and AD)
	Desmocollin 3	Basal and/or supra-basal layer of epidermis	IgA pemphigus (intra-epidermal neutrophilic type), pemphigus herpetiformis, pemphigus vulgaris	Hypotrichosis (AR)
Desmosomal plaque proteins	Desmoplakin I/II		Paraneoplastic pemphigus	Striate PPK (AD) Carvajal syndrome (AR): Diffuse PPK, wooly hair, left ventricular cardiomyopathy Lethal acantholytic epidermolysis bullosa (AR) Skin fragility–wooly hair syndrome (AR): PPK, wooly hair, and nail dystrophy
	Other plakins (envoplakin, periplakin)		Paraneoplastic pemphigus	
	Plakoglobin			Naxos disease (AR): Diffuse PPK, wooly hair, ARVC
	Plakophilin 1			Skin fragility and ectodermal dysplasia (AR)
	Plakophilin 2			ARVC (AD)
Stratum corneum desmosome protein	Corneodesmosin			Hypotrichosis simplex of the scalp (AD)

(AD: autosomal dominant; AR: autosomal recessive; ARVC: arrhythmogenic right ventricular cardiomyopathy; PPK: palmoplantar keratoderma)

the target antigen of IgA autoantibodies in the subcorneal pustular dermatosis (SCPD) type of IgA pemphigus. Serum IgA autoantibodies associated with reactivity against the desmosomal cadherins Dsc1 to 3 and Dsg1 and 3 are pathogenic in the intra-epidermal neutrophilic (IEN) variant of IgA pemphigus. Antibodies against Dsc1 to 3 have also been seen in patients of pemphigus herpetiformis and pemphigus vegetans. Several patients with Dsc-positive sera, particularly of pemphigus herpetiformis, showed no reactivity with Dsgs. The presence of DP autoantibodies is common to PV, PF, and bullous pemphigoid (BP). However, autoantibodies against envoplakin and periplakin on immunoblot, as well as autoantibodies to DP (on indirect immunofluorescence and rat bladder epithelium), appear to be sensitive and specific for PNP diagnosis. This has led to the development of an enzyme-linked immunosorbent assay (ELISA) that detects envoplakin as a diagnostic tool for PNP.

The desmosomal contacts between adjacent cells generate an intercellular KIF scaffold throughout the entire epidermal sheet. However, despite these critical roles in maintaining epidermal adhesion and integrity, desmosomes are not static structures. They are dynamic units that undergo regular remodeling, i.e., assembly and disassembly, to allow for cell migration within the epidermis in response to outside-in signaling during epidermal differentiation. Hence, the concept of pemphigus as a "desmosome-remodeling impairment disease" involving a mechanism of Dsg3 non-assembly and depletion from desmosomes through PV IgG-activated intracellular signaling events has been proposed. Two cell–cell adhesion states controlled by desmosomes have been recognized, which include "stable hyper-adhesion (Ca^{2+}-independent)" and "dynamic weak-adhesion (Ca^{2+}-dependent)" conditions. These conditions are mutually reversible through cell signaling events involving protein kinase C (PKC) and epidermal growth factor receptor (EGFR). The best example of this theory has been demonstrated in PV. Binding of IgG antibodies to Dsg3 causes its endocytosis from the cell surface, and results in specific depletion of Dsg3 from desmosomes, an event linked to acantholysis in the epidermis. This binding of anti-Dsg3 antibody to Dsg3 in the epidermal keratinocytes activates PKC, a signal-transducing non-receptor protein kinase (Src) and EGFR, which are linked to the generation of dynamic weak-adhesion desmosomes, followed by p38MAPK (mitogen-activated protein kinase)-mediated endocytosis of Dsg3, resulting in specific depletion of Dsg3 from desmosomes, and acantholysis. These weak-adhesion desmosomes appear to be the susceptible desmosomal state for Dsg3 depletion and cause pivotal and specific events leading to blistering in PV.

The disruption of the extracellular domain of Dsg1 has also been demonstrated as the basis of staphylococcal scalded skin syndrome and bullous impetigo in which Dsg1 is cleaved by the bacterial toxin. Similarly, mutations in various desmoglein proteins have been associated with different genodermatoses affecting the skin and other organs, depending on the distribution of affected desmoglein proteins, e.g., mutation in Dsg1 leads to striate palmoplantar keratoderma, mutation in Dsg2 and Dsc2 leads to arrhythmogenic right ventricular cardiomyopathy, and mutation in Dsg4 presents as hair abnormalities such as monilethrix or hypotrichosis. These have been enumerated in **Table 1.**

Besides playing a role in the pathogenesis of AIBDs, desmosomal proteins are associated with present and future paradigms in therapy. The B cell-depleting anti-CD20 antibody rituximab has been implemented as first-line therapy for moderate-to-severe PV/PF. Several trials are underway to test new treatment paradigms, including use of Dsg3-CAAR T cells, which have been successfully applied in experimental models of PV, to cause down-regulation of autoreactive T cells via Dsg3-coated nanoparticles, or targeting of FcRn function. It has been shown that targeting FcRn by efgartigimod rescued the loss of keratinocyte adhesion caused by recombinant monoclonal anti-Dsg3 antibodies derived from pemphigus mouse models or patients, and suggested that FcRn, besides controlling the autoantibody turnover, might also have direct effects on desmosomes. Phosphodiesterase 4 inhibitor apremilast, which was thought to mainly affect immune cells, also stabilizes keratin anchorage of desmosomes and is protective against PV-IgG-induced skin blistering.

Plakoglobin (PG)

PG, also known as gamma-catenin, is expressed throughout the layers of epithelium and in all types of epithelia. PG along with PKP is called armadillo family protein. The head end of PG binds to the desmosomal cadherins (Dsg and Dsc) and the tail end to DP, leading to attachment of Dsg and Dsc to DP **(Fig. 1)**. PGs are also responsible for recruitment of various proteins to desmosomes and might also modulate gene transcription.

Since PGs are present in multiple organs, its mutations present as palmoplantar keratoderma, cardiomyopathy, and woolly hair (Naxos syndrome) or lethal epidermolysis bullosa **(Table 1)**. Antibodies against this antigen are not found in AIBDs.

Desmoplakin (DP)

DP is part of the plakin gene family, which also includes BP antigen 1 and plectin. Among the two variants, DP I and II, DP I is mainly required for normal desmosomal functions. The head end of this protein (NH2- terminal) binds to PG, whereas the tail end (–COOH terminal) binds to KIF **(Fig. 1)**. Hence, DP acts as a major link between KIF and desmosomal plaque. Although antibodies against DP are found only in PNP, its mutation has been associated with various genodermatoses involving the skin, hair, nails, and heart **(Table 1)**.

Plakophilin (PKP)

Like PGs, PKPs also attach to the desmosomal plaque and KIF and are also associated with few transcription factors. They help in clustering of various desmosomal proteins and provide lateral support. Of the three known types, type 3 is present throughout the epidermis, type 1 is predominant in the basal layer, while type 2 is only expressed in the basal layer. Mutations in these proteins are associated with ectodermal dysplasia—skin fragility syndrome and cardiomyopathies **(Table 1)**.

Other Desmosomal Proteins

Envoplakin and periplakin are other desmosomal proteins which are incorporated during corneo-desmosome formation. Hence, they are mainly expressed in the upper layers of epidermis. Antibodies against these antigens have mostly been demonstrated in PNP.

ADHESION OF BASAL KERATINOCYTES WITH DERMIS

The dermo-epidermal junction is formed by a highly complex basement membrane complex, which begins from the lower surface of basal keratinocytes and extends upto the upper dermal layers **(Fig. 2)**. It is continuous along the epidermis and cutaneous appendages such as eccrine glands and hair follicles. The BMZ is composed of proteins derived from the keratinocytes of ectodermal origin as well as from dermal fibroblasts of mesodermal origin. The basal keratinocytes (ectoderm) produce hemidesmosomal components such as plectin, epidermal isoform of bullous pemphigoid antigen 1 (BPAG1e), bullous pemphigoid antigen 2 (BPAG2; collagen XVII), integrin α6 and β4, CD151 tetraspan, types IV and VII collagen, laminins 332 (α3β3γ2) and 311 (α3β1γ1), and heparan sulfate proteoglycans (HSPGs), to the epidermal basement membrane. The structures that originate from dermal fibroblasts include nidogen, types IV and VII collagen, and few other proteins that are translocated to the plasma membrane of basal keratinocytes where they condense and incorporate within the basement membrane. The BMZ can be divided into three distinct zones:

1. *From the lower surface of basal keratinocytes till lamina densa*: This zone consists of the keratin hemidesmosome complex, and lamina lucida containing anchoring filaments. The lower surface of basal keratinocytes contains various electron dense structures called hemidesmosomes, which connect KIFs present on the cytoplasmic side, to the anchoring filaments (made of collagen IV) present on the extracellular side. KIFs, 7–10 mm in diameter, are responsible for maintaining cell architecture, and are connected to the desmosomes (as described above) and hemidesmosomes. Below the basal keratinocytes, there is a 25–50 nm wide electron-lucent layer known as lamina lucida, which contains 2–8 nm wide anchoring filaments. Although anchoring filaments are present throughout, they are more concentrated around the hemidesmosomes. Various studies have questioned the in vivo existence of lamina lucida as it was not seen in skin prepared by high pressure preservation techniques. They have proposed that lamina lucida is an artifact created due to shrinkage of epidermal cells during processing. Despite these observations, it holds practical importance in scientific publications and helps in the visualization and description of anchoring filaments.

2. *Lamina densa*: It is an electron dense layer of 20–50 nm width, and has a granular fibrous appearance. It is formed by the molecular polymerization of various proteins like collagen IV, nidogen, laminins, and perlecans. Lamina densa acts as a structural scaffold of the dermo-epidermal junction. It is attached via anchoring filaments to the basal keratinocytes on one side and via anchoring fibrils to the dermal collagen on the other side.

3. *Sublamina densa*: It is composed of two micro-fibrillary structures; anchoring fibrils and fibrillins containing microfibrils (lamina fibro-reticularis).

   i. Anchoring fibrils (composed of collagen VII) are condensed fibrous aggregates of 20–75 nm diameter with a loosely woven frayed end. One end of these fibrils is attached to the lamina densa and the other end either gets attached to the fibrous network in the dermis or to the lamina densa after looping around dermal collagen.

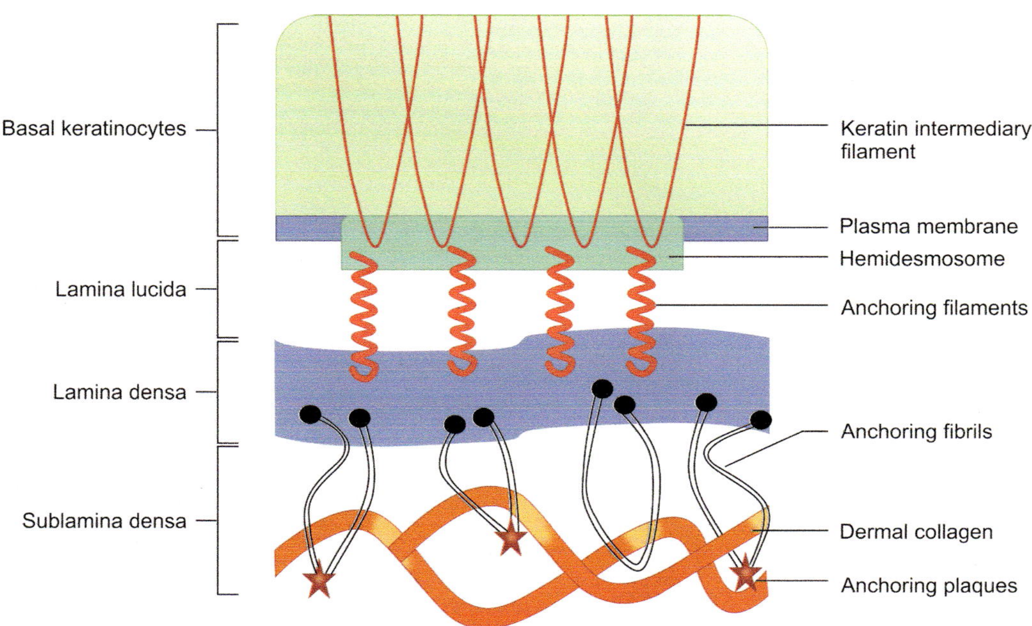

Fig. 2: Major ultrastructural subregions of the basement membrane zone.

ii. Microfibrils are 10–12 nm wide elastic tissue-related fibers. In the papillary dermis, microfibrillar elements insert vertically into the lamina densa and comprise of oxytalan fibers. At their inferior aspect, oxytalan fibers merge with microfibrillar elements oriented parallel to skin surface, designated as elaunin fibers. The network of oxytalan and elaunin fibers is contiguous with elastic fibers within the reticular dermis.

Epidermal-specific Basement Membrane Components

In this section, we will be discussing the ultrastructural components of hemidesmosomes and their clinical significance.

From Lower Surface of Basal Keratinocytes till Lamina Densa

Plectin

Plectin (500 kDa protein), a member of the plakin family, is a dumbbell-shaped dimeric protein found in the cytoplasmic plaque of hemidesmosome. Like other plakins, it is a multi-domain cytolinker which connects various cytoskeletal networks. The C-terminal of plectin binds to keratin and vimentin intermediary filaments and its N-terminal binds to the cytoplasmic part of integrin subunit β4, BP180 and actin **(Fig. 3)**. Mutations in the proteins encoding plectin are not associated with AIBDs, but occur in epidermolysis bullosa simplex (EBS) associated with muscular dystrophy, EBS Ogna type, and EBS with pyloric atresia **(Table 2)**. Sera from BP patients have shown autoantibodies binding to plectin, although it is a rare phenomenon and the pathogenicity of these antibodies is questionable.

Bullous Pemphigoid Antigen 1 (BPAG 1)

Since it was the first identified antigen against which pathological antibodies were present in BP, it was named BPAG1. BPAG1e (epidermal part) is also a plakin group of protein which resides in the cytoplasmic plaque of hemi-desmosomes and has a molecular weight of 230 kDa (also known as BP 230). It has a central coiled α helical rod domain with a globular carboxy terminal and an amino terminal. The central coiled rod domain has regular periodicity of acidic and basic amino acids, which causes its self-aggregation. Similarly, its carboxy terminal has periodic arrangement of specific amino acids, which help in its binding with KIFs. The N-terminal of BPAG1e attaches to the cytoplasmic domains of BPAG2, integrin subunit β4, and ERBIN **(Fig. 3)**. ERBIN interacts with the surface tyrosine kinase receptor, Erb-B2 and might provide a potential link between hemi-desmosome biology and tyrosine kinase (Erb-B2) signaling.

A neuronal form of BPAG1, BPAG1n (dystonin) has also been identified, which has a different N-terminal. This molecular association has also been used to explain the association of BP with neurological diseases like Alzheimer's disease. Although BPAG1 knocked-out mice have shown dystonia and ataxia along with epidermal fragility, they are not found in patients of EBS with homozygous missense mutations.

Bullous Pemphigoid Antigen 2 (BPAG2)

BPAG2 or collagen XVII is a transmembrane collagen with a cytoplasmic amino terminal containing many phosphorylation sites, and an extracellular domain containing multiple repeats of glycine-X-Y amino acids with intervening portion of other amino acids. Due to this amino acid sequence, the extracellular portion is referred to as collagenous domain, and it forms a globular head

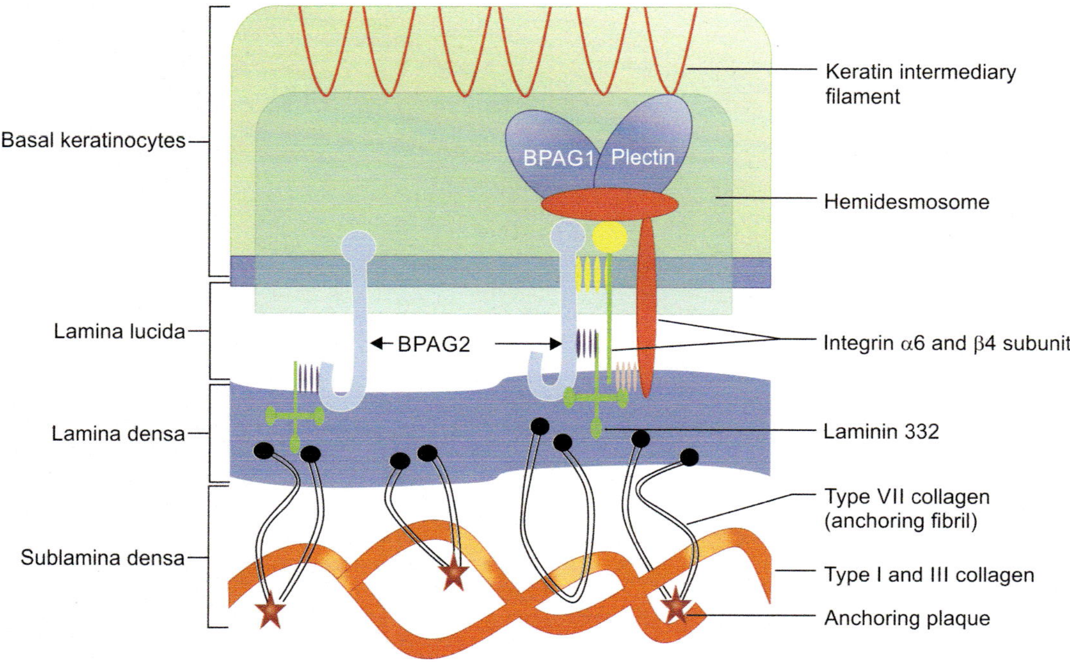

Fig. 3: Schematic diagram showing relationship of various dermo-epidermal junction components.

TABLE 2: Association of various diseases with components of basement membrane zone.

	Basement membrane zone component	Autoimmune disease	Genetic disease
Cytoskeletal proteins	Keratin 5 and 14		EBS
Hemidesmosomal plaque proteins	Bullous pemphigoid antigen 1/BP230	BP, MMP	EBS
	Plectin	BP, CP, LAD	• EBS-MD • JEB-PA
Other intracellular adhesion complex proteins	Kindlin-1		Kindler syndrome
Hemidesmosomal transmembrane components	Bullous pemphigoid antigen 2/Collagen XVII/BP180	BP, CP, LAD, PG, MMP	JEB-non-Herlitz
	• α6β4 integrin • CD151	BP, CP, MMP	• JEB-PA • Pre-tibial EB, nephritis, deafness
Anchoring filament proteins	Laminin 332	CP, MMP	JEB-Herlitz
	Ectodomain of collagen XVII	LAD, BP	JEB-non-Herlitz
	Collagen IV		• Alport syndrome—hematuria, renal failure, and sensory neural deafness • Goodpasture syndrome—pulmonary hemorrhage and glomerulonephritis
Anchoring fibril proteins	Collagen VII	EBA, MMP, bullous LE	DEB

(BP: bullous pemphigoid; CP: cicatricial pemphigoid; DEB: dystrophic epidermolysis bullosa; EBA: epidermolysis bullosa acquisita; EBS: epidermolysis bullosa simplex; EBS–MD: EBS with muscular dystrophy; JEB: junctional EB; JEB–PA: JEB with pyloric atresia; LAD: linear immunoglobulin A dermatosis; MMP: mucous membrane pemphigoid; PG: pemphigoid gestationis)

(containing Coll 1-15) with a flexible tail (Coll 1-14) and a core body (corresponding to Coll 15). Coll 15 rod domain inserts into the lamina densa and then its carboxy terminal loops back into lamina lucida **(Fig. 3)**.

Two isoforms of BPAG2 have been isolated; (1) full length 180 kDa protein and (2) an extracellular 120 kDa domain, which is shed from plasma membrane. Proteolysis of BPAG2 is performed by "sheddases"; the tumor necrosis factor-α-converting enzyme (TACE), and is inhibited by phosphorylation of BPAG2 by ecto-casein kinase, which modulates the adhesion and motility of keratinocytes.

In skin basement membrane, the extracellular portion of BPAG2 forms a trimer by cross-linking of its collagenous domains in a triple helix arrangement. At the amino-terminal, the helix is formed independently of collagen-forming amino acids, with the 16th non-collagenous portion (NC16) as nucleation site. This NC16 region is the first extracellular segment of BPAG2 and binds to integrin subunit α6. The cytoplasmic domain (amino terminal) of BPAG2 is associated with BPAG1e, integrin β4, and plectins, whereas the carboxy terminal is attached to laminin 332 **(Fig. 3)**.

Antibodies against NC16 domain of BPAG2 have been demonstrated in patients of BP, pemphigoid gestationis, and linear IgA bullous dermatosis (LABD), whereas antibodies targeting the carboxy terminal have been demonstrated in mucous membrane pemphigoid (MMP) **(Table 2)**. The main pathogenic effect of anti-BP180 autoantibodies appears to be mediated by FcγR but there is increasing evidence regarding the involvement of non-FcγR-mediated pathways. The pathogenicity of anti-BP180 autoantibodies also depends on the autoantibody iso-type, IgG sub-class, and glycosylation status, leading to a varying extent of complement activation at the dermoepidermal junction and attraction of inflammatory cells to the upper dermis. These differences in the pathogenicity of various antibodies might explain varied clinical morphology and variable association with neurological illnesses among BP patients. Mutations in BPAG2 encoding gene (COL17A1) leads to the development of junctional epidermolysis bullosa-non-Herlitz type with subepidermal blister, alopecia, enamel defect, and dystrophic nails **(Table 2)**.

Integrins

Integrins are transmembrane receptors which are formed by dimerization of α and β subunit. Both subunits have a hydrophobic transmembrane domain and a small cytoplasmic domain. The cytoplasmic domain binds to the intracellular cytoskeleton. Hemidesmosomes predominantly contain α6β4 integrin which binds to plectin and BPAG1 on the cytoplasmic side, and laminin 332 on the extracellular side **(Fig. 3)**. In the keratinocytes, focal adhesions between the actin cytoskeletal and extracellular matrix are formed by macromolecular complexes formed by integrins and other proteins like kindlin 1 and 2. Apart from cell adhesion, these molecules also play an important role in signal transduction, gene expression, and growth.

Mutation in the gene encoding kindlin 1 (*FERMT1*) leads to Kindler syndrome, manifesting as blistering, poikiloderma, photosensitivity, and increased risk of squamous cell carcinoma. The development of atrophy and malignancy in kindlin deficiency has been explained by a decreased integrin-mediated activation of transforming growth factor β and increased Wnt signaling in mouse models. Similarly, patients having mutation of α6 or β4 integrin subunit genes manifest as junctional epidermolysis bullosa with pyloric atresia.

Lamina Densa

Laminins

Laminins are heterotrimeric glycoproteins with 3 subunits (α, β, and γ,) connected to each other by disulfide bonds. Each subunit is encoded by a different gene, and till now, five α, three β, and three γ chains have been identified. Various combinations of the subunits create different types of laminins. Currently, they are named as 3-digit number, each digit signifying the type of α, β, and γ sub-unit in that laminin (e.g., laminin 332, previously known as laminin 5 or epiligrin, has α3, β3, and γ2 subunits). Predominant laminins at the dermoepidermal junction include laminin 332, 311, and 511. Laminins connect integrin and BPAG2 to type IV collagen of lamina densa and type VII collagen of sublamina densa **(Fig. 4)**. The subunits of laminin 332 are encoded by various genes such as LAMA3, LAMB3, and LAMC2. Mutations in these genes cause junctional epidermolysis bullosa, and often lead to early death.

Antibodies against laminin 332 manifest as MMP which is associated with solid organ malignancies (6–30% of patients in various studies). The indirect immunofluorescence assays such as laminin 332 biochip mosaic assay and laminin 332 footprint assay are easy-to-perform tests with excellent diagnostic accuracy. Their development might lead to the identification of MMP patients with antilaminin 332 antibodies, allowing early tumor screening in these patients.

Pathogenic antibodies against laminin γ1 (mainly against C-terminal) have been demonstrated in patients with anti-p200 pemphigoid. Although researchers were unable to produce clinical disease in mice with the administration of antilaminin γ1 containing sera, they could produce dermoepidermal separation in cryosection models. These patients have a clinical presentation similar to BP but show prompt response to treatment and have longer remission periods.

Type IV Collagen

It is a special collagen found specifically in basement membranes. Its molecular structure is similar to procollagen since it retains globular domains at carboxy- and amino terminals. Like other collagen molecules, it is made of 3α-chains which form a triple helical structure. Till now, six types of α-chains associated with type IV collagen have been identified [α1(IV)-α6(IV)], of which types 1, 2, 5, 6 are found in the skin basement membrane. Unlike other collagens, it is not helical throughout its length due to discontinuities in its glycine-X-Y repeats. These short discontinuations provide increased flexibility to collagen IV but make it susceptible to ordinary proteinases.

The macromolecular structure of this collagen resembles a hockey stick **(Fig. 4)**, where the blade corresponds to the retained globular domain near its amino-terminal (7S domain), handle corresponds to the triple helical portion and handle grip corresponds to the globular structure at amino-terminal (NC 1 domain). These molecules of type IV collagen arrange in a lattice structure resembling a spider, in which the 7S domain arranged at right angles to each other correspond to the body, and helix along with NC1 terminal corresponds to the legs of the spider. Such antiparallel

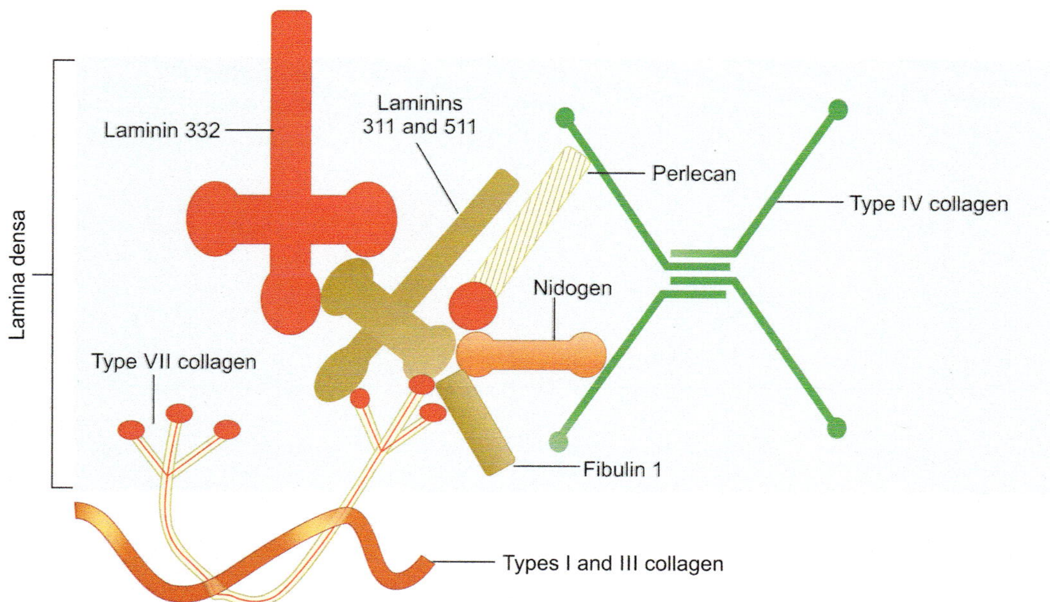

Fig. 4: Model of lamina densa showing binding of laminins, nidogen, and type IV collagen.

integration of type IV collagen forms a two-dimensional lattice which acts as key matrix within the lamina densa.

The defective formation of type IV collagen has been linked to Alport syndrome, characterized by hematuria, renal failure, and sensory neural deafness **(Table 2)**. Similarly, antibodies against this collagen are also seen in Goodpasture syndrome, manifesting as pulmonary hemorrhage and glomerulonephritis. Although such mutations or antibodies usually do not affect the skin, antibodies against $\alpha 5$ and $\alpha 6$ can cause glomerulonephritis with subepidermal blisters.

Nidogen

Nidogen is a glycoprotein found in lamina densa with two isoforms, type 1 and 2. The G3 domain of nidogen binds to cysteine-rich regions of $\gamma 1$ subunit containing laminins such as laminin 111, 311, and 511 **(Fig. 4)**, its G2 domain binds to type IV collagen, and the complex of laminin-nidogen binds to HSPGs and fibulin 1 and 2. Therefore nidogen acts as the main stabilizer for all macromolecules in the lamina densa. Similarly, nidogen 2 links fibulins to Heparan Sulphate Proteoglycans (HSPGs) as well as type 1 and IV collagen. No autoimmune or genetic disease has been identified due to nidogen. Surprisingly, even engineered mice lacking nidogen 1, do not show any overt abnormalities in the basement membrane. In such mutated mice, marked epidermal hyper-proliferation was seen in wound healing, but re-epithelialization was not altered.

Heparan Sulphate Proteoglycans (HSPGs)

These are a diverse group of macromolecules with a central protein core, with multiple glycosaminoglycans emerging from it in a "bottle brush" configuration. HSPGs of various types and configuration self-polymerize and also connect the various components of lamina densa. Of all HSPGs, perlecan is the most studied, which connects laminins and collagen IV-containing networks together. Besides providing stability, these molecules also restrict the permeability of basement membrane by providing negative charge to the lamina densa.

Anchoring Fibrils and Sublamina Densa

Type VII Collagen

It is found only in the sublamina densa of stratified squamous epithelium and forms a major component of anchoring fibrils. It consists of three identical α chains of 290 kDa. Its amino terminal has a large globular non-collagenous domain termed as NC1, and a smaller non-collagenous domain at the –COOH terminal, termed as NC2. During the assembly of anchoring fibrils, NC2 domains bind in anti-parallel manner via disulfide bonds. After proteolytic cleavage of the NC2 domain, a macromolecule with a central rod and a larger globular NC1 head is formed. Two such newly formed type VII collagens dimerize to from anchoring fibrils and its aggregated NC1 domains bind to the lamina densa of stratified squamous epithelium. NC1 domain has affinity for type 1 collagen in the dermis and type IV collagen in the lamina densa or anchoring plaques. Some studies have postulated that anchoring plaques in the sublamina densa

are dropped out portions of lamina densa during basement membrane remodeling, hence contain collagen IV. After the attachment of NC1 domain to lamina densa, anchoring fibrils either get attached to anchoring plaques in the dermis or loop around dermal collagen to get attached to lamina densa. This network of loops and tethers connects the dermis to lamina densa in the sublamina densa region **(Fig. 4)**.

Antibodies against the four immunodominant regions of NC1 domain of collagen VII have been identified in patients of epidermolysis bullosa acquisita (EBA) and bullous systemic lupus erythematosus (SLE). Although antibodies in both EBA and bullous SLE target the same antigenic site, bullous SLE has more inflammatory lesions and rapid progression of disease.

Mutation in the encoding gene of collagen VII (*COL7A1*) can cause both autosomal dominant and recessive forms of epidermolysis bullosa dystrophica (EBD). In the generalized recessive form of EBD (homozygous mutation), patients have premature termination of translation, leading to formation of nonsense mRNA. As no collagen VII is formed, these patients manifest as extreme skin fragility with scarring and risk of development of squamous cell carcinoma. Since carriers are able to produce sufficient amount of protein from a single allele, they do not have any manifestations of EBD. In patients with dominant dystrophic EBD, there is a missense mutation leading to formation of an abnormal protein chain. These abnormal α-chains trimerize with the normal α-chains to form abnormal looking collagen VII. Since these patients have both normal and abnormal anchoring fibrils, they manifest with a less severe clinical phenotype as compared to recessive EBD **(Table 2)**.

Microfibrils

Elastic fibers have two distinct components—(1) non-banded amorphous component, elastin and (2) regularly placed microfibrillary structures, fibrillins. Fibrillins have two types of fibers—oxytalan and elaunin fibers. Oxytalan fibers run perpendicular to the papillary dermis and connect the lamina densa to elaunin fibers in the dermis. Elaunin fibers have some amorphous components and run parallel to skin surface in the dermis. This network of oxytalan and elaunin fibers merges with the elastic fibers of the dermis and provides strength to the dermoepidermal junction.

CONCLUSION

The epidermis and dermal-epidermal junction are continuous with the extracellular matrix in the papillary dermis. The cell–cell and cell-basement membrane adhesion in the epidermis, and the cell-matrix adhesion in the dermis secure the attachment of the two skin layers and provide the skin with its resistance against environmental influences. The integrity of these adhesion structures is essential for the protection of the entire organ against mechanical, physical, or microbial insults. This is indirectly demonstrated by human disorders in which cutaneous adhesion structures are targeted by either genetic mutations or by pathogenic antibodies that perturb the function of target proteins, such as in epidermolysis bullosa or pemphigus. Tremendous advances have recently been made in discerning the molecular and functional details of epidermal and dermal adhesion, and in understanding the molecular pathology of skin fragility. This knowledge will facilitate design of therapeutic approaches not only for the rare genetic and common autoimmune adhesion disorders, but also for physiological processes such as skin aging.

TAKE HOME MESSAGE

- The adhesive structures in the skin include desmosomes, focal adhesions, hemidesmosomes, basement membrane, and dermal fibril network.
- The major components of desmosomes are the desmosomal cadherins (Dsg and Dsc), plakins (DP, envoplakin, and periplakin), and armadillo family proteins (PG and PKP).
- Basement membrane serves multiple functions such as acting as a substrate for attachment of cells, regulating permeability, providing a template for tissue repair and aiding in cell migration.
- The hemidesmosome, major dermoepidermal adhesion complex, comprises of plakin homologs, integrins, and collagenous transmembrane proteins.
- By transmission EM, the major ultrastructural subregions (from above downwards) of the epidermal basement membrane are—(1) the cytoskeleton, hemidesmosomal plaques, and plasma membranes of basal keratinocytes (2) an electron lucent region termed lamina lucida (3) lamina densa and (4) sublamina densa region of the papillary dermis.
- Acquired or inherited abnormalities in structural proteins within the epidermis and epidermal basement membrane often result in a disease phenotype characterized by blister formation.

MULTIPLE CHOICE QUESTIONS

1. **Which types of proteins are found in desmosomes?**
   - (a) Microfilaments
   - (b) Microtubules
   - (c) Keratin intermediary filaments
   - (d) Actin filaments

2. **What type of junction is a desmosome?**
   - (a) Tight junction
   - (b) Adherens junction
   - (c) Gap junction
   - (d) Desmosome junction

3. **What is the function of plakoglobin in skin desmosomes?**
   - (a) To anchor the intermediate filaments to the plasma membrane
   - (b) To provide mechanical strength to the desmosome
   - (c) To regulate the interaction between desmoglein and desmoplakin
   - (d) To regulate cell migration

4. **Mutation in plakophilin 1 leads to:**
   - (a) Naxos disease
   - (b) Carvajal syndrome
   - (c) Hypotrichosis simplex of scalp
   - (d) Skin fragility and ectodermal dysplasia

5. **Mutation in which of the following proteins does not lead to significant changes in skin?**
   - (a) Plakoglobin
   - (b) Nidogen
   - (c) Desmoglein
   - (d) Plakophilin

6. **Subcorneal pustular dermatosis type of IgA pemphigus is caused by a defect in which antigen?**
   - (a) Desmoglein 3
   - (b) Desmoglein 1
   - (c) BPAg1
   - (d) Desmocollin 1

7. **Anchoring fibrils are primarily composed of:**
   - (a) Type I collagen
   - (b) Type III collagen
   - (c) Type IV collagen
   - (d) Type VII collagen

8. **Regarding dermal-epidermal junction, which of the following statements is true?**
   - (a) There are no anchoring filaments in lamina lucida
   - (b) Lamina fibro-reticularis lies above lamina densa
   - (c) Lamina fibro-reticularis comprises of anchoring fibrils and the elastic microfibrils
   - (d) Blood vessels cross the dermal-epidermal junction to reach the epidermis

9. **Epidermolysis bullosa simplex (EBS), Weber–Cockayne type, is caused by which defect?**
   - (a) Collagen VII
   - (b) Alpha-6-beta-4 integrin
   - (c) Keratins 1 and 10
   - (d) Keratin 5

10. The main permeability barrier in lamina densa is:
(a) Heparan sulfate proteoglycan
(b) Collagen IV
(c) Laminin 5
(d) Nidogen

Answers

1. (c)   2. (d)   3. (c)   4. (d)   5. (b)   6. (d)   7. (d)   8. (c)   9. (d)   10. (a)

SUGGESTED READING

1. Uitto J, Richard G. Progress in epidermolysis bullosa: Genetic classification and clinical implications. *Am J Med Genet-Semin Med Genet*. 2004;131C:61-74.
2. Has C, Nyström A. Epidermal basement membrane in health and disease. *Curr Top Membr*. 2015;76:117-70.
3. Masunaga T. Epidermal basement membrane: Its molecular organization and blistering disorders. *Connect Tissue Res*. 2006;47:55-66.
4. Uitto J, Has C, Vahidnezhad H, Youssefian L, Bruckner-Tuderman L. Molecular pathology of the basement membrane zone in heritable blistering diseases: The paradigm of epidermolysis bullosa. *Matrix Biol*. 2017;57:76-85.
5. Bruckner-Tuderman L, Has C. Disorders of the cutaneous basement membrane zone: The paradigm of epidermolysis bullosa. *Matrix Biol*. 2014;33:29-34.
6. Qian H, Natsuaki Y, Koga H, Kawakami T, Tateishi C, Tsuruta D, et al. The second study of clinical and immunological findings in anti-laminin 332-type mucous membrane pemphigoid examined at Kurume University—diagnosis criteria suggested by summary of 133 cases. *Front Immunol*. 2021;12:77166.
7. Ahmed AR, Anwar S, Reche PA. Molecular basis for global incidence of pemphigoid diseases and differences in phenotypes. *Front Immunol*. 2022;13:807173.
8. Wang M, Li F, Wang X, Wang R, Chen T, Zhao J, et al. BIOCHIP mosaic for the diagnosis of autoimmune bullous diseases in Chinese patients. *Eur J Dermatol*. 2020;30:338-44.
9. Spindler V, Waschke J. Pemphigus—A disease of desmosome dysfunction caused by multiple mechanisms. *Front Immunol*. 2018;9:136.
10. Radine UK, Bumiller-Bini Hoch V, Boldt ABW, Zillikens D, Ludwig RJ, Hammers CM, et al. Electron microscopy of desmosomal structures in the pemphigus human skin organ culture model. *Front Med (Lausanne)*. 2022;9:997387.

CHAPTER 2

Principles of Immunology

Vishakha Hooda, Alpana Sharma

- Overview of innate and adaptive immunity
- Role of different immune cells
- Role of complement pathways and cytokine networks

INTRODUCTION

Autoimmune bullous diseases (AIBDs) are a group of complex immune-mediated disorders which affect the skin and mucosa. They are overwhelmed by innate and adaptive immunity. Innate immune cells act as early responders. They provide signals either by direct cell-to-cell contact or by secreting stimulatory molecules such as cytokines or chemokines to recruit both the cellular and humoral immune cells, i.e., T and B lymphocytes. B cells are crucial for autoantibody production, and along with other cells are involved in the recruitment and activation of T cells. T cells are involved in the bulk production of cytokines and in performing cytotoxic and effector functions.

INNATE AND ADAPTIVE IMMUNITY

The immune system protects the body against foreign pathogens. It consists of two arms of immunity—innate and adaptive. Innate immunity is also known as native immunity. It acts promptly and provides general, non-specific defense against the non-self. It prevents the microbes from breaching the skin and mucosal lining of the body. It consists of various immune cell types such as neutrophils, macrophages, monocytes, mast cells, dendritic cells (DCs), and natural killer (NK) cells. These cells recognize patterns such as the pathogen-associated molecular patterns (PAMPs), toll-like receptors (TLRs), or damage-associated molecular patterns (DAMPs), and act as effector as well as antigen presenting cells (APCs) that provide signals to the adaptive immunity to get activated. Adaptive immunity provides a specific response against the pathogens and creates a memory against them. A balance is required between both arms of the immunity for proper functioning. Variations in the frequency and functioning of these cells can create a diseased condition like autoimmunity.

Innate Immune Cells

Neutrophils

Neutrophils constitute around 40–70% of the total white blood cells (WBCs) and are the innate sentinels that act as one of the earliest cells in immune reactions. They function as phagocytes and secrete inflammatory cytokines and neutrophil extracellular traps (NETs), which are made of altered chromatin and "decorated" with cytoplasmic and granular bactericidal proteins that serve as a sticky NET to trap pathogens **(Fig. 1)**. In pemphigus vulgaris (PV), neutrophils are increased during the early stages of the disease while they are decreased during remission. Recently, Kowalska–Kępczyńska, *et al* showed NEUT-RI (neutrophil reactivity index) and NEUT-GI (neutrophil granularity index) as a potential diagnostic tool to detect the severity of pemphigus diseases. They showed an increase in both NEUT-RI and NEUT-GI in patients compared to healthy controls. This might be due to stimulation of interleukin (IL)-17 and IL-36 at the site of blisters, which attract the neutrophils at the site. NEUT-RI is significantly upregulated in pemphigus vegetans while NEUT-GI is upregulated in PV. NEUT-RI signifies a higher density of neutrophils in blisters and NEUT-GI shows a change in their internal morphology with increased granularity, which leads to the activation of neutrophil enzymes and production of reactive oxygen species (ROS) and an increase in degranulation. Few authors have shown a positive correlation of bullous pemphigoid (BP) severity with neutrophil and eosinophil count.

Macrophages

Macrophages are monocyte-derived cells that function as phagocytes and APCs and secrete both pro- and anti-inflammatory cytokines. Macrophages are categorized into two main subsets—(1) M1 macrophages (classically

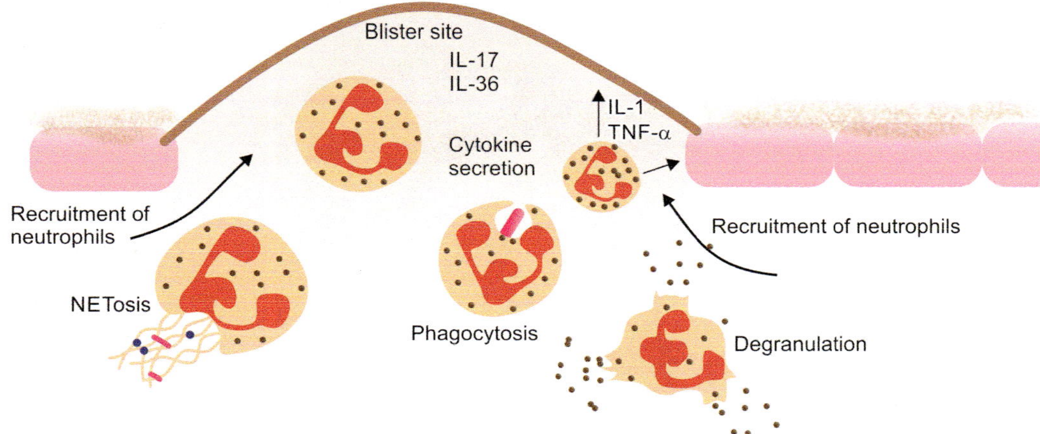

Fig. 1: Function of neutrophils at the site of blister in pemphigus: Recruitment of neutrophils at the site of blister in response to IL-17 and IL-36 leading to activation of neutrophils to perform phagocytosis, NETosis, degranulation, and secretion of cytokines such as IL-1 and TNF-α. (IL: interleukin; NET: neutrophil extracellular trap; TNF: tumor necrosis factor)

activated) which are pro-inflammatory in nature and (2) M2 macrophages (alternatively activated) which are anti-inflammatory in nature. M1 phenotype is induced by Th1-related cytokines like interferon γ (IFN-γ) and tumor necrosis factor α (TNF-α) or by the bacterial lipopolysaccharides, and is mediated by signal transducer and activator of transcription 1 (STAT1). These macrophages produce higher levels of pro-inflammatory cytokines such as TNF-α, IL-1α, IL-1β, IL-6, IL-12, IL-23, and cyclooxygenase-2 (COX-2), and low levels of IL-10. They possess tremendous microbicidal property and the ability to engulf a large number of pathogens. M2 macrophages are induced by Th2 cytokines IL-4 and IL-13 via activating STAT6 through the IL-4 receptor alpha (IL-4Rα). Besides IL-4 and IL-13, other cytokines such as IL-10 can govern M2 polarization via activating STAT3 through the IL-10 receptor (IL-10R). They play a role in tissue remodeling and repair, angiogenesis, and allergic reactions and are antiparasitic in nature.

CD206+ CD163+ M2 macrophages are abundantly present in both PV and BP. In 1979, a study using electron microscopy reported the abundance of macrophages penetrating the clefts between keratinocytes in PV patients. Some of these macrophages co-expressed Th2 homing receptor CCL17 with CD163. There is polarization of macrophages toward the M2 phenotype with a role in attracting Th2 cells to the lesional site. A sizeable number of IL-4+, IL-13+, pSTAT6+, and pSTAT1+ cells have been observed in the lesional skin of PV. Additionally, peripheral blood mononuclear cells (PBMCs) from PV patients with both mucosal and cutaneous lesions showed higher levels of CD14+ human leukocyte antigen (HLA) DR+ monocytes with high expression of iNOS (inducible nitric oxide synthase), with low CD4+ and high CD8 + T cells when compared to patients with only mucosal lesions, suggesting the involvement of M1 phenotype in the inflammation in PV. Our laboratory has also found an increase in macrophage-like monocytes in the peripheral blood of PV patients when compared to healthy controls. A recent transcriptome study has revealed a correlation of plasma cells (PC) with the M1 phenotype and DC abundance with the M2 phenotype. These findings support the Th1/Th2 theory in PV and allude to the involvement of both M1 and M2 macrophages in its pathogenesis.

Dendritic Cells (DCs)

DCs form a bridge between innate and adaptive immunity. They are professional APCs and are mainly of two types—(1) myeloid-derived DCs (mDCs) (CD1c+/CD141+) and (2) plasmacytoid DCs (pDCs) (CD303+/CD123+/CD304+). DCs present in the epidermis are langerhans cells (LC) (CD1a+/langerin+). In lesional skin of pemphigus foliaceus (PF), LCs and DCs are observed in high concentration, which also correlates with serum antibody titers. Epidermal LCs were found to be less abundant in lesional as compared to perilesional skin, while CD1a + dermal DCs were more prevalent in lesional skin. In PV, LCs are found abundantly in perilesional skin along with CD4+/CD8+ T cells. Normally, the pDCs are absent in the skin, but under diseased conditions like autoimmunity, they can be seen invading the tissues. Immunohistological studies have shown a plenitude of pDCs in PV blisters. Our group has reported increased number of both pDCs and mDCs in the peripheral circulation of PV patients, compared to healthy controls. Also, the relative mRNA expression of DC surface marker ILT3 and the expression of co-stimulatory molecules CD40 and CD80 responsible for the generation of appropriate immune response, was significantly up-regulated in PV. Furthermore, DC culture supernatants showed increased levels of IL-12 and TNF-α and decreased levels of IL-10 and IFN-γ. In BP, the overall frequency of LCs is increased in patients' skin, with redistribution of LCs toward the basal membrane.

Mast Cells

They are myeloid-derived immune cells. In BP, mast cells are found with increased frequency in the dermis, with loss of

TABLE 1: Summary of innate immune cell frequency, localization, and their secretory molecules in autoimmune bullous diseases.

Immune cell	Frequency	Localization	Secretory molecules
Neutrophils	Increased in PV, pemphigus vegetans and BP	Blister site	NETs and ROS
Macrophages	Increased M2 phenotype in BP lesions, increased macrophage-like monocytes in PV in blood	Clefts between keratinocytes, dermis and in basement membrane	IL-4, IL-13, iNOS, TGF-β and TNF-α
Dendritic cells	Increased in PV, PF and BP at lesional site and blood	• Epidermis • Dermis	IL-12, TNF-α
Mast cells	Increased in BP and PV	Dermis: Heavy accumulation near hair follicles and blood vessels	IL-1, IL-2, IL-5, IL-6, IL-8, TNF-α, eotaxin and IFN-γ
Natural killer cells	Increased in PV in blood	Dermis	IFN-γ, IL-6, IL-8

(BP: bullous pemphigoid; IFN: interferon; IL: interleukin; iNOS: inducible nitric oxide synthase; NET: neutrophil extracellular trap; PF: pemphigus foliaceus; PV: pemphigus vulgaris; ROS: reactive oxygen species; TGF: transforming growth factor; TNF: tumor necrosis factor)

their granular components. IgE antibodies that are present in high concentration in BP sera have receptors on mast cells that activate them. In addition, various cytokines such as IL-1, IL-2, IL-5, IL-6, IL-8, TNF-α, eotaxin and IFN-γ, and complement proteins are present in the blister fluid, which recruit and activate mast cells. The recombinant-humanized monoclonal antibody omalizumab prevents IgE from attaching to FcRI on the surface of mast cells and basophils, leading to amelioration of BP, including less pruritus and blistering, fewer urticarial plaques, and histologically, less eosinophilic inflammation. In the blister fluid in BP, IL-17 is present in increased amount, and according to a study by Nesmond, *et al*, an isoform of IL-17, IL-17RB, is expressed by mast cells which negatively correlates with disease severity. In PV, mast cells are found in the dermis, with a heavy accumulation near the hair follicles and blood vessels in the upper dermis.

Natural Killer (NK) Cells

They are innate cytotoxic cells that provide defense against non-self-antigens by recognizing major histocompatibility complex 1 (MHC 1) as a self-cell marker. They constitute 5–20% of the circulating lymphocytes. They are of two types based on the expression of their characteristic marker CD56, CD56 dim NK cells, and CD56 bright NK cells. The latter type is non-cytotoxic and produces inflammatory cytokines such as IFN-γ. In PV, NK cells are increased in peripheral circulation with a high expression of CD69 activation marker. A recent transcriptomic analysis has linked increased NK cell population in the dermis to B-cell proliferation. NK cells are also found to function as APCs in PV. Stern, *et al* provided evidence for this by finding considerable T cell proliferation while co-culturing NK cells and CD4+ T cells in the presence of desmoglein 3 (Dsg3). Additionally, IL-6, IL-8, and IFN-γ levels in NK cell culture supernatants increased. It is possible that NK cells are also prone to Th2-type regulation of disease development, given the rise in IL-10 mRNA expression and decrease in IL-12 signaling. In contrast, NK cells show a decrease in granzyme and perforin mRNA expression in PV, indicating their protective role in this disease. As a consequence, NK cells might demonstrate a dual functionality of both protective and pathogenic role in AIBDs.

A summary of the variation in frequency and localization of different innate immune cells with their secretory molecules in AIBDs is given in **Table 1**.

Adaptive Immune Cells

B Cells and their Phenotypic and Functional Determinants

B lymphocytes are an important component of humoral immunity. They are CD19+ cells with B-cell receptor (BCR) on their surface, which recognize the antigen and respond either dependently or independently of T cells. BCR plays a crucial role in the development of autoimmunity. BCR goes through development while B cells are produced from the hematopoietic stem cells. The different stages of BCR development gives rise to pro-, pre-, naïve and mature B cells **(Table 2)**. BCR undergoes cycles of rearrangements, somatic hypermutations, allelic exclusion, receptor editing, and class switching to give rise to receptors with different specificities toward non-self-cells. Although this is a tightly regulated process, any defect in this process leads to the formation of self-specific BCRs. This loss of self-tolerance can lead to formation of autoreactive B lymphocytes which give rise to PC and memory B cells, that contribute to the development of autoimmunity.

- *Conventional B cells or follicular B cells or B2 cells*: These cells are present in the peritoneal cavity and secondary lymphoid organs such as spleen and lymph nodes, where they give rise to plasma cells and memory B cells after interaction with the antigen. In AIBDs, disease severity correlates with the frequency of B cells.
- *Plasma cells*: After activation of the B2 cells, plasma B cells are rapidly generated in the germinal center or medullary cord of lymph nodes and are responsible for antibody production. They have the ability to produce autoantibodies even when antigen levels sink. This is due to the presence of its cytokine milieu—A proliferation-inducing ligand (APRIL), B lymphocyte stimulator (BLyS), and B-cell activating factor (BAFF), secreted at the inflammatory site by the adjacent immune cells and stromal cells which act as survival signals for the B cells. The lesional skin of pemphigus patients has shown considerable quantity of CD19+ B cells and CD138+

TABLE 2: Developmental markers of B cells and immunotherapy targets: Anti-CD20 monoclonal antibody (mAb)—rituximab, veltuzumab and ofatumumab target pre-, immature, mature, and memory B cells, while in patients resistant to rituximab, anti-CD19 inebilizumab is effective, which targets all types of B cells.

B cell stage	Ig	CD19	CD20	CD38	CD22	CD27	CD52	CD49d	CD138		
Pro B cell		+					+	+		**Anti-CD20 mAb** Rituximab Veltuzumab Ofatumumab	**Anti-CD19 mAb** Inebilizumab
Pre B cell		+	+				+	+			
Immature B cell	+	+	+				+	+			
Mature B cell	+	+	+	+/−	+		+	+			
Memory B cell	+/−	+	+		+	+	+	+			
Plasmablast	+/−	+		+		+	+	+	+		
Plasma cell		+/−		+		+	+	+	+		

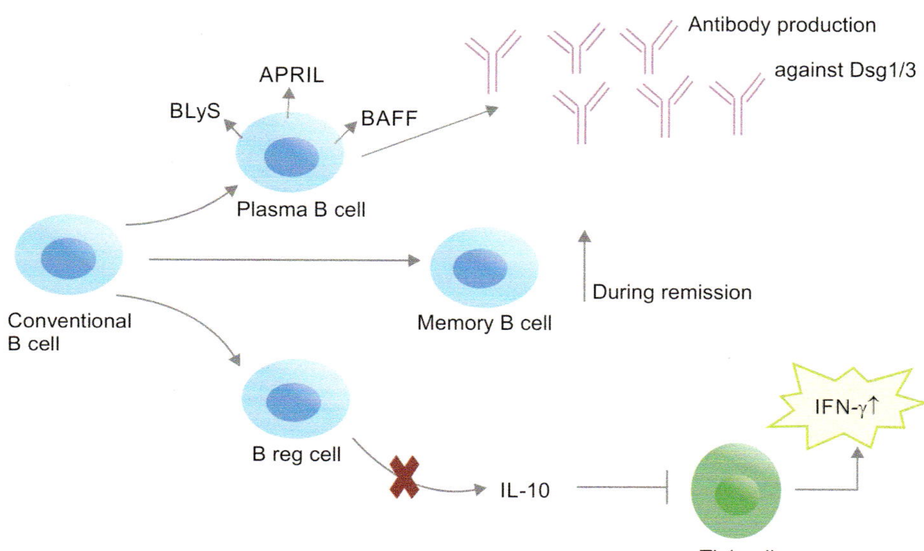

Fig. 2: Function of B cells and their subtypes in pemphigus: At the time of immune dysregulation, conventional B cells or B2 cells give rise to plasma and memory B cells. There is upregulation of markers such as APRIL, BLyS, and BAFF on plasma cells leading to production of auto-antibodies against Dsg1/3 which causes acantholysis and blister formation. Conventional B cells give rise to regulatory B cells which in pemphigus vulgaris have lost the ability to secrete IL-10, therefore, are unable to perform the protective function of downregulating IFN-γ, leading to inflammation.

(APRIL: A proliferation-inducing ligand; BAFF: B-cell activating factor; BLyS: B lymphocyte stimulator; Dsg: desmoglein; IFN-γ: interferon γ; IL: interleukin; reg: regulatory; Th: T-helper)

PCs. These lymphocytes produced pathogenic anti-Dsg1 and 3 antibodies in vitro.

- *Memory B cells*: B2 cells also give rise to memory B cells. These cells do not require BLyS and APRIL for their survival, which allows them to escape the therapeutics. The Dsg3-specific memory B cells have been found to be greatly enhanced in pemphigus patients during remission following immunosuppressive medication, which likely contributes to subsequent disease relapse.
- *Breg (regulatory) cells*: They are IL-10, TGF-β and IL-35 secreting cells. They are responsible for regulating immune reactions by suppressing inflammation and maintaining homeostasis. In pemphigus, although the frequency of Breg cells is found to be increased in peripheral blood, but their ability to produce IL-10 is impaired. Therefore, IFN-γ production by Th1 cells is not suppressed, leading to continual inflammation **(Fig. 2)**.

B cells are also involved in the formation of TLS (tertiary lymphoid structure) in the skin as they interact with T helper cells by presenting MHC class II and co-stimulatory molecules such as CD40 and CD80/86. Reports have also shown suppression of T cell activity by targeting B cells which act as APCs, thereby reducing disease severity.

T CELLS AND THEIR PHENOTYPIC AND FUNCTIONAL DETERMINANTS

T cells account for approximately 60% of the total lymphocytes present in blood. T cells function only after getting signal from antigens expressed by MHCs present on APCs or nucleated cells (majority of the cells in the body contain nucleus and are known as nucleated cells, while some cells such as platelets and red blood cells are non-nucleated cells).

- *CD8+ T cells* or *cytotoxic T lymphocytes* are activated by MHC class I molecules presented by nucleated cells. In pemphigus, CD8+ T cells are present in perivascular areas of the dermis. Studies have demonstrated the presence of Fas ligand (Fas-L) and caspases in sera of pemphigus patients. This indicates that the role of CD8+ T cells is perhaps through apoptotic pathways involving Fas/Fas-L. Analysis of the peripheral blood in BP patients revealed that they had less CD8+ T lymphocytes than younger adult controls. Another study however noted that the majority of CD8+ T cells in blood had dramatically increased and the number of CD4+ cells and the CD4/CD8 ratio had decreased both at baseline and after treatment in BP, when compared to healthy controls.
- *CD4+ T cells-Th1 and Th2*: CD4+ T cells are known as *helper T cells* and are categorized into various subsets depending on the cytokine milieu they secrete **(Fig. 3)**. In response to IFN-γ and IL-12, naïve T cells differentiate into *Th1 cells,* leading to activation of STAT 1 signaling which induces expression of T bet. T bet is a transcriptional regulator which promotes IFN-γ secretion from Th1 cells. *Th2 cells* are activated by IL-4 which activates the STAT6 pathway leading to induction of GATA3 (transcription factor that recognizes G-A-T-A nucleotide sequences in target gene promoters), which in collaboration with STAT5 produces the Th2 cytokines—IL-4, IL-5, IL-9, IL-13, IL-25, and thymic

stromal lymphopoietin (TSLP). IL-10 is secreted by both Th1 and Th2 cells. During autoimmune reactions, Th 2-derived cytokines like IL-4 encourage the proliferation of B cells, generation of antibodies, and shift of immunoglobulin class to IgE.

Early studies in PV had shown presence of Dsg reactive Th1 and Th2 cells in similar frequency in acute onset, chronic active and remittent disease. But later, according to a magnetic cell sorting cytokine secretion assay study, Th1 cells exceeded Th2 cells. Since Th2-derived cytokines are involved in autoantibody production by B cells, much importance has subsequently been given to Th2 cells, and it has been found that they are upregulated in PV patients compared to controls. In patients' sera, IL-4 and IL-10 were found to be upregulated while IFN-γ and IL-2 were found to be downregulated, indicating suppression of Th1 cytokines by Th2 cells. This suggests an imbalance of Th1/Th2 cells in PV pathogenesis.

In active BP, autoreactive Th1 and Th2 cells are present against the NC16A domain of BP180 antigen, but not in those who have attained remission or are receiving immunosuppressive medication. Th2 cytokines like IL-4 play an important role in the pathogenesis of BP. IL-4 and IL-5 are involved in eosinophil functionality (chemoattraction, maturation, and function). Both CD4+ and CD8+ T cells are present in lesional and perilesional skin of BP. Th2 cytokines with a moderate to strong IL-4 and IL-5 prevalence were noted in the perivascular area of upper dermis, while Th1 cytokine IFN-γ showed a moderate/focal expression at this site. A study revealed two major epitopes of Th2 cells for

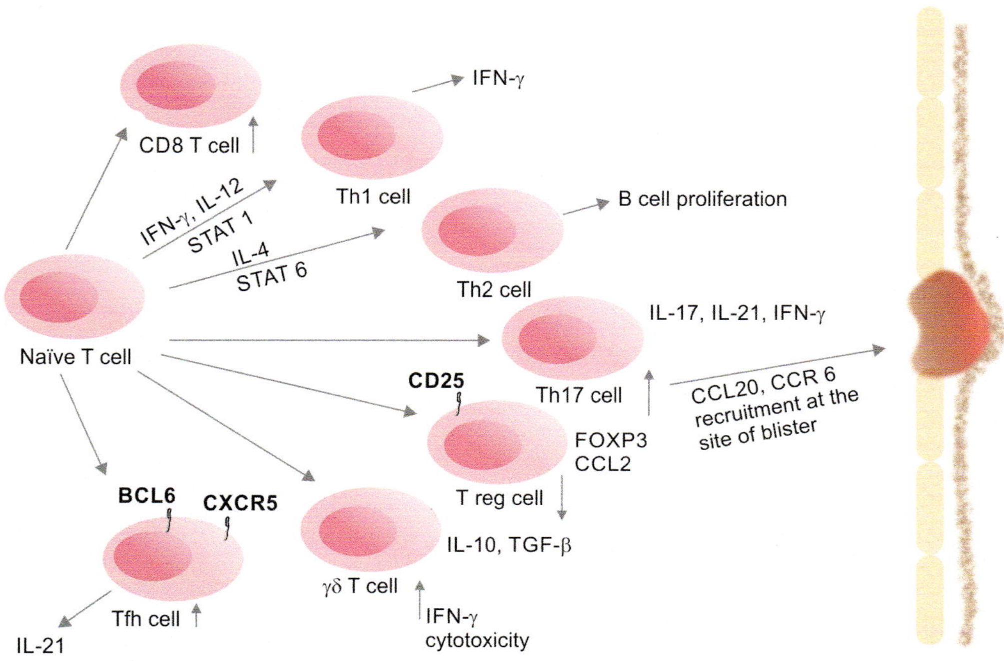

Fig. 3: Immune response of T cells and its subtypes in pemphigus.
(BCL: B-cell lymphoma; CCL: chemokine ligand; CCR: chemokine receptor; CXCR: chemokine receptor; FOXP3: forkhead box protein 3; IFN: interferon; IL: interleukin; ROR: retinoid-related orphan receptor; STAT: signal transducer and activator of transcription; Tfh: follicular T helper; Th: T helper; Treg: T regulatory)

NC16A-P2 (492–506 aa: VRKLKARVDELERIR) and P5 (501–515 aa: ELERIRRSILPYGDS), by ELISPOT assay. These epitopes are majorly involved in the activation of Th2 cells and secretion of IL-4 in BP.

- *Th17 cells*: They are a subset of CD4+ T cells. These cells produce pro-inflammatory cytokines like IL-17A/F, IL-21, IL-22, IFN-γ and granulocyte-macrophage colony-stimulating factor (GM-CSF). Naïve T cells in the presence of retinoid-related orphan receptor gamma T (RORγT) and STAT3 with IL-6 and transforming growth factor β (TGF-β) give rise to Th17 cells. In PV, Th17 cells are elevated in the peripheral circulation when compared to healthy controls both during the acute phase and active chronic phase, with elevated levels of IL-17A and chemokine ligand 20 (CCL20) in serum. Additionally, mRNA expression of RORγT and chemokine receptor 6 (CCR6), which is a receptor for CCL20, were amplified in PV. CCR6 is highly expressed on Th17 cells and the upregulation of both CCR6 and CCL20 results in recruitment of Th17 cells to the inflammatory sites in PV. IL-21 and IL-17A producing CD4+ cells have also been found in the lesional skin of PV.

  Th17 cells are found in the lesional skin of BP. They are also present with increased frequency in the peripheral blood of BP patients. The Th17-related cytokine IL-17, is found in both serum and blister fluid of BP. Recent research has revealed that IL-17 has a role in the tissue erosive process and inflammatory feedback loop in BP development. Matrix metalloproteinase 9 and neutrophil elastase, the two proteases implicated in blister formation, are expressed at higher levels when IL-17 is present, further illustrating the role of IL-17 in BP pathogenesis.

- *Regulatory T cells (Treg)*: These cells are a subset of CD4+ T cells which are CD25+ CD127– and FOXP3+ (forkhead box protein 3). Treg cells are an important component of the immune system that maintain self-tolerance and prevent autoimmunity. In PV, Tregs are decreased in frequency in peripheral blood. Dsg3-specific Treg cells are also found, which on signals from the auto-antigen, release the signature inhibitory cytokines IL-10 and TGF-β. In BP, studies have shown contrasting results, with some showing increased Tregs levels while the others showing decreased levels in both blood and lesional skin. Asothai, *et al* showed lower expression of CCR4-CCL22 in Treg cells in PV, which suggested a skin homing inefficiency of Tregs in this disease.

- *Follicular helper T cells (Tfh)*: Tfh cell is a type of CD4+ T cell that expresses BCL6 (B-cell lymphoma 6) and CXCR5 (chemokine receptor type 5). This cell type is involved in the generation of germinal centers and in providing co-stimulatory signals to B cells, thus helping them in antibody production. These cells express PD1 and CD40L, and secrete IL-21, which helps in B-cell development in the germinal centers. In both PV and BP, levels of Tfh cells are increased. According to co-culture studies, Tfh17 cells are principally incharge of causing B cells to produce Dsg-specific autoantibodies in PV.

- *Gamma delta T cells (γδ T cells)*: γδ T cells are a special class of T cells that recognize phosphoantigens (non-peptidic molecules that have undergone phosphory-lation and are metabolic intermediates in the formation of iso-prenoids) to get activated. They are increased in circulation in PV and decreased in BP patients. A study by Das, *et al* provided evidence of increased IFN-γ secretion and cytotoxicity by γδ T cells in PV patients when compared to controls. However, the exact mechanism by which these cells act is still unclear.

ROLE OF CYTOKINES IN PEMPHIGUS AND OTHER AIBDs

AIBDs are a nexus of several cytokines. These cytokines are necessary for activation and functioning of immune cells which drive the disease toward inflammation or anti-inflammation. There is an imbalance of these cytokines leading to improper functioning of immune cells. Some cytokines increase with disease severity while others either remain unaffected or decrease. **Table 3** summarizes the cytokine levels in various AIBDs.

COMPLEMENT-DEPENDENT PATHWAYS

Complement pathways are a series of proteolytic events that complement the innate system to perform effector functions against the pathogens. There are a group of approximately 50 proteolytic molecules present either in plasma or on the surface of various cells. The functions of complement pathways are opsonization, phagocytosis, cell lysis, and inflammation in order to attract other immune cells at the site of infection/inflammation. There are three main pathways that mediate the killing of pathogen—(1) classical pathway gets triggered only after the antibody binds to antigen, (2) alternative pathway recognizes C3b deposition on the microbe, and (3) the lectin pathway, which recognizes mannose-binding lectin (MBL) deposition. These pathways involve various molecules such as C1 to C9 and their proteolytic products such as C3a/b and C5a/b, which get deposited at the site of infection/inflammation. An imbalance in the complement molecules sometimes acts as a diagnostic tool for diseases **(Fig. 4)**.

In PV, autoantibodies mainly IgG1 and IgG4, of which IgG1 is a powerful activator of the complement pathway, are present against Dsg1 and Dsg3. The molecules of both the classical and alternative complement pathways, i.e., C1q, C3, C4, C5, C7, C9, ficolin, properdin, MBL, and membrane attack complex (MAC) are found in lesional skin especially in intercellular regions. Complement products are also found in the blister fluid of patients.

In endemic PF, patients in the El Bagre region of Colombia showed a robust presence of MAC in the lesions, which also positively correlated with autoantibody titers. CR1, a regulator of the complement system and

TABLE 3: Alteration of cytokine levels in pemphigus and bullous pemphigoid.

Cytokine	Pemphigus vulgaris		Bullous pemphigoid		Pemphigus foliaceus	
	Serum	*Blister*	*Serum*	*Blister*	*Serum*	*Blister*
IFN-γ	C	↑	C	↑	↓	
TNF-α	↑	No significant difference	No significant difference	↑		
TGF-β	C	No significant difference	C	C		
TSLP	No significant difference	No significant difference	↑	↑		
IL-1α	C	No significant difference	No significant difference	↓	↑	
IL-2	No significant difference	No significant difference	No significant difference	No significant difference but blister levels> serum levels	↓	
IL-4	C	No significant difference	No significant difference	↑	↓	
IL-5	C	No significant difference	↑	↑	No significant difference	
IL-6	↑	↑	No significant difference	↑	No significant difference	
IL-10	↑	↑	C	C	↑	
IL-12	C	No significant difference				
IL-17	↑		↑	↑	No significant difference	
IL-21	↑		↑			
IL-23	No significant difference		C	↑	↑	

(C: contrasting results in literature; IL: interleukin; TGF: transforming growth factor; TNF: tumor necrosis factor; TSLP: thymic stromal lymphopoietin)

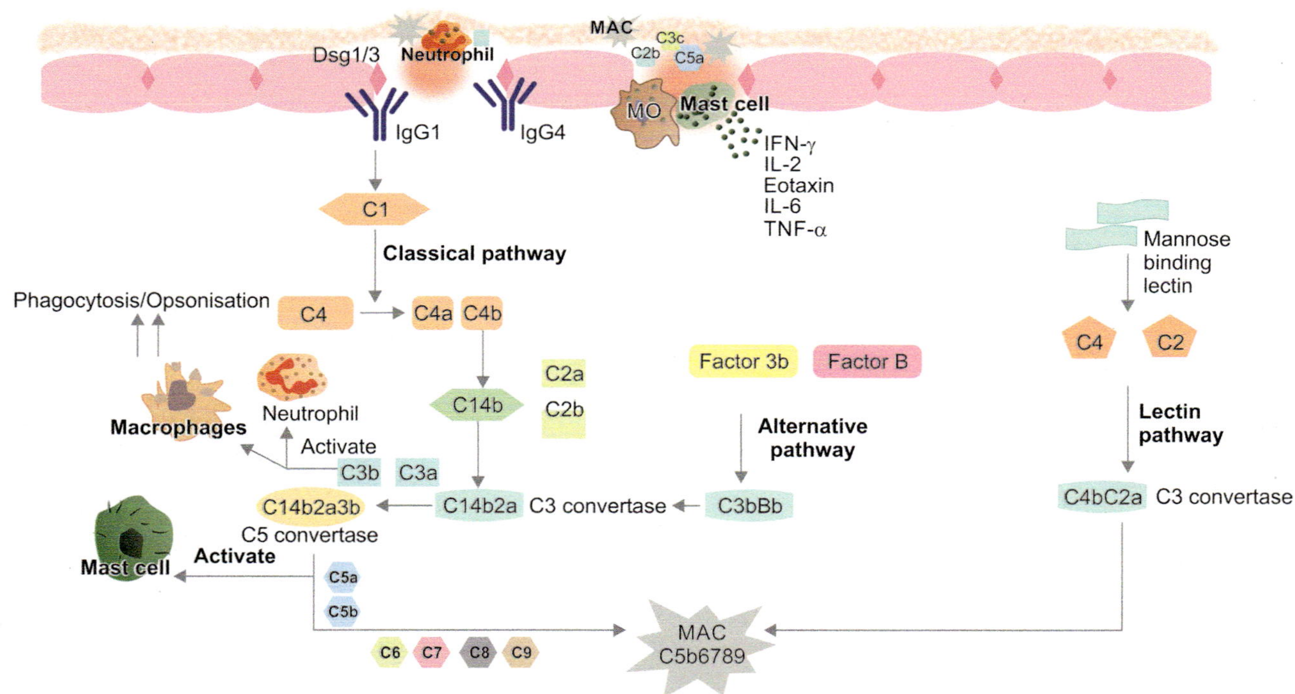

Fig. 4: Schematic overview of complement system and its molecules in autoimmune bullous diseases.
(Dsg: desmoglein; MAC: membrane attack complex; MO: macrophage)

anti-inflammatory in nature, is found in low levels in active disease in treatment naïve patients and in high levels in the lesions of patients undergoing treatment. This makes it a potential therapeutic target for the disease.

In BP, complement molecules of the classical pathway—C1, C3, C3d, properdin, C5, and MAC, are found in blisters, which may be responsible for the chemoattraction of several immune cells like mast cells and eosinophils.

CONCLUSION

Autoimmunity is a disease mediated by an imbalance of immune cells. Inflammatory and effector cells consistently have the upper hand in AIBDs, which leads to spread and recurrence of the disease. Published data suggests the role of altered antibody-mediated Th2 function along with involvement of Th17/Th1 with defective regulatory cells, activated Th1 cells, CD8 T cells, langerhan cells, NK cells, and mast cells in AIBDs. Although regulatory cells such as Bregs, Tregs, iNKT, and M2 macrophages have been identified, their functional activity needs further investigation. Despite the fact that various therapies have been shown to increase regulatory cells in AIBDs, none of them are effective enough to reverse the condition. This poses a need to study cross talk of several innate and adaptive immune cells in the diseased condition to elucidate the immunological networks and their significance in the pathogenesis. Further knowledge of pathways is required to identify novel therapeutic targets which might help in better management of this group of diseases.

TAKE HOME MESSAGE

- AIBDs are complex inflammatory diseases and the dysregulation of several immune cells may affect their crosstalk, which play a significant role in their immuno-pathogenesis.
- Neutrophils are increased in PV and BP as shown by NEUT RI and NEUT GI. They perform effector function by degranulation and ROS activity. They are responsible for the recruitment of other immune cells.
- In PV, there is an imbalance of M1 and M2 phenotype and involvement of both subtypes has been found, but in BP, the M2 phenotype is significantly involved which favors towards Th2 polarization.
- In PV and BP, both pDC and mDC are increased in both circulation and lesional skin. The expression of CD40 and CD80 is upregulated, which are responsible for co-stimulation.
- In PV and BP, mast cells are also increased along with IL-1, IL-2, IL-5, IL-6, IL-8, TNF-α, eotaxin, and IFN-γ.
- CD56 dim NK cells are increased in circulation with decreased levels of perforin and granzyme in PV and BP.
- BP is a Th2-mediated disease while PV is mediated by an imbalance of Th1/Th2 cells.
- Complement molecules which are proteolytic products involved in innate effector functions, are also present in the blisters of PV and BP, affecting the recruitment of several immune cells to the site.
- Immune cells and their stimulatory molecules can be used as therapeutic targets to combat AIBDs.

MULTIPLE CHOICE QUESTIONS

1. **In pemphigus vulgaris, autoantibodies are directed against which adhesion molecule?**
   - (a) Desmocollin 1
   - (b) Integrin
   - (c) Desmoglein 3
   - (d) Selectin

2. **Which of the following subtype of NK cells is cytotoxic in nature and is abundantly present in circulation?**
   - (a) CD56dim
   - (b) CD56high
   - (c) NKT
   - (d) Innate-induced NK cells

3. **The continuous production of antibodies by plasma B cells even after the removal of antigen is because of factors like:**
   - (a) BAFF and GATA3
   - (b) BLyS only
   - (c) BAFF, APRIL, and BLyS
   - (d) GATA3, BAFF and APRIL

4. **Regulatory immune cells like Bregs and Tregs secrete cytokines like:**
   - (a) IFN-γ, TNF-α, IL-10
   - (b) IL-10, TGF-β
   - (c) IL-17A, IL-17F, IL-23
   - (d) IL-4, IFN-γ, IL-21

5. **Cytotoxic T cells generally recognize antigens presented by:**
   - (a) Class II MHC
   - (b) Class I MHC
   - (c) Class III MHC
   - (d) HLA DR determinants

6. **Opsonization is a key feature of which of the following cells?**
   - (a) Macrophage
   - (b) Neutrophil
   - (c) Mast cell
   - (d) T cell

7. **Which of the following cytokine regulates T-cell-mediated immune responses?**
   (a) IL-4
   (b) TNF-α
   (c) TGF-β
   (d) MCSF

8. **Innate immune cells recognize which of the following markers on the pathogens to generate an immune response?**
   (a) TLRs
   (b) DAMPs
   (c) PAMPs
   (d) All of the above

9. **STAT3 and STAT6 are the transcription factors of which of the following cell types?**
   (a) Monocytes
   (b) Neutrophils
   (c) M1 macrophages
   (d) M2 macrophages

10. **Which cytokine is responsible for activation and proliferation of T cells after recognition of antigen by TCR and presence of co-stimulatory signals?**
    (a) IL-10
    (b) IL-2
    (c) MCSF
    (d) IL-15

Answers

1. (c)   2. (a)   3. (c)   4. (b)   5. (b)   6. (b)   7. (c)   8. (d)   9. (d)   10. (b)

SUGGESTED READING

1. Chiossi MPV, Costa RS, Roselino AMF. Dermal dendritic cell number correlates with serum autoantibody titers in Brazilian pemphigus foliaceous patients. *Braz J Med Biol Res.* 2004;37:337-41.
2. Fang H, Li Q, Wang G. The role of T cells in pemphigus vulgaris and bullous pemphigoid. *Autoimmun Rev.* 2020;19:102661.
3. Das D, Anand V, Khandpur S, Sharma VK, Sharma A. T helper type 1 polarizing $\gamma\delta$ T cells and scavenger receptors contribute to the pathogenesis of pemphigus vulgaris. *Immunology.* 2018;153:97-104.
4. Das D, Singh A, Antil PS, Sharma D, Arava S, Khandpur S, *et al.* Distorted frequency of dendritic cells and their associated stimulatory and inhibitory markers augment the pathogenesis of pemphigus vulgaris. *Immunol Res.* 2020;68:353-62.
5. Asothai R, Anand V, Das D, Antil PS, Khandpur S, Sharma VK, *et al.* Distinctive Treg associated CCR4-CCL22 expression profile with altered frequency of Th17/Treg cell in the immunopathogenesis of pemphigus vulgaris. *Immunobiology.* 2015;220:1129-35.
6. Das D, Akhtar S, Kurra S, Gupta S, Sharma A. Emerging role of immune cell network in autoimmune skin disorders: An update on pemphigus, vitiligo and psoriasis. *Cytokine Growth Factor Rev.* 2019;45:35-44.
7. Satyam A, Khandpur S, Sharma VK, Sharma A. Involvement of T(H)1/T(H)2 cytokines in the pathogenesis of autoimmune skin disease-pemphigus vulgaris. *Immunol Invest.* 2009;38:498-509.
8. Edwards G, Diercks GFH, Seelen MAJ, Horvath B, van Doorn MBA, Damman J. Complement activation in autoimmune bullous dermatoses: A comprehensive review. *Front Immunol.* 2019;10: 1477.
9. Kowalski EH, Kneibner D, Kridin K, Amber KT. Serum and blister fluid levels of cytokines and chemokines in pemphigus and bullous pemphigoid. *Autoimmun Rev.* 2019;18:526-34.
10. Tavakolpour S, Mahmoudi H, Mirzazadeh A, Balighi K, Darabi-Monadi S, Hatami S, *et al.* Pathogenic and protective roles of cytokines in pemphigus: A systematic review. *Cytokine.* 2020;129: 155026.
11. Bumiller-Bini V, Cipolla GA, de Almeida RC, Petzl-Erler ML, Augusto DG, Boldt ABW. Sparking Fire Under the Skin? Answers from the association of complement genes with pemphigus foliaceus. *Front Immunol.* 2018;9:695.

CHAPTER 3

Etiopathogenesis of Pemphigus

Sunil Dogra, Shikha Shah

- Genetics in relation to pemphigus
- Triggers
- Pathogenesis
- Animal models
- Future implications

INTRODUCTION

Pemphigus is a chronic and potentially life-threatening autoimmune bullous disease (AIBD) mediated by pathogenic autoantibodies against desmogleins (Dsgs), which results in acantholysis and consequent mucosal and cutaneous blistering. Understanding the etiopathogenesis of pemphigus remains a paradigm for better designing of disease evaluation tools and development of novel and targeted therapies.

The pathophysiology of pemphigus is summarized conceptually in **Flowchart 1**. The following sections aim to elucidate the intricacies of genetic factors, triggers, and exact pathogenic mechanisms behind the orchestration of this complex disease.

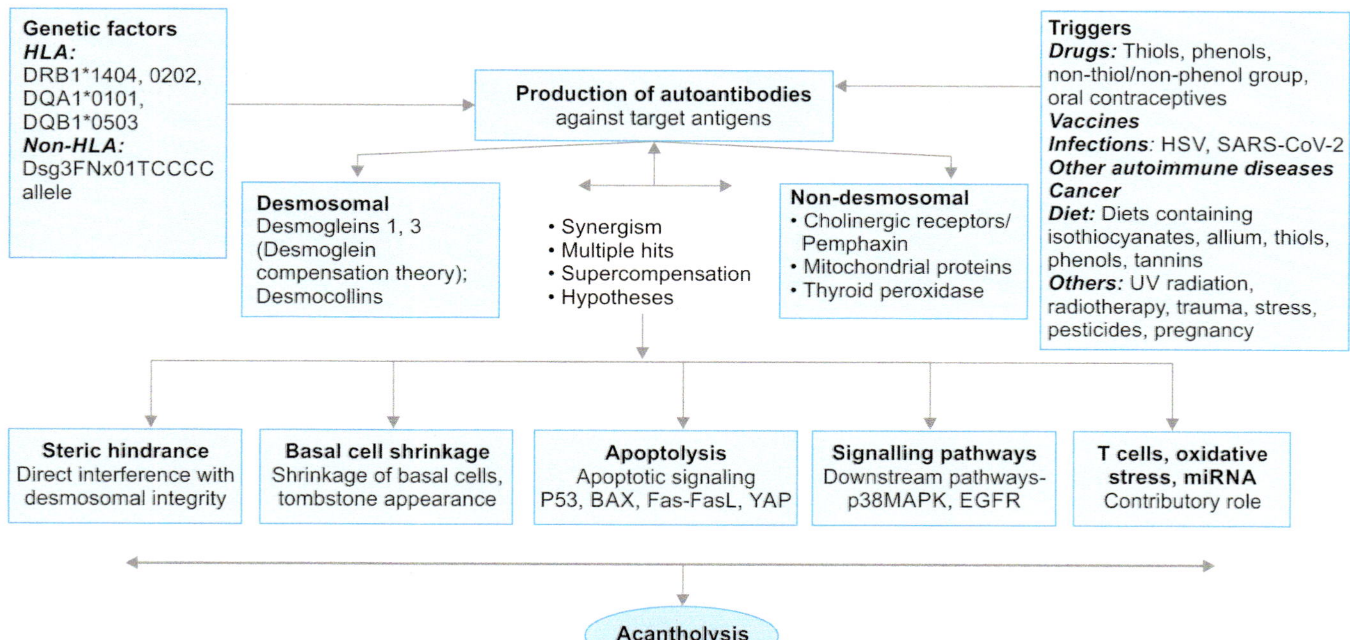

Flowchart 1: Pathophysiology of pemphigus: genetic and environmental factors trigger the production of autoantibodies to chiefly desmosomal but also to other non-desmosomal proteins. This in turn leads to acantholysis by synergy of various downstream mechanisms. (BAX: Bcl-2 associated X-protein; CoV: corona virus; Dsg: desmoglein; EGFR: epidermal growth factor receptor; HLA: human leukocyte antigen; HSV: herpes simplex virus; miRNA: microRNA; p38MAPK: p38 mitogen-activated protein kinase; SARS-CoV: severe acute respiratory syndrome-coronavirus; UV: ultraviolet; YAP: yes-associated protein)

GENETICS IN RELATION TO PEMPHIGUS

Genetic predisposition to pemphigus is evident in its ethnic susceptibility, occurrence of familial cases, presence of other autoimmune co-morbidities in patients and their family members as well as detection of anti-Dsg antibodies in asymptomatic relatives. Low titers of autoantibodies may be detected in about 15–31% of first-degree relatives of pemphigus patients, which may not be high enough to induce acantholysis per se, but makes them more susceptible to other triggers such as drugs or infections. PV is more common in the Jewish population and also shows a north–south gradient: more common in lower latitudes like Tunisia than northern countries like Finland. Genetic susceptibility with environmental factors can explain the disease dynamics.

Association studies that identify susceptibility genes by candidate–gene approach or genome-wide studies have revealed strongest association in Indian patients with type II human leukocyte antigen (HLA) alleles: DRB1*1404, 0202, DQA1*0101, and DQB1*0503. Among non-HLA genes, different haplotypes of autoantigen *Dsg3* gene were found in Indian patients. A higher incidence of PV and early age at onset for pemphigus seen in Indian population have been attributed to a higher frequency of Dsg3FNx01TCCCC in the Indian population.

TRIGGERS

Pemphigus is an organ-specific autoimmune disease which may potentially be triggered or exacerbated by various exogenous factors in susceptible individuals. A knowledge about these acantholytic triggers and their avoidance may prolong remission and/or prevent exacerbation.

Major Triggers

Drugs

Drugs are the most common reported triggers. The following groups are implicated:

- *Thiols*: Contain a sulfhydryl group (–SH) in their chemical structure; inhibit enzymes that aggregate keratinocytes and activate enzymes that disaggregate keratinocytes. They may themselves induce autoantibody formation (e.g., captopril, penicillamine).
- *Phenols*: Stimulate keratinocytes to release pro-inflammatory cytokines like tumor necrosis factor alpha (TNF-α) and interleukin-1 (IL-1), which modulate acantholysis (e.g., aspirin, rifampicin).
- *Non-thiol, non-phenol*: Can induce/flare-up of the disease by immune aberrations [(e.g., non-steroidal anti-inflammatory drugs (NSAIDs), angiotensin-converting enzyme inhibitors (ACEI)].

  Recently, use of oral contraceptives has also been shown to be associated with slightly increased rates of pemphigus than in controls.

It is prudent to elicit a detailed drug history in all new cases of pemphigus. The drug-induced pemphigus cases may resolve on drug discontinuation in almost 50% cases, especially those without the cell surface autoantibodies (classically described in pemphigus induced by thiols). However, some drugs may simply trigger the disease which is almost indistinguishable and follows a similar clinical course as idiopathic pemphigus. The readers are referred to Chapter 9 for a more detailed description of drug-induced pemphigus.

Vaccines

Vaccines are known to trigger autoimmune responses possibly by molecular mimicry and immune stimulation. There have been several reports in recent times of new-onset or exacerbation of pemphigus and other AIBDs with coronavirus disease 2019 (COVID-19) vaccination in susceptible individuals. Temporality is suggestive, however, direct cause–effect relation has not been proven.

Underlying Diseases

- *Infections*: Certain viral infections are considered to be indirect triggers for pemphigus by affecting the immune responses. Induction or worsening of pemphigus by herpes viruses and recently by severe acute respiratory syndrome coronavirus 2 (SARS-CoV-2) has been postulated.
- *Cancer*: Co-existence of different types of pemphigus, specially paraneoplastic pemphigus (PNP) and various cancers, suggests a complex role in causation. Checkpoint inhibition such as cytotoxic T-lymphocyte-associated protein 4 (CTLA-4) or programmed cell death-1 (PD-1) could break self-tolerance and induce autoimmunity.
- *Autoimmune diseases*: Autoimmune thyroiditis is the most common pemphigus-associated condition; with anecdotal evidence of co-existence with systemic lupus erythematosus, bullous pemphigoid, lichen planus, psoriasis, alopecia areata/universalis, and rheumatoid arthritis. A family history of autoimmune diseases can also be found.

Diet

Allium vegetables such as garlic and onion are well-known dietary triggers for inducing pemphigus. A diet rich in thiols, isothiocyanates, phenols, and tannins are also potential triggers. Among micronutrients, deficiency of vitamin D, selenium, copper, and zinc have been reported. Vitamin D has established immunoregulatory properties.

Radiotherapy

Pemphigus has sometimes been reported to occur with a dose of ionizing radiation as low as 70 Gy and the majority were related with breast cancer. A proper risk–benefit evaluation at the beginning of radiotherapy in pemphigus patients is warranted.

Pregnancy

Due to the perturbation in T helper 1 (Th1)/Th2 axis, pregnancy often results in disease flare-ups due to more immunoglobulin G (IgG) autoantibody production, as a consequence of an increase in Th2-associated cytokines. Delaying gestation until disease is in remission is recommended.

Stress

Emotional stress can alter glucocorticoid secretion and cytokine production, which in turn may induce or exacerbate pemphigus in susceptible patients. An underlying psychiatric co-morbidity, either primary or secondary to the disease, must be addressed to prevent disease flares.

Ultraviolet Radiation

Ultraviolet (UV) exposure leads to increase in pro-inflammatory cytokines, e.g., IL-1, IL-6, and TNF-α which in turn is known to induce and/or aggravate pemphigus. Particularly UVB is reported to trigger acantholysis in susceptible hosts.

Trauma

Trauma, burns, electrical injuries, and rarely honeybee stings are sometimes reported to trigger pemphigus by alteration of self-antigens or inducing systemic inflammatory responses.

Pesticides

Pesticides are known to trigger acantholysis by the estrogenic effects of organochlorines, decrease in receptor density (muscarinic, nicotinic) in the skin or decrease in regulatory T cells. Pesticides such as glyphosate and dichlorodiphenyltrichloroethane (DDT) have been implicated in contact pemphigus (pemphigus occurring at sites of local skin contact with chemicals).

Blood Group

No association between ABO or Rhesus groups with pemphigus has been conclusively found.

Seasonal Variation

Pemphigus is reported to be triggered or worsened around summer and spring; the role of UV light can be plausible here. However, winter exacerbations are also reported, which may peak along with increase in the incidence of respiratory infections that stimulate immune responses.

Smoking

Smoking has a protective role in pemphigus by its agonism on nicotinic acetylcholine receptors on keratinocytes to promote cell–cell adherence, stopping acantholysis, and stimulating the lateral spread of keratinocytes in erosion healing.

PATHOGENESIS

The basic premise of pemphigus lies in the term "acantholysis" coined by Auspitz in 1881, and derived from the Greek words "*Akantha*", meaning a thorn or prickle, and "*lysis*", i.e., loosening. It is a descriptor for the loss of cohesion between epidermal cells due to loss of intercellular bridges, i.e., desmosomes, eventuating into acantholytic cells which assume a round shape (smallest possible surface area for detached cells).

The various target autoantigens implicated in pemphigus are summarized in **Table 1**.

TABLE 1: Autoantigens implicated in pemphigus.

Desmosomal	Non-desmosomal
• Desmoglein 1, 3 • Desmocollin	• Cholinergic receptors [cholinergic receptor nicotinic alpha 9 (anti-CHRNα9) and anti-annexin A9 (ANXA9)/pemphaxin] • Mitochondrial proteins • Thyroid peroxidase • Peripheral myelin protein 22 (PMP22) • Human leukocyte antigen (HLA) proteins • Calcium-transporting adenosine triphosphatase (ATPase) type 2C member 1 (ATP2C1)

Evolution of Concepts for Acantholysis

Steric Hindrance Theory

The binding of autoantibodies to the mapped extracellular amino-terminals of desmosomes leads to direct interference and inhibition of cadherins, producing acantholysis. Apart from steric hindrance, autoantibodies also cause internalization and depletion of Dsg3 from the cell surface.

Desmoglein Compensation Hypothesis

This was the earliest concept postulated on the basis of differential expression of Dsg1 and Dsg3 in skin and mucosa to explain the localization of blistering across pemphigus subgroup of disorders. The nuances of this hypothesis have been discussed in **Table 2**.

TABLE 2: Desmoglein compensation hypothesis in pemphigus.

Postulate	Fallacy
Presence of only anti-Dsg3 antibodies:	
Expectation: Suprabasal acantholysis in mucosa	*Reality*: Can have both cutaneous and/or mucosal acantholysis
Presence of both anti-Dsg1 and anti-Dsg3 antibodies:	
Expectation: Suprabasal acantholysis in skin and mucosa	*Reality*: Can have only skin and/or mucosal acantholysis; on the other hand, patients without these antibodies also have skin and mucosal acantholysis
Presence of only anti-Dsg1 antibodies:	
Expectation: Superficial acantholysis in skin (pemphigus foliaceus)	*Reality*: Can have both cutaneous and/or mucosal acantholysis

Other fallacies in the Dsg-centric pathogenesis:
- Some patients having active disease may show undetectable anti-Dsg autoantibody levels.
- A lack of perfectly linear correlation between antibody titers and disease activity.
- Failure to explain disease heterogeneity.

This led to exploration of non-Dsg targets of auto-immunity and >50 such antigens have been identified by protein array technology.

Non-desmoglein Targets

Cholinergic receptors: The epidermis has both muscarinic and nicotinic cholinergic receptors with functional roles in mediating cell-to-cell adhesion. Smokers are said to have better therapeutic responses than non-smokers in pemphigus, re-instating the role of acetylcholine agonism in cellular adhesion. Antibodies identified against cholinergic receptors are: anti-cholinergic receptor nicotinic alpha 9 (anti-CHRNα9) and anti-annexin A9 (anti-ANXA9)/pemphaxin.

Mitochondrial proteins: Antimitochondrial antibodies have been identified in pemphigus patients which increase the reactive oxygen species (ROS) and may induce apoptosis. These antibodies are internalized within the keratinocytes via the neonatal fragment crystallizable (Fc) receptor which is expressed predominantly in basal keratinocytes. This may contribute to the localization of pemphigus blisters by explaining predominantly suprabasal acantholysis.

Non-Dsg adhesion molecules: Desmocollin 1 (Dsc1) is predominant in the superficial layers of epidermis, while Dsc3 in the suprabasal layers, akin to Dsgs. Anti-Dsc3 autoantibodies are postulated to be pathogenic. Other autoantibodies identified include anti-plakophilin and anti-E cadherin, which may contribute to acantholysis (refer to Table 1, Chapter 1).

Thyroid peroxidase: There is an increased risk of auto-immune thyroiditis in patients as well as first-degree relatives of pemphigus patients. Antithyroid peroxidase (TPO) antibodies, similar to Dsg-3 autoantibodies, can theoretically dissociate keratinocytes and activate the p38 mitogen-activated protein kinase (p38MAPK) signaling pathway.

Miscellaneous targets: Other potential antigens identified include peripheral myelin protein 22 (PMP22), HLA proteins, and calcium-transporting adenosine triphos-phatase (ATPase) type 2C member 1 (ATP2C1).

Multiple Hit Hypothesis

After the recognition of a plethora of autoantibodies, it was suggested that they work synergistically to mediate acantholysis by targeting different keratinocyte antigens, i.e., the concept of "multiple hits". It suggests that pemphigus is incited by at least three classes of autoantibodies directed against the desmosomal, non-desmosomal, mitochondrial, and other keratinocyte autoantigens.

Binding of autoantibodies results in activation of various downstream signaling pathways which include phospholipase C, protein kinase C, cyclin-dependent kinase 2, p38MAPK, epidermal growth factor receptor (EGFR), Src, c-Jun-N-terminal kinase, matrix metallopro-teinase 9 (MMP-9), c-Myc, glycogen synthase kinase beta, Fas/FasL, p53, BAX, and caspases 1, 3, and 8. The actual dissociation of keratinocytes is a plausible by-product of a combination of the following concepts:

Basal Cell Shrinkage Concept

This theory states that post binding of autoantibodies to the antigens, there is rupture of the cytoskeleton, resulting in collapse and shrinkage of the keratinocytes in the suprabasal layers.

Antibody-induced Apoptosis Theory; "Apoptolysis"

The binding of autoantibodies results in a pro-apoptotic milieu by increase in intracellular FasR, FasL, Bax, and p53 and a decrease in the level of B-cell lymphoma 2 (Bcl-2). This leads to activation of caspases, the resultant death-inducing signaling complex mediates acantholysis. The basal cells, therefore, do not die but rather *shrink,* rendering a "tombstone" appearance.

Supercompensation Theory

In light of the identification of multiple new target antigens, it has been postulated that binding of specific auto-antibodies to epidermal antigens in varying combination results in specific downstream signaling pathways and acantholysis only if addition of these effects exceeds an established threshold. This threshold can be overcome by highly pathogenic autoantibodies (e.g., anti-Dsg3) or varying combinations of sub-pathogenic and pathogenic autoantibodies. This evolving concept of specific auto-antibody profiles is expected to explain the clinical heterogeneity and differential phenotypes of PV, a complex disease.

Role of T-cells in the Pathogenesis of Pemphigus

Not only B cells, but T cells too contribute to the patho-genesis of pemphigus, which may serve as future thera-peutic targets. Dsgs as autoantigens in PV are identified by langerhans cells in the epidermis which act as antigen-presenting cells (refer to Chapter 2). These peptides are presented to CD4+ T cells leading to their activation. Various subsets of T cells are also dysregulated in the circulation:

- Th1 cells produce interferon gamma (IFN-γ) and enable Th2 cells to produce more IL-4 and autoantibodies.
- Th17 cells secrete IL-17 which potentiate inflammation.
- Tfh cells (follicular helper T cells) produce IL-21 which facilitates production of antibodies.
- Gamma delta (γδ) T cells have cytotoxic activity.
- A decrease in regulatory T (Treg) cells leads to unchecked production of autoreactive T cells.

Hence, Th2 and Tfh cells cause autoreactive B-cell survival and autoantibody production, and Th1 and Th17 produce cytokines causing inflammation.

Role of Oxidative Stress in Pemphigus

In vitro studies have demonstrated the accumulation of yes-associated protein (YAP) in cells affected by pemphigus along with an increase in ROS, which may also contribute to acantholysis. This opens further avenues for research in the potential use of antioxidants in pemphigus therapy.

Salient Points in the Pathogenesis of other Pemphigus Variants

Pemphigus Foliaceus

Endemic pemphigus foliaceus (PF) (fogo selvagem) resembles the sporadic variant but affects children and young adults predominantly in rural areas of Brazil and Tunisia. Most patients reside near rivers and there has been implication of black flies (*Simulium* species) in their pathogenesis whose salivary proteins (LJM11) are found to cross-react with Dsg1. This may trigger an initial auto-immune response which by epitope spreading eventuates into evident clinical disease. The pathogenic anti-Dsg1 autoantibodies here target the extracellular N-terminal domain.

Paraneoplastic Pemphigus

In PNP, multiple epitopes are targeted including the plakin family, and antibodies can be IgG, IgA, or both. There is a role of cell-mediated cytotoxicity as well as direct infiltration of Dsg-specific T cells in the epidermis, leading to interface dermatitis. This explains the polymorphous lesions resembling erythema multiforme or lichen planus and recalcitrance of mucosal lesions. There are several autoantigens implicated in the pathogenesis of PNP, which include envoplakin, periplakin, bullous pemphigoid (BP) 230, epiplakin, plectin, p200, desmosomal cadherins (Dsg1, 3; Dsc1, 2, 3) and alpha-2-macroglobulin-like antigen-1 (α2ML1). The potential pathomechanisms of this paraneoplastic autoimmunity include:

- *Breakdown of central tolerance*: Improper negative selection process in thymus (e.g., in thymomas), can result in a clone of autoreactive T cells escaping central tolerance, leading to autoimmunity.
- *Breakdown of peripheral tolerance*: There is an imbalance of Tregs and IL-6 in PNP, which may induce autoimmunity.
- *Molecular mimicry*: There is cross-reactivity of T cells directed against the tumor-derived neoantigens with desmosomal and hemidesmosomal self-proteins. Epitope spreading may further explain multiple self-antigens in PNP.

Immunoglobulin A (IgA) Pemphigus

IgA autoantibodies predominantly target desmocollins in the epidermis. The difference here lies in the IgA–Fc receptors (CD89) they possess, which recruits plenty of neutrophils and causes massive inflammation, leading to the clinical picture of pustule formation.

ANIMAL MODELS

Ex Vivo Model

Ex vivo model uses the human skin organ culture (HSOC) assay. IgG fractions prepared from pemphigus patients' sera (PV IgG), or other engineered anti-Dsg3 and/or Dsg1 antibodies are injected subcutaneously into human skin culture and the histopathology shows blistering after 24 hours. This assay preserves the normal architecture of the skin and can also be used to study the efficacy of various drugs in preventing this blistering.

In Vitro Models

The desmosomal cadherins internalization assay was based on the finding of internalization of Dsg3 after binding of autoantibodies, with eventual collapse of keratin cytoskeleton. This assay uses normal human epidermal keratinocytes (NHEK) or HaCaT cells. By exposure to specific Ca^{2+} levels, there is formation of cellular contact and differentiation of keratinocytes post which they are exposed to PV IgG and internalization of Dsg3 is assessed using the principles of immunofluorescence.

The other in vitro model is the dispase-based keratinocyte dissociation assay which studies the dissociation of keratinocytes in cellular monolayer on exposure to autoantibodies [PV IgG, single-chain variable fragment (scFv), or AK23] on NHEK or HaCaT lines.

These in vitro and ex vivo assays can be used to test novel therapeutic agents as well as generate detailed information on signaling pathways. For example, it was observed that cutaneous blistering can be prevented by inhibition of p38MAPK signaling, while in mucosa, PV IgG and AK23 induce blisters via a p38MAPK-independent pathway.

In Vivo Models

These models aim to study disease progression in living organisms. There are two types of models: passive and active. In the *passive* model, PV IgG or other engineered anti-Dsg3 antibodies are injected subcutaneously or intraperitoneally into newborn mice. The mice develop blisters in 24–36 hours, which show the typical histology as seen in patients. The limitations of the passive model include lack of long-term follow-up of animals and their inability to produce antibodies themselves.

In *active* models, the autoantibodies are produced by animals themselves. Dsg3 null mice are not tolerant against Dsg3 (never exposed to the immune system). After adoptive transfer of naive lymphocytes from Dsg3 null mice, Rag2$^{-/-}$ immunodeficient mice produce anti-Dsg3 IgG antibodies that result in PV phenotype. In an alternative model, Dsg3 null mouse is repeatedly immunized with recombinant Dsg3. The receiving Rag2$^{-/-}$ mouse will develop blisters and hair loss (intercellular adhesion of mice follicular epidermis is mainly mediated by Dsg3). The other models include induction of tolerance breakdown in WT mice by high breakage of antigen. The animal models are discussed in more detail in Chapter 4.

Animal models also suggest a role of MMPs in the pathogenesis of pemphigus. It is observed that anti-Dsg3 autoantibodies mediate acantholysis by ADAM10, a member of the ADAM family of MMPs by activating the EGFR pathway. On the other hand, there is upregulation of other MMPs and downregulation of tissue inhibitors of metalloproteinases via the non-Dsg autoantibodies. The translation of this finding in clinical practice is yet to be made in pemphigus, in contrast with pemphigoid disorders where drugs like tetracyclines, which inhibit MMPs are used in its treatment.

FUTURE IMPLICATIONS

Identification of specific clusters of autoantibody signatures has led to the questioning of the age-old Dsg compensation theory as the sole pathogenic mechanism. By delving into molecular pathogenesis, there can be future research into finding relevant disease biomarkers and designing more targeted therapies for this autoimmune malady.

CONCLUSION

There is better understanding of non-desmoglein targets and mediators of acantholysis in recent times. The pathogenesis of pemphigus is evolving and advances continue to improve our understanding of the disease.

TAKE HOME MESSAGE

- PV is chiefly mediated by autoantibodies against Dsgs that are intercellular adhesion molecules of the cadherin family.
- There is a genetic predisposition to the disease in terms of HLA type II alleles as well as non-HLA genes, e.g., Dsg3.
- There are various triggers for initiation and/or exacerbation of the disease such as drugs, vaccines, trauma, and UV light.
- The underlying key pathogenetic mechanism is "acantholysis". To explain the pathophysiology, the earliest concept was "Dsg compensation theory", based on differential expression of Dsg3 and Dsg1 in mucosa and skin.
- After identification of other potential autoantibodies against cholinergic receptors, mitochondrial proteins, TPO, etc., it has been suggested that acantholysis is the result of various insults that culminate into a blistering threshold.
- The direct inhibition of Dsgs by autoantibodies as a solo process is insufficient to produce dyscohesion in a stand-alone manner. Various signaling pathways (e.g., p38MAPK) orchestrate the acantholysis in PV.
- Animal models for research into molecular pathogenesis include ex vivo, in vitro, and in vivo approaches.
- Further research into immune signatures and correlation with varying clinical phenotypes is warranted.

MULTIPLE CHOICE QUESTIONS

1. **Autoantibodies to which of the following autoantigen(s) is implicated in the pathogenesis of pemphigus vulgaris?**
   - (a) Anti-Dsg3
   - (b) Pemphaxin
   - (c) Anti-TPO
   - (d) All of the above

2. **Which of the following drugs contains a sulfhydryl group which activates enzymes that disaggregate keratinocytes and result in drug-induced pemphigus?**
   - (a) Rifampicin
   - (b) NSAIDs
   - (c) Penicillamine
   - (d) ACE inhibitors

3. **Contact pemphigus and protective effect of smoking on pemphigus can be explained by which of the following signalling?**
   - (a) Adrenergic
   - (b) Cholinergic
   - (c) Histaminergic
   - (d) Dopaminergic

4. **Binding of autoantibodies resulting in a pro-apoptotic milieu leads to activation of caspases, mediating acantholysis. The basal cells hence do not die but rather shrink, rendering a tombstone appearance. This theory of pemphigus pathogenesis is referred to as:**
   - (a) Necrolysis
   - (b) Necroptosis
   - (c) Apoptolysis
   - (d) Apoptosis

5. **Which of the following is an active in vivo animal model for pemphigus vulgaris?**
   - (a) Dsg internalization assay
   - (b) HSOC assay
   - (c) Keratinocyte dissociation assay
   - (d) Dsg3 null and Rag2$^{-/-}$ assay

Answers

1. (d)   2. (c)   3. (b)   4. (c)   5. (d)

SUGGESTED READING

1. Vodo D, Sarig O, Sprecher E. The genetics of pemphigus vulgaris. *Front Med (Lausanne)*. 2018;5:226.
2. Kanwar AJ, De D. Pemphigus in India. *Indian J Dermatol Venereol Leprol*. 2011;77:439-49.
3. Tavakolpour S. Pemphigus trigger factors: special focus on pemphigus vulgaris and pemphigus foliaceus. *Arch Dermatol Res*. 2018;310:95-106.
4. Madala J, Bashamalla R, Kumar MP. Current concepts of pemphigus with a deep insight into its molecular aspects. *J Oral Maxillofac Pathol*. 2017;21:260-3.
5. Sinha AA, Sajda T. The evolving story of autoantibodies in pemphigus vulgaris: Development of the "Super Compensation Hypothesis". *Front Med (Lausanne)*. 2018;5:218.
6. Didona D, Maglie R, Eming R, Hertl M. Pemphigus: current and future therapeutic strategies. *Front Immunol*. 2019;10:1418.
7. Lotti R, Atene CG, Zanfi ED, Bertesi M, Zanocco-Marani T. In vitro, ex vivo, and in vivo models for the study of pemphigus. *Int J Mol Sci*. 2022;23:7044.
8. Calabria E, Canfora F, Mascolo M, Varricchio S, Mignogna MD, Adamo D. Autoimmune mucocutaneous blistering diseases after SARS-CoV-2 vaccination: A Case report of Pemphigus Vulgaris and a literature review. *Pathol Res Pract*. 2022;232:153834.
9. Costan VV, Popa C, Hâncu MF, Porumb-Andrese E, Toader MP. Comprehensive review on the pathophysiology, clinical variants and management of pemphigus (Review). *Exp Ther Med*. 2021;22:1335.
10. Cirillo N, Prime SS. A scoping review of the role of metallo-proteinases in the pathogenesis of autoimmune pemphigus and pemphigoid. *Biomolecules*. 2021;11:1506.
11. Fang H, Li Q, Wang G. The role of T cells in pemphigus vulgaris and bullous pemphigoid. *Autoimmun Rev*. 2020;19:102661.
12. Hannah R, Ramani P, Tilakaratne WM, Sukumaran G, Ramasubramanian A, Krishnan RP. Critical appraisal of different triggering pathways for the pathobiology of pemphigus vulgaris: A review. *Oral Dis*. 2022;28:1760-9.
13. Rehman A, Huang Y, Wan H. Evolving mechanisms in the pathophysiology of pemphigus vulgaris: a review emphasizing the role of desmoglein 3 in regulating p53 and the yes-associated protein. *Life (Basel)*. 2021;11:621.
14. Kim JH, Kim SC. Paraneoplastic pemphigus: paraneoplastic autoimmune disease of the skin and mucosa. *Front Immunol*. 2019;10:1259.

CHAPTER 4

Etiopathogenesis of Autoimmune Bullous Diseases excluding Pemphigus

Laxmisha Chandrashekar

- Animal models in autoimmune bullous diseases
- Pathogenesis of:
  - Bullous pemphigoid
  - Pemphigoid gestationis
  - Lichen planus pemphigoides
  - Epidermolysis bullosa acquisita
- Mucous membrane pemphigoid
- Dermatitis herpetiformis
- Linear IgA dermatosis
- Bullous systemic lupus erythematosus
- Anti p200 pemphigoid (anti-laminin γ1 pemphigoid)

INTRODUCTION

Autoimmune bullous diseases (AIBDs) are characterized by blisters and erosions which involve the skin and mucosae. The subepidermal AIBDs are characterized by autoantibodies against components of the basement membrane zone (BMZ). Central to the pathogenesis is the loss of immunological tolerance leading to the production of autoreactive T and B cells. Loss of immune tolerance could be due to a genetic predisposition or infections, drugs, malignancies, etc. There are also associated abnormalities in T regulatory cells. Autoreactive B cells produce pathogenic antibodies against components of the BMZ. Activation of complement results in activation and recruitment of effector cells which release inflammatory mediators and cytokines, leading to tissue damage. In some cases, complement-independent blistering can also occur.

ANIMAL MODELS IN AUTOIMMUNE BULLOUS DISEASES

As discussed in Chapter 3, the animal models are of two types—(1) passive disease model and (2) active model.

Passive Model

Neonatal and Adult Mice

The animal is injected with autoantibodies (either from serum of patients with disease, or from generation of auto-antibodies in rabbit). This is useful for understanding the antibody-mediated effects and tissue damage **(Figs. 1A to C)**.

Administering immunoglobulin G (IgG) from individuals with pemphigus vulgaris (PV) into newborn BALB/c mice caused the mice to develop blisters. This is an example of passive model. However, it is not ideal for studying long-term effects or therapeutic interventions.

Passive models involve both neonatal and adult mice. The quantity of antibodies needed to elicit a reaction in adult mice is higher compared to neonatal mice.

Human Skin/Humanized Mice

This enables the replication of human disease. This is done either by using a humanized mouse or by transplantation of human skin in immunodeficient mice with severe combined immunodeficiency (SCID). This technique is used to study the role of anti-laminin 332 antibodies in disease pathogenesis. Human anti-bodies fail to bind to the skin of neonatal mice. Hence, SCID mice with transplanted human skin from a healthy volunteer are used. The injection of either rabbit anti-laminin 332 or patient IgG results in blisters without inflammation.

Active Model

Active models include transgenic models, forced immunization models, and autoreactive lymphocyte transfer.

- *Transgenic model*: These are genetically modified mice. These include the introduction of human autoantigens, knockout of its genes and change of function of endogenous genes, e.g., the production of XVII collagen by transgenic mice. This skin when grafted to syngeneic wild mice produces autoantibodies to collagen XVII.
- *Forced immunization model*: Here, the wild or transgenic mice are injected with an autoantigen to generate an immune response to produce antibodies, e.g., the injection of the NC-1domain of murine collagen into

mice. With further boosts, autoantibody is produced against collagen VII in the mice **(Figs. 2A to C)**.

- *Autoreactive lymphocyte transfer*: These models are used to overcome self-tolerance which prevents the mouse's immune system from reacting with the human antigen, e.g., the generation of a knockout mouse lacking the autoantigen followed by immunization with the autoantigen. The splenocytes containing both B and T cells are transferred to Rag2 (immunocompromised mice) knockouts expressing the autoantigen, which initiates an immune response.

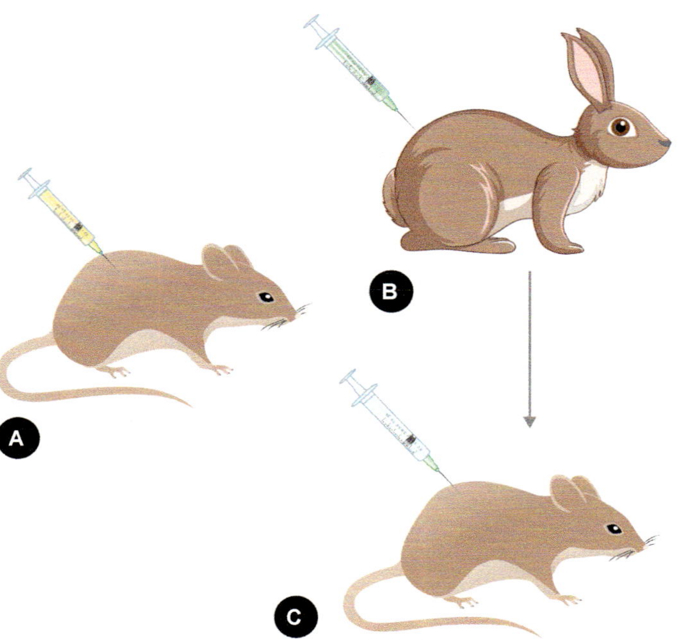

Figs. 1A to C: Passive animal model: (A) mouse is being injected with human IgG, (B) rabbit is injected with murine antigen (C) antibody to the murine protein is injected in to the mouse.

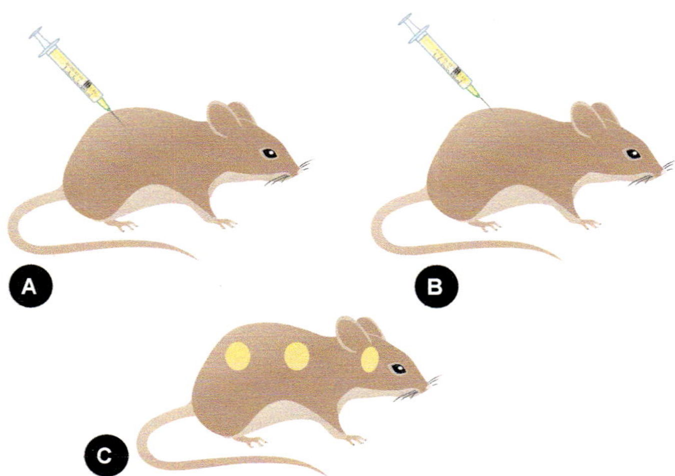

Figs. 2A to C: Active animal model: (A and B) Mouse is injected with repeat dose of autoantigen to produce autoantibodies (C) erosions and blisters noted over the mouse following development of autoantibodies.

PATHOGENESIS OF AUTOIMMUNE BULLOUS DISEASES

Bullous Pemphigoid (BP)

In bullous pemphigoid (BP), the blisters are caused by autoantibodies directed against the hemidesmosome components.

- *Genetic factors* include human leukocyte antigen (HLA) DQB1*0301 in Caucasians and DRB1*04, DRB1*1101, and DQB1*0302 among the Japanese. Gene polymorphisms [cytokine genes interleukin-8 (IL-8) and IL-1β, MT-ATP8] are also associated with BP.
- *Triggers*: Drugs, vaccines, viral infections, radiotherapy, and neurological and neuro-degenerative diseases are associated with BP.
- *Antigens*: BP180 (NC16A) and BP 230 are the antigens.

  BP180 or collagen XVII is a transmembrane protein with the N-terminal within the hemidesmosome plaque and the C-terminal in the lamina lucida. The non-collagenous domain (NC16A) is the target of most autoantibodies. BP 230 belongs to the plakin family and connects the keratin intermediate filaments with the hemidesmosomes **(Figs. 3 and 4)**.

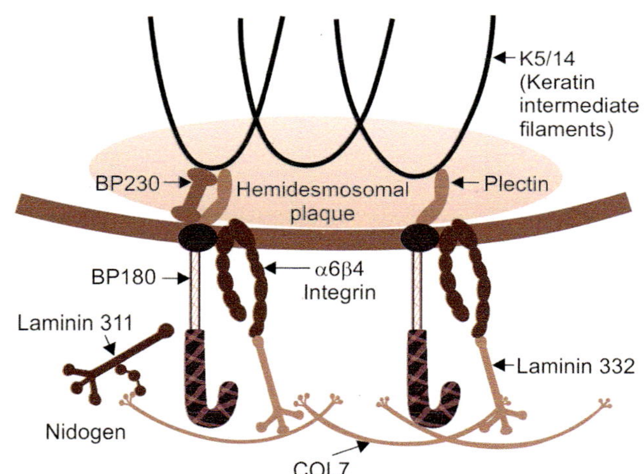

Fig. 3: Structure of basement membrane zone.

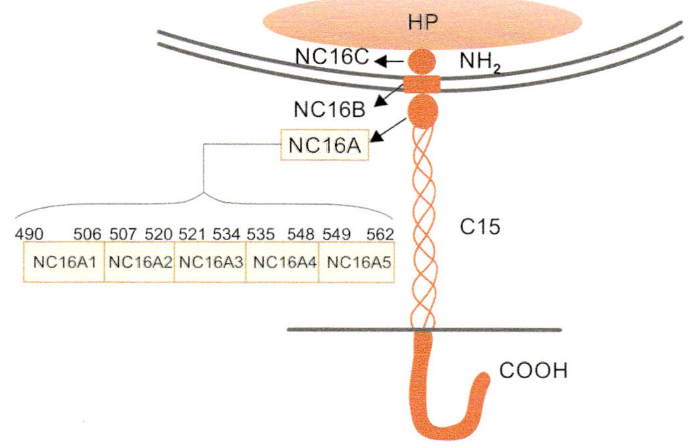

Fig. 4: Structure of BP180 showing the main antigen target (NC16A). (HP: hemidesmosomal plaque; NC: non-collagenous)

- *Autoantibodies*: IgG and/or IgE directed against BP180 (NC16A) and BP 230.

Mouse Models

Passive model: The major limitation of using patient serum is the lack of cross-reactivity between the human BP 180 and the murine analog. To overcome this, rabbits are first immunized with the murine fusion protein (mus 180A). This leads to antibody production in the rabbit, which is injected into neonatal mice. This results in the development of redness and slight epidermal change on mild pressure. Histology of the skin reveals a subepidermal blister, and there is deposition of IgG and complement at the BMZ.

Cobra venom was used to study the effect of complement. When mice complement was depleted by cobra venom and then injected with the murine antibody, there were no skin changes. The disease could not be replicated in knockout models of C5 deficient and FcyR111 (receptor on neutrophils) mice. This highlights the role of complement and neutrophils in disease pathogenesis.

Active model: One of the limitations of animal models is that they are transient and cannot fully replicate human disease. This is overcome through the use of an active model using knockouts and adoptive transfer.

Steps

- Rag2 deficient mice crossed with COL XV11-humanized mice (lack mouse COL XV11, but have human XV11).
- Produce Rag2-/-/COL XV11 humanized mice.
- Grafting (immunization) is performed from COLXVII-transgenic mice onto matched 6-week-old wild-type mice.

- Isolation of splenocytes from the grafted wild-type mice.
- Injection of these splenocytes into the Rag2-/-/COL XV11 humanized mice.
- Recipient mice produce antibodies to collagen XV11 and develop blisters.
- Depletion of CD4+ cells results in no antibody production to collagen XV11.

Steps in Disease Pathogenesis (Fig. 5)

Complement Dependent Pathway:
- Loss of immune tolerance.
- This leads to the production of autoantibodies against BP180 and 230.
- IgG1 and IgG3 autoantibodies along with complement activate effector cells (neutrophils and eosinophils).
- IgE antibodies to NC16A activate and recruit eosinophils, causing them to degranulate and help in blister formation.
- Release of proteolytic enzymes [matrix metalloproteinase-9 (MMP-9) and neutrophil elastase], cytokines, and chemokines.
- Inflammation and blister formation.

The classical and alternate pathways (lesser extent) are involved in blister formation. IL-17 is elevated in the serum of patients and plays a vital role in inducing blister formation. Eosinophils activate tissue factors which further activate the coagulation pathway, contributing to blister formation. Monocytes increase the capacity of neutrophils to release MMP-9. Among the other proteolytic enzymes, granzyme B also has been reported to be elevated in BP and contributes to blistering.

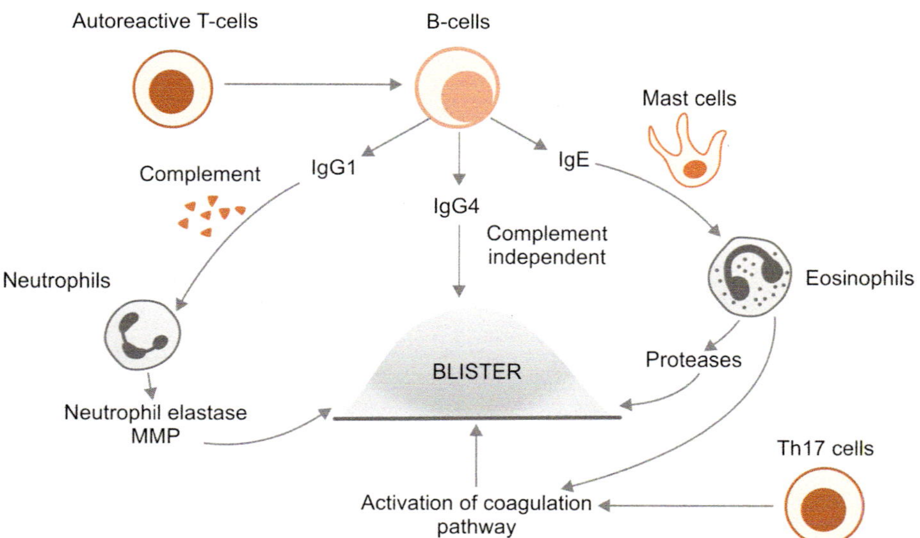

Fig. 5: Pathogenesis of bullous pemphigoid: Showing both complement-mediated and independent mechanisms of blistering. *Image courtesy*: Dr Vinupriya S, Assistant Professor, Department of Dermatology, KMCH Institute of Sciences and Research, Coimbatore, Tamil Nadu, India.

(MMP: matrix metalloproteinase; Th17: T helper 17)

Complement-independent Mechanisms

Macropinocytosis, and proteasome- and ubiquitin-mediated degradation of BP 180-The production of anti-BP180 induces internalization of the antigen complexed with antibody through pinocytosis, which eventually leads to blister formation **(Fig. 6)**.

Probable steps:
- Internalization of BP180 with antibody by pinocytosis
- Weakening of BMZ
- Degradation of these by proteasomes and/or lysosomes
- Release of cytokines (IL-6 and IL-8) by keratinocytes which help in blister formation. IL-8 released from keratinocytes recruits and activates neutrophils. IL-6 contributes to tissue damage.
- *IgE and eosinophils*: Anti BP180 IgE and BP180-IgE complexes bind to the BMZ and FcεR1 receptors on mast cells, eosinophils, and basophils. This causes degranulation and release of pro-inflammatory mediators [eosinophil granule proteins and reactive oxygen species (ROS)]. Keratinocytes also release eotaxin-1 and IL-5 resulting in a positive loop contributing to inflammation and blister formation.
- IgG4 antibodies are capable of inducing non-inflammatory BP in the absence of complement.

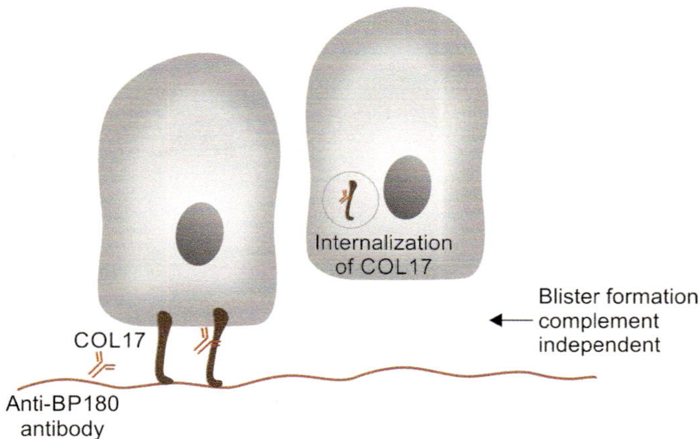

Fig. 6: Pathogenesis of bullous pemphigoid: Production of anti-BP180 induces internalization of the antigen complexed with antibody through pinocytosis, which eventually leads to blister formation.

Associations

- *Neurologic diseases:* Patients with neurologic diseases have a higher risk of developing BP. One hypothesis is that in neurologic diseases, there is a loss of self-tolerance to BP 180, and a degree of crosstalk exists between brain BP180 and skin BP180.
- *Thrombosis*: There is an increased risk of thrombosis and thrombo-embolism among patients with BP. Inflammation in BP triggers the coagulation cascade. D-dimer and prothrombin fragment (F1+2) have been reported to increase in patients with BP and parallel autoantibody BP180 level.

- *Vitamin D deficiency*: Patients with BP have a higher prevalence of vitamin D deficiency.

Drug-induced Pemphigoid (Dipeptidyl Peptidase-4 Inhibitors)

Dipeptidyl peptidase-4 (DPP) inhibitors, also known as gliptins, are commonly used anti-diabetic medications. Numerous studies have established a link between drug use and risk of BP.

DPP-4 (CD26) is part of the prolyloligopeptidase group of enzymes, which breaks down numerous bioactive peptides. It is widely expressed in different cell types, including keratinocytes and T-lymphocytes. Studies have reported that the expression of DPP-4/CD26 is increased in BP patients regardless of prior treatment with gliptins. Inhibition of DPP-4 increases the pro-inflammatory cytokines with eosinophilic stimulation, and an impact on plasminogen activation and plasmin formation.

Among the Japanese, specific unique immunological characteristics have been described. They are predominantly non-inflammatory and associated with the HLA-DQB1*03:01 allele. However in Europeans, no such differences have been reported.

Pemphigoid Gestationis

It is a specific pregnancy dermatosis. It typically appears during the third trimester but can also occur in the second trimester or after delivery. It is mostly self-limiting and disappears by 6 months post-delivery. If a woman has pemphigoid gestationis (PG) during one pregnancy, there is a 90% chance that it will recur in future pregnancies and be more severe. However, if the woman changes partner, the risk of the condition occurring in subsequent pregnancy drops to 5%. It is associated with hyperthyroidism, molar pregnancy, trophoblastic tumors, and choriocarcinoma.

Genetic Factors

- *Major histocompatibility complex (MHC):* MHC class II plays a crucial role in the development of PG. Maternal HLA-DRB1*0301 and DRB1*0401/040X alleles are strongly associated with PG. Both haplotypes are reported in 45% of cases and 3% of controls. Trophoblast and stromal amniochorionic cells express these haplotypes.
- *Aberrant complement system*: C4*QO is present in 90% of PG cases which may hinder the removal of immune complexes and facilitates deposition. This allele is in strong linkage disequilibrium with the DR-3 and DR-4 alleles; hence, pathogenicity is in doubt.
- *Autoantibody target*: IgG antibodies (predominantly IgG1 subclass) directed against NC16A BP180. Antibodies to full-length BP180 and BP230 have also been reported.
- *Modulation*: Progesterone and estrogen modulate disease activity. Disease severity decreases in late pregnancy on account of high progesterone. Postpartum disease severity increases accompanied by reduced progesterone and increased estrogen levels.

Steps in disease pathogenesis:
- Loss of immune privilege of the fetoplacental unit
- BP180 is presented to MHC class II
- Recognized as foreign
- Formation of autoantibody
- Autoantibody binds to amniotic membrane.
- The placental basement membrane undergoes structural changes.
- Anti-BP180 antibodies are deposited at the dermo-epidermal junction (DEJ).
- Activate complement
- Recruit effector cells (eosinophils and neutrophils)
- Proteases are released.
- Blister formation

The primary event starts with loss of immune privilege due to aberrant maternal MHC class II expression. BP180 is presented to MHC complex in the presence of paternal MHC class II allele. BP180 is recognized as foreign, producing anti-BP180 antibodies that affect the placenta and skin. In addition to anti-BP180, antibodies against paternal MHC antigens are also produced, the significance of which is unclear. The anti-BP180 antibodies are deposited at the DEJ which results in complement activation and effector response. The activated eosinophils and neutrophils degranulate releasing proteases leading to blister formation.

Lichen Planus Pemphigoides

It is a subepidermal bullous disorder showing overlap of lichen planus and BP. It is first characterized by lichenoid inflammation, followed by the development of sub-epidermal blisters. The bullae develop over both lichenoid areas and normal skin. Medication has been reported to trigger lichen planus pemphigoides (LPP). Recently, it has been reported as a complication of programmed cell death protein and programmed death-ligand 1 inhibition checkpoint blockage.

Autoantibody targets: BP180 (NC16A, C terminal epitope), BP230, desmoglein-1, 130 kDa, and 200 kDa.

Steps in disease pathogenesis:
- Cytotoxic CD8+ cells (lichen planus)
- Apoptosis of basal cells
- Exposure of DEJ antigens
- Autoantibodies against collagen XVII
- Activation of both complement and non-complement blistering mechanisms
- Effector cell activation
- Activation of proteases
- Bulla formation

Anti-BP180 (NC16A) and anti-BP230 antibodies are associated with a clinical presentation similar to BP; however, those with anti-BP180 (C-terminal portion of BP180) have predominant mucosal lesions akin to mucous membrane pemphigoid (MMP).

Epidermolysis bullosa Acquisita

Epidermolysis bullosa acquisita (EBA) is characterized by autoantibodies to collagen VII. It clinically presents as inflammatory or non-inflammatory forms.

Structure of Collagen VII

Collagen VII is essential for skin stability. Anchoring fibrils contain collagen VII which bind molecules in the basal lamina to the underlying connective tissue. It has a central collagenous domain flanked by a large non-collagenous domain (NC1) and a smaller non-collagenous domain (NC2) **(Fig. 7)**. NC1 binds to other proteins such as laminin 332, collagen 1, and collagen IV.

Autoantigen

The predominant antigen is the epitope in NC1 domain of collagen VII. Rarely, reactivity to NC2 and collagen domain has been reported.

Autoantibody Type

IgG (most common), followed by IgA (10%), and rarely IgE and IgM are the autoantibodies seen.

These are pathogenic, based on clinical and experimental data. In an ex vivo human model, it was observed that anti-collagen VII (COLVII) could recruit neutrophils resulting in DEJ separation. In both passive transfer (antibody to COLVII) and injection mouse models (COLVII antigen), it was possible to replicate the inflammatory EBA-like presentation. Anti-COLVII (NC1) antibodies correlate with disease activity among EBA patients.

Genetic Factors

Association with HLA-DR2, HLA-DRB1*13 and HLA-DRB1*15:03, has been reported. Supporting evidence also comes from the immunization mouse model. There is a strong association of disease susceptibility (inflammatory EBA) with the MHC H2s haplotype.

Cutaneous Microbiome

Rich and diverse skin microbiome prior to immunization in mice can prevent or modulate blister formation. In an immunized genetically identical mouse model (SJL/J), 20%

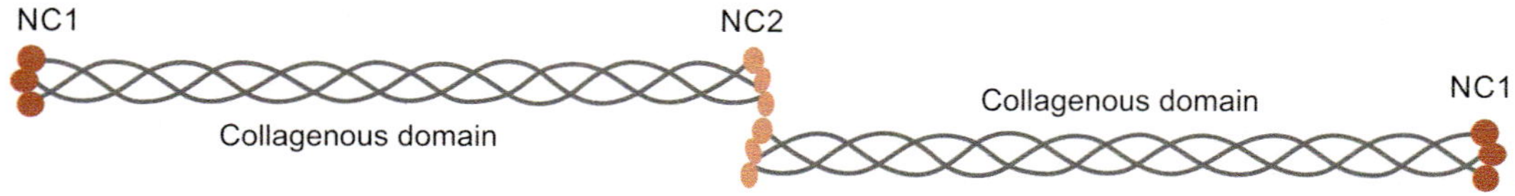

Fig. 7: Structure of collagen VII.
(NC: non-collagenous)

of the mice failed to produce blisters. It is postulated that the effect of innate immune response (skin microbiome) modulates this effect.

Associations

Diabetes mellitus, autoimmune thyroiditis, inflammatory bowel disease, rheumatoid arthritis, and hepatitis C infection

Steps in Disease Pathogenesis (Fig. 8)

- Loss of immune tolerance (genetic and environmental causes)
- Afferent phase: Production of autoantibodies against COLVII
- Maintenance of autoantibody
- Efferent phase: Activation of complement and recruitment of neutrophils followed by activation of proteases leading to inflammation.

Experimental Data

Data from the immunization mouse model suggests that anti-COLVII antibody production is T cell-dependent. Mice deficient in T cells do not produce these autoantibodies. Depletion of CD4+ cells in mouse models delays autoantibody production and clinical disease. In an immunization mouse model (injected with COLVII) depleted of B cells, CD4+ T cell response to the antigen was not observed. Development of these COLVIICD4+ cells needs B cells, dendritic cells, and macrophages. Autoantibodies were not observed in granulocyte macrophage colony-stimulating factor (GM-CSF)-depleted mice and with neutrophil depletion, suggesting their key role in autoantibody production.

Maintenance of Autoantibody

Disease activity and progression are affected by the autoantibody's half-life and immunoglobulin pathogenicity.
- *Neonatal Fc receptor (FcRn)*: It controls the half-life of autoreactive antibodies. It prevents the catabolism of IgG. This has been demonstrated with intravenous immunoglobulin (IVIg), which inhibits FcRn, thereby reducing autoantibody level **(Fig. 9)**.
- *Differential glycosylation*: It affects the pathogenicity of the autoantibody. Agalactosylated IgG antibodies are pro-inflammatory. In contrast, sialylated IgG antibodies are anti-inflammatory.

Efferent Phase

- Activation of complement (C3a and C5a)
- Recruitment of neutrophils and mast cells to the skin (upregulation of CD18 and ICAM 1)
- Bind Fc domain of IgG through Fc gamma receptor (FcgR) expressed on the cell surface of neutrophils **(Fig. 10)**.
- Neutrophil activation
- Release of elastase and gelatinase
- Activates matrix metalloproteinases and produces reactive oxygen species.
- Damage to the BMZ and bullae formation.
- Inflammation at BMZ further activates keratinocytes and mast cells.
- Production of inflammatory cytokines and chemokines
- Perpetuate inflammation

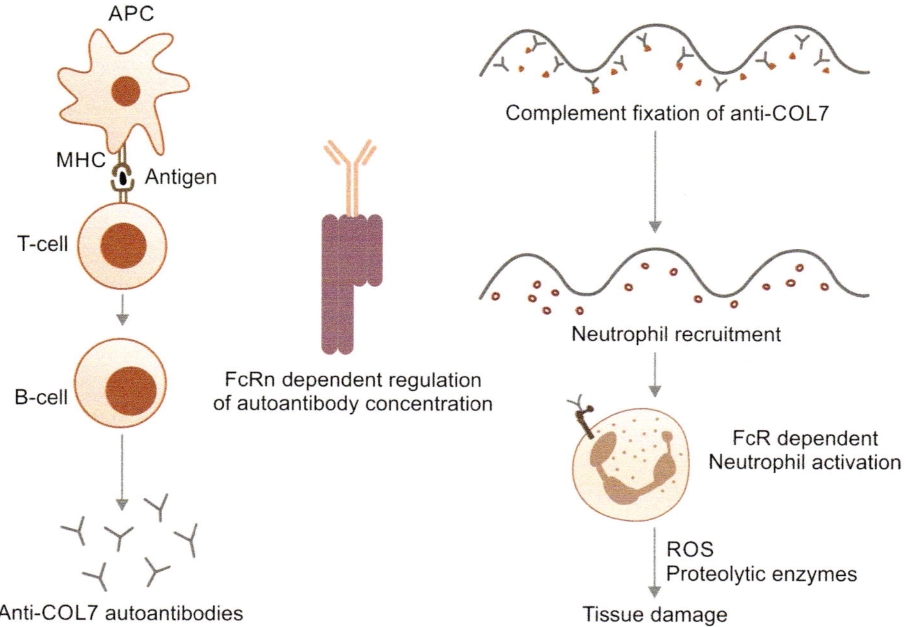

Fig. 8: Pathogenesis of epidermolysis bullosa acquisita (EBA): Loss of tolerance, followed by an afferent phase, maintenance of autoantibody, and efferent phase.

(APC: antigen presenting cell; COL7: collagen 7; FcRn: neonatal crystallizable fragment receptor; MHC: major histocompatibility complex; ROS: reactive oxygen species)

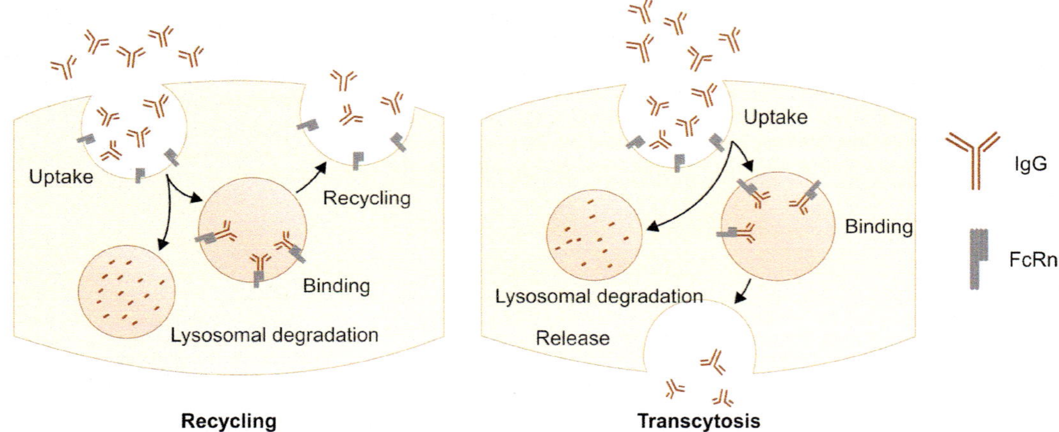

Fig. 9: Fc neonatal receptor (FcRn) and epidermolysis bullosa acquisita (EBA): Neonatal Fc receptor preventing catabolism of autoantibodies.

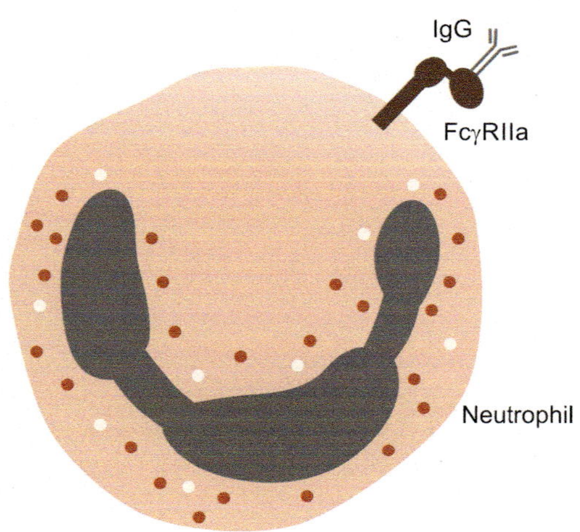

Fig. 10: Fcγ receptor and epidermolysis bullosa acquisita (EBA): IgG antibody binding to neutrophil induces crosslinks in FcγR.

FcγR and EBA

FcγR plays an essential role in the pathogenesis of EBA **(Fig. 10)**. Autoantibody binding to effector cells (neutrophils) induces crosslinks in the FcγR. This results in a downstream cascade leading to inflammation. In an inflammatory milieu, activating FcγR (FcγRI, FcγRIII, and FcγRIV) are upregulated, and inhibitory FcγRIIB are down-regulated. In a passive transfer mouse model, mice deficient in the common gamma chain of the activating FcγR region, failed to develop the disease even in the presence of anti-COLVII antibodies. In a knock-out mice model, only mice with knock-out FcγR1V failed to produce any clinical or histological evidence of disease.

Resolution

Flightless I, an actin-remodeling protein, modulates skin blistering in experimental EBA. Expression of flightless 1 is accompanied by a decrease in the tight junction (claudin 1 and 4) expression, resulting in delayed healing.

Mucous Membrane Pemphigoid

It predominantly affects the mucosae. The conjunctival and oral mucosae are commonly involved. It is characterized by both blistering and scarring. The difficulties in diagnosis of MMP are due to multiple antigen targets and low titers of circulating autoantibodies.

Genetic Factors

HLA-DQB1*0301 has been reported to be associated with MMP. In ocular MMP, association with HLA-DR4, HLA-DQw3 and HLA-DQβ*10301 has been reported.

Target Antigens

BP180 (C terminal), BP 230, Laminin 332, type VII collagen, and α6-β4 integrin are the various antigen targets.

Autoantibodies

They belong to IgG and IgA subtypes.

Pathophysiology

Laminin 332 Variant of MMP

- *Associations*: Vaccination (diphtheria-tetanus vaccine), tumors (pancreatic, colonic, gastric tumors, and lymphoma), mercury poisoning, and amalgam teeth procedures
- *Pathogenic steps*:
  o Loss of immune tolerance to laminin 332
  o Inflammation
  o Decreased adhesion to the basement membrane

In an antibody transfer mouse (anti-laminin 332 antibody transfer) model experiment, it was reported that mice injected with the recombinant antibody showed erosions and crusts predominantly on the head and neck along with oral involvement. Control mice who received rabbit IgG did not develop clinical or histological alteration. Histology of the experimental mouse showed a subepithelial separation and inflammatory cells in the upper dermis. In addition, the experimental group had a greater density of collagen fibers. The role of complement is not clearly established in mouse models. In another mouse model, injection of rabbit anti-laminin 332 against the immuno-dominant region produced lesions similar to MMP, which was both Fc and complement-dependent.

COL17-type MMP

COL17 directly binds to COL4 in the keratinocytes from skin and oral mucosa.

Pathogenic steps (Fig. 11):
- IgG produced against C-terminal of COL17
- Disrupts binding of COL17 to COL4
- Non-inflammatory blister formation

Another mechanism probably is due to internalization of COL17 on autoantibody binding to the C-terminus of collagen 17. This plays a vital role in MMP; however, all anti-MMP antibodies did not show this.

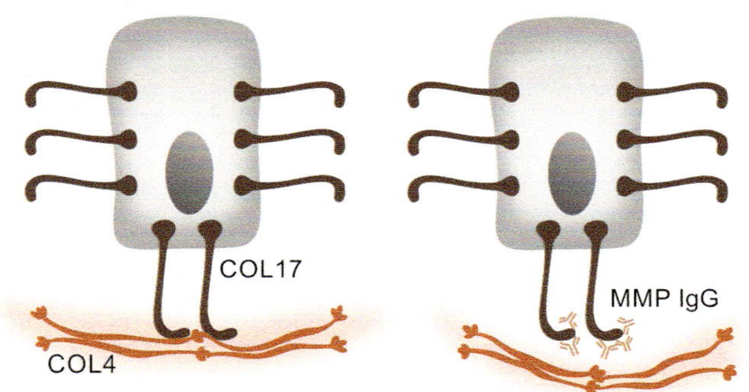

Fig. 11: Pathogenesis of mucous membrane pemphigoid (MMP): Disruption of COL17-COL4 binding by autoantibody, leading to non-inflammatory blister formation.
(COL: collagen; MMP: mucous membrane pemphigoid)

Ocular MMP

- *Genetic association*: DQw7, HLA A2, HLA B*49, HLA B*35, HLA B*8, DR-2, and DR-4 have been reported with ocular MMP.
- *Associations*: Topical timolol, pilocarpine, epinephrine, and practolol, have been reported with ocular MMP.
- *Antigen targets*: They include α6β4 integrin, BP180, laminin 332, COLVII.
- *Autoantibody*: They belong to IgG and IgA class.

Pathogenesis: There are three steps in the pathogenesis of ocular MMP **(Fig. 12)**. It includes the injury phase, inflammatory phase, and fibrotic phase. A two-hit hypothesis has been proposed to explain the findings in ocular MMP. The first hit is the genetic predisposition and the second hit is probably an unknown trigger.

1. *Injury phase*: It is characterized by the following processes:
   a. Two-hit process
   b. Autoantibodies against target antigens
   c. Produce specific B cell clones
   d. Production of autoantibodies which target BMZ
   e. Activate complement
2. *Inflammatory phase*: It is characterized by the activation of effector cells resulting in cell damage and activation of fibrosis.
   a. Activation of inflammatory cells (granulocytes, mast cells, T lymphocytes and macrophages)
   b. Migrate to substantia propria
   c. Tissue damage and release of inflammatory and profibrotic cytokines (Th1 and Th2)
   d. Cell damage and stimulation of fibroblasts

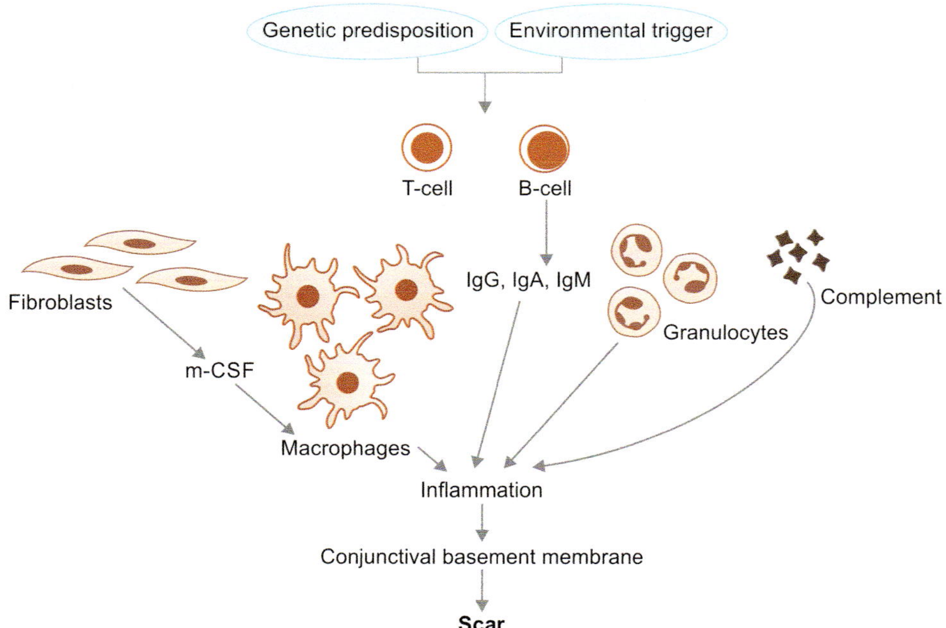

Fig. 12: Pathogenesis of ocular mucous membrane pemphigoid (MMP): Injury phase, inflammatory phase, and fibrotic phase.
(m-CSF: macrophage-colony stimulating factor)

3. *Fibrotic phase*: It is characterized by activation of fibroblasts that results in inflammation and scarring. Steps in the process are:
   a. Activated conjunctival fibroblasts
   b. Produce cytokines and extracellular matrix components
   c. Endothelial cells proliferate and form fibrotic granulation issue
   d. Subconjunctival scarring

Dermatitis Herpetiformis

It is an AIBD characterized by associated gluten sensitivity. It is a specific manifestation of celiac disease, presenting as itchy polymorphic lesions which are symmetrically distributed over the extensor aspects.

- *Genetic factors*: Dermatitis herpetiformis (DH) is associated with HLA-DQ2 (85% of cases) and DQ8 (15%).
- *Triggers*: They include gluten, potassium iodide, gastrointestinal surgery, drugs, gastrointestinal infection, and hormonal therapy.
- *Autoantigen*: Epidermal transglutaminase (eTG or TG3)—it is usually expressed in the spinous layers and is involved in the terminal differentiation of keratinocytes. Tissue transglutaminase (tTG or TG2) is the primary autoantigen of celiac disease.
- *Autoantibodies*: They belong to the IgA class directed against eTG. There is conflicting literature regarding pathogenicity. Passive transfer (SCID mouse model with human skin grafts) using anti-eTG or human serum from DH patients failed to elicit any blisters, though granular IgA deposits were detected.

Steps in Disease Pathogenesis (Fig. 13)

- tTG/TG2 catalyzes the deamidation of gluten
- Increased gluten peptide binding to HLA-DQ2 and DQ8 expressed on the antigen presenting cells (APC).

- Immune response against tTG and gliadin. This response is mediated by both Th1 and Th2.
- Gut inflammation (formation of anti-tTG IgA deposits and increased IL-8 enhanced selectin and GM-CSF)
- Autoimmunity against eTG/TG3 is probably due to epitope spreading

Epitope spreading: The development of autoantibodies targeting eTG is unclear in patients with celiac disease. It could be due to epitope spreading in view of the homology between tTG and eTG. Other observations in support of this hypothesis include a low prevalence of these antibodies in children compared to adult cases of DH.

Formation of skin eTG/IgA aggregates: One hypothesis is that epidermal trauma leads to eTG shedding into the dermis, where it binds to circulating anti-eTG IgA. Another hypothesis is that these aggregates (eTG/IgA) exist as circulatory immune complexes.

- eTG/IgA in skin activates fibrin found at the tips of dermal papillae.
- This results in blister formation and activates effector cells (predominantly neutrophils).
- Activated neutrophils migrate to the skin.
- Release granzyme B and elastase.
- Cleave collagen BMZ at lamina lucida (probably through destruction of laminin 332).
- Further release of proteases from basal keratinocytes.
- Blister formation and pruritus (mediated by neuropeptides, corticotropin-releasing factor, and IL-31).

Linear IgA Dermatosis

It is characterized by linear deposits of IgA along the BMZ. It occurs both in children and adults.

There are three patterns of IgA deposition in linear IgA dermatosis (LAD)—(1) lamina lucida type (most common),

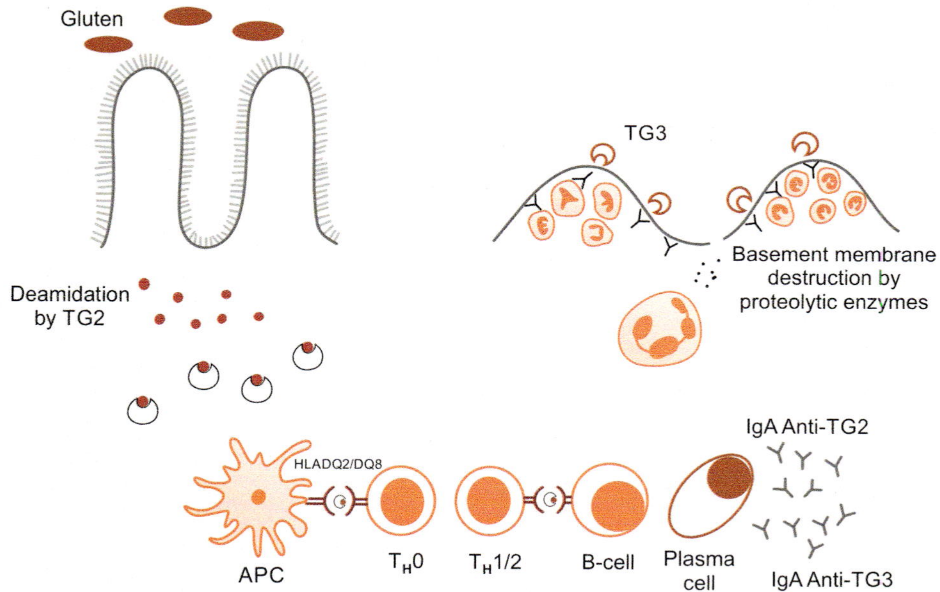

Fig. 13: Pathogenesis of dermatitis herpetiformis.
(APC: antigen presenting cell; TG2: tissue transglutaminase; TG3: epidermal transglutaminase; T$_H$: T helper)

(2) sublamina densa type, and (3) combined pattern. There is significant overlap with BP, MMP, and EBA.

Genetic Factors

Associated with HLA-B8, HLA-CW7, DR3, and tumor necrosis factor 2 (TNF2).

Triggers

They include infections, drugs (vancomycin-50% of cases), vaccination, and autoimmune disorders (Crohn's disease, ulcerative colitis, and autoimmune lymphoproliferative disorders).

Antigen Targets

- *Lamina lucida type*: linear IgA antigen 1 (LAD-1, 120 kDa), linear IgA bullous dermatosis antigen (LABD97, 97 kDa), BP230, BP180, collagen VII, and laminin 332.
- *Sublamina densa type*: Probably collagen VII.

Autoantibody Type

They belong predominantly to IgA1 and sometimes IgG.

Steps in Disease Pathogenesis

- Genetic background with stressors (infections, drugs, vaccination, etc.)
- Production of aberrant IgA1 antibodies
- Bind to antigens at the DEJ (ectodomain of BP180, LAD-1, and LABD 97)
- Activation of neutrophils by these autoantibodies
- Cross-linking of FcαRI on neutrophils with IgA immune complexes
- Release of leukotriene B4, elastase, and reactive oxygen species
- Accumulation of predominantly neutrophils and few eosinophils independent of complement in the skin
- Inflammation and blister formation

Neoepitope Formation

The primary antigenic stimulus is the processed extracellular part of BP180 ectodomains. Proteolytic cleaving of BP180 by ADAM (a disintegrin and metalloprotease) 9, 10, 17 and plasmin produces the soluble ectodomain LAD-1 and LABD 97. The N terminals of both LAD-1 and LABD97 are present within the NC16A domain **(Fig. 14)**. Sera of most react with cleaved BP180 and not the full-length BP180.

Intermolecular Epitope Spreading Phenomenon

Disease progression and inflammation could result in the exposure of intracellular BP230-producing autoantibodies to BP230. These were more frequently detected when BP180 autoantibodies were present (LAD-1 and NC16A).

Complement activation: IgA immune complex can activate neutrophils by binding to and crosslinking with FcαRI, which is complement-independent. IgA activates complement weakly unlike IgG or IgM. Moreover, as it lacks a C1q binding site, it cannot activate the classical complement pathway. However, it can activate the alternate and lectin pathways.

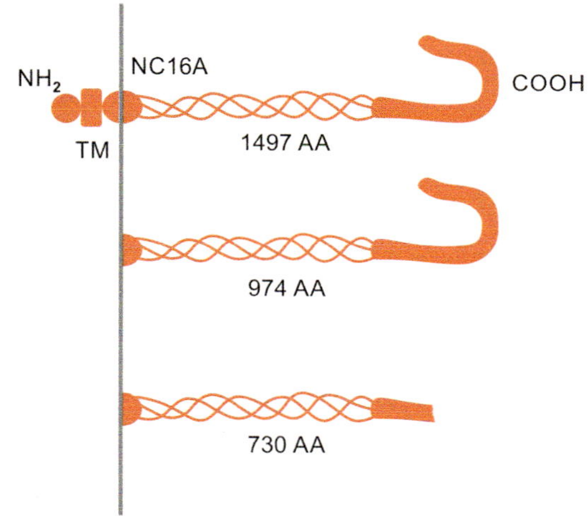

Fig. 14: Pathogenesis of linear IgA dermatosis: Neoepitope formation-proteolytic cleaving of BP180 by ADAM 9, 10, 17, and plasmin produces the soluble ectodomain LAD-1 and LABD 97.

Bullous Systemic Lupus Erythematosus

Bullous lupus erythematosus (BSLE) is a rare AIBD characterized by a subepidermal blister which usually heals without milia or scarring. It occurs in patients with SLE.

Genetic Factors

BSLE has been reported to be associated with HLA-DR2.

Drugs

Methimazole and nivolumab can trigger BSLE.

Antigen Targets

They include type VII (NC1 and NC 2 domain). Other antigens reported are laminin 332, laminin 311, and BPAg1. These are probably due to epitope spreading.

Autoantibody Type

They belong predominantly to IgG2 and IgG3, followed by IgA and IgM.

The autoantibodies are pathogenic. This has been demonstrated in a human cryosection model. Incubation with patient sera in the presence of neutrophils induced a subepidermal split. In this model, the autoantibodies did not fix complement.

Steps in Pathogenesis

- Autoantibodies (predominantly IgG) are produced against collagen VII
- They bind to both NC1 and NC2
- Recruitment of neutrophils and activation of complement
- Blister formation occurs

Anti p200 Pemphigoid (Anti-laminin γ1 Pemphigoid)

It is a rare subepidermal AIBD characterized by autoantibodies against the 200 kD protein present in the lamina lucida.

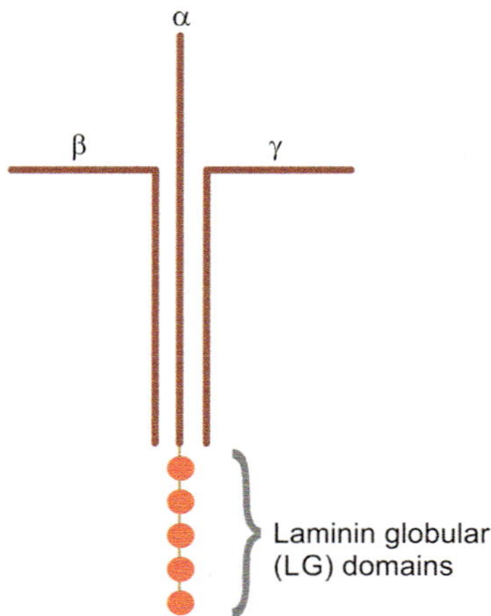

Fig. 15: Structure of laminin heterotrimer.

Antigen Targets

Laminin γ1 (C terminus) is the main antigen. Other antigens reported include BP180, laminin 332, BP230, and COL7 (in about 25% of cases). This is most likely due to epitope spreading. Laminin γ1 is a 200 kD protein. It is part of the laminin heterotrimer **(Fig. 15)** which serves to maintain adhesion outside the hemidesmosome. The C-terminal portion binds to integrins and the arm part binds to nidogen through which it anchors to the BMZ.

Autoantibody Types

They belong to IgG4 type. The antibodies detected in antilaminin γ1 pemphigoid are pathogenic.

Associations

It is associated with psoriasis. It is hypothesized that there is an alteration of the extracellular matrix in psoriatic skin on account of the rapid cell cycle and turnover, which stimulates the production of autoantibodies against the 200 kD protein.

CONCLUSION

The interplay between different components of the innate and adaptive immunity and complement system directed against the components of the basement membrane zone is responsible for various subepidermal AIBDs. Its thorough understanding helps the clinician recognize specific clinical manifestations, undertake relevant investigations and prescribe specific treatment directed against the various pathomechanisms responsible for the disease.

TAKE HOME MESSAGE

- AIBDs are characterized by loss of tolerance either due to a genetic cause or an environmental trigger. Loss of tolerance is associated with activation of the immune system, production of autoantibodies, recruitment of inflammatory cells, and inflammation. These processes are predominantly complement-mediated.

- These blistering disorders are studied with the use of various animal models and sometimes with ex vivo human skin cryosections. These models include both passive and active models.

- In BP, NC16A of BP180 is the predominant antigen target. Pathogenic antibodies are predominantly of IgG and IgE class. There are both complement-dependent and independent mechanisms of blister formation. The main effector cells are eosinophils and neutrophils which release protease and cationic proteins, which contribute to inflammation and blister formation.

- In PG, the primary event starts with loss of immune privilege due to aberrant maternal MHC class II expression. This results in BP180 being presented to the MHC complex in the presence of paternal MHC class II allele. BP180 is recognized as foreign, resulting in the production of anti-BP 180 antibodies that affect both the placenta and skin.

- In LAD, the primary antigenic stimulus is the processed extracellular part of BP180 ectodomain. Proteolytic cleaving of BP180 by ADAM 9, 10, 17, and plasmin produces the soluble ectodomain LAD-1 and LABD 97. In the presence of a genetic background and trigger, aberrant IgA1 antibodies are produced toward the antigen targets. These activate neutrophils which release ROS, leukotriene B4, and elastase, resulting in inflammation and blister formation. IgA1 weakly activates complement.

- In EBA, NC1 domain of COL7 is the main autoantigen. IgG to NC1 is the most common autoantibody. These antibodies are pathogenic. The development of EBA is characterized by loss of immune tolerance, an afferent phase characterized by autoantibodies to COL7, maintenance of autoantibody, and an efferent phase characterized by activation of complement and recruitment of neutrophils followed by activation of proteases leading to inflammation.

  Autoantibody binding to effector cells (neutrophils) induces crosslinks in the FcgR. This results in a downstream cascade leading to inflammation. In an inflammatory milieu, activating FcgR (FcgRI, FcgRIII, and FcgRIV) is upregulated and inhibitory FcgR11B is downregulated.

- In MMP, laminin 332, BP180 (C terminal), BP230, COL7, and α6-β4 integrin, are the autoantigens. Autoantibodies belong to IgG and IgA subclass. There are three steps in the pathogenesis of ocular MMP—(1) injury phase, (2) inflammatory phase, and (3) fibrotic phase. A two-hit hypothesis has been proposed to explain the findings in ocular MMP. The first hit is genetic predisposition and the second hit is probably an unknown trigger.

- In BSLE, COL7 (NC1 and NC2 domain) are the main antigenic targets. Others reported are laminin 332, laminin 311, and BPAg1. These are probably due to epitope spreading. Pathogenic autoantibodies belong predominantly to the IgG2 and IgG3 class, followed by IgA and IgM. Binding of autoantibodies results in activation of complement and recruitment of neutrophils, which then leads to blister formation.

- In anti p200 pemphigoid (anti-laminin γ1 pemphigoid), the target antigen is laminin γ1 (C terminus). Others reported include BP180, laminin 332, BP230, and COL7 (in about 25% of cases). This is most likely due to epitope spreading. The pathogenic antibodies belong to IgG4 type.

MULTIPLE CHOICE QUESTIONS

1. **Which of the following antibody binds weakly to complement?**
   (a) IgG1
   (b) IgG3
   (c) IgM
   (d) IgA

2. **Which of the following is an active mouse model?**
   (a) Injection of patient serum containing IgG into mice
   (b) Injection of rabbit serum containing IgG into mice
   (c) Injection of NC-1 domain of murine collagen 7 into mice
   (d) Injection of patient serum containing IgG to SCID mice transplanted with human skin

3. **Which of the following antibodies is associated with malignancies?**
   (a) Anti-laminin γ1
   (b) Anti-NC16A BP180
   (c) Anti-laminin 332
   (d) Anti-α6-β4 integrin

4. **Which of the following is true regarding neonatal Fc receptor?**
   (a) It is associated with catabolism of IgG
   (b) IVIg stimulates FcRn
   (c) It stands for neonatal crystallizable fragment receptor
   (d) FcRn stimulators are used to treat autoimmune diseases

5. **Autoantibodies in dermatitis herpetiformis predominantly belong to which class?**
   (a) IgG
   (b) IgA
   (c) IgM
   (d) IgE

6. **What is internalization of antigen followed by destruction called?**
   (a) Osmosis
   (b) Pinocytosis
   (c) Transcellular elimination
   (d) Diffusion

Answers

1. (d)   2. (c)   3. (c)   4. (c)   5. (b)   6. (b)

SUGGESTED READING

1. Pollmann R, Eming R. Research techniques made simple: mouse models of autoimmune blistering diseases. *J Invest Dermatol.* 2017;137:e1-e6.

2. Bieber K, Sun S, Ishii N, Kasperkiewicz M, Schmidt E, Hirose M, *et al.* Animal models for autoimmune bullous dermatoses. *Exp Dermatol.* 2010;19:2-11.

3. Genovese G, Di Zenzo G, Cozzani E, Berti E, Cugno M, Marzano AV. New insights into the pathogenesis of bullous pemphigoid: 2019 Update. *Front Immunol.* 2019;10:1506.

4. Cole C, Vinay K, Borradori L, Amber KT. Insights into the pathogenesis of bullous pemphigoid: the role of complement-independent mechanisms. *Front Immunol.* 2022;13:912876.

5. Yang M, Wu H, Zhao M, Chang C, Lu Q. The pathogenesis of bullous skin diseases. *J Transl Autoimmun.* 2019;2:100014.

6. Ujiie H, Shibaki A, Nishie W, Sawamura D, Wang G, Tateishi Y, *et al.* A novel active mouse model for bullous pemphigoid targeting humanized pathogenic antigen. *J Immunol.* 2010;184:2166-74.

7. Sadik CD, Lima AL, Zillikens D. Pemphigoid gestationis: Toward a better understanding of the etiopathogenesis. *Clin Dermatol.* 2016;34:378-82.

8. Schauer F, Mai S, Hofmann SC, Mai Y, Izumi K, Kern JS, *et al.* Autoreactivity to BP180 neoepitopes in patients with pemphigoid gestationis. *JAMA Dermatol.* 2022;158:212-4.

9. Hübner F, Langan EA, Recke A. Lichen planus pemphigoides: From lichenoid inflammation to autoantibody-mediated blistering. *Front Immunol.* 2019;10:1389.

10. Papara C, Danescu S, Sitaru C, Baican A. Challenges and pitfalls between lichen planus pemphigoides and bullous lichen planus. *Australas J Dermatol.* 2022;63:165-71.

11. Koga H, Prost-Squarcioni C, Iwata H, Jonkman MF, Ludwig RJ, Bieber K. Epidermolysis bullosa acquisita: The 2019 update. *Front Med (Lausanne).* 2019;5:362.

12. Kamaguchi M, Iwata H. The diagnosis and blistering mechanisms of mucous membrane pemphigoid. *Front Immunol.* 2019;10:34.

13. Branisteanu DC, Stoleriu G, Branisteanu DE, Boda D, Branisteanu CI, Maranduca MA, *et al.* Ocular cicatricial pemphigoid (Review). *Exp Ther Med.* 2020;20:3379-82.

14. Antiga E, Maglie R, Quintarelli L, Verdelli A, Bonciani D, Bonciolini V, *et al.* Dermatitis herpetiformis: novel perspectives. *Front Immunol.* 2019;10:1290.

15. Kemppainen E, Salmi T, Lindfors K. Missing insight into T and B cell responses in dermatitis herpetiformis. *Front Immunol.* 2021;12:657280.

16. Mori F, Saretta F, Liotti L, Giovannini M, Castagnoli R, Arasi S, *et al.* Linear immunoglobulin A bullous dermatosis in children. *Front Pediatr.* 2022;10:937528.

17. Edwards G, Diercks GFH, Seelen MAJ, Horvath B, van Doorn MBA, Damman J. Complement activation in autoimmune bullous dermatoses: a comprehensive review. *Front Immunol.* 2019;10:1477.

18. Contestable JJ, Edhegard KD, Meyerle JH. Bullous systemic lupus erythematosus: a review and update to diagnosis and treatment. *Am J Clin Dermatol.* 2014;15:517-24.

19. Florea F, Bernards C, Caproni M, Kleindienst J, Hashimoto T, Koch M, *et al.* Ex vivo pathogenicity of anti-laminin γ1 autoantibodies. *Am J Pathol.* 2014;184:494-506.

20. Kridin K, Ahmed AR. Anti-p200 pemphigoid: A systematic review. *Front Immunol.* 2019;10:2466.

Clinical Aspects of Pemphigus and other Autoimmune Bullous Diseases

CHAPTER 5

Clinical Classification of Pemphigus and other Autoimmune Bullous Diseases

Atiya Yaseen

- Classification of autoimmune bullous diseases
- Intraepidermal autoimmune bullous diseases
  - Pemphigus
  - Classification of pemphigus
- Subepidermal autoimmune bullous diseases
  - Pemphigoid diseases
  - Classification of pemphigoid diseases
- Other subepidermal autoimmune bullous diseases

INTRODUCTION

Immunobullous diseases are distinct organ-specific autoimmune blistering disorders, pathogenetically caused by circulating antibodies that target structural elements of the skin such as the adhesion molecules of the epidermis (pemphigus group), proteins in the hemidesmosomes, and basement membrane zone (BMZ) (pemphigoid group) and epidermal and tissue-type transglutaminases [dermatitis herpetiformis (DH)]. This classifies autoimmune bullous diseases (AIBDs) into 3 groups: (1) intraepidermal, (2) subepidermal (lamina lucida/densa), and (3) sublaminal. They can be further classified based on their target autoantigens and antibody profile. However the classification is being upgraded, with rarer and newer variants being added. This is attributed to the progress in understanding of the pathogenesis of AIBDs based on immunoblotting, immunofluorescence, and flow cytometry.

Classification of AIBDs (based on the level of the split) is shown in **Figure 1**.

INTRAEPIDERMAL AUTOIMMUNE BULLOUS DISEASES

Pemphigus (Greek: Pemphix—Blister)

Pemphigus includes a group of severe AIBDs which if not treated can be life-threatening. There are two dominant variants of pemphigus based on the level of split: the *superficial forms* grouped under pemphigus foliaceus (PF) and the *deep forms* under pemphigus vulgaris (PV); and *other variants* such as paraneoplastic pemphigus (PNP), pemphigus herpetiformis (PH), drug-induced pemphigus (DIP), and IgA pemphigus.

Classification of Pemphigus

- *Pemphigus vulgaris (PV)*:
  - Mucosal dominant
  - Mucocutaneous
  - Cutaneous dominant

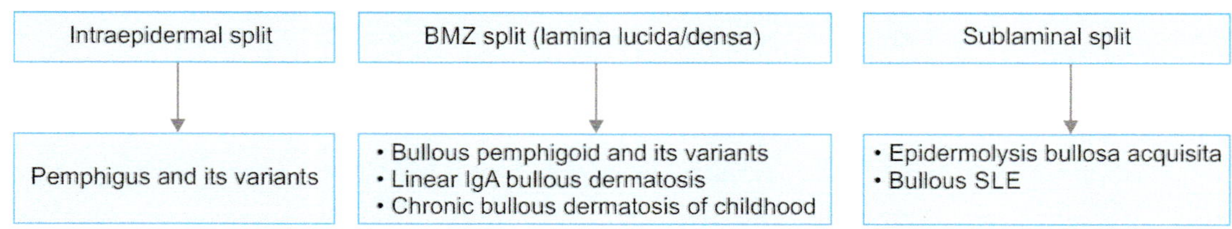

Fig. 1: Classification of autoimmune bullous diseases based on the level of split in the skin.
(BMZ: basement membrane zone; IgA: immunoglobulin A; SLE: systemic lupus erythematosus)

- o *Pemphigus vegetans*:
    - – Neumann type
    - – Hallopeau type
- *Pemphigus foliaceus (PF)*:
    - o Endemic type (fogo selvagem)
    - o Non-endemic type
    - o Pemphigus erythematosus (PE) (Senear–Usher syndrome)
- Paraneoplastic pemphigus *(PNP)*/paraneoplastic auto-immune multiorgan syndrome (PAMS)
- *IgA pemphigus*:
    - o Subcorneal pustular dermatosis-type
    - o Intraepithelial neutrophilic IgA dermatosis
- Pemphigus herpetiformis
- Drug-induced pemphigus

Pemphigus Vulgaris

This is the most prevalent subtype of pemphigus with mucosal and mucocutaneous involvement respectively. Depending on their phenotype, most PV patients demons-trate IgG4 and IgG1 antibodies against Dsg3 (mucosal) or both Dsg1 and 3 (mucocutaneous). Almost all patients with PV have painful erosions in the oral mucosa. More than half develop erosions on the skin (mucocutaneous PV).

Pemphigus vegetans is a subtype of PV with lesions presenting in the body folds (axillae, submammary region, and groins) and periorificial areas (lips, anus). It is further divided into two subtypes: (i) pustular variant (Hallopeau); and (ii) papillomatous and more severe variant (Neumann) **(Fig. 2)**.

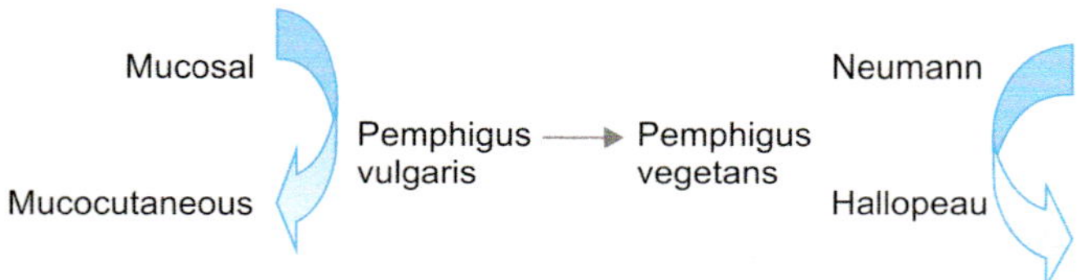

Fig. 2: Subtypes of pemphigus vulgaris.

Pemphigus Foliaceus

This subtype of pemphigus is characterized by the loss of keratinocyte adhesion in the subcorneal layer of the epidermis due to circulating IgG antibodies against Dsg1, and presenting clinically as superficial cutaneous blisters and erosions typically in seborrheic areas without mucosal involvement. It is classified into two types: endemic (fogo selvagem) and non-endemic PF. The two differ in their geographical distribution, age of onset, and high familial incidence of the endemic variant. The other variant of PF is PE (Senear–Usher syndrome) with clinical features of both PF and lupus erythematosus (LE). However, the inclusion of PE as a subtype of PF is somewhat controversial as the autoantibody profile in PE seems to be more diverse **(Fig. 3)**.

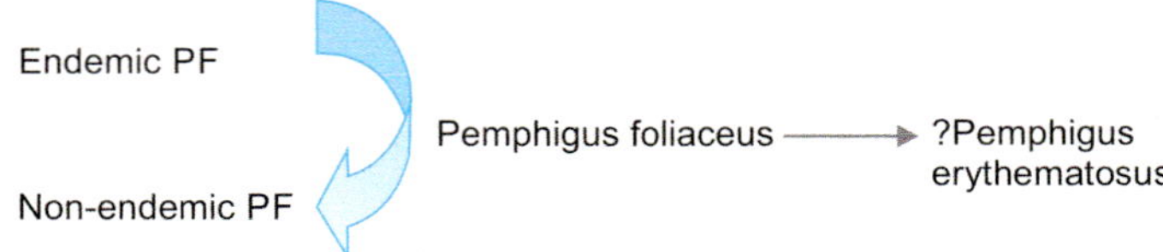

Fig. 3: Clinical variants of pemphigus foliaceus (PF).

Paraneoplastic Pemphigus/Paraneoplastic Autoimmune Multiorgan Syndrome

This rare subtype of pemphigus is an autoimmune multiorgan syndrome associated with benign or malignant neoplasms. It presents with a polymorphous cutaneous eruption and desquamative gingivitis. The autoantibody response in PNP is more diverse compared to PV and PF including IgG against desmoplakin, envoplakin, periplakin, plectin, 230 kDa bullous pemphigoid (BP) antigen 1, and the recently discovered 170 kDa antigen protease inhibitor alpha-2-macroglobulin like-1. Consequently, direct immunofluorescence (DIF) of tissues from these patients has features of pemphigus as well as basement membrane labeling.

Immunoglobulin A (IgA) Pemphigus

It is characterized by tissue-bound IgA autoantibody deposited on the keratinocyte surface. Two subtypes of IgA pemphigus are identified based on clinical, histopatho-logical, and immunofluorescence studies **(Fig. 4)**.

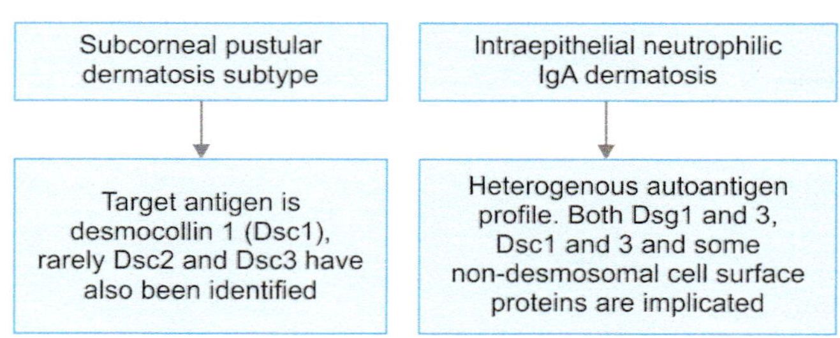

Fig. 4: Subtypes of immunoglobulin (IgA) pemphigus.
(Dsc: desmocollin; Dsg: desmoglein)

Pemphigus Herpetiformis

This is a rare variant of pemphigus clinically resembling DH, with pruritus, annular erythema and peripheral vesicles, or grouped vesicles on erythematous base. IgG autoantibodies are directed against Dsg1 and in some cases against Dsg3. However, non-Dsg desmosomal targets such as Dsc1, 2 and 3 have also been identified in few cases.

Drug-induced Pemphigus (DIP)

Three main groups of drugs have been associated with DIP: (1) thiol group, (2) phenol group and (3) non-thiol/non-phenol group. Some topical drugs such as imiquimod, cantharidin, and ophthalmic ointments have been attributed to cause "contact pemphigus". Clinical presentations of DIP include PV, followed by PF and in few cases manifestations of PE, PH, IgA pemphigus, PNP, pemphigus–pemphigoid overlap, and unclassified cases.

A summary of the various types of pemphigus with their target antigens and antibodies and level of split is depicted in **Table 1**.

TABLE 1: **Classification of pemphigus showing the target antigens and autoantibodies in each subtype along with the level of split.**

Pemphigus subtype	Antigen targeted	Circulating antibody	Level of split
Pemphigus vulgaris	Desmoglein 3 ± 1	IgG (occasionally IgM, IgA), complement	Suprabasal
Pemphigus foliaceus	Desmoglein 1, occasionally desmocollins	IgG, complement	Subcorneal
Paraneoplastic pemphigus	Plakins, plectins, desmogleins, BP230, α2ML1	IgG	Suprabasal and subepidermal
IgA pemphigus	Desmocollins, desmoglein 1 and 3	IgA	Subcorneal and intraepidermal
Pemphigus herpetiformis	Desmoglein 1 and sometimes 3, occasionally desmocollins 1-3	IgG, IgA, complement	Intraepidermal

(α2ML1: alpha-2-macroglobulin like-1; BP: bullous pemphigoid; IgA: immunoglobulin A; IgG: immunoglobulin G; IgM: immunoglobulin M)

SUBEPIDERMAL AUTOIMMUNE BULLOUS DISEASES

These can be classified as follows:
- Bullous diseases with binding above the lamina densa with antibodies against the hemidesmosomal components, e.g., pemphigoid diseases
- Sublamina densa-binding diseases caused by autoantibodies against collagen type VII, e.g., epidermolysis bullosa acquisita (EBA) and bullous systemic lupus erythematosus (BSLE)

Pemphigoid Diseases (Greek: Pemphix—Blister; Eidos—Form)

Pemphigoid group of AIBDs are characterized by circulating autoantibodies targeting structural proteins of the dermo-epidermal junction, which link the basal keratinocytes to the extracellular matrix of the dermis. Some prominent target antigens include BP120 (the intracellular plaque protein of hemidesmosomes) and BP180/collagen XVII (extracellular matrix protein), BP230, p200/laminin γ1, and laminin 332. The classification of pemphigoid diseases includes several subtypes based on clinical symptoms, target antigens, and autoantibodies.

Classification of pemphigoid diseases:
- *Bullous pemphigoid (BP)*
- *Mucous membrane pemphigoid (MMP)*:
  - Oral pemphigoid
  - Ocular pemphigoid
  - Anti-laminin 332 MMP
- *Pemphigoid gestationis (PG)*
- *Anti-p200/laminin γ1 pemphigoid*
- *Other pemphigoid disorders*
  - Lichen planus pemphigoides (LPP)
  - Cicatricial pemphigoid
  - Anti-type IV collagen pemphigoid
  - Anti-105 kDa antigen pemphigoid
- Linear IgA disease/linear IgA bullous dermatosis (LAD/LABD)
- Chronic bullous dermatosis of childhood (CBDC)

Bullous Pemphigoid

This is the most common AIBD of adults especially the elderly. It is characterized by IgG autoantibodies against two hemidesmosomal proteins BP180 and BP230. After a prodrome of pruritus and urticated and erythematous lesions, it progresses to tense vesicles and bullae. It predominantly affects the skin, with mucous membrane involvement seen in only 10–25% of the cases.

Non-bullous Pemphigoid

Approximately 20% of BP patients do not show blistering, a variant termed non-bullous pemphigoid (NBP). As compared to BP, NBP shows predominant reactivity to BP230 and less frequent complement activation, which might render it the characteristic clinical presentation. The term encompasses pruritic NBP, pemphigoid nodularis, papular pemphigoid, prodromal BP, and BP incipiens.

Pemphigoid Gestationis (PG)

PG is a rare autoimmune pregnancy dermatosis typically occurring in the second-to-third trimester as pruritic urticarial papules and plaques with overlying tense blisters, on the abdomen periumbilically and then spreading to involve the entire abdomen and thighs. Circulating autoantibodies IgG1 and IgG3 target BP180 more commonly than BP230.

Mucous Membrane Pemphigoid (MMP)

MMP is a chronic, subepidermal AIBD with predominant mucosal involvement characterized by autoreactivity to BP180 and less often to BP230 and α6 and β4 subunits of integrins. It most commonly affects the oral cavity followed by conjunctivae, skin, nasal cavity, anogenital areas, pharynx, larynx, and esophagus. Depending on the site of involvement, it has been subdivided as:
- Oral pemphigoid
- Ocular pemphigoid
- *Anti-laminin 332 (formerly epiligrin, laminin 5) MMP*: Characterized by scarring mucosal lesions and increased relative risk of malignancies especially adenocarcinoma

Anti-p200/Laminin γ1 Pemphigoid

It is characterized by autoantibodies against a 200 kDa protein (p200) of the dermo-epidermal junction. Presentation is similar to BP and the inflammatory subtype of EBA but with greater palmoplantar, cephalic, and mucosal involvement and an early age of onset compared to classical BP. Scarring or milia formation, though rare, has sometimes been observed.

Other Pemphigoid Disorders

Lichen planus pemphigoides: It is characterized by lesions of lichen planus with additional blistering on both LP lesions and normal skin (BP). An autoimmune response directed against BP180 has been implicated in the pathogenesis.

Cicatricial pemphigoid: This entity was previously used to describe patients with MMP. But currently the term is restricted to a variant of pemphigoid disease where skin lesions heal with scarring but mucous membranes are not predominantly affected. Brunsting–Perry pemphigoid is a clinical subtype of cicatricial pemphigoid sans mucosal involvement with multiple target antigens: type VII collagen, BP180, BP230, laminin 332, and desmoplakin I/II.

Linear IgA Bullous Dermatosis and Chronic Bullous Dermatosis of Childhood

It is a subepidermal blistering disorder with IgA deposition at the dermo-epidermal junction. It occurs both in adults and children with the latter being termed as chronic bullous disease/dermatosis of childhood (common between 6 months and 1 year of age). The major target antigens are LABD97 and LAD-1 antigens, which are cleaved products of BP180. Other less common ones are BP230, LAD 285, and collagen VII. Clinical presentation is heterogenous with tense hemorrhagic blisters on an erythematous base or normal skin. Mucosal involvement is more common in adults.

OTHER SUBEPIDERMAL AUTOIMMUNE BULLOUS DISEASES

- Epidermolysis bullosa acquisita (EBA)
- Bullous systemic lupus erythematosus (BSLE)

Epidermolysis Bullosa Acquisita

EBA is characterized by IgG (mainly IgG1 and IgG4) and rarely IgA autoantibodies against type VII collagen, located in the anchoring fibrils of the BMZ. Two subtypes are identified:

1. *Classic mechanobullous*: Presenting with blisters, scarring and milia formation at trauma-prone areas
2. *Inflammatory variant*: Resembling pemphigoid diseases

Bullous Systemic Lupus Erythematosus

Two immunologically distinct subsets of BSLE are identified:

1. Type 1 with type VII collagen autoantibodies (similar to EBA)
2. *Type 2 without such antibodies*: Caused by severe vacuolar alteration of the dermo-epidermal junction and dermal edema. However, some cases of type 2 BSLE have been recognized as having antibodies against BP180, BP230, and laminin 332.

The various subepidermal AIBDs with their specific antigens and antibodies are depicted in **Table 2**.

TABLE 2: Immunopathologic classification of subepidermal autoimmune bullous diseases.

Subepidermal bullous disease	Antigen targeted	Circulating antibody
Lamina lucida disorders		
Bullous pemphigoid	BP180, BP230, LAD, plectin	IgG, complement
Mucous membrane pemphigoid	BP180, BP230, LAD, laminin 332, integrin α6β4, collagen 7	IgG, IgA, complement
Pemphigoid gestationis	BP180	IgG, complement
Anti-p200/laminin γ1 pemphigoid	p200	IgG, complement
Lichen planus pemphigoides	BP180	IgG, complement
Cicatricial pemphigoid	BP180, BP230, laminin 332	IgG, complement
Linear IgA disease	LABD97 & LAD-1 (cleaved products of BP180), LAD 285, BP230, collagen VII, plectin	IgA
Lamina densa disorders		
Epidermolysis bullosa acquisita	Collagen type VII	IgG, IgA, complement
Bullous SLE	Collagen type VII, BP180, BP230, laminin 332	IgG, IgM, IgA, complement

(BP: bullous pemphigoid; IgA: immunoglobulin A; IgG: immunoglobulin G; IgM: immunoglobulin M; LAD: linear IgA disease; SLE: systemic lupus erythematosus)

DERMATITIS HERPETIFORMIS (DUHRING–BROCQ DISEASE)

DH is the cutaneous manifestation of celiac disease. An autoantibody population against tissue transglutaminase (tTG) characterizes celiac disease. Since subclinical gluten sensitivity is obligated to develop in DH, these patients develop another autoantibody population against epidermal transglutaminase (eTG) in addition to tTG. eTG are localized at the BMZ in the papillary tips and are targeted by IgA auto-antibodies. In contrast to other AIBDs, DH has no circulating autoantibodies. The pathological IgA is bound to eTG, but these enzymes are not present in the papillary dermis of healthy skin. Therefore, some consider DH as a gluten-induced eTG-IgA immune complex disease of the skin. Clinical manifestations include an intensely pruritic rash predominantly affecting the extensor surfaces. The vesicular eruption is not evident as that is destroyed by excoriations.

CONCLUSION

The classification of pemphigus and other AIBDs is based on clinical, histopathological, and immunopathological criteria. The differentiation of these disorders assumes importance since specific treatment options are now available. Moreover, certain AIBDs are associated with malignancy; hence, it is vital to screen individuals diagnosed with these disorders.

TAKE HOME MESSAGE

- Autoimmune bullous diseases are chronic skin diseases primarily affecting the adults, with considerable impact on their quality of life.
- Their classification is based on the level of skin blister formation as intraepidermal and subepidermal.
- The classification of immunobullous diseases is important as this differentiation is a guide to treatment options which are now widely available and specifically target different subsets of diseases.
- With progress in our understanding of the pathogenesis of these disorders, the classification system is constantly being updated with newer additions being made to the existing ones.

MULTIPLE CHOICE QUESTIONS

1. **Pemphigus vegetans is a subtype of:**
   - (a) Paraneoplastic pemphigus
   - (b) Pemphigus herpetiformis
   - (c) Pemphigus vulgaris
   - (d) IgA pemphigus

2. **Senear–Usher syndrome is synonymous with:**
   - (a) Subcorneal pustular dermatosis
   - (b) Pemphigus erythematosus
   - (c) Chronic bullous dermatosis of childhood
   - (d) Dermatitis herpetiformis

3. **Which of the following is not a pemphigoid disorder?**
   - (a) Linear IgA disease
   - (b) Mucous membrane pemphigoid
   - (c) Cicatricial pemphigoid
   - (d) Dermatitis herpetiformis

4. **BP incipiens is a subtype of:**
   - (a) Bullous pemphigoid
   - (b) Mucous membrane pemphigoid
   - (c) Non-bullous pemphigoid
   - (d) Cicatricial pemphigoid

5. **Which of the following autoimmune bullous diseases is a lamina densa disorder?**
   - (a) Bullous pemphigoid
   - (b) Chronic bullous disease of childhood
   - (c) Bullous SLE
   - (d) Dermatitis herpetiformis

6. **Ocular pemphigoid is a subtype of:**
   - (a) Cicatricial pemphigoid
   - (b) Bullous pemphigoid
   - (c) Mucous membrane pemphigoid
   - (d) Lichen planus pemphigoides

Answers

1. (c)   2. (b)   3. (d)   4. (c)   5. (c)   6. (c)

SUGGESTED READING

1. Hertl M, Schuler G. [Bullous autoimmune dermatoses. 1: Classification] *Hautarzt*. 2002;53:207-19; quiz 220-1.
2. Murrell DF. Blistering diseases: Clinical features, pathogenesis, treatment. Germany: Springer-Verlag Berlin Heidelberg; 2015.
3. Horváth B. Autoimmune bullous diseases, 2nd edition. Switzerland: Springer Nature Switzerland AG; 2022.

Intraepidermal Autoimmune Bullous Diseases

CHAPTER 6

Pemphigus Vulgaris

Rhea Ahuja, Sujay Khandpur

- Epidemiology of pemphigus vulgaris
- Associated co-morbidities
- Clinical manifestations
- Involvement of special sites
- Bedside tests
- Prognosis and disease outcome
- Psychological co-morbidity
- Diagnostic modalities and treatment options

INTRODUCTION

Pemphigus is a group of intraepidermal autoimmune bullous diseases. Its name is derived from the Greek word "pemphix," meaning 'blister' or 'bubble'. Broadly, it can be characterized into pemphigus foliaceus (PF), pemphigus vulgaris (PV), immunoglobulin A (IgA) pemphigus, drug-induced pemphigus, and paraneoplastic pemphigus (PNP). In this chapter, we shall be focusing on the clinical aspects of PV.

EPIDEMIOLOGY

PV represents the most common form of pemphigus, accounting for up to 70% cases. In India too, PV is recognized as the most prevalent variant, and forms 75–92% of total pemphigus patients.

Although the disease is reported worldwide, there are significant variations with respect to geographical distribution and ethnicity. The annual incidence rates vary from <0.76 per million population in Finland to 4.4 per million in India and 16.1 per million in Israel. Further, there is a disproportionate overrepresentation of the disease in certain ethnic groups such as the Ashkenazi Jews and those of Mediterranean origin. Simon, *et al* have reported the frequency of PV in North America to be 32 per million population in people of Jewish origin compared to 4.2 per million population in other ethnic groups. This ethnic variation is possibly due to the presence of several human leukocyte antigen (HLA) class II genes namely *HLA-DRB1*04* and *HLA-A*10* among Ashkenazi Jew pemphigus patients.

It has also been shown that the proportion of subjects with anti-desmoglein 1 (Dsg1) antibody profile in PV is significantly higher in patients of Indian origin (75%) as compared to those of North European descent (46%).

The presence of these anti-Dsg1 antibodies is predictive of a potentially more severe cutaneous phenotype.

The disease commonly affects individuals between 40 and 60 years of age. However, the age of presentation is highly variable, ranging from 36.5 years in Kuwait to 72.4 years in Bulgaria. In India, most patients are <40 years of age, in contrast to the rest of the world, where PV has a late age of onset, usually between 40 and 60 years. Mascarenhas, *et al* and Singh, *et al* observed a significant proportion of their patients being <40 years of age; similarly, Sehgal VN reported a higher disease prevalence between 21 and 40 years. Interestingly, the age of presentation depends more on ethnic origin, rather than the geographical distribution after migration. An epidemiological study in Israel showed the mean age of onset among Arab patients to be significantly lower than that of native Jewish population (44.3 ± 15.4 vs. 54.5 ± 15.6 years, respectively), being comparable to the age of onset in other Middle Eastern and Arab countries.

The gender ratio is almost equivalent, with no specific predilection. However, many contrasting results have been reported in literature, with some studies showing a female preponderance (F:M—5:1), while others have reported a higher proportion of male patients (M:F—3:1).

ASSOCIATED CO-MORBIDITIES

Both cross-sectional and controlled studies have found an association of PV with other autoimmune diseases. The prevalence of autoimmune thyroid disease (AITD), rheumatoid arthritis, and type 1 diabetes mellitus (T1DM) was higher in PV patients compared to their first-degree relatives or the general population. Interestingly, clustering of two different sets of autoimmune diseases with PV (autoimmune diathesis) was proposed: AITD, rheumatoid arthritis, and T1DM, and systemic lupus erythematosus

(SLE), AITD, and rheumatoid arthritis, possibly as a result of shared genetic susceptibility to these different diseases. Another cross-sectional study reported a two-fold increased risk of diabetes, with an increased prevalence of hypothyroidism and inflammatory bowel disease (standardized prevalence ratio ~1.5) in PV patients.

AITD is perhaps the most extensively studied co-morbidity, with prevalence rates varying between 0% and 13.4%. Though the frequency of antithyroid peroxidase and antithyroglobulin antibodies has been reported to be higher in PV patients, the difference with respect to general population is not statistically significant. Moreover, it does not necessarily translate to clinical hypothyroidism, so currently routine screening of patients for thyroid antibodies is not indicated.

Some case reports have also shown an association between PV and psoriasis. This association may be biologically plausible in accordance with the epitope spreading phenomenon in which inflammation from one skin disease leads to a favorable environment for the expression of intraepidermal antigens and subsequent generation of an immune response. Further, elevated levels of plasminogen activator have been noted in psoriatic lesions, and plasminogen activation is known to play a role in acantholysis. Kridin, *et al* critically analyzed this association and found Israeli pemphigus patients to be associated with a 2.6-elevated odds of psoriasis [95% confidence interval (CI) 1.9–3.6]. They concluded that the association was significant, and clinicians should be aware of this rare co-morbidity.

The association between bullous pemphigoid and neurological diseases is well known; recent literature suggests its co-existence with PV as well. A retrospective, population-based cross-sectional study found a two-fold higher prevalence of epilepsy, dementia, and Parkinson's disease among PV patients compared with matched controls. Dsg1 is expressed not only on the skin epithelial surface but also in corpus callosum and in oligodendrocytes, explaining the possible occurrence of cross-reactivity to antibodies. It is worthwhile to note that both pemphigus and Parkinson's disease are commonly reported among the Ashkenazi Jews, underlining an inherent genetic susceptibility.

PV has also been found to be associated with malignancies, both solid organ and hematological, and this is independent of the distinct PNP, where a malignancy follows, precedes, or occurs concurrently with the diagnosis. Compared to controls, an increased prevalence of esophageal and laryngeal cancers has been reported. Similarly, a higher frequency of chronic leukemia, multiple myeloma, and non-Hodgkin's lymphoma is noted in these patients. While certain immunosuppressive agents like azathioprine may increase the risk of a hematological malignancy, the more likely hypothesis is chronic immune stimulation in an inflammatory disease leading to a random introduction of pro-oncogenic mutations in rapidly multiplying cells.

CLINICAL MANIFESTATIONS

Most PV patients present with mucosal involvement, and oral erosions are often the first manifestation preceding cutaneous lesions. Oral lesions have been noted in up to 84% of PV patients, and they are the first manifestation in 66% cases. Within the oral mucosa, the disease most commonly manifests in areas prone to frictional trauma, like the buccal mucosa along the occlusion plane, palate and gingival mucosa **(Figs. 1 to 3)**. Oral lesions manifest as painful, irregularly shaped (jagged margins) erosions or ulcers with surrounding inflammation, covered with whitish-gray necrotic slough, with less tendency to heal spontaneously. There may be superimposed candidal infection.

The upper and lower gingivae may show superficial erythematous desquamative gingivitis, and the retromolar trigone may be frequently involved **(Fig. 4)**, especially in those with persistent disease. Kumar, *et al* highlighted

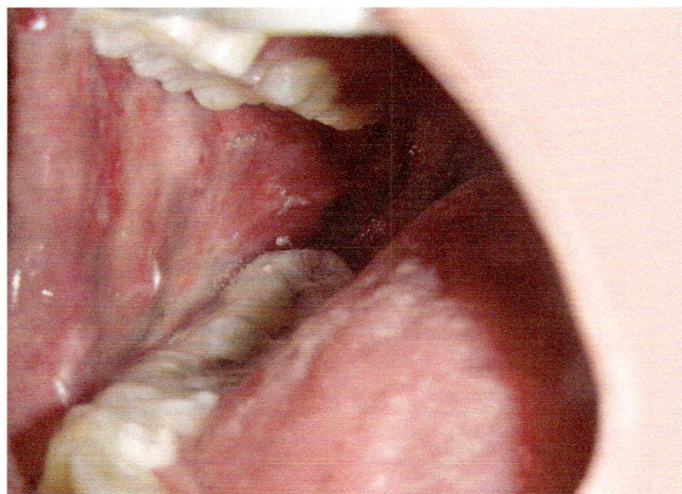

Fig. 1: Oral pemphigus vulgaris: Multiple erosions on the buccal mucosa.

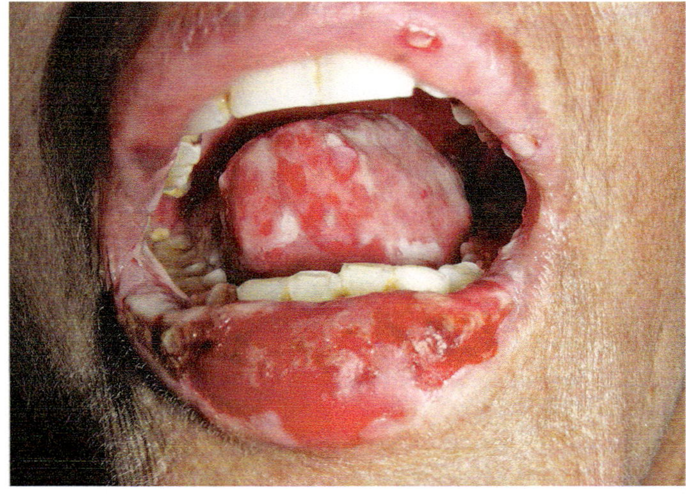

Fig. 2: Oral pemphigus vulgaris: Multiple, discrete-to-confluent erosions involving the tongue, labial and buccal mucosae.

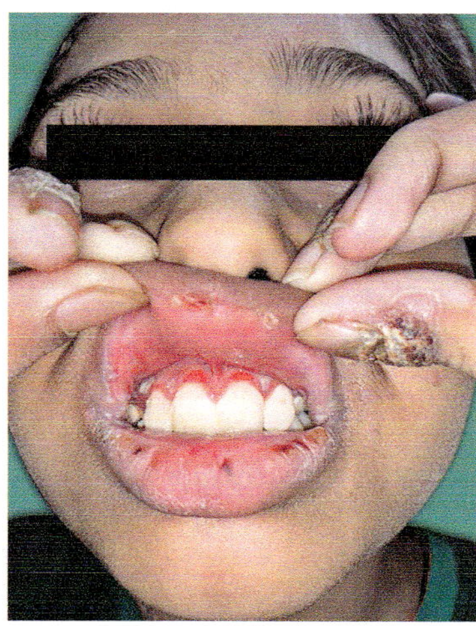

Fig. 3: Oral pemphigus vulgaris: Involvement of gingival and labial mucosae.

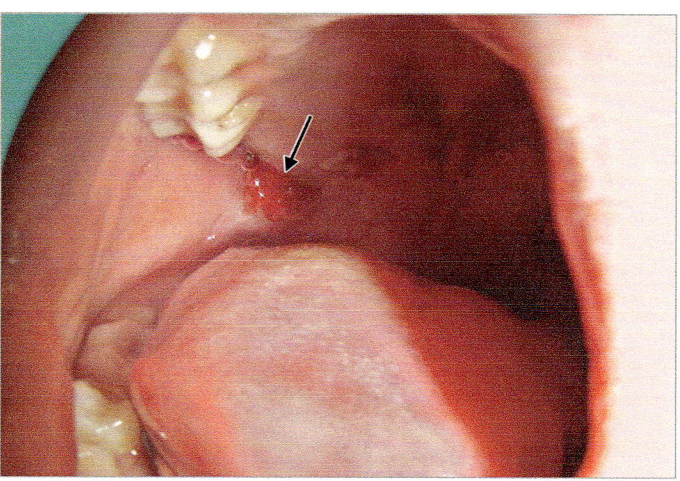

Fig. 4: Oral pemphigus vulgaris: A non-healing erosion in the retromolar trigone (arrow) along with many palatal erosions.

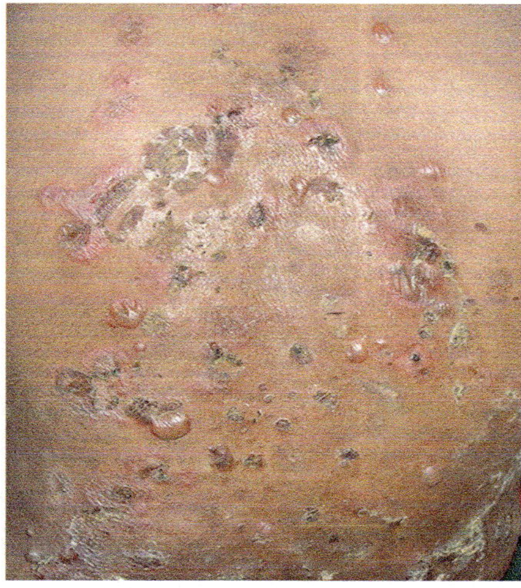

Fig. 5: Pemphigus vulgaris: Multiple flaccid vesicles and bullae, erosions and crusted plaques on normal and erythematous skin on the back.

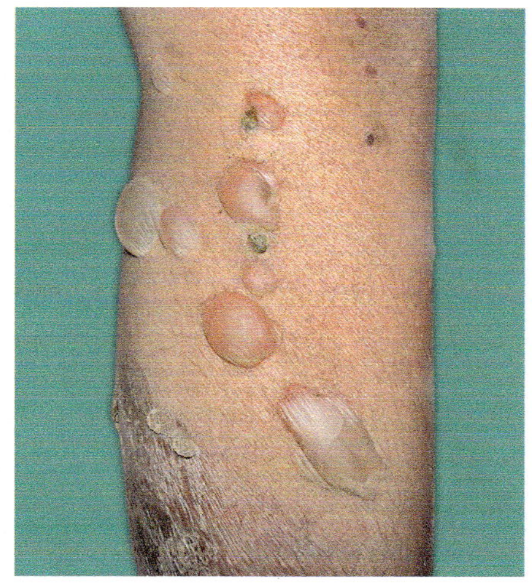

Fig. 6: Pemphigus vulgaris: Large bullae containing clear-to-turbid fluid, present on normal skin.

certain factors associated with refractoriness to treatment of oral lesions, such as lesions occurring along the occlusion line on buccal mucosa, on retromolar trigone, lesions which are deep and have a lichenoid hue, and long-standing lesions. It has been observed that disease onset in the oral mucosa has a 10 times higher chance of relapse.

Oral lesions usually persist longer, require a longer treatment course, and are associated with significant morbidity resulting in impaired quality of life. It is important not only to examine the extent of erosions and their number but also to assess the subjective discomfort [as in the recently devised POLIS (Pemphigus Oral Lesions Intensity Score) scale] before deciding treatment, and for subsequent follow-up.

Cutaneous lesions manifest as flaccid vesicles or bullae on normal-appearing or erythematous skin. They rupture to form painful erosions that extend peripherally, form oozy and crusted plaques, with little tendency to heal spontaneously **(Figs. 5 to 7)**. Any cutaneous site may be affected, with predilection for the trunk, groins, axillae, face, and scalp **(Figs. 8 and 9)**; however, there is often sparing of the palms and soles.

Rarely, despite the presence of both anti-Dsg1 and 3 antibodies, mucous membrane involvement is not observed. This exclusive cutaneous presentation is referred to as "cutaneous-type/pure cutaneous PV." Clinical findings in this rare variant may show a seborrheic distribution similar to PF **(Fig. 10)**, may have features reminiscent of linear IgA bullous disease and eczema, or the presentation is akin to the skin lesions noted in muco-cutaneous PV.

Lesions with atypical morphologies have also been observed. Folliculocentric papulovesicular and papulopustular lesions can occur on the chest, back, and arms **(Fig. 11)**. These have been noted in patients who are on oral steroids and have subsequently developed a flare. Other morphologies include targetoid lesions coalescing into an annular configuration **(Fig. 12)**, pustules with surrounding

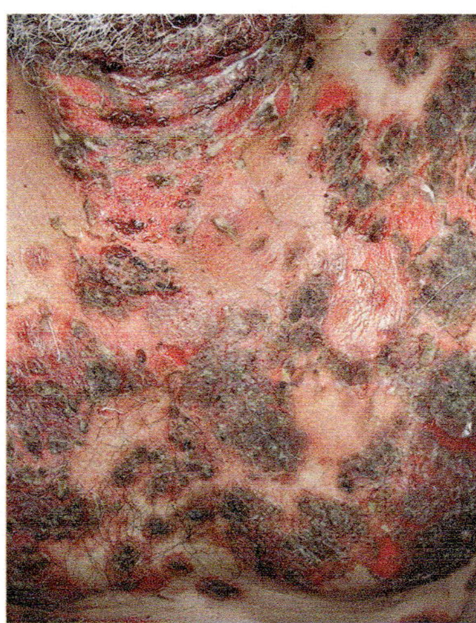

Fig. 7: Pemphigus vulgaris: Confluent erosions and crusted plaques on the chest.

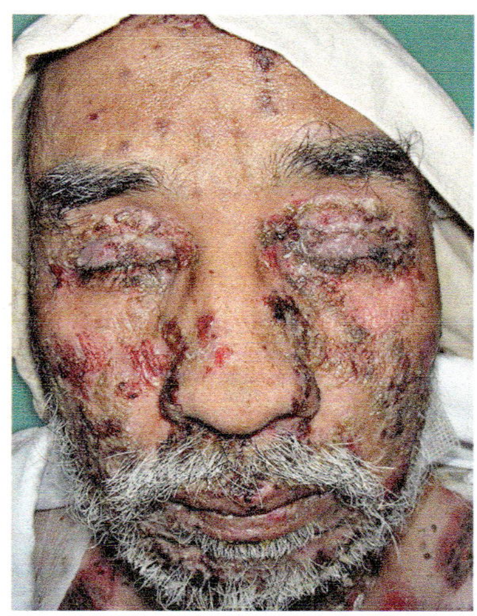

Fig. 8: Pemphigus vulgaris: Erosions and crusted plaques on the face.

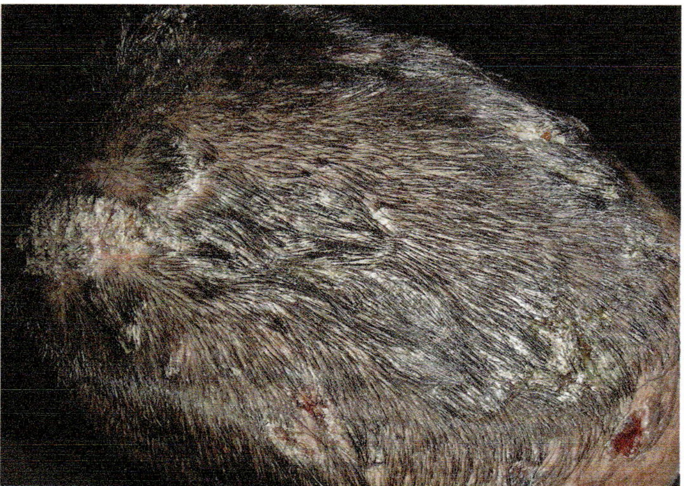

Fig. 9: Pemphigus vulgaris: Extensive crusted plaques on the scalp.

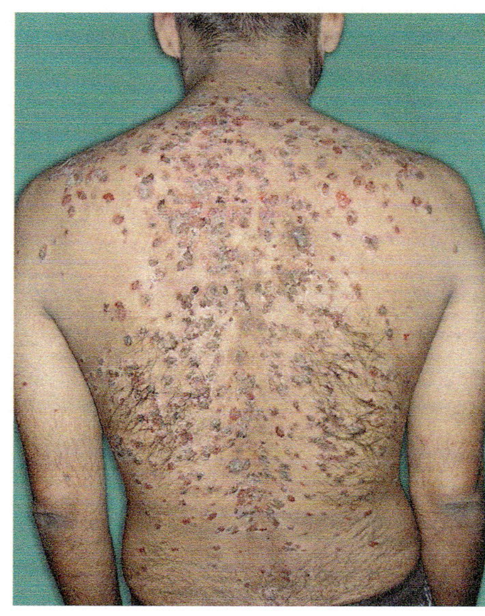

Fig. 10: Pure cutaneous pemphigus vulgaris: Multiple erosions and crusted plaques in seborrheic distribution on the back resembling pemphigus foliaceus.

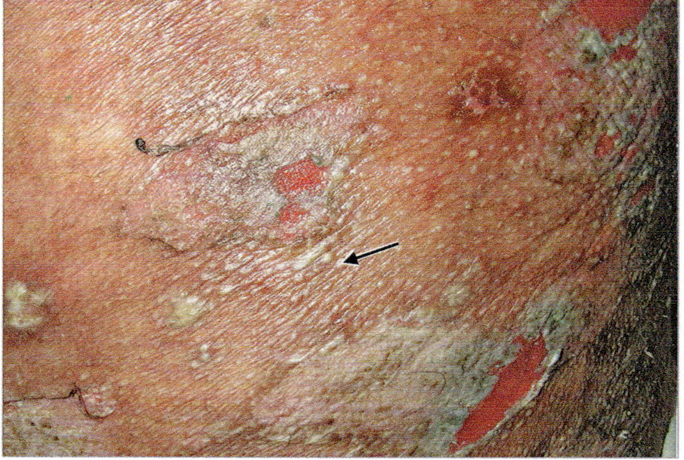

Fig. 11: Pemphigus vulgaris: Multiple follicular pustules (arrow) on the trunk.

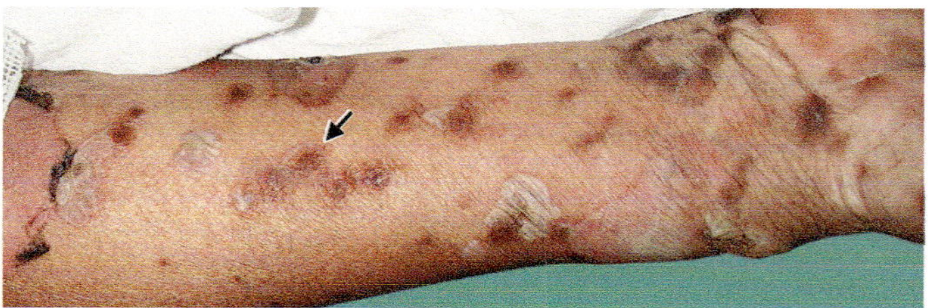

Fig. 12: Pemphigus vulgaris: Targetoid lesions (arrow) on the right forearm.

erythema, and a diffuse desquamation simulating toxic epidermal necrolysis **(Fig. 13)**. While the clinical implication and long-term prognosis of patients with these atypical morphologies are not clear, presence of targetoid lesions may raise a suspicion of PNP.

Rarely, patients may present with localized PV, a relatively benign subset, with lesions usually limited to the sun-exposed areas, sites of trauma, and surgical scars. It usually involves the face **(Figs. 14 and 15)**, scalp, and/or oral mucosa. Localized PV has been found to remain confined to a particular area for variable periods ranging from 5 months to 7 years. While some authors attribute this localization to Koebner-like phenomenon, others believe that ultraviolet radiation may act as a triggering factor. Regional variation in Dsg antigens and absent or low rates of circulating anti-Dsg antibodies have also been postulated to play a role in localized PV. It usually shows good response to topical steroids alone, without the need of systemic agents.

Pruritus is not uncommon in pemphigus and has been reported in around 80% of patients, with the mean Bullous Pemphigoid Disease Area Index (BPDAI) pruritus score being comparable to bullous pemphigoid. Further, the impact on quality of life by itch as measured by the Autoimmune Bullous Disease Quality of Life (ABQoL) score, has been found to be similar between pemphigus and bullous pemphigoid. The presence of pruritus also increases the chances of subsequent relapse, and new-onset itch in remission indicates impending disease reactivation.

PV usually heals with transient hyperpigmentation without residual scarring. There may be development of hyperpigmented, verrucous plaques resembling seborrheic keratosis, known as post-pemphigus acanthomata **(Fig. 16)**.

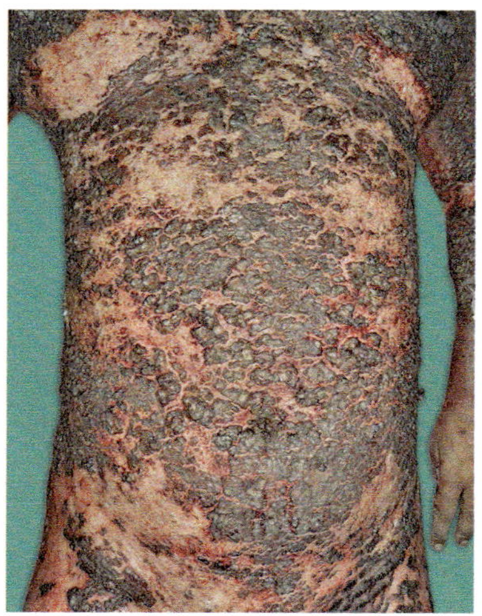

Fig. 13: Pemphigus vulgaris: Severe disease mimicking toxic epidermal necrolysis. *Image courtesy*: Dr Vinay Keshavamurthy.

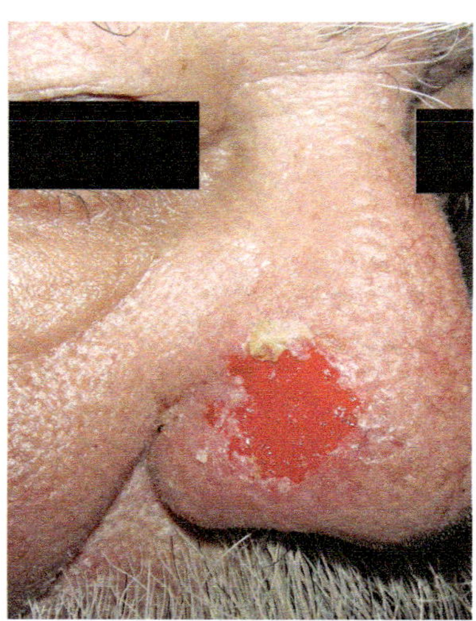

Fig. 14: Localized pemphigus vulgaris: A single erosion on the right ala of the nose.

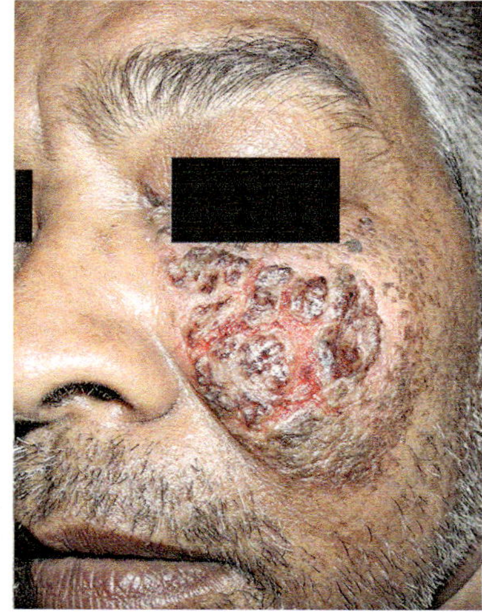

Fig. 15: Localized pemphigus vulgaris: A crusted plaque on the left cheek.

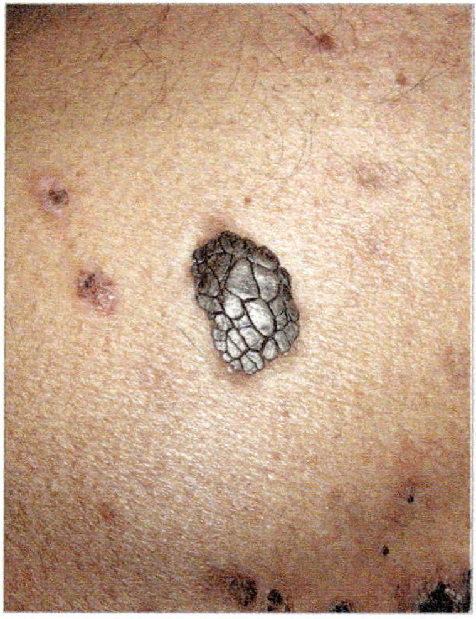

Fig. 16: Post-pemphigus acanthomata: Black crusted plaque resembling seborrheic keratosis.

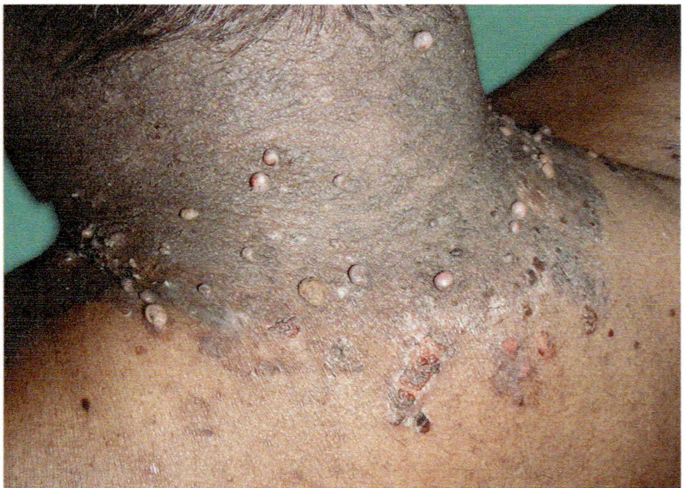

Fig. 17: Acrochordon-like papules: Formed after healing of pemphigus vulgaris.

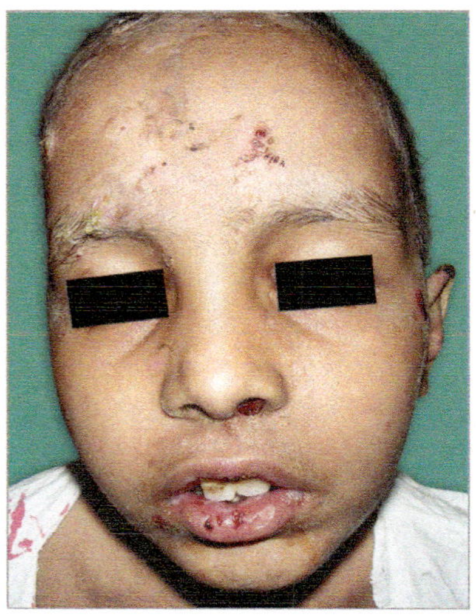

Fig. 18: Childhood pemphigus vulgaris: Mucocutaneous erosions in a child.

These lesions histopathologically show intraepidermal clefting and positivity on direct immunofluorescence (DIF), suggesting persistent clinical activity. Rarely, extensive keloidal scarring of pemphigus lesions, acrochordon-like papules **(Fig. 17)**, and acanthosis nigricans-like residual lesions have also been reported.

PV may rarely occur in children (0.1–0.5 cases/100,000 children/year). It usually affects adolescents in the age group of 13–19 years and shares similar clinical, histological, and immunological features with adult PV **(Figs. 18 and 19)**. Most of the children have both mucosal and skin involvement, with oral lesions being the first manifestation. Ocular involvement leading to conjunctivitis with hyperemia and mucoid discharge, has also been reported in this age group. The diagnosis of PV is often delayed, and initially these children may be misdiagnosed as having impetigo, herpes simplex infection, or epidermolysis bullosa. The overall prognosis in childhood PV is better than in adult disease.

Neonatal PV is a self-limiting bullous dermatosis caused by the passive transplacental transfer of IgG antibodies from the mother to her fetus. A physiological variation in Dsg distribution is present in neonates; both Dsg1 and 3 are present in the upper layers, while only Dsg3 is present in the suprabasal layers, so there is a greater chance in a pregnant woman with PV delivering an affected child than a pregnant woman with PF. The antibody titer of the mother or her clinical presentation at the time of delivery does not predict the severity of neonatal PV, which can range from only oral involvement to widespread denuded skin. It follows a transitory course, and the lesions usually resolve within 3 weeks of birth as the maternal antibodies are metabolized.

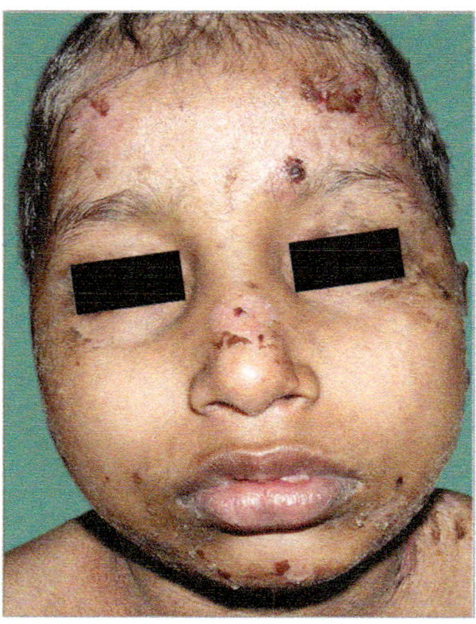

Fig. 19: Childhood pemphigus vulgaris: Healing erosions on the face and neck.

SPECIAL SITES OF INVOLVEMENT

Scalp Involvement

There is presence of Dsgs (Dsg1–4) in the hair follicles; Dsg1 is expressed in the inner root sheath (IRS) and the innermost layers of the outer root sheath (ORS), Dsg2 is present in the bulge and bulb matrix cells, Dsg3 is expressed throughout the ORS, while Dsg4 is extensively present in the matrix and IRS. Thus, scalp is a commonly affected site in PV, in 16–60% cases **(Fig. 9)**. It may sometimes be the first site of involvement in 9–15% of patients. Scalp involvement can cause both non-scarring and scarring alopecia and may also lead to tufted folliculitis. Delmonte, *et al* had demonstrated that anagen hair with intact root sheaths can be easily pulled out from both lesional and non-lesional scalp skin in PV patients. This has been referred to as "normal anagen effluvium" and is regarded as the equivalent of Nikolsky sign on the skin. In a study on 52 newly diagnosed PV patients, the degree of anagen hair loss showed significant correlation with the concentration of anti-Dsg antibody as well as scalp and skin pemphigus disease area index (PDAI) scores. Scalp lesions in most patients tend to be recalcitrant, and in >60% patients, scalp is the site of residual lesions.

Palmoplantar Involvement: Dyshidrosiform Pemphigus

Involvement of the palms and soles in PV has been rarely described **(Fig. 20)**. The lesions begin as a vesicobullous eruption that mimic bullous tinea pedis or pompholyx, with subsequent crusting, with or without nail involvement. It is usually associated with more severe disease and is a poor prognostic marker.

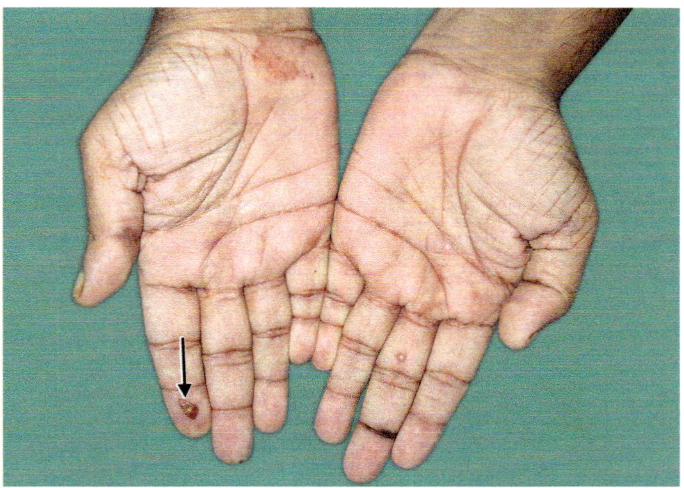

Fig. 20: Dyshidrosiform pemphigus vulgaris: Tense vesicles (arrow) and erosions on the palms.

Nail Involvement

Dsg1 and 3 are normally expressed in the proximal nail fold, nail matrix, and hyponychium. Ungual lesions in pemphigus are secondary to vesiculation in the nail bed/nail matrix or due to acantholysis in the nail fold. Nail involvement in PV is relatively uncommon but a study estimated the frequency of nail changes to be around 22% in their patients. Commonly, paronychia **(Fig. 21)** and onychomadesis **(Fig. 22)** are seen, and recurrent paronychia may rarely be the only manifestation. Beau lines can also be noted and their distance from the proximal nail fold serves as an indirect marker about the time of disease onset, and their number indicates the number of relapses.

There is a direct correlation between nail involvement and disease duration and severity. This is because the proximal nail matrix is an immune-privileged site and gets involved only later in the disease course as a result of prolonged inflammation.

Involvement of Other Mucosae

Dsg3 is present on the entire ocular surface, i.e., cornea, bulbar and palpebral conjunctiva, and also in deeper layers like the retina. The frequency of ocular involvement in PV is estimated to be 7–16.5%. It commonly affects the eyelids and conjunctiva **(Fig. 23)**, and mild-to-moderate non-cicatrizing conjunctivitis is the most frequent ocular involvement. Patients usually complain of redness, photophobia, pain, and ocular irritation but visual acuity is not affected. Usually full recovery occurs without sequelae.

Genital mucosa may also be involved. Involvement of the esophageal mucosa can occur in PV. In a study, 57% patients complained of dysphagia and 21.4% of odynophagia, while hematemesis was reported in only 3.5% patients. Sometimes patients may vomit out a cast of the mucosal lining of esophagus, referred to as "esophagitis dissecans superficialis" or "exfoliative esophagitis".

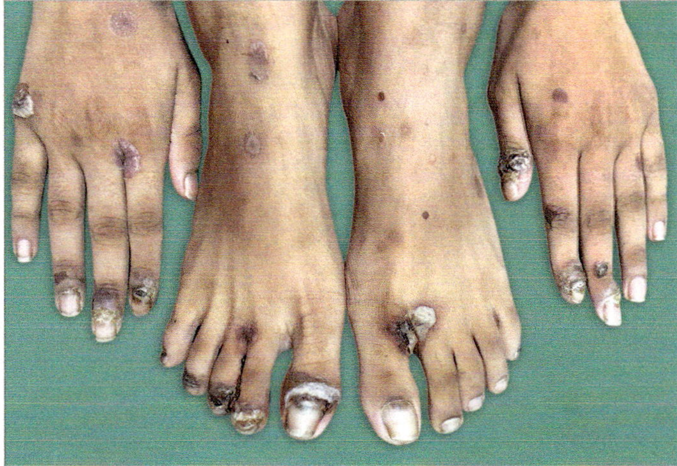

Fig. 21: Nail involvement in pemphigus vulgaris: Multiple finger and toe nails showing paronychia.

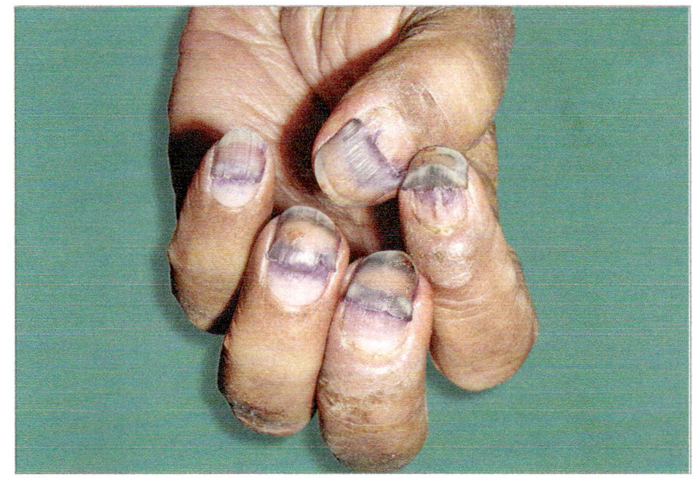

Fig. 22: Nail involvement in pemphigus vulgaris: Onychomadesis of the nail plates. Nail discoloration is due to gentian violet application.

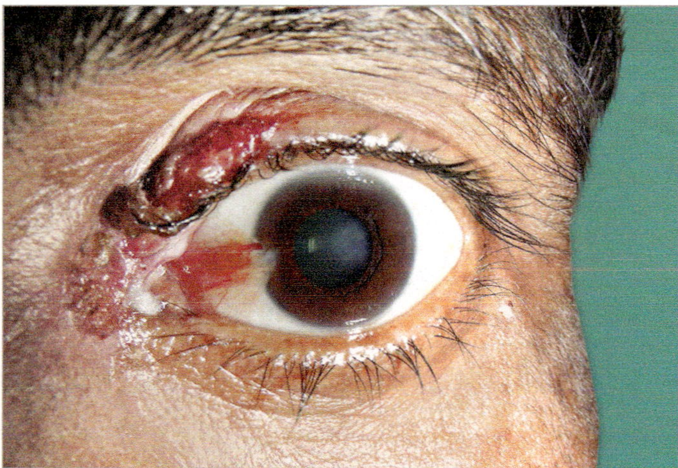

Fig. 23: Eye involvement in pemphigus vulgaris: Erosions present on the eyelid with associated pterygium.

PV may also involve the larynx. In a prospective study on 40 PV patients, nearly half of them reported pharyngeal or laryngeal symptoms, and upon endoscopic evaluation, the proportion of these patients having laryngeal involvement was approximately 95%. Epiglottis was the most common site of involvement, and this may sometimes be misdiagnosed as viral or bacterial laryngitis. Symptom severity can vary from hoarseness of voice to frank airway impairment requiring tracheostomy. Intubation is often avoided because of the fragility of laryngeal mucosa, which could be seriously injured. Instituting therapy early is important to prevent worsening of epiglottic edema, and preserving the upper airway is of utmost importance as mucosal sloughing by positive Nikolsky sign may prove to be lethal.

The clinical variants of PV are enlisted in **Table 1**.

TABLE 1: Clinical variants of pemphigus vulgaris (PV).

- Classic PV: Mucocutaneous PV
- Pure mucosal PV
- Cutaneous type/pure cutaneous PV
- Rare types
  - *Folliculocentric papulopustules/papulovesicles*
  - *Pustules with surrou nding erythema*
  - *Targetoid lesions with annular configuration*
  - *TEN-like lesions*
- Localized PV: Lesions limited to sun-exposed areas, trauma sites and surgical scars
- Special sites of involvement
  - *Scalp*
  - *Palms and soles*: Dyshidrosiform PV
  - *Nails*: Paronychia, onychomadesis, Beau lines
  - *Other mucosae*: Ocular, genital, nasal, esophageal, pharynx, larynx
- Childhood PV
- Neonatal PV

Pemphigus Vegetans

Pemphigus vegetans is a rare subtype of PV characterized by vegetating verrucous lesions predominantly localized to the intertriginous areas. Its prevalence varies from 1 to 2% among all pemphigus patients. Like PV, it results from autoantibodies to transmembrane proteins, more commonly anti-Dsg3 than anti-Dsg1.

There are two recognized clinical subtypes based on the initial presentation and disease course—Hallopeau and Neumann. The former starts as pustules and has a relatively benign course, while the latter begins as flaccid vesicles and shows a clinically unremitting course with a poorer response to therapy. Both these subtypes evolve to develop hyperkeratotic vegetative plaques with a predilection for flexural areas **(Figs. 24 to 26)**. Oral mucosal involvement is also commonly noted, in up to 60–80% cases, often at disease onset. Cerebriform tongue is an eponymous clinical sign described in up to 50% cases of pemphigus vegetans, with grooves on the dorsal aspect resembling the sulci and

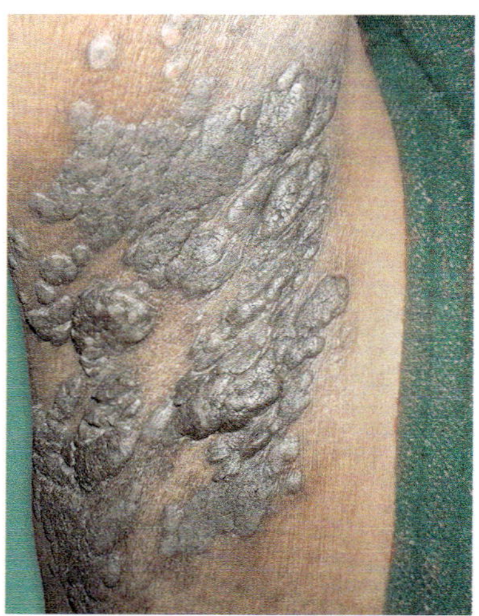

Fig. 24: Pemphigus vegetans: Hyperpigmented verrucous vegetative plaques in the axilla.

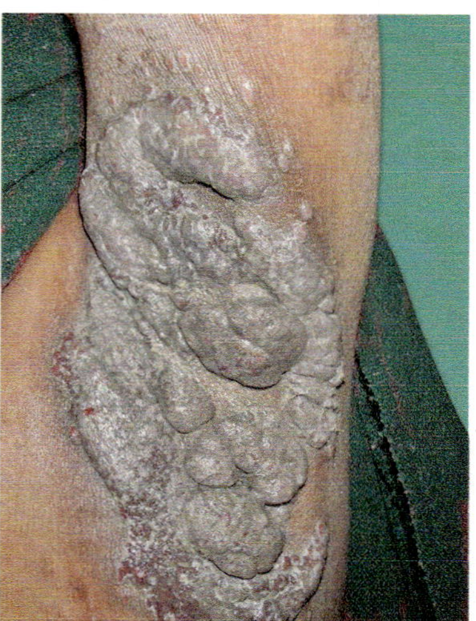

Fig. 25: Pemphigus vegetans: Vegetative, nodular, eroded plaques in the axilla.

gyri in the brain **(Fig. 27)**. Rarely, the lesion may be localized to the scalp **(Fig. 28)**, face, vermilion border of lips **(Figs. 29 and 30)**, dorsa of hands, fingers and feet **(Figs. 31 to 33)**, peri-anal region and nail folds.

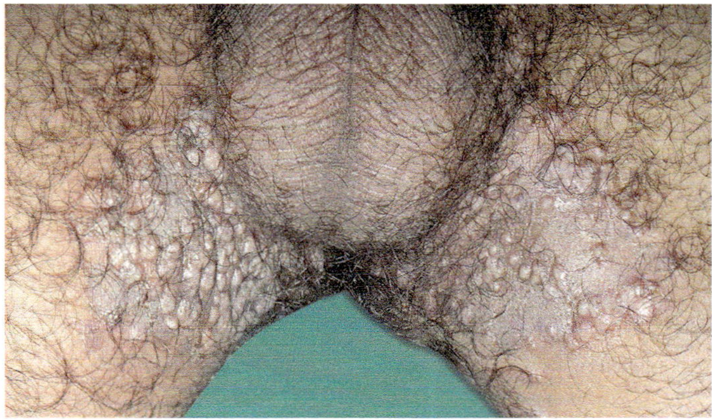

Fig. 26: Pemphigus vegetans: Vegetative plaques on both groins.

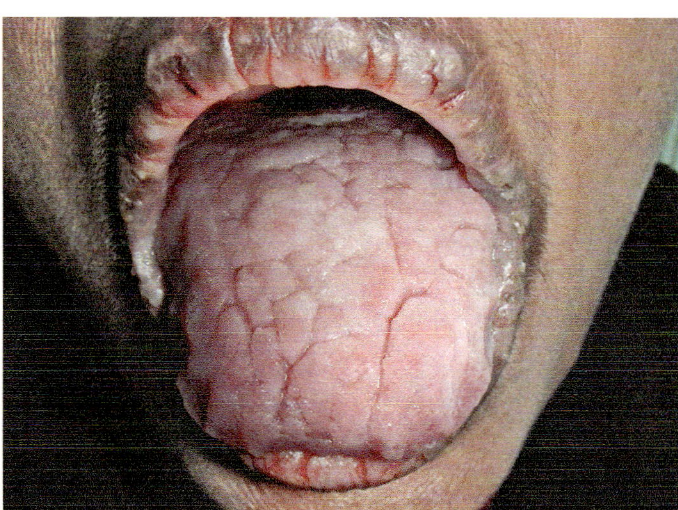

Fig. 27: Pemphigus vegetans: Grooves on dorsum of tongue suggestive of cerebriform tongue.

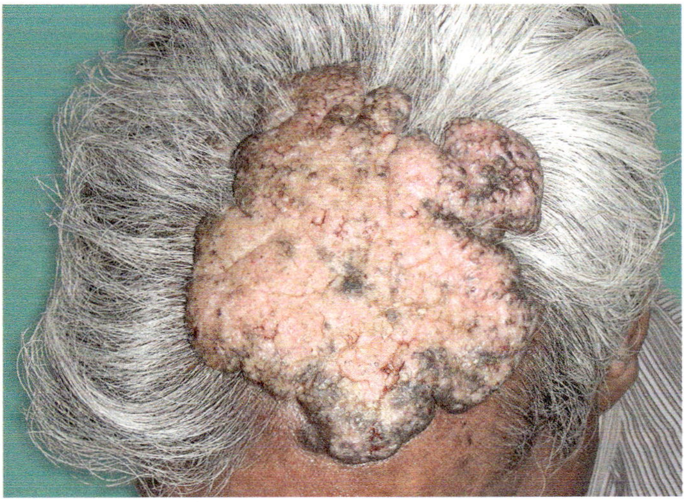

Fig. 28: Pemphigus vegetans: Fleshy plaque on scalp.

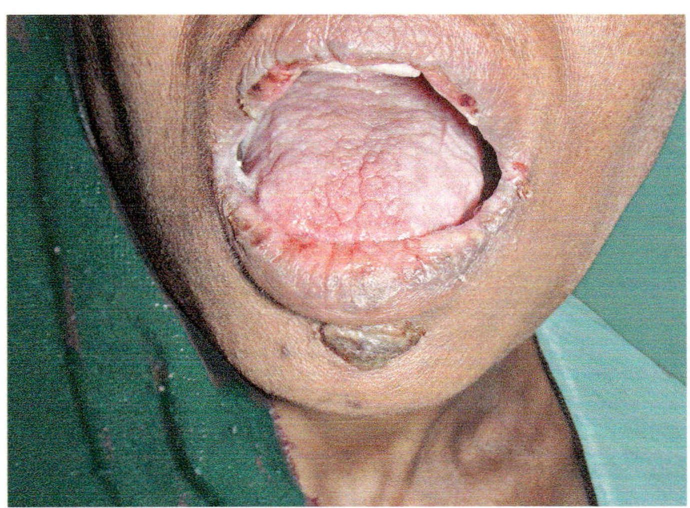

Fig. 29: Pemphigus vegetans: Crusted, vegetative plaque on lower lip with erosions on lip mucosa.

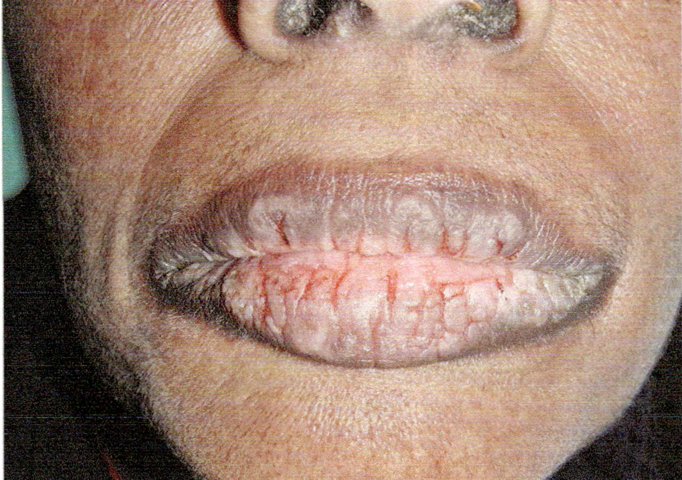

Fig. 30: Pemphigus vegetans: Verrucous plaques with grooves on both lips.

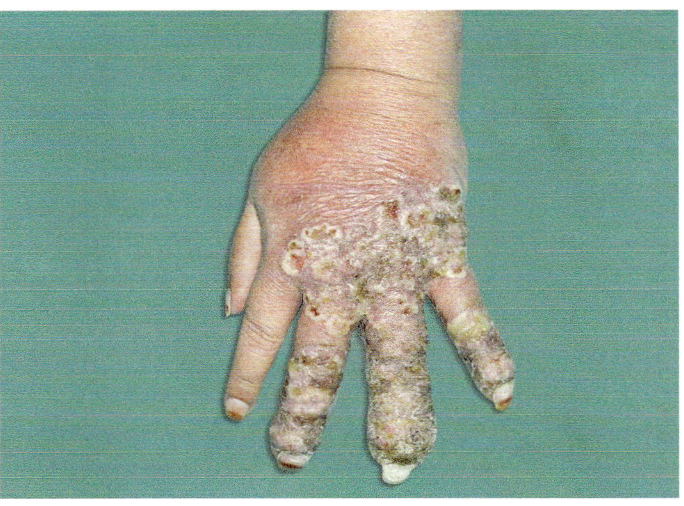

Fig. 31: Pemphigus vegetans: Crusted (purulent), scaly plaque on dorsum of the hand.

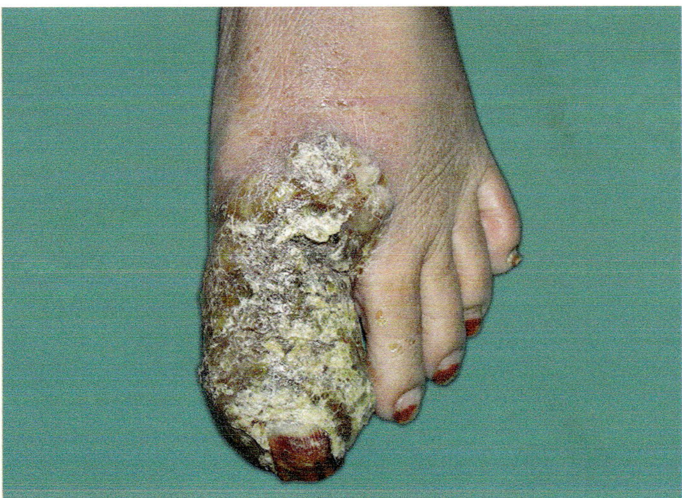

Fig. 32: Pemphigus vegetans: Crusted (purulent), scaly plaque on great toe.

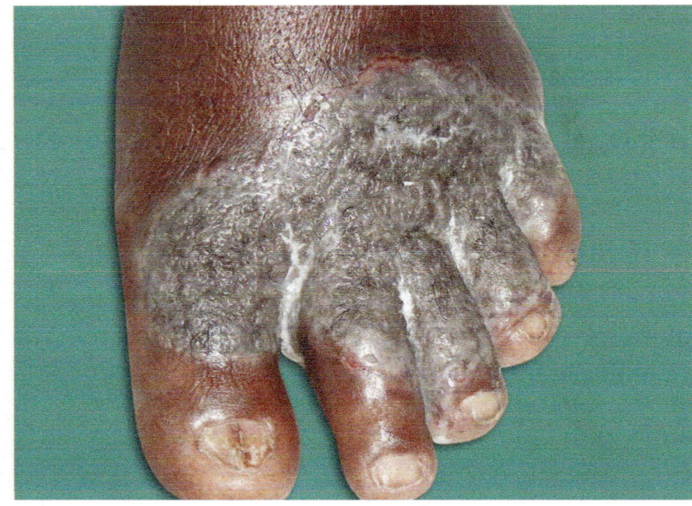

Fig. 33: Pemphigus vegetans: Hyperpigmented, vegetative plaque on dorsum of foot.

BEDSIDE TESTS

Nikolsky Sign

Nikolsky sign was first described in pemphigus by Dr Pyotr Vasilyewich Nikolsky in 1896, who explained that weakening of connections between the skin layers (acantholysis) results in the extension of erosions under shear stress on apparently unaffected skin. It is elicited by applying tangential or lateral pressure with the thumb in perilesional skin (indirect or marginal Nikolsky sign), or normal distant skin far from the lesions (direct Nikolsky), leading to shearing off of the epidermis **(Figs. 34A and B)**. A study done to evaluate the specificity and sensitivity of the Nikolsky sign found that it was positive in 19.5% patients. While the direct Nikolsky sign (38%) had a lower sensitivity than the indirect one (69%), it had a higher specificity (100%) compared to the indirect one (94%) in the diagnosis of pemphigus. It was concluded that a positive Nikolsky sign, especially the direct sign, is moderately sensitive but highly specific for the clinical diagnosis of PV. Further, a positive sign indicates active disease, and it becomes negative when the patient receives appropriate immunosuppressive therapy. Its reappearance during the course of treatment signifies a relapse, necessitating increase in the dosage of the immunosuppressant or the introduction of new drugs.

Other subtypes include the wet and dry Nikolsky signs, depending on the type of eroded floor left after lateral pressure: moist and glistening or dry, respectively. In patients with active PV, wet sign is demonstrated, while the dry sign signifies a re-epithelializing lesion, indicative of healing. Its subclinical equivalent is known as the microscopic Nikolsky sign wherein classical microscopic changes of PV are noted on a skin biopsy after application of lateral pressure. The microscopic Nikolsky sign can be seen in >70% of the patients after applying tangential pressure.

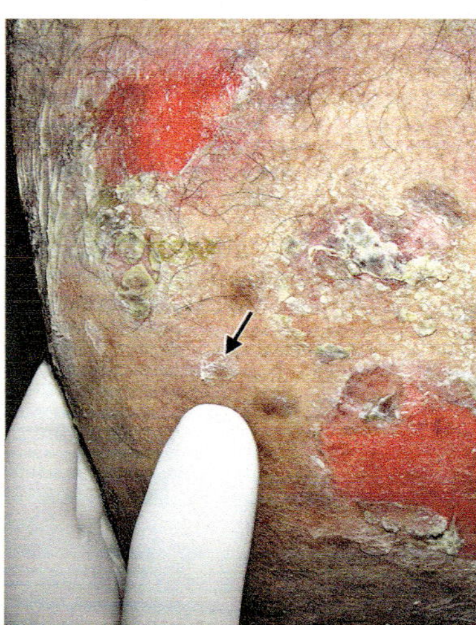

Fig. 34A: Nikolsky sign (indirect) in pemphigus vulgaris: Shearing off of skin in perilesional area (arrow) on applying tangential pressure.

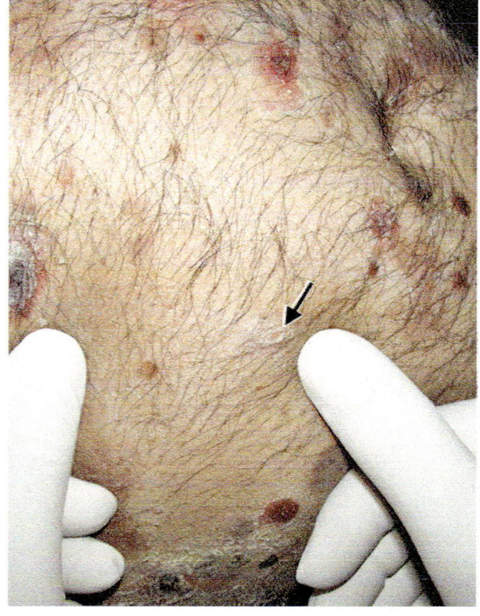

Fig. 34B: Nikolsky sign (direct) in pemphigus vulgaris: Shearing off of skin in distant normal skin (arrow) on applying tangential pressure.

The sign can also be elicited in the oral mucosa. Here, a firm sliding force is applied to the mucosal surface (usually the gingival mucosa) using a dental instrument (periodontal probe). It has been shown to be highly specific in mucosal PV.

Bulla Spread Sign or Lutz Sign

Bulla spread sign or Lutz sign is elicited by applying unidirectional mechanical pressure on the roof of the intact blister, resulting in peripheral extension of the bulla beyond the marked margin, with an irregular angulated border **(Fig. 35)**. Its variation is known as the Asboe-Hansen sign, where pressure is applied directly on the center of the intact roof in case of a small bulla.

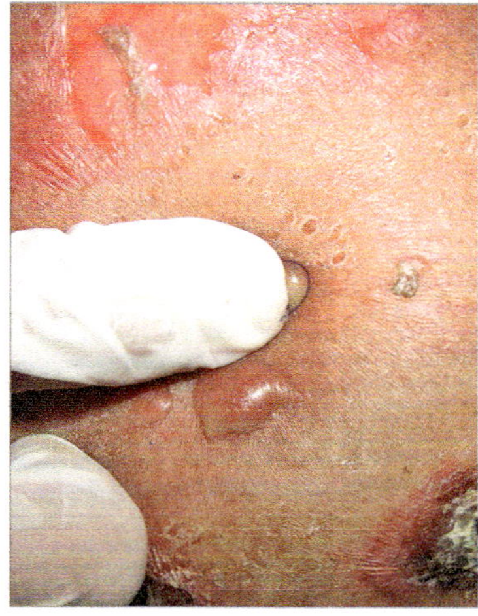

Fig. 35: Bulla spread sign in pemphigus vulgaris: Peripheral extension of the vesicle on applying lateral pressure.

Tzanck Smear

Tzanck smear is a simple and point-of-care diagnostic cytology technique. In this, an intact blister is deroofed, the roof folded along one side and the floor gently scraped. Scraping may also be taken from the undersurface of the roof and also an oral erosion. The tissue obtained is smeared onto a clean glass slide and allowed to air dry. It is then stained with diluted Giemsa stain (diluted 1:10 with distilled water), which is kept for 15 minutes. After rinsing with water, it is examined under the microscope. The cell nuclei stain reddish purple to pink while the cytoplasm appears bluish.

In PV, the diagnostic finding is the presence of acantholytic cells. These are large, round keratinocytes, about 16–20 µm in diameter, with a high nuclear:cytoplasmic ratio and abundant basophilic cytoplasm. The basophilia appears more prominent peripherally on the cell membrane due to peripheral condensation of cytoplasm ("mourning edged" cells), leading to a perinuclear halo **(Figs. 36A and B)**. Other less common findings include "Sertoli rosette," which is a cluster of cells with an epithelial cell at the center, peripherally surrounded by leukocytes, and "streptocytes," which are chains of leukocytes adhered together by a glue-like material. In a study, the sensitivity and specificity of Tzanck smear for the diagnosis of pemphigus, in comparison with histopathology, was 85% and 83.3%, respectively.

Some authors have also performed DIF on Tzanck smears, which is a minimally invasive and easy-to-operate technique, that can assist in rapid and accurate diagnosis. Aithal, *et al* showed DIF positivity in 40% PV patients on Tzanck smear compared to 46.67% on a skin biopsy, when diagnosed within 3 months of disease onset. The patients

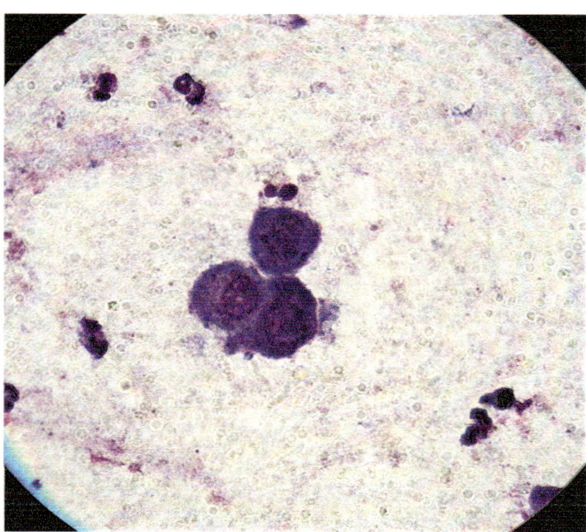

Fig. 36A: Tzanck smear in pemphigus vulgaris showing acantholytic cells: large, round keratinocytes with large, round nuclei, a perinuclear halo, and peripheral condensation of cytoplasm (Giemsa stain, ×40).

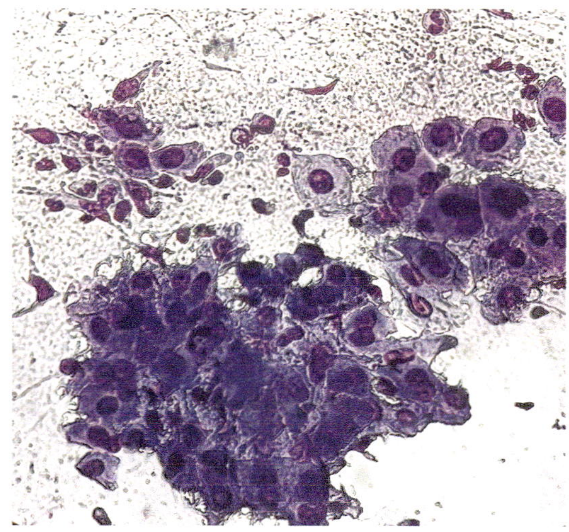

Fig. 36B: Tzanck smear in pemphigus vulgaris showing clusters of acantholytic cells (Giemsa stain, ×40).

presenting beyond 3 months of their illness showed only 20% positivity on Tzanck smear compared to 100% positivity on skin biopsy.

PROGNOSIS AND DISEASE OUTCOME

PV is a chronic disorder that requires prolonged treatment and regular follow-up. There has been a marked improvement in mortality rates and overall prognosis with use of appropriate treatment. Mortality among PV patients drastically reduced from 75% to 30% following the introduction of oral corticosteroids in the early 1950s and to <10% after the addition of conventional immunosuppressants.

The expected duration of treatment has further shortened, and overall prognosis has improved with the advent of targeted therapies like rituximab.

The case fatality rate has varied from 7.65% to 15.74%. A poor prognosis and increased mortality are associated with a higher age at disease onset (cutoffs: 50/65 years), extensive disease with scalp or oral erosions, higher intercellular antibody titers (on indirect immunofluorescence) and higher baseline anti-Dsg3 antibody levels [on enzyme-linked immunosorbent assay (ELISA)], treatment defaulters, and the presence of concomitant coronary artery disease. The most common cause of death is septicemia followed by pneumonia, peptic ulcer disease, and cardiovascular events.

Psychological Morbidity

PV is a chronic disease that features painful oral and cutaneous erosions, significantly impairing the quality of life. In a study, the mean Dermatology Life Quality Index (DLQI) score of PV patients was 10.9 ± 6.9, being next only to atopic dermatitis. The scores were higher in patients with involvement of the nasal mucosa and pharynx, those with extensive skin involvement and a positive Nikolsky sign, and in patients who reported itching. A longer disease duration also contributed to worsening of DLQI scores. Concomitant depression and anxiety has been observed in 30–77% patients.

Overall prevalence of psychiatric co-morbidity in PV patients as assessed by the screening general health questionnaire, has ranged between 41% and 73.7%, while the proportion of definite cases has been estimated to be about 33%, as analyzed by the Structured Clinical Interview for Diagnostic and Statistical Manual of Mental Disorders, fourth edition (DSM-IV) axis I disorder.

These psychiatric morbidities have shown a positive correlation with higher clinical disease activity, number of days spent in hospital, and a shorter duration of clinical remission.

PV also affects the quality of life of caregivers. In a study, the mean family DLQI (FDLQI) score was 13 ± 7 for the caregivers and showed a positive correlation with the patients' disease extent and severity, age of the caregiver, and his marital status (higher in married caregivers).

DIAGNOSTIC MODALITIES AND TREATMENT OPTIONS

The various diagnostic modalities and therapeutic options for PV will be discussed in detail in subsequent chapters. They are summarized in **Tables 2 and 3**.

TABLE 2: Various diagnostic modalities for pemphigus vulgaris.

- *Histopathology*: Biopsy from entire intact small bulla or lesion margin
- *Direct immunofluorescence*: Biopsy from perilesional skin
- *Indirect immunofluorescence*: Patient's serum sample
- *ELISA for anti Dsg1 and 3 antibodies*: Patient's serum sample
- *Other techniques*:
  - Immunoblot assay
  - Immunoprecipitation
  - Immune-electron microscopy
- *Newer modalities*:
  - BIOCHIP mosaic
  - Lateral flow immunoassay

(Dsg: desmoglein; ELISA: enzyme-linked immunosorbent assay)

TABLE 3: Various treatment options for pemphigus vulgaris.

- *Systemic steroids*: Daily/Pulse (parenteral and oral)
- *Conventional immunosuppressants and anti-inflammatory agents*:
  - Azathioprine
  - Mycophenolate mofetil
  - Methotrexate
  - Cyclophosphamide
  - Dapsone
- *Biologicals and small molecules*:
  - CD20 blockers:
    - *First generation*: Rituximab, ofatumumab, veltuzumab
    - *Second generation*: Tositumomab, obinutuzumab
  - CD19 blockers:
    - Blinatumomab, inebilizumab
  - CD22 modulator:
    - Epratuzumab
  - Anti-BAFF:
    - Belimumab
  - Anti-APRIL:
    - Atacicept
  - Bruton tyrosine kinase inhibitors:
    - Ibrutinib
  - FcRn antagonists:
    - Efgartigimod, rozanolixizumab
- Intravenous immunoglobulins
- *Other therapeutic modalities*:
  - Immunoadsorption
  - Plasmapheresis
  - Extracorporeal photopheresis
  - CAAR-T cells

(APRIL: a proliferation-inducing ligand; BAFF: B-cell activating factor; CAAR: chimeric autoantibody receptor; FcRn: neonatal Fc receptor)

CONCLUSION

PV is the most common type of pemphigus with predominantly mucocutaneous form of the disease. It produces significant physical and psychological morbidity and even mortality necessitating prompt management.

TAKE HOME MESSAGE

- PV accounts for over 70% of all subtypes of pemphigus and is commoner in Ashkenazi Jews and people of Mediterranean origin. In India, the age of onset is earlier, being around 40 years of age or younger.
- Increased association with various co-morbidities is being reported, such as hematologic and solid organ malignancies (esophageal and laryngeal cancer), other autoimmune diseases (AITD, T1DM, rheumatoid arthritis, SLE), psoriasis, and neurologic diseases (dementia, epilepsy, and Parkinson's disease).
- Oral mucosal lesions are noted in up to 84% of the patients and precede skin lesions in 66% cases.
- Cutaneous lesions manifest as flaccid vesicles or bullae, which rupture to form painful erosions and crusted plaques, with little tendency to spontaneous healing. Cutaneous type PV has only skin lesions, despite the presence of antibodies to both Dsg1 and 3.
- Scalp involvement is common due to the presence of Dsgs (Dsg1–4) in the hair follicles. It is often recalcitrant to treatment.
- Nail changes can be seen in >20% cases and commonly manifest as recurrent paronychia and onychomadesis.
- Positive Nikolsky sign, especially the direct sign, is moderately sensitive but highly specific for the clinical diagnosis of PV.
- Sensitivity and specificity of the Tzanck smear, for diagnosis of pemphigus, on comparison with histopathology was 85% and 83.3%, respectively. An acantholytic cell is a large, round keratinocyte, about 16–20 μm in diameter with a high nuclear:cytoplasmic ratio, abundant basophilic cytoplasm pushed to the periphery, and a perinuclear halo.
- Current case fatality rate for PV varies from 7.65% to 15.74%, and has dramatically reduced from the previously reported rate of 75%.
- Poor disease prognosis is associated with higher age at disease onset, extensive disease with scalp or oral erosions, higher intercellular antibody titer and Dsg antibody levels, treatment defaulters, and the presence of concomitant coronary artery disease.
- Overall prevalence of psychiatric co-morbidity in PV ranges between 41% and 73.7%, most common association being mild-to-moderate anxiety and/or depression.

MULTIPLE CHOICE QUESTIONS

1. **PV is disproportionately overrepresented in which ethnic population?**
   - (a) Indian brahmins
   - (b) Ashkenazi jews
   - (c) Australian aborigines
   - (d) Native Americans

2. **Patients with PV having higher anti-Dsg1 titers are potentially:**
   - (a) At a higher risk for severe cutaneous involvement
   - (b) At a lower risk for severe cutaneous involvement
   - (c) At a higher risk for severe mucosal involvement
   - (d) No such association

3. **Involvement of which of the following sites in PV is not a poor prognostic marker?**
   - (a) Scalp
   - (b) Flexure
   - (c) Nail
   - (d) Palms and soles

4. **Which of the following is an incorrect statement?**
   - (a) Direct Nikolsky has lower sensitivity compared to marginal Nikolsky
   - (b) Direct Nikolsky has lower specificity compared to marginal Nikolsky
   - (c) A dry Nikolsky signifies a re-epithelializing lesion
   - (d) A positive Nikolsky signifies active disease

5. **Which of the following is described as an oral mucosal manifestation in pemphigus vegetans?**
   - (a) Geographic tongue
   - (b) Strawberry tongue
   - (c) Cerebriform tongue
   - (d) Bald tongue

6. **DIF on Tzanck smear:**
   - (a) Has a higher specificity than DIF on tissue smear
   - (b) Has higher sensitivity than DIF on tissue smear
   - (c) Has same sensitivity and specificity as DIF on tissue smear
   - (d) Sensitivity depends on the duration of disease

7. **Which of the following is not correct regarding scalp involvement in PV?**
   - (a) It is often the site of residual lesions
   - (b) Anagen effluvium in PV patients is regarded as equivalent of Nikolsky sign in skin
   - (c) Like skin, only Dsg1 and 3 are present in hair follicles
   - (d) Scalp lesions can heal with both scarring and non-scarring alopecia

8. **Which of the following is not a sequelae of PV?**
   - (a) Scarring
   - (b) Hyperpigmentation
   - (c) Acrochordon-like lesions
   - (d) Acanthomata-like lesions

9. Which of the following psychiatric co-morbidities is most commonly associated with PV?

(a) Bipolar disorder

(b) Anxiety and depression

(c) Schizophrenia

(d) Somatoform disorder

10. Which of the following is incorrect regarding bulla spread sign?

(a) It is also known as Lutz sign

(b) In case of small vesicles, the Asboe-Hansen sign is used

(c) Pressure is applied in the center of an unruptured bulla

(d) An angular advancement of bulla beyond the marked margin is seen in PV

Answers

1. (b)   2. (a)   3. (b)   4. (b)   5. (c)   6. (d)   7. (c)   8. (a)   9. (b)   10. (c)

SUGGESTED READING

1. Kridin K. Pemphigus group: overview, epidemiology, mortality, and comorbidities. *Immunol Res*. 2018;66:255-70.

2. Kanwar AJ, Ajith C, Narang T. Pemphigus in North India. *J Cutan Med Surg*. 2006;10:21-5.

3. Leshem YA, Katzenelson V, Yosipovitch G, David M, Mimouni D. Autoimmune diseases in patients with pemphigus and their first-degree relatives. *Int J Dermatol*. 2011;50:827-31.

4. Daneshpazhooh M, Behjati J, Hashemi P, Shamohammadi S, Mortazavi H, Nazemi MJ, et al. Thyroid autoimmunity and pemphigus vulgaris: is there a significant association? *J Am Acad Dermatol*. 2010;62:349-51.

5. Guliani A, De D, Handa S, Mahajan R, Sachdeva N, Radotra BD, et al. Identification of clinical and immunological factors associated with clinical relapse of pemphigus vulgaris in remission. *Indian J Dermatol Venereol Leprol*. 2020;86:233-9.

6. Chams-Davatchi C, Valikhani M, Daneshpazhooh M, Esmaili N, Balighi K, Hallaji Z, et al. Pemphigus: analysis of 1,209 cases. *Int J Dermatol*. 2005;44:470-6.

7. Gupta LK, Singhi MK. Tzanck smear: a useful diagnostic tool. *Indian J Dermatol Venereol Leprol*. 2005;71:295-9.

8. Pasricha JS, Khaitan BK, Raman RS, Chandra M. Dexamethasone-cyclophosphamide pulse for pemphigus. *Int J Dermatol*. 1995; 34:875-82.

9. De D, Bishnoi A, Handa S, Mahapatra T, Mahajan R. Effectiveness and safety analysis of rituximab in 146 Indian pemphigus patients: a retrospective single-center review of up to 68 months follow-up. *Indian J Dermatol Venereol Leprol*. 2020;86:39-44.

10. De D, Kumar S, Handa S, Mahajan R, Singh SM. Psychological morbidity in pemphigus patients in clinical remission and its relation with clinico-demographic parameters. *J Dtsch Dermatol Ges*. 2022;20:26-33.

CHAPTER 7

Pemphigus Foliaceus

Ajithkumar Kidangazhiathmana, Geethanjali S

- History
- Epidemiology
- Pathophysiology
- Clinical features
- Differential diagnoses
- Diagnosis
- Treatment
- Prognosis

INTRODUCTION

Pemphigus foliaceus (PF) is a variant of the pemphigus group of autoimmune bullous diseases characterized by intraepidermal acantholysis due to autoantibodies directed against the desmoglein 1 (Dsg1) antigen which is densely expressed in the upper layers of the epidermis. This results in separation of the epidermis in the stratum granulosum, leading to superficial blister formation which rupture easily to leave scaling and crusting.

There are different types of PF, of which the classical, sporadic or idiopathic PF and endemic or fogo selvagem (FS) type are the most common. Other rarer forms include pemphigus erythematosus (PE) and drug-induced PF.

HISTORY

The term *pemphigus foliaceus* is derived from the words "pemphix" and "folia" which mean blister and leaf, respectively. This condition was first described by Cazenave in 1844. Civatte showed that similar to pemphigus vulgaris (PV), acantholysis occurs in PF too; hence, he classified pemphigus into two types. Hebra too agreed to this and classified pemphigus into PV and PF.

FS is an endemic type of PF seen in Brazil, Tunisia, and Finland. The word is derived from Portuguese language and means "uncontrolled fire." It was described first in Brazil by Caramuru Paes Leme, and the description of the disease matched with Cazenave's original description. The histopathology of FS was described by Viera.

Another geographically restricted type of endemic PF was described among the people of a mining town in the El Bagre area in Colombia. This is called El Bagre-endemic PF or pemphigus Abreu–Manu. Inter-racial outbreeding practices causing genetic predisposition, along with environmental triggers, have been postulated to be associated with the endemicity of this disease.

In 1925, Senear and Usher described PE, which has combined features of pemphigus, lupus erythematosus (LE), and seborrheic dermatitis. In 1968, using the immunofluorescence technique, Chorzelski and co-workers established PE as a separate type of pemphigus, which shares immunological and clinical features with LE. They demonstrated deposition of immunoglobulins at both the dermoepidermal junction and intercellular regions of the epidermis.

EPIDEMIOLOGY

PF is a rare disease with an annual incidence of about 0.04 per 100,000 population, whereas in endemic countries such as Tunisia, it is around 6.7 per million. Classical PF is seen in the age group of 40–60 years, with no specific gender predilection as opposed to its onset in the second and third decades in FS.

Pemphigus Abreu–Manu predominantly affects men in their fourth decade. FS is seen mainly among young rural workers living near water bodies and forests, the habitat of black flies (*Simulium*). Other hematophagous insects such as kissing bugs, sandflies, and bed bugs are also implicated in the development of FS. The development of the disease is considered to be a result of molecular mimicry. The salivary antigens from these insects trigger an antibody response which cross-reacts with the Dsg1 antigen because of same conformational epitopes.

PATHOPHYSIOLOGY

PF is caused by autoantibodies directed against Dsg1. Dsg1 is a transmembrane cell adhesion molecule expressed on the surface of keratinocytes, with a molecular weight of 160 kDa. The binding of autoantibodies leads to acantholysis due to loss of intercellular adhesion and finally subcorneal blister formation. Dsg1 is expressed more in the upper layers of epidermis and its expression is very low in the mucosa, accounting for the absence of mucosal lesions in PF.

Non-desmoglein antigens have also been recognized in PF. In pemphigus Abreu–Manu, an endemic form of PF, autoantibodies against the molecules of plakin family, myocardial zonula adherens protein, armadillo repeat gene deleted in velo-cardio-facial syndrome (ARVCF) and p0071, have been demonstrated. These additional antigens are also expressed in the cell junctions in multiple organs, which might be the cause of multiple-organ involvement including cardiac conduction abnormalities, renal damage, neurological manifestations such as axonopathy, and optic nerve sheath involvement in this type of PF.

The risk of development of the disease is linked to *HLA-DRB1*04:01*, *HLA-DRB1*04:06*, *HLA-DRB1*14*, and *HLA-DRB1*01:0* in various studies. *HLA-DRB1* alleles *04:04, *14:02, *14:06, and *01:02 are specifically associated with FS.

CLINICAL FEATURES

The clinical variants of PF phenotype include:
- Classic/sporadic PF
- Endemic PF
- Pemphigus erythematosus
- Drug-induced PF

Classic Pemphigus Foliaceus

Hebra classically described PF as a disease with small bullae and less fluid, so they are always flaccid. The roof of the bullae dry up into a flat crust. The erosions resulting from fall of the crusts do not show a tendency to heal and spread to contiguous areas of the skin and, in some cases, involve the entire skin (erythroderma).

Since blisters are very superficial, the patient may not notice intact blisters and presents with erosions, scaling, and crusting **(Figs. 1 and 2)**. The scales are characteristically described as "puff pastry" or "cornflake" like. It typically involves the seborrheic sites such as face, scalp, and upper trunk **(Figs. 3 to 6)**. The lesions that begin at seborrheic sites can extend to cause widespread involvement and even progress to erythroderma **(Fig. 7)**. PF presents with skin lesions without mucosal involvement unlike PV.

Patients complain of pain and burning sensation associated with the lesions. Skin fragility can be demonstrated by a positive Nikolsky sign. A direct Nikolsky sign is suggestive of generalized skin involvement.

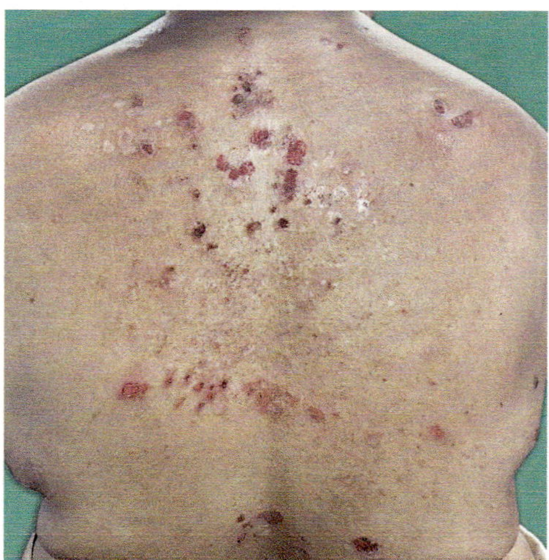

Fig. 1: Pemphigus foliaceus: Crusted erosions on the back.

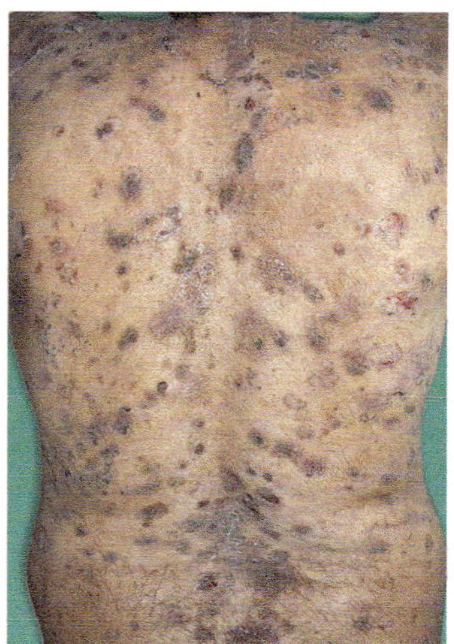

Fig. 2: Pemphigus foliaceus: Crusted and scaly plaques and erosions on the back. *Image courtesy*: Dr Sujay Khandpur.

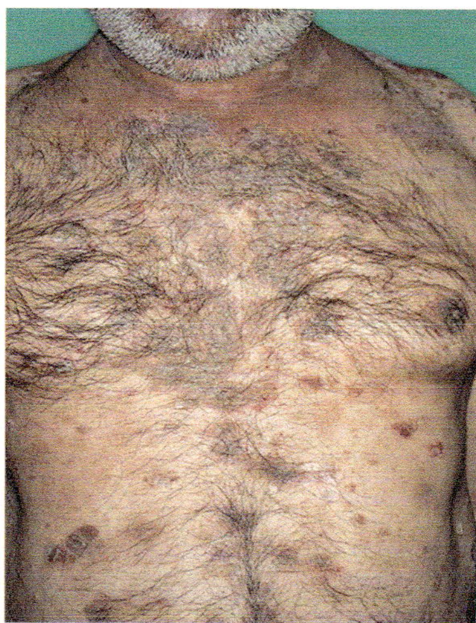

Fig. 3: Pemphigus foliaceus: Crusted and scaly plaques on the chest predominantly on presternal area. *Image courtesy*: Dr Sujay Khandpur.

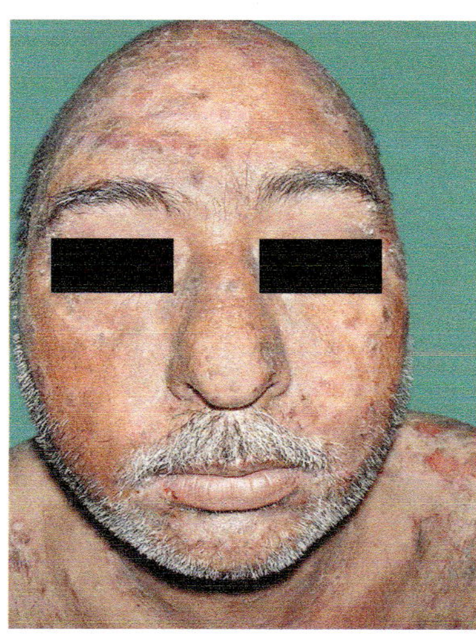

Fig. 4: Pemphigus foliaceus: Crusted and scaly plaques on face involving the seborrheic sites. *Image courtesy*: Dr Sujay Khandpur.

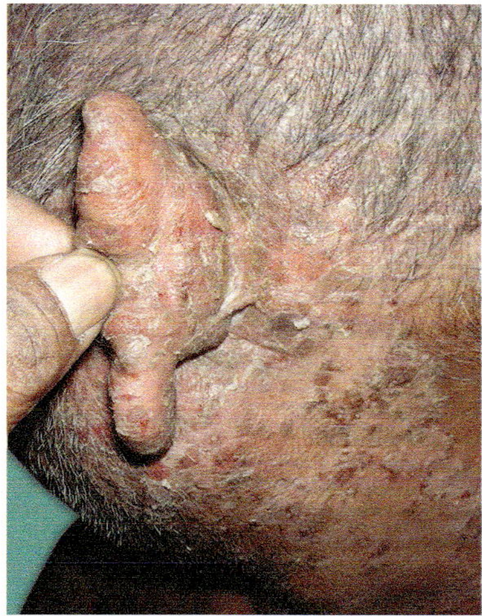

Fig. 5: Pemphigus foliaceus: Crusted and scaly plaques on the ear, retroauricular area, and scalp. *Image courtesy*: Dr Sujay Khandpur.

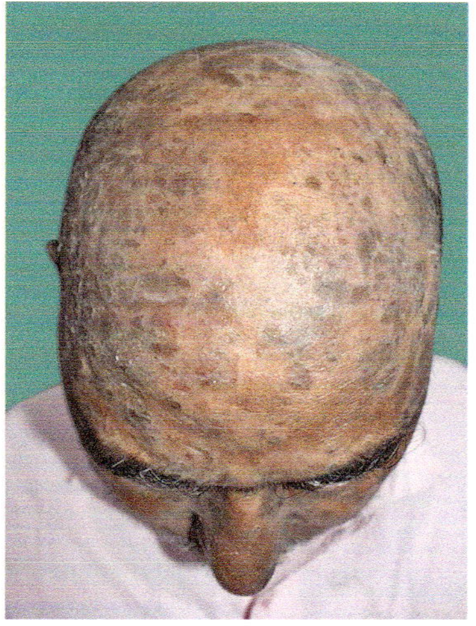

Fig. 6: Pemphigus foliaceus: Healing erosions on the scalp. *Image courtesy*: Dr Sujay Khandpur.

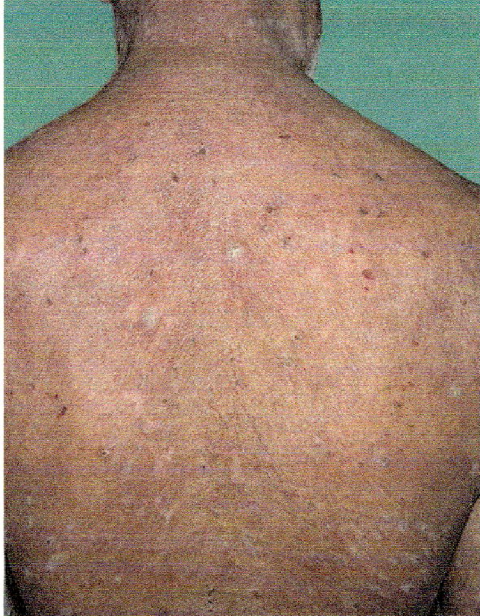

Fig. 7: Erythrodermic pemphigus foliaceus: Extensive involvement with generalized erythema and crusting. *Image courtesy*: Dr Sujay Khandpur.

Endemic Pemphigus Foliaceus (Fogo Selvagem)

FS can present with localized or disseminated disease. Localized disease is similar to the sporadic form. The lesions are associated with intense pain, hence the name wildfire. Disseminated forms of FS are classified into four types:

1. *Vesiculobullous or bullous-exfoliative*: This type is characterized by sudden onset of blisters and erosions. They occur in an annular or circinate pattern, which later erode, form crusts, and resemble tinea imbricata.
2. *Erythrodermic*: The entire skin is affected.
3. *Keratotic*: This is a rare, treatment-resistant variant characterized by keratotic lesions.
4. *Herpetiformis*: It is considered a type of FS as well as PV and sporadic PF. Here, superficial blisters are arranged in a grouped pattern. They may arise on urticated skin.

The yellowish discoloration of nails, as if they are dipped in iodine, is known as the "Viera sign" and is described in FS.

Pemphigus Abreu–Manu/El Bagre-endemic PF

This type of endemic PF can present as a localized form resembling PE, or as a generalized form with systemic manifestations. It can have multiple episodes of relapses. In about one-third of the patients, systemic involvement can occur, especially renal involvement.

Less Common Presentations of Pemphigus Foliaceus

These include lesions similar to seborrheic keratoses with an acute onset of pigmented hyperkeratotic lesions, impetigo-like lesions, and scaly erythema of the scalp, mistaken for seborrheic dermatitis. Pemphigus seborrheicus is characterized by superficial blisters and extensive erythematous plaques and erosions on seborrheic sites.

Childhood Pemphigus Foliaceus

It is rare, except in endemic areas, and presents with annular, circinate, or polycyclic lesions. Erythrodermic PF in children can also occur **(Fig. 8)**.

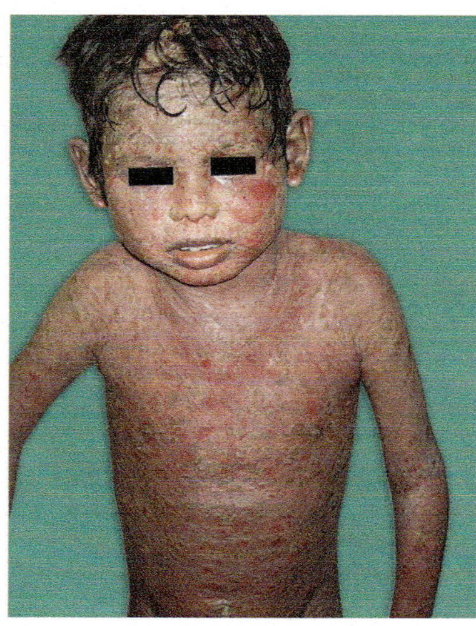

Fig. 8: Childhood pemphigus foliaceus: Erythrodermic involvement by pemphigus foliaceus in a child. *Image courtesy*: Dr Sujay Khandpur.

Pemphigus Erythematosus

PE (Senear–Usher syndrome) is a type of PF, which presents with overlapping features of LE. However, it is now clear that manifestations of LE are often subclinical in these patients.

Patients present with erythematous scaly or crusted erosions on the face in a "butterfly" distribution **(Fig. 9)**, and on the scalp, with or without involvement of other seborrheic sites. Even though mucosal involvement does not occur in PF, it has been reported in PE. Patients give a history of photosensitivity and worsening of skin lesions on sun exposure. PE shows a female preponderance. Many patients test positive for antinuclear antibody.

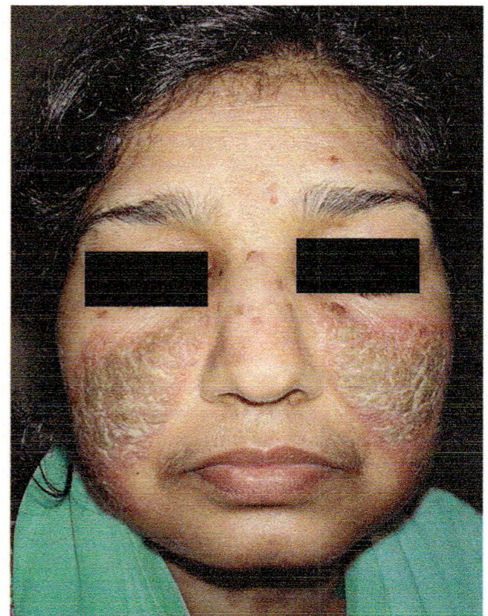

Fig. 9: Pemphigus erythematosus: Erythematous crusted and scaly plaques on the "butterfly area" of the face. *Image courtesy*: Dr Sujay Khandpur.

Drug-induced Pemphigus Foliaceus

Drug-induced pemphigus most often presents morphologically as PF. It presents within months of exposure to the culprit drug and can go into remission on discontinuation of the drug. Most commonly, the thiol group of drugs such as penicillamine and captopril have been implicated.

DIFFERENTIAL DIAGNOSES

PF can be mistaken for bullous impetigo, IgA pemphigus, drug eruption, subcorneal pustular dermatosis, seborrheic dermatitis, and LE (in PE cases).

When PF presents as erythroderma, other causes of erythroderma including psoriasis and pustular psoriasis need to be ruled out.

DIAGNOSIS

The various diagnostic modalities are described in **Table 1**.

TREATMENT

The main objectives of treatment are to control blister formation, reach drug-free remission if possible, and improve the quality of life of patients with agents causing the least drug-related complications.

Based on the body surface area of involvement and pemphigus disease area index (PDAI), similar to PV, PF is classified into mild (body surface area < 5% or PDAI < 15), moderate (PDAI between 15 and 45), and severe (PDAI > 45) disease, for the purpose of treatment.

There is a paucity of trials in the treatment of PF alone. Most studies have combined different subtypes of pemphigus. Treatment of PF is extrapolated from these combined studies and also from case reports and series. An international consensus of recommendations by Murrel, *et al* based on Delphi survey has suggested systemic

TABLE 1: Diagnostic modalities in pemphigus foliaceus.

Tzanck smear:
- It shows acantholytic cells
- PF shows fewer acantholytic cells than PV

Histopathology:
- Lesional biopsy from a fresh vesicle shows subcorneal split with few acantholytic cells
- The earliest change is eosinophilic spongiosis or epidermal microabscesses and intercellular vacuole, followed by formation of a subcorneal cleft
- The number of acantholytic cells are less compared to PV
- Dyskeratotic granular keratinocytes are seen
- The split does not involve hair follicles unlike PV
- In older lesions, hyper- and parakeratosis, acanthosis, and papillomatosis are seen
- Inflammatory infiltrate composed of neutrophils, eosinophils, and lymphocytes may be present in both the blister and dermis

Histopathological patterns include:
- Eosinophilic spongiosis
- Subcorneal blister with few acantholytic cells
- Subcorneal blister with dyskeratotic keratinocytes

Direct immunofluorescence:
- A perilesional biopsy shows intercellular deposit of immunoreactants IgG and C3 in the epidermis in a "honeycomb" or "chicken wire" or "fish net" appearance. There may be increased intensity of staining in upper epidermis
- PE shows both intraepidermal and basement membrane zone staining

Serology:
- ELISA
- Indirect immunofluorescence
Autoantibodies against Dsg1 in the serum can be demonstrated

Immunoblot assay:
- A 160 kDa band is highlighted

(Dsg1: desmoglein 1; ELISA: enzyme-linked immunosorbent assay; PE: pemphigus erythematosus; PF: pemphigus foliaceus; PV: pemphigus vulgaris)

TABLE 2: Treatment options for pemphigus foliaceus according to updated S2K guidelines.

Topical steroids:
- Class III or IV steroids alone, in case of very limited lesions

Systemic steroids:
- Mild disease: 0.5–1 mg/kg/ day of prednisolone
- Moderate-to-severe disease: 1–1.5 mg/kg/day of prednisolone

Adjuvants:
- Rituximab: 1 g, 2 doses, 2 weeks apart and then additional doses as required
- Dapsone: Up to 1.5 mg/kg/day, usually along with topical steroids in milder cases
- Azathioprine: 1–2 mg/kg/day
- Mycophenolate mofetil: 2 g/day or mycophenolate Na: 1,440 mg/day

In refractory cases:
- Cyclophosphamide 50 mg/day or as pulse
- Intravenous immunoglobulin 2 g/kg/cycle every 4 weeks

Source: Adapted from Joly P, *et al*. Updated S2K guidelines on the management of pemphigus vulgaris and foliaceus initiated by the European Academy of Dermatology and Venereology (EADV). *J Eur Acad Dermatol Venereol*. 2020;34: 1900-13.

Other options such as cyclophosphamide, intravenous immunoglobulin, intravenous steroid pulses, and immunoadsorption are used in refractory cases **(Table 2)**.

PROGNOSIS

PF runs a chronic course. Though it is a milder disease compared to PV and generally controlled with milder immunosuppression, it needs longer treatment to achieve drug-free remission. Frequent relapses with mild breakthrough of disease are common in PF.

The prognosis is good with adequate therapy, and it is considered a benign disease especially if localized. The main complications include secondary skin infection and erythroderma, and complications related to immunosuppressive agents.

CONCLUSION

PF is one of the pemphigus group of AIBDs, characterized by very superficial blisters in the subcorneal layer. The disease can have varying presentations, and may be mistaken for other dermatoses, especially in early stages. The definite diagnosis is made with histopathology and direct immunofluorescence. PF follows a chronic course even with treatment, with frequent recurrences.

TAKE HOME MESSAGE

- PF occurs due to auto antibodies against Dsg1.
- It runs a prolonged recurring and relapsing course.
- PF is amenable to treatment with systemic steroids or rituximab with or without adjuvant immunosuppressants.
- A lifelong follow-up is required because of the chronic and relapsing disease course.

steroids and rituximab as first-line treatment for pemphigus in general, and azathioprine and mycophenolate mofetil as first-line adjuvants.

Systemic steroids remain the mainstay of treatment for PF. Adjuvants such as azathioprine, mycophenolate mofetil, and dapsone are also recommended.

Dapsone and topical steroids are used for mild disease.

Rituximab is now considered the first-line option for PF, especially in moderate-to-severe cases, even though there is 50% chance of relapse. Rituximab in combination with short-term steroids is safer and superior to treatment with systemic steroids alone.

According to the new updated S2K guidelines by the European Academy of Dermatology and Venereology, the treatment options for mild cases of PF include dapsone, topical steroids, systemic corticosteroids, or rituximab. If the patient is initially treated with dapsone or topical steroids, then rituximab or systemic steroids with or without adjuvants are considered as second-line options. In moderate-to-severe disease, rituximab or systemic corticosteroids are considered first line treatment.

MULTIPLE CHOICE QUESTIONS

1. **Which of the following is the target antigen in pemphigus foliaceus?**
   (a) Desmoglein 1
   (b) Desmoglein 3
   (c) BPAG1
   (d) Envoplakin

2. **All are true regarding pemphigus foliaceus, *except*:**
   (a) Lesions are seen predominantly in the seborrheic sites
   (b) Mucosal lesions are common
   (c) Intact vesicles are rarely seen
   (d) Erythroderma can be a manifestation

3. **Yellowish discoloration of nails seen in endemic PF is known as:**
   (a) Nikolsky sign
   (b) Brocq sign
   (c) Viera sign
   (d) Abreu–Manu sign

4. **Scales in PF are characteristically described as:**
   (a) Mica-like
   (b) Furfuraceous
   (c) Puff pastry-like
   (d) Collarette-like

5. **Which of the following is false?**
   (a) Systemic steroids are the mainstay of treatment in pemphigus foliaceus
   (b) Rituximab combined with steroids can be used as a first-line treatment option in PF
   (c) Mild disease involves <5% body surface area or PDAI <15
   (d) Dapsone is used alone in the treatment of severe cases

6. **Pemphigus Abreu–Manu is described from which country?**
   (a) Columbia
   (b) Tunisia
   (c) Brazil
   (d) Finland

7. **What is Senear–Usher syndrome?**
   (a) Pemphigus vulgaris
   (b) IgA pemphigus
   (c) Pemphigus herpetiformis
   (d) Pemphigus erythematosus

8. **All of the following are the histological patterns seen in pemphigus foliaceus, *except*:**
   (a) Eosinophilic spongiosis
   (b) Subcorneal blister with few acantholytic cells
   (c) Subcorneal blister with dyskeratotic cells
   (d) Suprabasal blister

9. **What is the molecular weight of desmoglein 1?**
   (a) 130 kDa
   (b) 160 kDa
   (c) 180 kDa
   (d) 230 kDa

10. **Pemphigus foliaceus can clinically mimic:**
    (a) Histiocytosis
    (b) Seborrheic dermatitis
    (c) Porphyria
    (d) Diffuse cutaneous mastocytosis

Answers

1. (a)   2. (b)   3. (c)   4. (c)   5. (d)   6. (a)   7. (d)   8. (d)   9. (b)   10. (b)

SUGGESTED READING

1. Hans-Filho G, Aoki V, Bittner NRH, Bittner GC. Fogo selvagem: endemic pemphigus foliaceus. *Ann Bras Dermatol.* 2018;93: 638-50.

2. Joly P, Horvath B, Patsatsi A, Uzun S, Bech R, Beissert S, et al. Updated S2K guidelines on the management of pemphigus vulgaris and foliaceus initiated by the European Academy of Dermatology and Venereology (EADV). *J Eur Acad Dermatol Venereol.* 2020;34: 1900-13.

3. Joly P, Maho-Vaillant M, Prost-Squarcioni C, Hebert V, Houivet E, Calbo S, et al. First-line rituximab combined with short-term prednisone versus prednisone alone for the treatment of pemphigus (Ritux 3): a prospective, multicentre, parallel-group, open-label randomized trial. *Lancet.* 2017;389:2031-40.

4. Palacios-Álvarez I, Riquelme-Mc Loughlin C, Curto-Barredo L, Iranzo P, García-Díez I, España A. Rituximab treatment of pemphigus foliaceus: A retrospective study of 12 patients. *J Am Acad Dermatol.* 2021;85:484-6.

5. Murrell DF, Peña S, Joly P, Marinovic B, Hashimoto T, Diaz LA, et al. Diagnosis and management of pemphigus: Recommendations of an international panel of experts. *J Am Acad Dermatol.* 2020;82: 575-85.

6. Abreu-Velez AM, Upegui-Zapata YA, Valencia-Yepes CA, Upegia-Quiceno E, Yi H, Vargas Florez A, et al. A new variant of endemic pemphigus foliaceus in Colombia, South America. *Our Dermatol Online.* 2020;11:284-99.

Paraneoplastic Pemphigus (Paraneoplastic Autoimmune Multiorgan Syndrome)

Vishal Gaurav, Deepika Pandhi, Kyle T Amber

- Epidemiology
- Etiology
- Pathogenesis
  - Autoantibodies
  - Humoral immunity
  - Cellular immunity
  - Pathogenesis of bronchiolitis obliterans
  - Pathomechanisms of paraneoplastic autoimmunity
    - Breakdown of central tolerance
    - Breakdown of peripheral tolerance
    - Treg imbalance and IL-6
    - Molecular mimicry
- Clinical features
  - History
  - Mucosal lesions
- Cutaneous lesions
- Nail changes
- Ocular lesions
- Pulmonary involvement
- Musculoskeletal involvement
- Other organ system involvement
- Associated malignancies
- Differential diagnoses
- Investigations
- Diagnostic criteria
- Management
- Complications
- Prognosis

INTRODUCTION

Paraneoplastic syndromes are characterized by a group of signs and symptoms that occur either due to an abnormal immune response to tumor cells or due to the biologic effects of substances produced by tumor cells, and not due to metastasis or tumor invasion. Paraneoplastic dermatoses encompass all mucocutaneous paraneoplastic syndromes that point toward an underlying internal malignancy. Autoimmune bullous paraneoplastic dermatoses classically include paraneoplastic pemphigus (PNP) and antilaminin 332 mucous membrane pemphigoid.

PNP is a rare but life-threatening mucocutaneous syndrome mediated by paraneoplastic autoimmunity. It was first described by Anhalt, *et al* in 1990 in five patients presenting with painful mucosal erosions, polymorphous skin lesions, and underlying lymphoproliferative neoplasms [malignant lymphoma, chronic lymphocytic leukemia (CLL), thymoma, and sarcoma]. Since multiorgan involvement in not frequent in pemphigus but is seen commonly in PNP, Czernik, *et al* introduced a more inclusive nomenclature "paraneoplastic autoimmune multiorgan syndrome (PAMS)". However, Mahajan, *et al* suggested the term "paraneoplastic autoimmune multiorganopathy"

to be more precise and unambiguous, encompassing the heterogeneous manifestations of this distinct paraneoplastic process.

EPIDEMIOLOGY

Incidence and Prevalence

Given the rarity of PNP, its exact incidence and prevalence is unknown at present. Less than 500 cases have been reported globally. A 10-year retrospective study from 13 regions in France estimated that PNP accounts for nearly 5% of pemphigus cases. In a retrospective study from Japan, 25 out of 496 pemphigus patients (5%) had an internal malignancy. Twelve patients [out of 100,000 patients with non-Hodgkin's lymphoma (NHL) and CLL] were found to have PNP in an adverse event reporting analysis. Only 3 of these 12 were identified by the reporting physician, highlighting the difficulty in diagnosis due to varied clinical manifestations.

Age

PNP usually occurs in individuals aged 45–70 years, with an average age of 50 years at diagnosis. However, Chinese patients present at a younger age of about 30 years due to the relatively frequent association of Castleman disease in children with PNP and a high frequency of this neoplasm in the Chinese population. In a series of 14 cases of childhood PNP (<18 years) reported by Mimouni D, *et al*, 12 had Castleman disease. In a retrospective case series of 8 patients from South India, the mean age at presentation was 31 years (8–46 years), suggesting that PNP may present earlier in India due to geographical and genetic variations.

Gender

There is no sex predilection. Both genders seem to be equally affected with a female-to-male ratio of 1.09:1.

Ethnicity

Caucasians and Han Chinese patients are at an increased risk due to the presence of human leukocyte antigen (HLA)-class II DRB1*03 and HLA-class I Cw*14 alleles, respectively.

ETIOLOGY

PNP is associated with an underlying lymphoproliferative disorder (NHL and CLL) in 70–80% of the patients **(Table 1)**. However, Castleman disease is the most frequently associated neoplasm in China and South Korea as well as in children. The association with Castleman disease is striking, given its rarity in the general population. Castleman disease is a non-clonal lymphoproliferative disease affecting the lymph nodes of various body regions; while unicentric Castleman disease (UCD) is localized or uni-focal and common, multicentric Castleman disease has an aggressive course, presenting in a generalized or multifocal

manner. Pathological subtypes include hyaline vascular type, plasma cell type, mixed type, and human herpes virus 8-associated Castleman disease. In a retrospective study from China including 114 patients with Castleman disease, 37 patients were diagnosed with PNP using specific auto-antibodies. Non-hematologic neoplasms associated with PNP include sarcoma, thymoma, squamous cell carcinoma, adenocarcinoma, and malignant melanoma. Interestingly, the more common solid organ tumors like adenocarcinoma of the breast, bowel and lung, or cutaneous malignancies like basal cell and squamous cell carcinoma are very infrequently associated with PNP. Rarely, malignancy may not be identified at the time of diagnosis, necessitating extended clinical follow-up to detect any occult neoplasm. Additionally, in a small number of patients, malignancy does not seem to occur even with more prolonged follow-up, raising the potential for a separate non-paraneoplastic subtype.

PATHOGENESIS

Autoantibodies

A range of autoantibodies directed against the different components of desmosomes and hemidesmosomes are detected in PNP **(Table 2)**. Antiplakin autoantibodies are the most characteristic and specific for PNP. Plakins are large proteins (molecular weight: 200–800 kDa) that cross-link cytoskeletal structural proteins and also anchor the cytoskeletal proteins to the plasma membrane at specific sites (refer to Chapter 1). The presence of plakin domain

TABLE 1: Neoplasms associated with paraneoplastic pemphigus.

Neoplasm	
Hematological	70–80%
Non-Hodgkin lymphoma	40%
Chronic lymphocytic leukemia	7–18%
Castleman disease	15–37%
Waldenström macroglobulinemia	4%
Hodgkin lymphoma, monoclonal gammopathy	<1%
Non-hematological	16–25%
Thymoma (malignant and benign)	8%
Sarcoma (liposarcoma, leiomyosarcoma, malignant nerve sheath tumor, poorly differentiated sarcoma, dendritic cell sarcoma, reticulum cell sarcoma, retroperitoneal sarcoma, inflammatory myofibroblastic sarcoma)	7%
Squamous cell carcinoma (of the skin, tongue, and vagina)	9%
Adenocarcinoma (gastric and colonic)	<1%
Others (renal, bladder, and breast)	<1%
Poorly differentiated carcinoma (lung)	2%
Malignant melanoma	0.6%

TABLE 2: Target antigens of paraneoplastic pemphigus with their molecular weights.

Antigens	Molecular weight (kDa)
Plakin family	
Plectin	500
Epiplakin	500
Desmoplakin 1	250
Desmoplakin 2	210
BPAG1/BP230	230
Envoplakin	210
Periplakin	190
Cadherin family	
Desmoglein 1	160
Desmoglein 3	130
Desmocollin 1	100
Desmocollin 2	100
Desmocollin 3	100
Other proteins	
α-2-macroglobulin-like antigen-1 (A2ML1)	170
BPAG2/BP180	180
p200	200

(consisting of two pairs of spectrin repeats separated by a putative Src-homology-3/SH3 domain) is the defining feature of all plakin family members. It consists of seven members, including desmoplakins (Dpks: Dpk1 and Dpk2), plectin, BP230, microtubule-actin crosslinking factor 1, envoplakin, periplakin, and epiplakin. Amongst the plakin proteins, autoantibodies to envoplakin and periplakin are the most characteristic and specific to PNP. Other target antigens include BP180, p200, protease inhibitor α-2-macroglobulin-like antigen-1 (A2ML1), desmosomal cadherins, i.e., desmogleins (Dsgs—Dsg1 and Dsg3) and desmocollins (Dscs—Dsc1, Dsc2, and Dsc3).

Immunopathogenesis

The immunopathogenesis of PNP is complex. The humoral immune response in PNP is immunoglobulin G (IgG) mediated and since the plakin molecules are located intracellularly and IgG cannot penetrate the cell membrane, the pathophysiologic mechanism of antiplakin autoantibodies is unclear at present. There is a definitive role of cell-mediated cytotoxicity in the pathogenesis of recalcitrant stomatitis and polymorphous cutaneous lesions. The specific role of humoral and cell-mediated immunity is discussed below.

Humoral Immunity

Autoantibodies to desmosomal cadherins can cause suprabasal acantholytic blisters in PNP as these are the only exposed desmosomal components. Anti-Dsg3 autoantibodies from PNP patients induce blisters in neonatal mice. However, some patients of PNP develop mucosal erosions, and skin blisters in the absence of circulating anti-Dsg antibodies. Some of these patients have circulating anti-Dsc3 antibodies instead of anti-Dsg3 antibodies. Similarly, anti-A2ML1 autoantibody decreases keratinocyte adhesion by activating plasmin. The IgG subclass is also different in PNP. While, anti-Dsg IgG4 is the dominant IgG subclass in PV and pemphigus foliaceus (PF), anti-Dsg IgG1 is the dominant subclass in PNP. Since Th1 immune response is IgG1 predominant and Th2 response is IgG4 predominant, the above observation suggests that Th1 is the dominant immune response in PNP. Anti-Dsg3 antibodies from PNP patients react with all the five extracellular subdomains (EC) of human Dsg3, while anti-Dsg3 autoantibodies from sera of PV patients bind to EC1 and EC2 domains. These observations confirm that the mechanism of acantholysis in PNP is different from that of PV and also varies amongst PNP patients, thereby accounting for PNP cases without any identifiable autoantibodies. Antibodies to BP230, BP180, and p200 are also seen.

Cellular Immunity

Lichenoid dermatitis on histology is seen in most biopsies from the skin, mucosa, and bronchial epithelium in patients with bronchiolitis obliterans, indicating the involvement of cell-mediated immune response in the pathogenesis. Both CD8+ and CD4+ T cells are involved. Since lichenoid dermatitis may be the only sign of PNP or may develop before the appearance of blisters, it is suggested that infiltration by autoreactive T cells leading to interface dermatitis and keratinocyte apoptosis might lead to exposure of self-antigens, thereby inducing autoantibody production. Dsg3-specific CD4+ T cell-derived interferon-γ is a crucial inducer of interface dermatitis. Autoreactive CD8+ T cells induce apoptosis in keratinocytes and are frequently observed in the epidermis of PNP, suggesting that they also contribute to the interface dermatitis. The significance of CD56+ cells, expressed by both CD8+ T cells and natural killer cells in the infiltrate, is not understood at present.

Pathogenesis of Bronchiolitis Obliterans

Though direct immunofluorescence demonstrates both intercellular and linear deposition of IgG at the basement membrane zone (BMZ) in bronchial biopsies from patients with bronchiolitis obliterans, it is still uncertain which type of autoantibodies are pathogenic, as desmosomal cadherins, in particular Dsg1 and 3, are not expressed in the normal respiratory epithelium. However, Dsg3 is expressed ectopically in lungs with squamous metaplasia. Squamous metaplasia of the respiratory epithelium can occur in patients with systemic inflammation as is evident in patients with malignancy. Therefore, anti-Dsg3 antibodies might be pathogenic for bronchiolitis obliterans. Recently, acantholysis was demonstrated in the murine respiratory epithelium following injection of anti-epiplakin antibodies, suggesting their potential role in the pathogenesis of bronchiolitis obliterans. Adoptive transfer of Dsg3-specific CD4+ T cells in RAG2$^{-/-}$ mice induces ectopic Dsg3 expression and pulmonary inflammation. Similarly, injection of IgG from PNP sera into Dsg3$^{-/-}$ mice leads to marked infiltration of CD8+ T cells in the respiratory epithelium and lungs. These findings suggest that both humoral and cell-mediated immunity may be involved in the pathogenesis of bronchiolitis obliterans in PNP patients. Injury to the bronchial epithelium leads to plugging of terminal bronchioles, resulting in airflow obstruction, and ventilation-perfusion abnormalities that damage the alveolar epithelium resulting in a diffusion barrier that causes intractable hypoxia.

Pathomechanisms of Paraneoplastic Autoimmunity

Breakdown of Central Tolerance

In health, autoreactive T cells undergo negative selection in the thymus. However, defective selection due to a tumor of the thymus, i.e., thymoma, may lead to breakdown of central tolerance, leading to spillage of autoreactive T cells into peripheral circulation. Thymoma induces many autoimmune responses and is associated with several other autoimmune disorders, e.g., myasthenia gravis. Myasthenia gravis often accompanies thymoma-associated PNP. The role of autoimmune regulator (*AIRE*) gene has been suggested.

Breakdown of Peripheral Tolerance

Some autoreactive T cells escape to the periphery from the thymus under normal circumstances. Their activation is prevented via several mechanisms, viz., T-cell anergy and deletion and suppression by regulatory T cells (Tregs) that are important for peripheral tolerance. Normally, CD28, a co-stimulatory molecule expressed by T cells, interacts with its ligands CD80 and CD86 expressed by professional antigen presenting cells (APCs). However, B cells derived from lymphomas express CD80 and/or CD86 which induce T-cell proliferation and prevent T-cell anergy. CLL derived B cells upregulate these co-stimulatory molecules leading to activation of autoreactive T cells after escape from peripheral tolerance.

Treg Imbalance and Interleukin-6

Treg imbalance has been proposed to lead to the induction of paraneoplastic autoimmunity. Interleukin (IL)-6 is a pro-inflammatory cytokine that inhibits Treg differentiation, FoxP3 expression and suppressive function of Tregs. IL-6 also promotes the function and differentiation of follicular T helper cells that further induce B cell proliferation, differentiation, and isotype switching. IL-6 is markedly elevated in the sera of PNP patients. Interestingly, significant amount of IL-6 is released into the circulation from NHL, CLL, and Castleman tumor. Like thymomas, Castleman tumors are also associated with autoimmune diseases including myasthenia gravis and autoimmune cytopenia. IL-6 is also frequently elevated in patients with Castleman tumor, especially in idiopathic multicenter Castleman disease. These findings suggest that IL-6 might be a crucial inducer of paraneoplastic autoimmunity.

Molecular Mimicry

The tumor antigens mimicking self-antigens can be expressed by tumor cells due to mutation. When these are attacked by antitumor immune response, both the tumor cells as well as normal tissue are damaged, leading to the development of autoimmune diseases. Further, tissue damage-induced epitope spreading explains the presence of autoantibodies to multiple self-antigens in PNP patients.

CLINICAL FEATURES

History

A pre-existing malignancy or history of cancer is present in 41% of the patients at presentation. However in remaining patients, malignancy is detected during work-up or even later. As mentioned previously, a small percentage of patients appear to never develop a malignancy despite long term follow-up.

Mucosal Lesions

Intractable stomatitis is the most common and consistent feature of PNP, seen in almost all (98.9%) patients. Erosive mucositis is usually the first manifestation, preceding the skin lesions by days, weeks, or months, is frequently painful and florid, and characteristically involves the vermilion of lips **(Figs. 1 to 3)**. Other sites of involvement include oro- and nasopharynx, nasal mucosa, tongue (especially the lateral borders), esophagus, stomach, duodenum, intestines, respiratory epithelium, conjunctiva **(Fig. 4)**, and the anogenital region **(Table 3)**. Isolated mucosal involvement is seen in 13% of the patients.

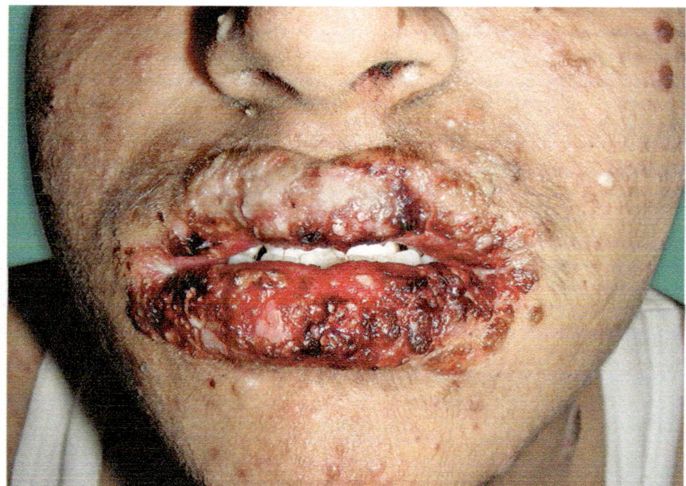

Fig. 1: Paraneoplastic pemphigus: Erosive stomatitis involving the vermilion border of lips in a patient with renal cell carcinoma-induced PNP.

Fig. 2: Paraneoplastic pemphigus: Confluent erosions on labial mucosa. *Image courtesy*: Dr Sujay Khandpur.

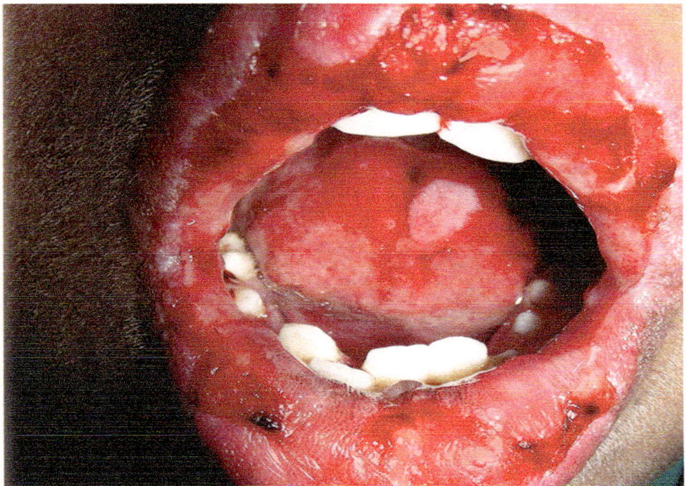

Fig. 3: Paraneoplastic pemphigus: Confluent erosions on labial mucosa, tongue, and oral mucosa. *Image courtesy*: Dr Sujay Khandpur.

Fig. 4: Paraneoplastic pemphigus: Hyperemia of the conjunctiva along with confluent lip erosions. *Image courtesy*: Dr Sujay Khandpur.

TABLE 3: Mucosal involvement in paraneoplastic pemphigus.

Site	Percentage
Oral	93–99%
Ocular	41%
Nasal	12%
Genital	27%

Cutaneous Lesions

Cutaneous lesions are polymorphic and usually appear after the onset of mucosal lesions. They are present in about 85% of patients. These include vesicles, bullae, erosions, papules and plaques **(Fig. 5)**, targetoid **(Fig. 6)**, and lichenoid lesions **(Figs. 7A and B)**. The varied clinical morphologies were classified by Nguyen, *et al* **(Table 4)**. Scalp is usually spared and palms and soles are often involved **(Fig. 8)** in PNP. Two cases of PNP presenting as erythroderma, one with exfoliative erythroderma and the other with erythrodermic lichenoid dermatitis, have been reported. Onset after systemic interferon or radiotherapy, as well as lesions localized to the radiation field, have also been reported. The occurrence of annular lesions and overlap with IgA pemphigus is also known. A clinical and immunological overlap with mucous membrane pemphigoid was seen in a patient with three malignancies (thyroid carcinoma, clear cell carcinoma of the kidney, and follicular dendritic cell sarcoma) and anti-laminin 332 autoantibodies.

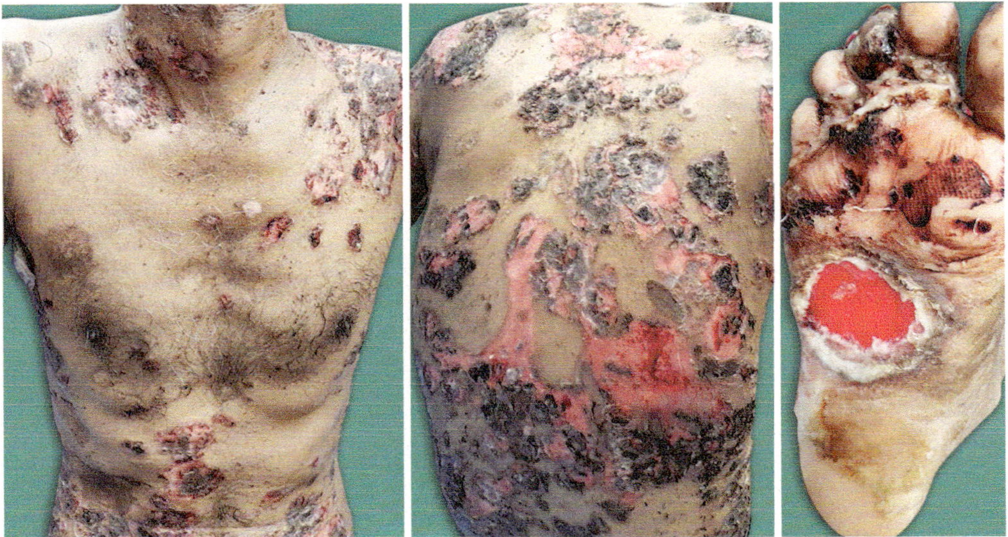

Fig. 5: Paraneoplastic pemphigus: Extensive erosions, vesicles, and crusted plaques on the trunk and sole in a patient with non-Hodgkin lymphoma.

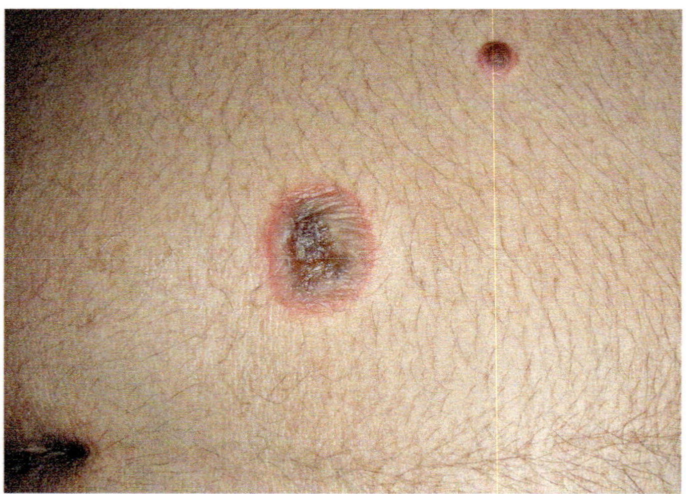

Fig. 6: Paraneoplastic pemphigus: Targetoid lesions on trunk. *Image courtesy*: Dr Sujay Khandpur.

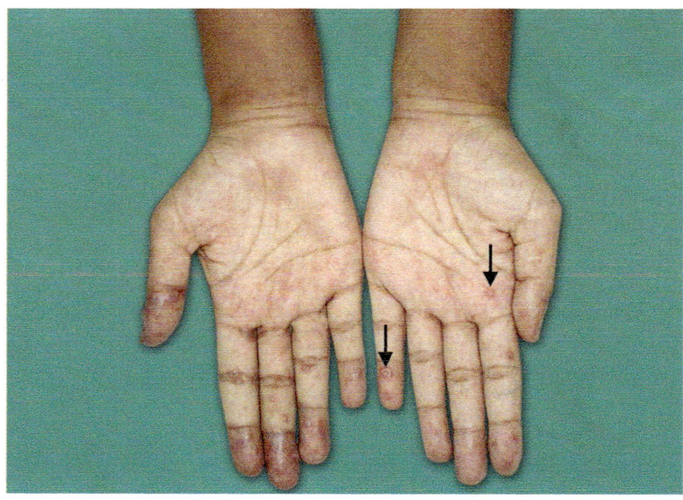

Fig. 8: Paraneoplastic pemphigus: Multiple vesicles and targetoid lesions (arrows) on palms.

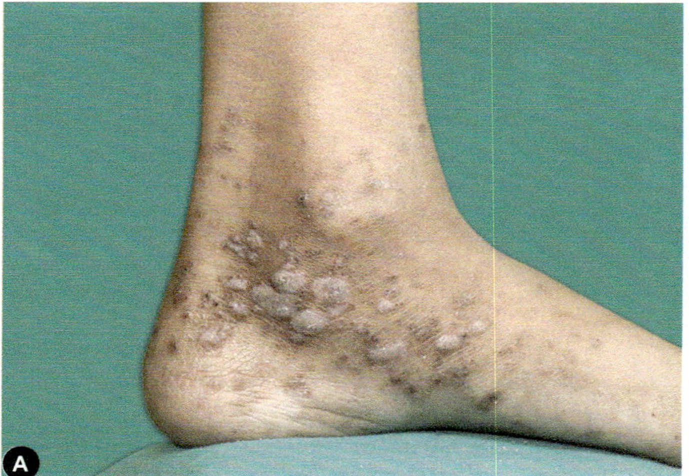

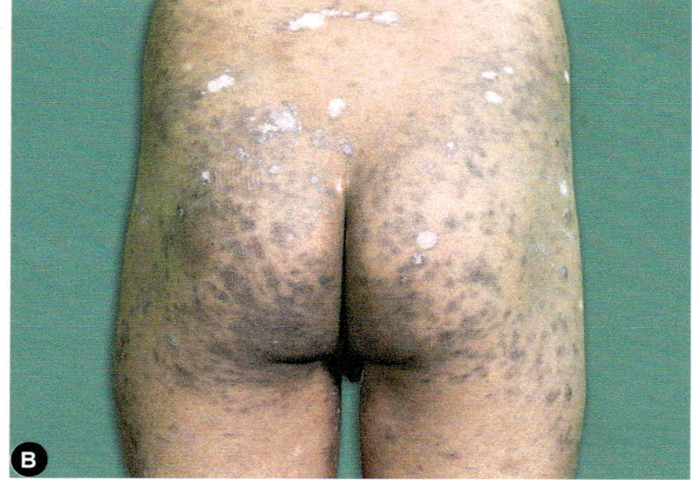

Figs. 7A and B: (A) Paraneoplastic pemphigus: Lichenoid lesions on the foot and lower leg. (B) Paraneoplastic pemphigus: Lichenoid lesions on the lower back and buttocks. *Image courtesy*: Dr Vinay Keshavamurthy.

TABLE 4: Classification of cutaneous lesions in paraneoplastic pemphigus.

Category	Description	Percentage
Pemphigus-like (foliaceus, vulgaris and vegetans)	Flaccid blisters, erosions, crusts and erythema **(Fig. 5)**	41%
Bullous pemphigoid-like	Scaly erythematous papules and sero-hemorrhagic tense vesicles and bullae, more common on the extremities	3%
Erythema multiforme-like	Targetoid erythematous papules, and plaques with central blister, distributed over trunk and extremities, resembling erythema multiforme **(Fig. 6)**, or toxic epidermal necrolysis in more advanced cases. Polymorphic changes, mainly erythematous peeling pellets with erosions and sometimes recalcitrant ulcerations	56%
Graft-versus-host disease (GVHD)-like	Scattered dusky red scaly papules	Rare
Lichen planus (pemphigoides, and erosive)-like	Flat, red-brown scaly papules and plaques on the trunk and extremities **(Figs. 7A and B)**, rapidly extending to the face and neck, accompanied by palmoplantar lesions and severe stomatitis, more commonly seen in children	13%
Cicatricial pemphigoid-like	Gingival soreness, erosive gingivostomatitis, and conjunctivitis	Rare
Linear IgA dermatosis-like	Tense bullae arranged in annular configuration with mucosal involvement	Rare

Nail Changes

Commonly, nail units are involved in PNP. Both scarring and non-scarring nail changes have been described. The non-scarring changes include periungual erosions and edema (paronychia) **(Fig. 9)**, onycholysis, longitudinal ridging, and splitting, while the scarring nail changes include dorsal pterygium, onychomadesis, and anonychia.

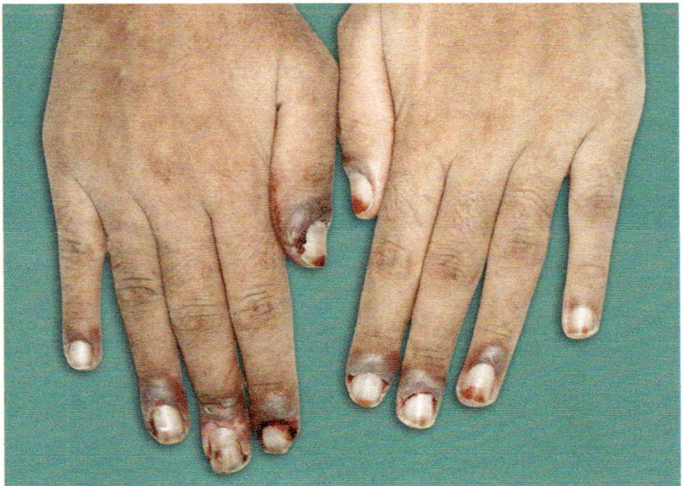

Fig. 9: Paraneoplastic pemphigus: Paronychia in all finger nails. *Image courtesy*: Dr Sujay Khandpur.

Ocular Lesions

Ocular involvement is seen in 41–70% of PNP patients. The common symptoms include eye pain, burning, discharge and diminution of vision. The findings include bilateral conjunctival hyperemia **(Fig. 4)** and erosions, pseudomembranous conjunctivitis, bilateral corneal erosions/ulcerations and melting, symblepharon and pterygium formation, shortening of fornix, and thickening of palpebral margin.

Pulmonary Involvement

Pulmonary involvement is seen in 30–90% of PNP patients, especially in those with Castleman disease. Progressive dyspnea is the earliest manifestation which may be accompanied by non-productive cough. Chest radiography does not show any changes at this stage. Pulmonary function test shows an obstructive pattern with involvement of both large and small airways. Pulmonary function deteriorates in most cases despite immunosuppressive therapy and eventually progresses to bronchiolitis obliterans. Spirometry demonstrates airflow obstruction that does not reverse with inhaled bronchodilator challenge. Forced expiratory volume in one second (FEV1) is reduced, and the ratio of FEV1 to forced vital capacity (FVC) is also reduced. Secondary pneumonia is commonly associated, increasing the mortality.

Musculoskeletal Involvement

Evidence of musculoskeletal disease characterized by muscle weakness is seen in 39% patients, with 35% eventually developing myasthenia gravis. This occurs due to the presence of autoantibodies directed against the components of the neuromuscular junction or muscle itself, including acetylcholine receptor, acetylcholine esterase, muscle specific kinase, ryanodine receptor, and titin. These autoantibodies are further elevated in sera of PNP patients with dyspnea. As expected, patients with thymoma have a higher frequency of myasthenia symptoms.

Involvement of other Organ Systems

PNP-associated mucositis may involve the gastrointestinal tract. Multifocal colonic and gastric erosions have been reported. Renal and neurological involvement in the form of glomerulosclerosis and paraneoplastic neurological syndrome have also been reported.

Common Malignancies associated with Paraneoplastic Pemphigus

In about 10% of patients, the neoplasm is detected during the course of the disease. Since majority of PNP patients have associated hematologic malignancies (84% in some studies), one must be familiar with the common clinical presentations of these disorders in addition to B symptoms (fever, weight loss, night sweat, extreme fatigue, and early satiety). NHL, CLL, and Castleman disease are the most common hematologic disorders associated with PNP. NHL is a neoplasm of the lymphoid tissues originating from B-cell precursors, mature B cells, T-cell precursors and mature T cells. Both nodal and extranodal diseases are known to occur. This includes involvement of the Waldeyer's ring (tonsils, base of tongue, and naso-pharynx), cervical, supraclavicular, axillary, inguinal, femoral, mesenteric, and retroperitoneal nodal sites. It may also involve orbital structures (eyelids, extraocular muscles, lacrimal apparatus, and conjunctiva), mediastinum (persistent cough, chest discomfort, and superior vena cava syndrome), retroperitoneal, mesenteric and pelvic nodes (presenting as ascites or lymphedema), liver, and spleen (hepatosplenomegaly). The most common sites of primary extranodal disease are the gastrointestinal tract, followed by skin. CLL is a chronic lymphoproliferative disorder characterized by monoclonal B cell proliferation. It generally presents as localized or generalized lympha-denopathy involving the cervical, supraclavicular and axillary lymph nodes, hepatosplenomegaly, and/or leukemia cutis. As discussed earlier, Castleman disease is a rare, non-clonal lymphoproliferative disorder which occurs as a result of impaired immuneregulation leading to abundant proliferation of B lymphocytes and plasma cells in the lymphoid organs. The unicentric type presents as a slow-growing, non-malignant painless solitary mass at a single anatomic site that is asymptomatic initially but gradually starts producing symptoms when the surrounding structures get compressed. Multicentric Castleman disease presents with generalized lymphadenopathy, hepatosplenomegaly, deep vein thrombosis, edema, ascites, pleural and pericardial effusion, and rarely with generalized anasarca. The readers can refer to other sources for clinical presentations of other rare sarcomas and carcinomas.

DIFFERENTIAL DIAGNOSES

The clinical heterogeneity of PNP lends itself to multiple differential diagnoses. These are summarized in **Table 5**.

TABLE 5: Differential diagnosis of paraneoplastic pemphigus.

Differential diagnosis	Differentiating points
Pemphigus vulgaris	• Mucosal involvement is less diffuse • Absence of polymorphous lesions • Palmoplantar lesions are uncommon • Paronychial lesions are less common • Frequent scalp involvement
Stevens–Johnson syndrome/toxic epidermal necrolysis	• Confluent erosive lesions • Rapid evolution • Temporal association with drug intake
Erythema multiforme	• Rapid evolution • Temporal association with drug or herpes simplex virus infection
Bullous pemphigoid	• Absence of polymorphous lesions • Absence of hemorrhagic stomatitis • Palmoplantar lesions are uncommon
Mucous membrane pemphigoid	• Desquamative gingivitis healing with mucosal scarring • Isolated epithelial tags
Oral erosive lichen planus	It is generally focal and involvement of vermilion lip is uncommon
Chemotherapy-induced mucositis	• Develops 5–14 days after chemotherapy • Less severe • Mucosal erythema and aphthous-like ulcers are common
Major aphthous stomatitis	• Recurrent well-circumscribed ulcers with central necrotic fibrinous exudate surrounded by erythematous halo • Spares the vermilion lip
Mucocutaneous reactions of immune checkpoint inhibitors	• Less severe stomatitis • Mucocutaneous lesions respond to topical steroids and cessation of drug • Interstitial pneumonitis rather than bronchiolitis obliterans

INVESTIGATIONS

Histopathology

The variability in clinical presentation results in significant histologic differences. Biopsies from oral lesions show non-specific changes of inflammation and ulceration to lichenoid mucositis **(Fig. 10)** with variable degree of epidermal necrosis and suprabasal acantholysis. The histologic features of cutaneous lesions also vary with the clinical morphology of lesions **(Table 6)**. While suprabasal acantholysis is prominent in vesiculobullous lesions, lichenoid or vacuolar interface dermatitis are prominent in erythematous maculopapular lesions. Lesions with overlapping clinical features demonstrate mixed histological features of suprabasal acantholysis and lichenoid/interface dermatitis **(Table 7)**.

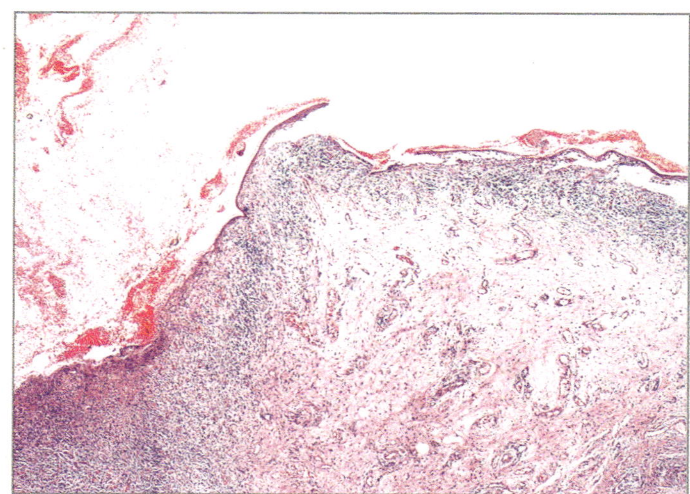

Fig. 10: Paraneoplastic pemphigus: Biopsy from oral mucosa showing a lichenoid infiltrate at the dermo-epidermal junction (H&E, ×40).

TABLE 6: Histological patterns of interface dermatitis in paraneoplastic pemphigus.

Histological pattern	Epidermal changes
Lichen planus-like	Lichenoid band-like infiltrate at the dermo-epidermal junction with basal layer degeneration (squamatization)
Erythema multiforme or graft-versus-host disease like	• Individual keratinocyte necrosis • Lymphocytic exocytosis
Cutaneous lupus erythematosus or dermatomyositis like	• Vacuolar interface change • Sparse lymphocytic exocytosis in the basal layer

TABLE 7: Histopathologic features of paraneoplastic pemphigus.

Histopathologic feature	Percentage (%)
Lichenoid/vacuolar interface dermatitis + suprabasal acantholysis	42
Suprabasal acantholysis	29
Lichenoid/vacuolar interface dermatitis	21

Source: Adapted from Svoboda SA, *et al*. Paraneoplastic pemphigus: Revised diagnostic criteria based on literature analysis. *J Cutan Pathol*. 2021;48:1133-8.

Immunopathology

Direct Immunofluorescence

Granular or linear deposits of IgG and C3 along the BMZ in combination with intraepidermal intercellular immuno-staining in a fish-net pattern, is characteristic of PNP **(Fig. 11)**. However, intraepidermal staining may be negative in up to 50% of cases, presumably due to predominant activation of cellular immunity **(Table 8)**. The sensitivity can be improved by carefully examining the adnexal structures, which may be the only site of immunopositivity.

Indirect Immunofluorescence

Indirect immunofluorescence (IIF) studies show inter-cellular binding of IgG autoantibodies to the cell surface, throughout the epidermis of stratified squamous, columnar, and transitional epithelia. Apart from this staining pattern, cytoplasmic staining as well as strong staining of the basal mucosal cells is also seen. Since monkey and guinea pig esophagus are used as substrates to demonstrate the presence of anti-Dsg1 and 3 auto-antibodies, they lack specificity for the diagnosis of PNP. Hence, rat bladder

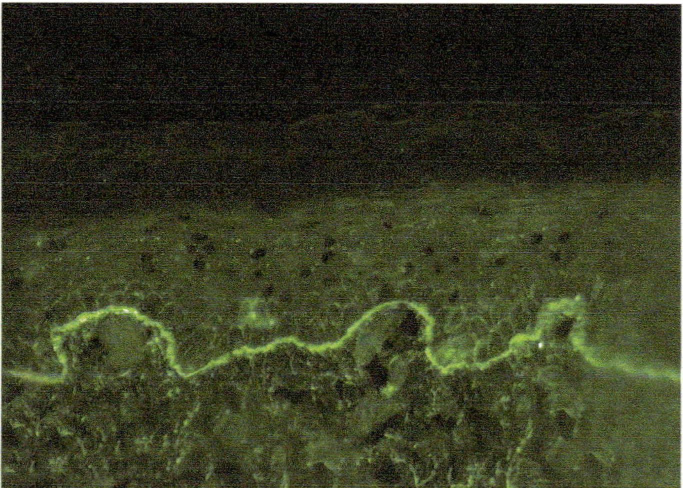

Fig. 11: Paraneoplastic pemphigus: DIF showing linear deposition of IgG along dermoepidermal junction and intercellular supra-basal deposition of IgG in a fishnet pattern (FITC; ×40). Note that the intercellular deposition is fainter than linear BMZ deposition.
(BMZ: basement membrane zone; DIF: direct immunofluorescence; IgG: immunoglobulin G)

TABLE 8: Reported proportion of cases with positive immunological features in paraneoplastic pemphigus.

Immunological test	Percentage (%)
Direct immunofluorescence	78
Intercellular and junctional (IgG and/or C3)	43
Intercellular (IgG and/or C3)	28
Intercellular deposition within adnexal epithelium only	1.1
Junctional (basement membrane zone) (IgG and/or C3)	4.5
Evidence of anti-plakin antibody	77
IIF positivity on transitional epithelia	67
ELISA test	4.2
Immunoblot assay	40
Immunoprecipitation	31

(DIF: direct immunofluorescence; ELISA: enzyme-linked immunosorbent assay; IgG: immunoglobulin G; IIF: indirect immunofluorescence)

Source: Adapted from Svoboda SA, *et al*. Paraneoplastic pemphigus: Revised diagnostic criteria based on literature analysis. *J Cutan Pathol*. 2021;48:1133-8.

urothelium (transitional epithelium) is the preferred substrate, as it expresses plakins, but not Dsg1 and Dsg3. Ideally, both substrates should be used to increase the sensitivity and specificity. The most characteristic IIF pattern on rat bladder is the urothelial cell-surface staining, often with cytoplasmic immunostaining. A strong cytoplasmic staining of all epidermal layers on salt-split skin is very specific for PNP. Despite its relatively low sensitivity (86%), IIF using rat bladder is a highly specific (98%) method to differentiate PNP from other immunobullous disorders. However, not all PNP patients have antibodies against all the antigens of the plakin complex. In addition to PNP, anti-plakin autoantibodies have been detected in other diseases as well, such as anti-desmoplakin autoantibodies in PV and erythema multiforme, anti-periplakin autoantibodies in PF and toxic epidermal necrolysis, and rarely, anti-envoplakin autoantibodies in PF and PV.

Enzyme-linked Immunosorbent Assay

Enzyme-linked immunosorbent assay (ELISA) using the recombinant N-terminal domain and linker subdomain of envoplakin and the linker subdomain of periplakin has 75% sensitivity and 92–99% specificity. In addition, auto-antibodies to Dsg1 and 3, Dsc1, 2, and 3, and BP180 antigens are also seen in PNP. Multiplex ELISA containing precoated envoplakin antigen besides Dsg1/3, BP180 and 230, and collagen VII, may be used. ELISA scores demonstrate parallel fluctuations with disease activity and hence are useful in monitoring disease activity, planning schedules for tapering corticosteroids, and predicting flares or relapse. Chemiluminescent enzyme immunoassay (CLEIA) is a more sensitive and rapid technique for detecting IgG autoantibodies in PNP patients.

Immunoblot Assay and Immunoprecipitation

Immunoblot (IB) assay against the epidermal cell extracts can effectively detect antibodies against envoplakin, periplakin, and desmoplakin.

Immunoprecipitation (IP) is the most sensitive and specific test to detect anti-plakin antibodies in PNP. Radio-active and non-radioactive IP has a sensitivity of 95% and 100%, respectively. IP is considered superior to IB in detecting antibodies that react with conformational epitopes (epitopes dependent on three-dimensional structure), while IB detects antibodies against the linear epitopes (epitopes that are preserved even after denaturation).

Special Tests

Intra-abdominal and intrathoracic malignancies such as intra-abdominal lymphoma, intrathoracic or retro-peritoneal Castleman tumors and retroperitoneal sarcomas are usually undetectable by physical examination or routine investigations. Computed tomography scan (CT), magnetic resonance imaging (MRI), or positron emission tomography (PET)-CT using fluorodeoxyglucose, from the neck to the base of the bladder, are used for screening.

DIAGNOSTIC CRITERIA

The heterogeneity of clinical signs and symptoms in PNP makes it a diagnostic challenge for clinicians. The original diagnostic criteria based on key clinical, histological, and immunological features were proposed by Anhalt, *et al* in 1990. These were subsequently revised by Camisa and Helm in 1993 to make them more robust. However, these criteria may still fail to capture a significant proportion of PNP cases as nearly 30% of patients develop PNP prior to the diagnosis of malignancy. Also, with the advent of newer diagnostic techniques such as IP, IB, and ELISA to detect antiplakin antibodies, these criteria were revised in 2021 by Svoboda, *et al* to make them more inclusive. Overall, 89.4% of cases meet the revised diagnostic criteria proposed by Svoboda, *et al*, compared to the Camisa and Helm diagnostic criteria that are met by 71.2% of cases. The more recent S2K guidelines are built on these diagnostic criteria **(Table 9)**.

TREATMENT

The treatment of PNP is undefined at present. The reason for the refractory nature of disease compared to PV and other autoimmune diseases is unknown. Early diagnosis and treatment of the underlying malignancy are vital. When associated with benign or encapsulated tumors such as Castleman disease or thymoma, excision can induce remission in nearly half of the patients. Since autoantibodies can be produced post-operatively in these individuals by sensitized B cells, continued immunosuppression in the form of prednisolone and rituximab may be required for 1–2 years following surgery. Measures aimed at preventing hematogenous spread of autoantibodies from the tumor

TABLE 9: Diagnostic criteria for paraneoplastic pemphigus adapted from the S2k guidelines.

Clinical criteria	
1	Chronic erosive mucositis
2	Polymorphic skin lesions such as flaccid or tense vesicles, lichenoid lesions and erythema multiforme-like lesions
3	Underlying neoplasm such as lymphoproliferative or hematologic malignancy
Laboratory criteria	
Major criteria	
1	IIF showing intercellular staining on rat bladder epithelium
2	Positivity on ELISA test, immunoblot assay or immunoprecipitation for anti-plakin (anti-envoplakin, anti-desmoplakin, or anti-periplakin) or anti-A2ML1 antibody
Minor criteria	
1	Histopathology showing lichenoid interface dermatitis, acantholysis and keratinocyte necrosis, either alone or in combination
2	IIF and DIF showing cytoplasmic cell membrane staining of keratinocytes and linear or granular IgG and/or C3 deposits along the dermo-epidermal junction
3	ELISA, immunoblot assay, or immunoprecipitation showing positivity for anti-desmoglein antibodies and at least one of the following autoantibodies: anti-desmocollin, anti-epiplakin, anti-plectin, anti-BP180, or anti-BP230

Diagnosis of PNP/PAMS is considered "confirmed" with 2 clinical criteria + 1 major laboratory criterion, or 2 clinical criteria + 2 minor laboratory criteria. Diagnosis of PMP/PAMS is considered "possible" with 2 clinical criteria + 1 minor laboratory criterion. If a neoplasm is not detected, 2 clinical criteria, 2 major laboratory criteria or 1 major laboratory criterion and 2 minor laboratory criteria are needed to make a "provisional" diagnosis of PNP/PAMS. In this case, monitoring is recommended to exclude a possible occult tumor

(ELISA: enzyme-linked immunosorbent assay; IIF: indirect immunofluorescence; PAMS: paraneoplastic autoimmune multiorgan syndrome; PNP: paraneoplastic pemphigus)

Source: Adapted from Antiga E, *et al*. S2k guidelines on the management of paraneoplastic pemphigus/paraneoplastic autoimmune multiorgan syndrome initiated by the European Academy of Dermatology and Venereology (EADV). *J Eur Acad Dermatol Venereol*. 2023;37:1118-34.

should be used, in addition to surgery. These include embolization of tumor vessels to reduce blood supply, minimal intraoperative manipulation and infusion of high-dose intravenous immunoglobulin (IVIG) before and after surgery. These measures also prevent the development of bronchiolitis obliterans, as surgery is not helpful in allevia-ting pulmonary symptoms, if already present. Therefore, in children with lung disease, lung transplantation may be required.

However in cases associated with unresectable or metastatic disease, treatment of the underlying neoplasm does not necessarily lead to improvement in the disease course. The prognosis is very poor in cases associated with NHL or CLL, leading to death within 2 years of diagnosis.

No randomized therapeutic trials have been performed due to rarity of this disease and the available data is limited to case reports and case series. High-dose corticosteroids are considered first-line agents. Cutaneous lesions typically respond well to therapy (within 12 weeks), however, stomatitis and pulmonary disease are refractory to treatment. Cyclosporine, cyclophosphamide, azathioprine, mycophenolate mofetil, thalidomide, ibrutinib, pyridostigmine bromide, IVIG, rituximab, and plasmapheresis have been used with limited success. Rituximab has unpredictable results and complete response is rarely seen. It has no effect on the progression of bronchiolitis obliterans and many cases of PNP have been described in patients who were previously on treatment with rituximab as part of a chemotherapy regimen for the underlying lymphoproliferative neoplasm **(Table 10)**.

Since PNP develops due to the interplay of both humoral and cell-mediated immunity, other agents targeting T cells and/or B cells have also been used. These include alemtuzumab (humanized monoclonal antibody against CD52, expressed on T- and B-cell surface) which has been used in hematologic malignancy-associated PNP. Similarly, daclizumab and basiliximab (non-depleting monoclonal antibody against CD25 on T cell) have shown promising results. The recent S2K guidelines provide several treatment recommendations **(Table 10)**.

PNP is a multiorganopathy, and should be managed by a multidisciplinary team comprising of dermatologists, oncologists, oncosurgeons, ophthalmologists, pulmonologists, infectious disease specialists, gastroenterologists, and urologists/gynecologists.

Wound care is important to prevent infection. Occlusive hydrating dressings not only prevent wound infection but also prevent fluid and electrolyte loss. Low adhesive wound dressings such as petroleum jelly impregnated-gauze, silver dressings, or bioengineered dressings may be used.

Pain management is important as frequently stomatitis is very painful, leading to inability to eat or drink. It can be managed by using topical corticosteroids and/or analgesics. However systemic opioids may be required.

TABLE 10: Treatment recommendations for paraneoplastic pemphigus from the S2k guidelines.

- Initial recommendations
  - Treatment of underlying malignancy
  - Oral corticosteroids: 0.5mg/kg-1.5 mg/kg/day
  - Topical therapy: clobetasol propionate ointment, topical antiseptics, local wound care of skin and mucosal lesions
  - Anti-B-cell agents in the presence of underlying B-cell proliferative malignancies
- Additional options
  - Steroid-sparing agents: azathioprine, mycophenolate mofetil, methotrexate, cyclosporine, cyclophosphamide
  - Rituximab (in patients with or without underlying B-cell malignancy)
  - High dose intravenous immunoglobulin
  - Immunoadsorption, plasmapheresis

Source: Adapted from Antiga E, *et al.* S2k guidelines on the management of paraneoplastic pemphigus/paraneoplastic autoimmune multiorgan syndrome initiated by the European Academy of Dermatology and Venereology (EADV). *J Eur Acad Dermatol Venereol.* 2023;37:1118-34.

Infection can be prevented by using antiseptic baths and topical antimicrobials. Systemic infection warrants systemic antibiotics.

COMPLICATIONS

Sepsis, dehydration, electrolyte imbalance, multiorgan failure, gastrointestinal bleeding, ocular complications, bronchiolitis obliterans, and malnutrition can complicate PNP.

PROGNOSIS

The prognosis is poor with a mortality rate of 75–90%. Overall survival rates at the end of 1, 2, and 5 years are 49%, 41%, and 38%, respectively, with death occurring due to respiratory failure, infection, gastrointestinal bleeding, multiorgan failure, and evolution of neoplasm. However, prognosis is good when the underlying neoplasm is localized and amenable to excision.

The outcome of PNP does not necessarily parallel the course of the underlying neoplasm, rather, the complications of PNP and its treatment contribute significantly to morbidity and mortality. Like mucositis, pulmonary disease in PNP is usually unresponsive to medical therapy and hence dyspnea and hypoxia are ominous prognostic signs. No definite correlation exists between tumor burden and the severity of autoimmune syndrome in patients with malignant neoplasms, therefore treatment of the primary malignancy has no bearing on the autoimmune disease activity.

CONCLUSION

PNP is a rare life-threatening mucocutaneous disease associated with internal malignancy. Recalcitrant stomatitis is the most characteristic feature of the disease with variable cutaneous and systemic manifestations. Histology, DIF, IIF, ELISA, and investigations directed toward specific malignancy help in confirmation of the diagnosis. However, internal malignancy may not always be apparent at presentation. Early diagnosis and treatment of underlying malignancy are vital. The response to treatment is variable, with cutaneous lesions responding within weeks; however, stomatitis and bronchiolitis obliterans are usually refractory to treatment. The prognosis is poor with high mortality.

TAKE HOME MESSAGE

- PNP is a rare but life-threatening mucocutaneous paraneoplastic syndrome mediated by paraneoplastic autoimmunity.
- It is also called "PAMS" or "paraneoplastic auto-immune multiorganopathy" due to involvement of multiple organs, viz., lungs, eyes, gastrointestinal tract, thyroid, and kidneys.
- PNP accounts for up to 5% of pemphigus cases.

- It usually occurs in individuals aged 45–70 years, with an average age of 50 years at diagnosis. There is no sex predilection.
- Certain HLA alleles increase the risk of PNP.
- PNP is associated with an underlying lymphoproliferative disorder (NHL, CLL, and Castleman disease) in 70–80% of the patients.
- A range of autoantibodies directed against the different components of desmosomes and hemidesmosomes are detected in PNP. Antiplakin autoantibodies are the most characteristic and specific for PNP.
- The immunopathogenesis of PNP is complex with involvement of both humoral and cellular immunity. Immune injury also involves the respiratory epithelium leading to development of bronchiolitis obliterans. Many mechanisms have been proposed to explain the pathology of paraneoplastic autoimmunity.
- Malignancy can be present before, at or detected after the diagnosis of PNP.
- Intractable stomatitis is the most common and consistent feature, seen in almost all patients.
- Cutaneous lesions are polymorphic and include pemphigus-like, pemphigoid-like, erythema multiforme-like, graft-versus-host disease-like, and lichen planus-like lesions, with erythema multiforme-like presentation being the most common.
- Pulmonary, musculoskeletal, renal, and neurological involvement is seen in PNP.
- Differential diagnosis includes lichen planus, erythema multiforme, bullous pemphigoid, pemphigus vulgaris, graft-versus-host disease, and Stevens–Johnson syndrome.

- Immunoprecipitation is the most sensitive and specific test to detect antiplakin antibodies in PNP. However, IB, IIF, and ELISA can also be used.
- The variability in clinical presentation results in significant histologic variability. Variable degree of suprabasal acantholysis and/or lichenoid/interface dermatitis is seen on histology.
- CT or MRI from neck to the base of the bladder is used for malignancy screening with PET-CT being used to detect occult lymphoma.
- The original diagnostic criteria proposed by Anhalt, *et al* have been revised by many researchers to increase the sensitivity and specificity of these criteria. The modified diagnostic criteria proposed by Svoboda, *et al* are met by 89.4% of PNP cases.
- There are no guidelines for the management of PNP; hence, early diagnosis and management of the underlying neoplasm are of paramount importance.
- The tumor should be minimally manipulated during surgery to avoid hematogenous dissemination of auto-antibodies. Alternatively, IVIG can be used before surgery.
- Medical management options include corticosteroids, biologics (rituximab, alemtuzumab, daclizumab, and basiliximab), IVIG, and conventional steroid-sparing agents, though they have not been found to be uniformly effective.
- The outcome of PNP does not necessarily parallel the course of the underlying neoplasm, rather, the complications (especially, bronchiolitis obliterans) and its treatment contribute significantly to morbidity and mortality. Prognosis is poor with a mortality rate of 75–90%.

MULTIPLE CHOICE QUESTIONS

1. **The malignancy least likely to be associated with PNP is:**
   - (a) Non-Hodgkin lymphoma
   - (b) Chronic lymphocytic leukemia
   - (c) Waldenström macroglobulinemia
   - (d) Malignant melanoma

2. **The most characteristic and specific autoantibodies for PNP are directed against:**
   - (a) Epiplakin
   - (b) Desmoplakin
   - (c) Envoplakin
   - (d) Plectin

3. **The most common cutaneous lesions of PNP are:**
   - (a) Pemphigus-like
   - (b) Bullous pemphigoid-like
   - (c) Lichen planus-like
   - (d) Erythema multiforme-like

4. **The most sensitive and specific test to detect antiplakin antibodies in PNP is:**
   - (a) Indirect immunofluorescence
   - (b) Immunoblotting
   - (c) Immunoprecipitation
   - (d) Enzyme-linked immunosorbent assay (ELISA)

5. **Anti-CD25 monoclonal antibody used for the treatment of PNP is:**
   - (a) Basiliximab
   - (b) Dostarlimab
   - (c) Loncastuximab
   - (d) Amivantamab

6. **Bronchiolitis obliterans in PNP is commonly associated with which malignancy?**
   - (a) Non-Hodgkin lymphoma
   - (b) Castleman disease

    (c)   Chronic lymphocytic leukemia/lymphoma

    (d)   Multiple myeloma

7. The most common musculoskeletal involvement in PNP is:

    (a)   Arthritis

    (b)   Myositis

    (c)   Osteitis

    (d)   Myasthenia gravis

8. The histology of maculopapular lesions in PNP shows:

    (a)   Spongiotic tissue reaction

    (b)   Lichenoid tissue reaction

    (c)   Psoriasiform tissue reaction

    (d)   Vesiculobullous tissue reaction

9. Which of the following signs and symptoms of PNP responds poorly to oral steroids?

    (a)   Stomatitis

    (b)   Cutaneous lesions

    (c)   Myasthenia gravis

    (d)   Ocular involvement

10. Which of the following treatments has shown improvement in mucositis in PNP?

    (a)   Rituximab

    (b)   Thalidomide

    (c)   Tumor removal

    (d)   Both (b) and (c)

Answers

1. (d)   2. (c)   3. (d)   4. (c)   5. (a)   6. (b)   7. (d)   8. (b)   9. (a)   10. (d)

SUGGESTED READING

1. Didona D, Fania L, Didona B, Eming R, Hertl M, Di Zenzo G. Paraneoplastic dermatoses: A brief general review and an extensive analysis of paraneoplastic pemphigus and paraneoplastic dermatomyositis. *Int J Mol Sci*. 2020;21:2178.

2. Anhalt GJ, Kim SC, Stanley JR, Korman NJ, Jabs DA, Kory M, *et al*. Paraneoplastic pemphigus. An autoimmune mucocutaneous disease associated with neoplasia. *N Engl J Med*. 1990;323:1729-35.

3. Czernik A, Camilleri M, Pittelkow MR, Grando SA. Paraneoplastic autoimmune multiorgan syndrome: 20 years after. *Int J Dermatol*. 2011;50:905-14.

4. Mahajan VK, Sharma V, Chauhan PS, Mehta KS, Sharma AL, Abhinav C, *et al*. Paraneoplastic pemphigus: a paraneoplastic autoimmune multiorgan syndrome or autoimmune multiorganopathy? *Case Rep Dermatol Med*. 2012;2012:207126.

5. Amber KT, Valdebran M, Grando SA. Paraneoplastic autoimmune multiorgan syndrome (PAMS): Beyond the single phenotype of paraneoplastic pemphigus. *Autoimmun Rev*. 2018;17:1002-10.

6. Lee J, Bloom R, Amber KT. A systematic review of patients with mucocutaneous and respiratory complications in paraneoplastic autoimmune multiorgan syndrome: Castleman's disease is the predominant malignancy. *Lung*. 2015;193:593-6.

7. Sathishkumar D, Agrawal P, Baitule AM, Thomas M, Eapen A, Kumar S, *et al*. Paraneoplastic autoimmune multiorgan syndrome: A retrospective study from a Tertiary Care Center in South India. *Indian Dermatol Online J*. 2021;12:572-6.

8. Liu Q, Bu DF, Li D, Zhu XJ. Genotyping of HLA-I and HLA-II alleles in Chinese patients with paraneoplastic pemphigus. *Br J Dermatol*. 2008;158:587-91.

9. Gaurav V, Pandhi D, Sharma S, Rastogi S. Renal cell carcinoma-induced paraneoplastic pemphigus. *Indian Dermatol Online J*. 2022;13:407-10.

10. Maruta CW, Miyamoto D, Aoki V, Carvalho RGR, Cunha BM, Santi CG. Paraneoplastic pemphigus: a clinical, laboratorial, and therapeutic overview. *An Bras Dermatol*. 2019;94:388-98.

CHAPTER 9

Other Variants of Pemphigus

Saritha Mohanan, C Udayashankar

- Immunoglobulin A (IgA) pemphigus
- Immunoglobulin G/Immunoglobulin A (IgG/IgA) pemphigus
- Drug-induced pemphigus including contact pemphigus
- Pemphigus herpetiformis

INTRODUCTION

The most common types of pemphigus are pemphigus vulgaris (PV) and pemphigus foliaceus (PF). Another morbid variant is paraneoplastic pemphigus. These have been dealt with in previous chapters. In this chapter, the rarer variants of pemphigus will be discussed.

IMMUNOGLOBULIN A (IgA) PEMPHIGUS

(Synonyms: Intraepidermal Neutrophilic IgA Dermatosis, Intercellular IgA Dermatosis, Intercellular IgA Vesiculopustular Dermatosis, Intraepidermal IgA Pustulosis, IgA Pemphigus Foliaceus, IgA Herpetiform Pemphigus)

Immunoglobulin A (IgA) pemphigus was first reported by Varigos, *et al* in 1979. The blister formation is due to acantholysis caused by circulating antibodies against the desmosomes. It is classically divided into two types—(1) intraepidermal neutrophilic (IEN) type (2) subcorneal pustular dermatosis (SPD) type. The autoantigen is desmocollin 1 in the SPD type and desmoglein 1 and 3 and desmocollin 2 and 3 in the IEN type.

Hashimoto, *et al* proposed the term "intercellular IgA dermatosis" and classified the disease into 6 subtypes—(1) SPD type, (2) IEN type, (3) IgA pemphigus vegetans, (4) IgA PF, (5) IgA PV, and (6) unclassified type. A common pathophysiology for all the types has not yet been described.

Epidemiology

IgA pemphigus is a rare entity. In a systematic review, the age of patients ranged from 1 month to 94 years (mean age 51.5 ± 21 years). A slight female preponderance was also noted. IgA pemphigus has also been reported in children.

Clinical Manifestations

Clinical manifestations include vesicles, pustules, and circinate plaques with herpetiform vesicles, predominantly involving the flexures, proximal extremities, and trunk. Symptoms include pruritus in half of the affected patients, and occasionally pain. IgA pemphigus does not involve the oral mucosa.

The IEN type **(Figs. 1 and 2)** is characterized by pustules distributed in an annular configuration, variously

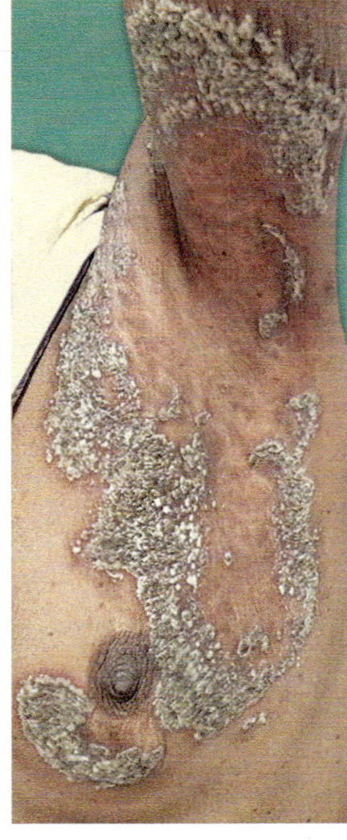

Fig. 1: IgA pemphigus: Annular arrangement of pustules in intraepidermal neutrophilic (IEN) type of IgA pemphigus.

described as "flower-like" or "sunflower-like" appearance. The SPD type shows erythematous lesions with pustules, sometimes with a fluid level called 'hypopyon' **(Fig. 3)**, erosions, and scaling. The SPD type is more common than the IEN type. There are few reports of IgA pemphigus occurring in association with linear IgA dermatosis. Compared to PV, IgA pemphigus has a milder course.

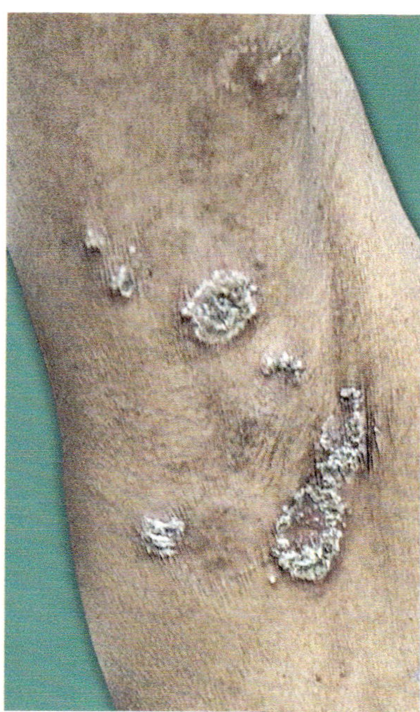

Fig. 2: IgA pemphigus: 'Sunflower-like' pattern in Intraepidermal neutrophilic (IEN) type of IgA pemphigus.

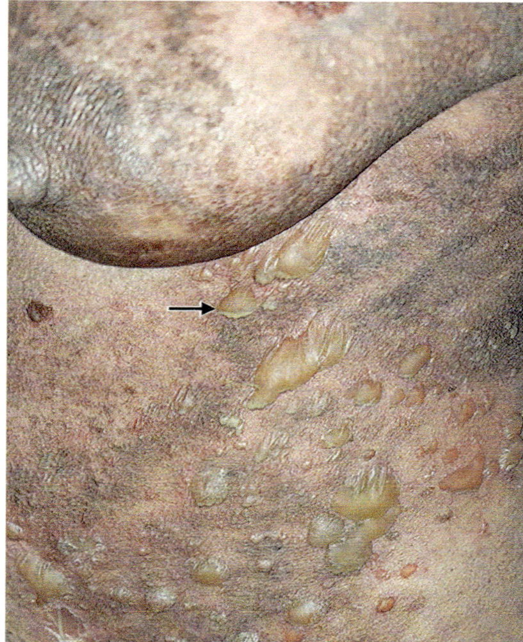

Fig. 3: IgA pemphigus: Pus-filled vesicles with 'hypopyon' formation (arrow). *Image courtesy*: Dr Sujay Khandpur.

Associations

IgA pemphigus is associated with malignancies such as lung cancer and IgA gammopathy. Gastrointestinal diseases such as Crohn's disease and gluten-sensitive enteropathy have also been reported. A systematic review reported other conditions such as Sjögren's syndrome, myasthenia gravis, rheumatoid arthritis, and ulcerative colitis. HIV infection and thiol group of drugs have also been implicated.

Diagnosis

- *Histopathological examination*: It shows neutrophilic infiltration in the epidermis. There is minimal acantholysis. In the SPD type, pustules are present in the subcorneal layer. The IEN type is characterized by a cleft confined to the mid or entire epidermis.
- *Direct immunofluorescence (DIF)*: In the SPD type, IgA deposition is limited to the upper epidermal cell surfaces, while in the IEN type, intercellular IgA staining is seen either throughout the epidermis or restricted to the lower epidermis. Absence of IgA deposit can differentiate SPD (Sneddon–Wilkinson disease) from the SPD variant of IgA pemphigus, since clinical and histopathological features of both the entities are similar. A systematic review found circulating IgA antibodies in only 66.7% of IgA pemphigus patients, although DIF found intercellular IgA antibody deposition in 97% of the patients.

Management

There are no consensus guidelines regarding management of IgA pemphigus. It has a milder course, and first-line treatment is systemic corticosteroids (prednisolone 1 mg/kg/day) supplemented with dapsone. Dapsone at a dose of 25–125 mg/day, is reported to produce clinical response in 2–3 days. The other potentially effective treatments include colchicine, mycophenolate mofetil, isotretinoin, acitretin, adalimumab, and even plasmapheresis.

Prognosis

The clinical course of IgA pemphigus is benign and milder compared to PV. In malignancy-associated disease, prognosis is related to the malignancy.

IMMUNOGLOBULIN G/IMMUNOGLOBULIN A (IgG/IgA) PEMPHIGUS

IgG/IgA pemphigus is a rare variant described by Nishigawa, *et al* in 1987. It is defined by the presence of epidermal intercellular antibodies of both the IgG and IgA types on DIF, displaying similar clinical and histopathological features to the other subtypes of pemphigus. The level of the cleft may be subcorneal, intraepidermal (most common), or suprabasal. The target antigens include Dsg1 or 3 and desmocollins 1, 2, and 3.

Pathophysiology

The occurrence of IgG and IgA antibodies to the Dsgs and desmocollins has been attributed to epitope spreading, although class switching of antibodies does not occur in this phenomenon. Another theory is that IgA antibodies are seen in the initial stages of IgG pemphigus; however, below the level of detection by DIF.

Epidemiology

Age of onset is highly variable and ranges from 11 to 81 years. It has been reported more commonly in women.

Clinical Features

Two types of lesions have been described; annular or arciform pattern of erythema with overlying blisters, or discrete vesicles and erosions as in pemphigus. Trunk and extremities are the most frequently involved sites. Patients may experience pain or pruritus. Mucosal involvement has been reported.

This variant is sometimes considered a type of IgA pemphigus. However in one analysis, the clinical features resembled IgG pemphigus, i.e., PV rather than IgA pemphigus. Hashimoto, *et al* reported mixed features of IgG and IgA pemphigus and coined a new term "intercellular IgG/IgA dermatosis" and opined that it is a distinct entity. There are reports of cases without IgA deposition on DIF or indirect immunofluorescence (IIF) but having circulating IgA antibodies against Dsg1 and 3, detected by enzyme-linked immunosorbent assay (ELISA). Hence, this entity can be seen as occupying a spectrum, with features of PV at one end to mixed features, and to features of IgA pemphigus at the other end.

Associations

Many authors have postulated that IgG/IgA pemphigus may be associated with malignancies of the lung, ovary, gall bladder, pancreas and endometrium, thymoma, and IgA gammopathy. Solid organ tumors are related to IgA pemphigus in contrast to paraneoplastic pemphigus, which is usually associated with lymphoproliferative malignancies.

Histopathology

Most cases show a neutrophilic infiltrate in the epidermis. Acantholysis is commonly reported, though not seen in all cases. Nakajima, *et al* have suggested that dyskeratosis of acantholytic cells and neutrophilic infiltrate in the epidermis can be considered diagnostic of this disease.

Treatment

The ideal treatment of IgG/IgA pemphigus is not defined. Varying combinations of drugs like dapsone, low dose steroids, colchicine, minocycline, retinoids and topical steroids have been tried, with variable response. The prognosis is usually good; however, Toosi, *et al* observed that moderate-to-high dose of steroids is required for disease control.

DRUG-INDUCED PEMPHIGUS

The drugs causing pemphigus can be grouped into the thiol group, phenol group, and non-thiol non-phenol group. The thiol group of drugs contain a sulfhydryl group (-SH). In this group, the common drugs implicated are penicillamine, captopril, lisinopril, thiopronine/tiopronin, and bucillamine. Phenol drugs include aspirin, rifampicin, and levodopa. The non-thiol non-phenol drugs are non-steroidal anti-inflammatory agents and calcium channel blockers. There have been reports of pemphigus occurring after therapy with biologics especially secukinumab and tocilizumab. Some vaccines are also reported to induce pemphigus (**Table 1**).

TABLE 1: Drugs causing pemphigus.

Thiol	Penicillamine, captopril, penicillin, piroxicam, lisinopril, thiopronine/tiopronin, and bucillamine
Phenol	Rifampicin, cefadroxil, levodopa, aspirin, heroin, and phenobarbital
Non-thiol non-phenol	Glibenclamide, calcium channel blocker, progesterone, non-steroidal anti-inflammatory drugs (NSAIDs), secukinumab, and tocilizumab

Pathogenesis

The mechanism by which medications trigger pemphigus is biochemical and immunological. Drugs with the thiol group activate proteolytic enzymes such as plasminogen activator, inhibit enzymes causing keratinocyte aggregation, interfere with cell-to-cell adhesion of the keratinocytes by forming disulfide bond in the adhesion molecules, bind to Dsg1 and 3, and induce antigenicity in the Dsgs. The phenol group causes acantholysis by interfering with the regulation and synthesis of complement and proteases, and by stimulation of the keratinocytes to produce tumor necrosis factor-α and interleukin-1. These agents may also cause acantholysis through alternative pathways such as activation of autoantibodies or altering the target antigen structure on the keratinocytes.

Epidemiology

A recent systematic review found the mean age of these patients to be 57.12 ± 16.9 years (range 8–105 years), with a female to male ratio of 1.3. The most common implicated drugs were penicillamine, captopril, and bucillamine. The most common clinical subtype was PV, followed by PF and paraneoplastic pemphigus. Other clinical subtypes included pemphigus herpetiformis, pemphigus vegetans, combined features of pemphigus and pemphigoid, polymorphic pemphigus, IgA pemphigus, pemphigus erythematosus, and unclassified form. Although PV is the most common clinical subtype, the three most implicated drugs, i.e., penicillamine, captopril, and bucillamine, induce a PF subtype most commonly. In penicillamine-induced pemphigus, PF:PV type of morphology occurs in a ratio of 4:1. The mean interval between drug initiation and disease onset was 154.27 ± 277.5 days, with a median of 60 days.

It was observed that penicillamine-induced pemphigus required the longest healing time.

Diagnosis

Drug-induced pemphigus presents a diagnostic challenge since clinical and histopathological findings are like idiopathic pemphigus. A thorough treatment history of the patient helps in identifying the causative drug. Histopathology may show suprabasal or subcorneal cleft. Drug-induced pemphigus should be considered if significant eosinophils are present in the biopsy section. DIF and IIF findings are similar to classic pemphigus; however, negative IF reports are not uncommon in this variant. Serology (ELISA) shows presence of antibodies against Dsg1, 3, or both.

Treatment

The first step in the management is to stop the offending drug. In a recent systematic review it was observed that 25% of the reported cases improved with drug cessation alone. The remaining patients required further treatment, including systemic steroids, azathioprine, methotrexate, mycophenolate mofetil, intravenous immunoglobulin (IVIg) or plasmapheresis.

Prognosis

Among all the variants of pemphigus, drug-induced pemphigus has the best prognosis. It is better in those patients who do not have circulating autoantibodies. Some studies have shown better prognosis with the thiol group, though a recent review did not find any difference in outcome between the thiol and non-thiol drugs.

Contact Pemphigus

PV has been triggered in certain cases due to skin contact with a chemical substance **(Fig. 4)**. It has been reported with multiple agents such as tincture of benzoin, topical phenols, garlic, pesticides, cosmetic procedures such as chemical peels, and drugs, specifically imiquimod and nickel. They trigger an altered local response and acantholytic reaction in the skin or mucosa when in contact with the skin. Distant sites too can be affected due to enhanced allergic contact hypersensitivity.

PEMPHIGUS HERPETIFORMIS

It is a rare form of pemphigus that resembles dermatitis herpetiformis clinically and pemphigus vulgaris histopathologically. The term pemphigus herpetiformis was introduced by Jablonska, *et al* in 1975.

Pathogenesis

The target antigen is Dsg1 more commonly, and in some, it is Dsg3. Antibodies against desmocollins 1, 2, or 3 may also be present. Some patients have IgA autoantibodies against these antigens. The change in targets of autoimmune response, as shown in animal models, could be responsible for the clinical heterogeneity of this disease. The pathogenic blister-inducing activity of IgG antibodies in pemphigus herpetiformis is weaker than in PV.

Clinical Features

It is characterized by vesicles arranged in annular pattern, or grouped vesicles on an erythematous base, associated with intense itching **(Fig. 5)**. Occasionally, it can evolve into PV or PF. In a retrospective study comprising 26 patients, a positive Nikolsky sign was seen in 38% patients and mucosal involvement in 23% of the patients.

Diagnosis

Costa, *et al* have proposed the following diagnostic criteria for this disease:
- *Clinical*: (1) Pruritic herpetiform intact blisters with/without erosions; and/or (2) pruritic annular or urticarial erythematous plaques with/without erosions;

Fig. 4: Contact pemphigus: Erosion induced by topical retinoid in a patient of pemphigus vulgaris in remission.

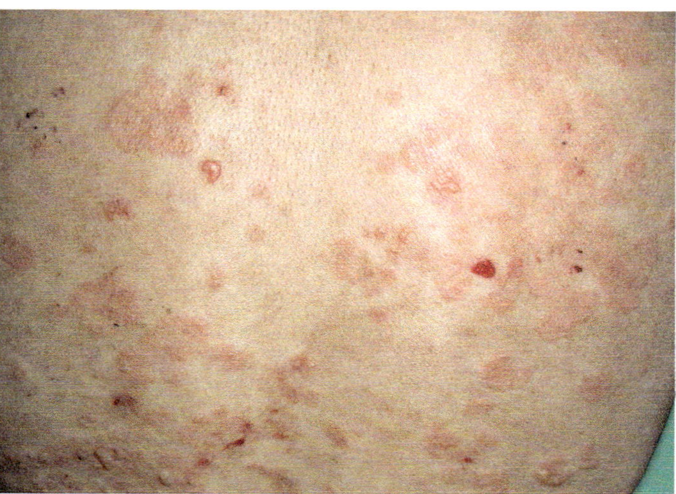

Fig. 5: Pemphigus herpetiformis: Annular and grouped arrangement of vesicles on erythematous base. *Image courtesy*: Dr Sujay Khandpur.

- *Pathologic*: (1) Intraepidermal eosinophils or neutrophils, or both; and/or (2) intraepidermal split with/without acantholysis;
- *Immunologic*: (I) DIF showing IgG with/without C3 intercellular deposits; (2) IIF showing IgG to epithelial cell surface; and/or (3) detection of serum autoantibodies against Dsg1 or 3 or desmocollins 1, 2, 3, or both.

Treatment

Treatment includes dapsone and systemic corticosteroids.

Prognosis

It has a better prognosis than PV. In a study, relapse rate was found to be 27%.

CONCLUSION

IgA pemphigus, IgG/IgA pemphigus, and pemphigus herpetiformis are rare variants of pemphigus. They have a better prognosis as compared to PV. Drug-induced pemphigus is caused by thiol, phenol or non-thiol non-phenol group of drugs. A careful history and physical examination can aid

in picking up these variants. Knowledge of these variants is important because there are slight variations which are important to note, in treatment, associations and prognosis when compared to classical pemphigus.

TAKE HOME MESSAGE

- Rare variants of pemphigus include IgA pemphigus, IgG/IgA pemphigus, pemphigus herpetiformis, and drug-induced pemphigus.
- IgA pemphigus presents in two forms—(1) IEN type and (2) SPD type.
- IgG/IgA pemphigus is a part of a spectrum ranging from PV to IgA pemphigus.
- While these rarer variants have a better prognosis compared to PV, they can be associated with internal malignancy especially IgA monoclonal gammopathy.
- Drug-induced pemphigus presents clinically as PF or PV and has a good prognosis.
- Pemphigus herpetiformis presents clinically like dermatitis herpetiformis and histopathologically like pemphigus vulgaris.

MULTIPLE CHOICE QUESTIONS

1. **Autoantigen in SPD type of IgA pemphigus is:**
   - (a) Desmoglein 3
   - (b) Desmocollin 1
   - (c) Desmoglein 1
   - (d) Desmocollin 3

2. **Dyskeratosis of acantholytic cells can be seen in:**
   - (a) Pemphigus vulgaris
   - (b) Herpetiform pemphigus
   - (c) IgA pemphigus
   - (d) IgG/IgA pemphigus

3. **Drug-induced pemphigus with the longest healing time is seen due to:**
   - (a) Rifampicin
   - (b) Captopril

   - (c) Penicillamine
   - (d) Piroxicam

4. **Most common clinical type seen in drug-induced pemphigus is:**
   - (a) Pemphigus vulgaris
   - (b) Pemphigus herpetiformis
   - (c) Pemphigus foliaceus
   - (d) IgA pemphigus

5. **Which drug is commonly used along with systemic steroids in the treatment of pemphigus herpetiformis?**
   - (a) Colchicine
   - (b) Dapsone
   - (c) Azathioprine
   - (d) Rituximab

Answers

1. (b)   2. (d)   3. (c)   4. (a)   5. (b)

SUGGESTED READING

1. Hashimoto T, Teye K, Ishii N. Clinical and immunological studies of 49 cases of various types of intercellular IgA dermatosis and 13 cases of classical subcorneal pustular dermatosis examined at Kurume University. *Br J Dermatol*. 2017;176:168-75.

2. Nishikawa T, Shimizu H, Hashimoto T. Role of IgA Intercellular Antibodies: Report of Clinically and Immunopathologically Atypical Cases. Proceedings of the XVII World Congress Dermatology. Berlin, Germany: Springer-Verlag; 1987. pp. 383-4.

3. Hashimoto T, Teye K, Hashimoto K, Wozniak K, Ueo D, Fujiwara S, *et al*. Clinical and immunological study of 30 cases with both IgG and IgA anti-keratinocyte cell surface autoantibodies toward the definition of intercellular IgG/IgA dermatosis. *Front Immunol*. 2018;9:1-8.

4. Toosi S, Collins JW, Lohse CM, Wolz MM, Wieland CN, Camilleri MJ, *et al*. Clinicopathologic features of IgG/IgA pemphigus in comparison with classic (IgG) and IgA pemphigus. *Int J Dermatol*. 2016;55:e184-90.

5. Kridin K, Patel PM, Jones VA, Cordova A, Amber KT. IgA pemphigus: A systematic review. *J Am Acad Dermatol*. 2020;82:1386-92.

6. Ghaedi F, Etesami I, Aryanian Z, Kalantari Y, Goodarzi A, Teymourpour A, *et al*. Drug-induced pemphigus: A systematic review of 170 patients. *Int Immunopharmacol*. 2021;92:107299.

7. Wang YM, Mao XM, Zhao WL, Wang YH, Zuo YG, Jin HZ, *et al*. The clinical, immunological, and pathological features for relapse of pemphigus herpetiformis: a univariate analysis of 26 cases. *Br J Dermatol*. 2020;182:802-4.

8. Gualtieri B, Marzano V, Grando SA. Atypical pemphigus: autoimmunity against desmocollins and other non-desmoglein autoantigens. *Ital J Dermatol Venereol*. 2021;156:134-41.

Subepidermal Autoimmune Bullous Diseases

CHAPTER 10

Bullous Pemphigoid and the Pemphigoids

Geeti Khullar, Luca Borradori

- Epidemiology
- Associated diseases/co-morbidities
- Bullous pemphigoid
  - Clinical manifestations
  - Non-bullous pemphigoid and other clinical variants
  - Infantile and childhood pemphigoid
- Drug-induced bullous pemphigoid
  - Dipeptidyl peptidase-4 inhibitor-induced bullous pemphigoid
- Differential diagnoses
  - Pemphigoid gestationis
  - Lichen planus pemphigoides (LPP)
  - Anti-p200 pemphigoid
  - Anti-p105 pemphigoid
- Prognosis and disease outcome
- Psychological morbidity
- Management of bullous pemphigoid: Objectives and principles

INTRODUCTION

The term "pemphigoid" comes from an ancient Greek word (*pemphix*) meaning "blister" or "pustule". In 1953, Walter Lever differentiated pemphigoid from pemphigus based on clinical and histological features.

Bullous pemphigoid (BP) is the most common sub-epidermal autoimmune bullous disease (sAIBD) worldwide. It mainly affects the elderly population. It typically presents with intense itching and tense blisters on both normal appearing and erythematous inflamed skin. Immunologically, BP is characterized by the production of IgG autoantibodies directed against two distinct structural components of the hemidesmosomes along the epidermal basement membrane zone (BMZ), the BP antigen 230 (BP230, also called BPAG1, epidermal isoform) and the BP antigen 180 (BP180, also called BPAG2 or type XVII collagen). BP180 is regarded as the major pathophysiologically important target autoantigen in BP.

EPIDEMIOLOGY

In both retrospective and prospective studies, the incidence of BP in Europe has been estimated to be 4.5–14 new cases per million population per year. Higher incidences of 23 and 43 per million per year have been reported in France and UK, respectively. Evidence exists that the incidence has increased two- to fourfold in the last two decades. This increase is most likely related to a higher proportion of older adults in the population, the increasing use of drugs potentially triggering BP such as dipeptidyl peptidase-4

inhibitors (DPP-4i) and immune checkpoint inhibitors, a better diagnosis of the non-bullous presentations, and possibly the availability of more performant laboratory diagnostic tools. In Asia, estimates of BP incidence range from 2.6 to 7.5 cases per million per year. There is paucity of epidemiological data in the Indian subcontinent. Although BP is reported to represent the most common sAIBD in India accounting for 40% of the cases, this percentage is much lower than in Western countries. The median age at onset ranges from 60 to 75 years and the incidence increases rapidly beyond 80 years of age. In India, BP seems to occur in a younger population, with a mean age between 59 and 62.5 years as reported in two studies. Men are twice more commonly affected than women. Infantile and childhood forms of BP are rare. However and intriguingly, in a study from Israel, the incidence in infants was estimated to be 23.4 cases per million per year. Affected infants usually have peculiar clinical features.

ASSOCIATED DISEASES/CO-MORBIDITIES

Case-control and population-based studies from different world regions have unequivocally reported that patients with neurological disorders including stroke, dementia, multiple sclerosis, and Parkinson's disease, have a significantly increased risk of developing BP. The reported odds ratios (ORs) are up to 3.3, 6.4, 13.6, and 9, respectively. Approximately 22–46% of BP patients suffer from at least one neurological condition. Neuropsychiatric disorders such as bipolar disorder have also been found more frequently in these cases. BP usually occurs at an interval of few months to 5 years after the onset of the neurological disease.

Although these associations imply a causal association, the so called population attributable fraction calculated for each neurological disease and BP remains below 7%, an observation indicating that neurological diseases can explain only a small proportion of cases.

Although neuronal isoforms of BPAG1 are expressed in the central and peripheral nervous system, there is little validated experimental data which has unequivocally demonstrated cross-reactivity between the epithelial and neuronal isoforms of BPAG1. The expression of BP180 (BPAG-2) in the brain is also a matter of controversy, with inconclusive data.

Among the cutaneous dermatosis, BP has been associated with psoriasis (OR: 2.02) in some studies. Chronic cutaneous inflammation may favor an autoreactive immune response. The use of coal tar or psoralens with ultraviolet (UV) therapy may also act as a trigger. Recently, it has been suggested that interleukin-17 (IL-17)-mediated inflammation represents a common causal driver in both diseases.

The association of BP with malignancies does not seem causally relevant in the vast majority of patients. Although some reports suggested an increased risk of hematological, gastric, and other solid organ malignancies, in a large national record linkage study with a cohort of 2,873,720 individuals with various malignancies, there was no increased risk of concurrent or subsequent BP compared to the cohort without a record of malignant cancer. This study, however, found the risk of BP to be increased in few specific cancers, most notably renal cancer. Since BP typically occurs in older patients, the possibility of finding an associated neoplasm on aggressive screening is very likely. A targeted screening for malignancies should primarily be based on patient's history, presence of distinct risk factors and clinical examination.

BP has been anecdotally reported in association with various autoimmune diseases such as systemic lupus erythematosus, rheumatoid arthritis, Hashimoto thyroiditis, Graves' disease, Crohn's disease, and ulcerative colitis. While a British case–control study found no increased risk of autoimmune disorders, the analysis of a large US registry of hospitalized patients recently indicated that BP patients had a mild increased risk [OR 1.35; 95% confidence interval (CI) 1.24–1.48] of association with one or more autoimmune disorders, including unspecified autoimmune diseases, vitiligo, and chronic urticaria, the practical relevance of which is doubtful.

A retrospective study from India on 96 BP patients (constituting 7.5% of all AIBDs), reported co-morbidities in 83.3% of cases, most frequently type 2 diabetes mellitus (T2DM) (38.5%) and hypertension (36.4%). Neurological diseases such as stroke and epilepsy were present in 16.7% of the cases. Less frequent co-morbidities included coronary artery, thyroid and respiratory diseases, and malignancies.

CLINICAL MANIFESTATIONS

The early stage of BP is typically characterized by the development of intense pruritus with excoriations **(Fig. 1)**, urticarial **(Fig. 2)** and/or eczematous plaques, which may either affect one body site such as the trunk or legs, or be generalized. These features may persist for weeks or months before the occurrence of vesicles and bullae on both inflamed and normal appearing skin **(Fig. 3)**. The lesions are distributed symmetrically, mainly on the lower abdomen **(Fig. 4)**, axillary and inguinal areas, upper arms, and thighs. The Nikolsky sign is negative. The bullae which are serous, rarely hemorrhagic, persist for some

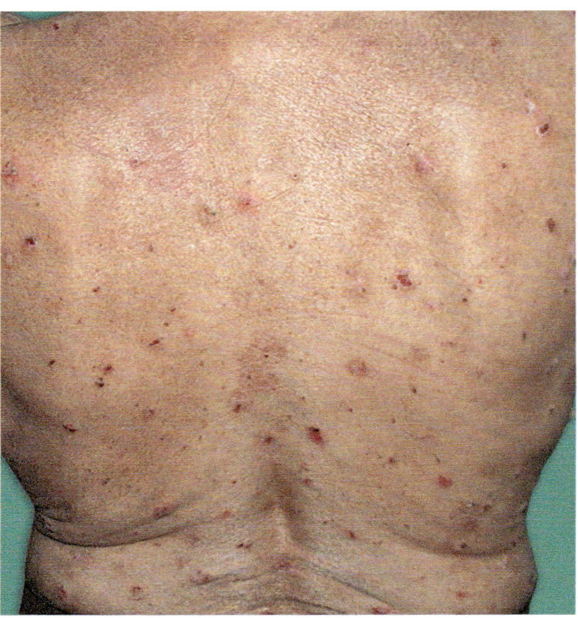

Fig. 1: Bullous pemphigoid variant characterized by the presence of excoriations and prurigo-like lesions. *Image courtesy*: Dr Sujay Khandpur.

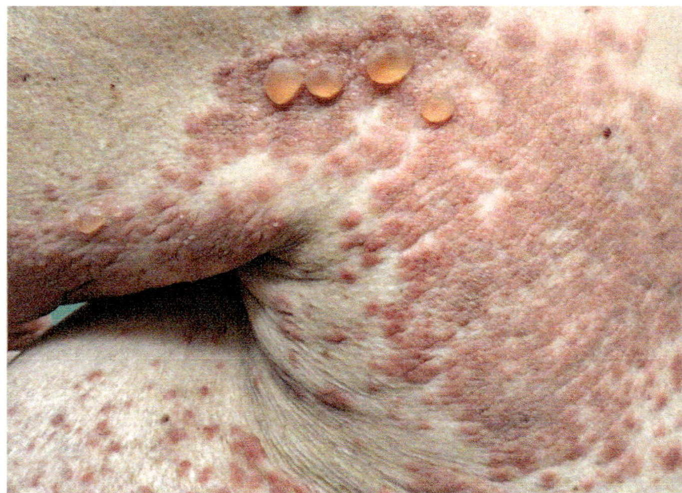

Fig. 2: Bullous pemphigoid: Typical features with urticarial and eczematous plaques and tense blisters.

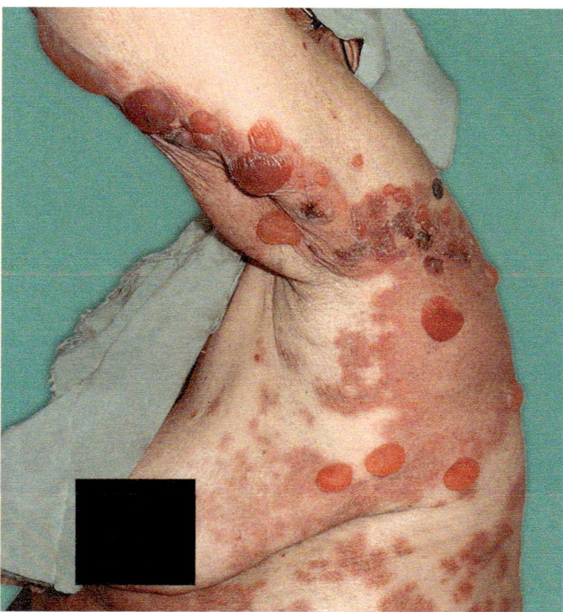

Fig. 3: Bullous pemphigoid: Tense bullae filled with sero-hemorrhagic fluid arising on an urticarial base. *Image courtesy*: Dr Vinay Keshavamurthy.

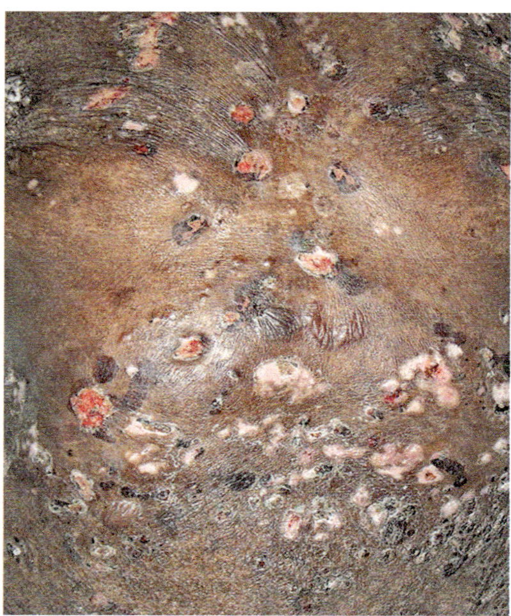

Fig. 4: Bullous pemphigoid: Symmetrically distributed bullae, erosions and crusts on the chest and abdomen. *Image courtesy:* Dr Sujay Khandpur.

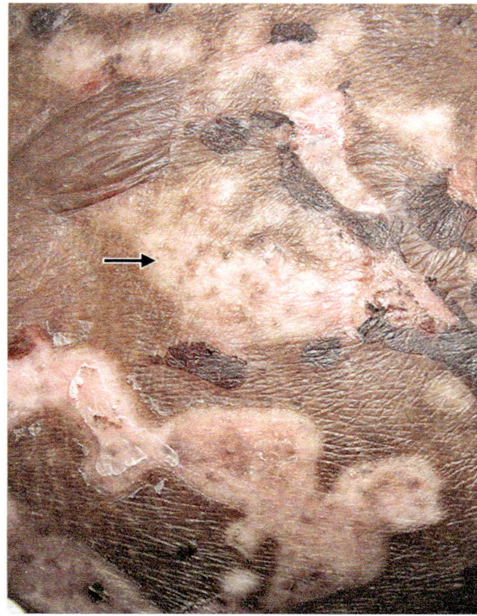

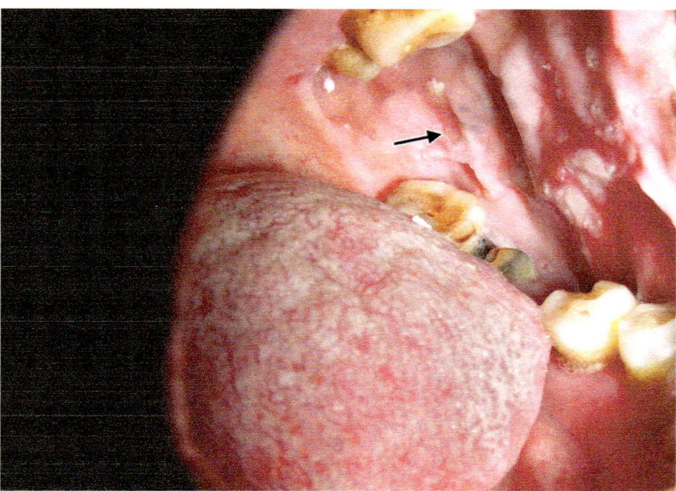

Fig. 6: Bullous pemphigoid (oral): Erosions and ulcerations in the buccal mucosa. *Image courtesy*: Dr Sujay Khandpur.

Fig. 5: Bullous pemphigoid: Lesions healing with dyspigmentation with follicular hyperpigmentation (arrow). *Image courtesy:* Dr Sujay Khandpur.

days before rupturing, resulting in erosions. They heal with hyper- or hypopigmentation, sometimes with follicular hyperpigmentation **(Fig. 5)**, and may rarely have an atrophic appearance with milia formation. Mucous membrane involvement occurs in 10–25% of cases, is usually mild and affects mainly the oral mucosa, with a tendency to spare the lips **(Fig. 6)**. The ocular, nasal, pharyngeal, and anogenital mucosae are usually not affected. Nonetheless, there are cases of BP in which various mucosal sites are involved. These are transitional forms with features reminiscent of mucous

membrane pemphigoid. Nail changes are uncommon—longitudinal ridging, Beau's lines, onychomadesis, or pterygium formation may be observed. Although majority of cases have generalized involvement, in localized BP, the skin lesions may be limited to one or few areas—pretibial region **(Fig. 7)**, umbilicus, sites of previous trauma such as radiotherapy, surgery, burns, UV and photodynamic therapy, around fistulas, or colostomy sites. Unilateral involvement with lesions confined only to the hemiplegic side, rarely occurs.

The Bullous Pemphigoid Disease Area Index (BPDAI) is a useful clinical scoring system to measure disease activity as well as sequelae (post-inflammatory pigmentation). The disease activity score is the sum of scores calculated

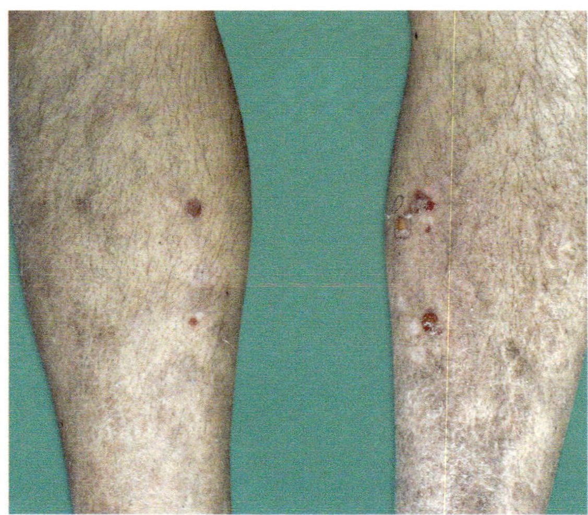

Fig. 7: Bullous pemphigoid: Vesicles and erosions localized to pretibial region.

Pemphigoid nodularis is characterized by excoriated hyperkeratotic nodules. Pemphigoid vegetans shows vegetating papillomatous lesions predominantly in intertriginous areas. Vesicular BP presents as multiple, small, grouped vesicles on erythematous base, resembling dermatitis herpetiformis **(Fig. 9)**. Other variants include erythrodermic, ecthyma gangrenosum-like, intertrigo-like, lymphomatoid papulosis-like, and toxic epidermolysis-like BP **(Table 1)**.

It has been questioned whether it is conceptually appropriate to differentiate so many "distinct" variants. The underlying immunological and genetic factors responsible for the wide spectrum of BP presentations remain so far unclear. It is likely that future studies may reveal distinct inflammatory signatures which may account for this phenotypic variability.

separately for the skin (blisters/erosions and urticarial lesions/erythema) and mucosae (range 0–360). A subjective component of BPDAI measures the severity of pruritus using visual analog scale (range: 0–30). It has been found that BPDAI score correlates well with the titers of anti-BP180 antibodies but not with anti-BP230 antibodies.

Non-bullous Form of BP and Other Variants

A significant proportion of BP patients, up to 20%, develop pruritic, eczematous, urticarial, or prurigo-like lesions, which remain for months or years as the only presenting feature of the disease. An Indian study has shown non-bullous forms of BP in approximately 16% of the patients.

BP lesions may have an annular, figurate, targetoid, or herpetiform arrangement. Dyshidrosiform BP is associated with vesicles and bullae on the palms and soles mimicking pompholyx **(Figs. 8A and B)**. These lesions rarely remain localized and invariably subsequently generalize.

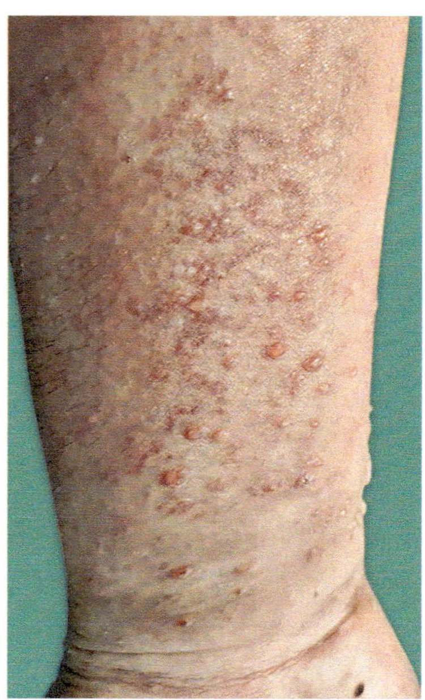

Fig. 9: Bullous pemphigoid—vesicular: Grouped tense vesicles on the forearm.

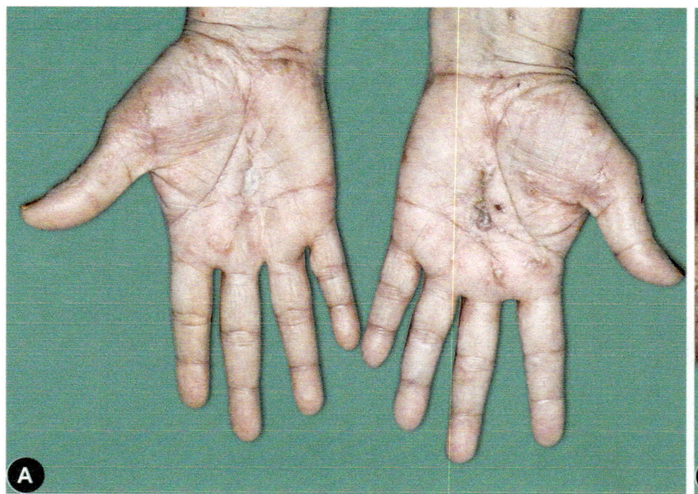

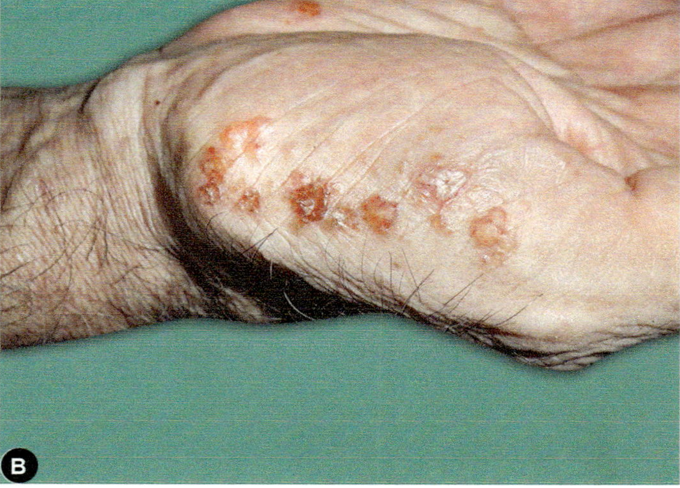

Figs. 8A and B: (A) Bullous pemphigoid-dyshidrosiform: Multiple vesicles on both palms mimicking pompholyx. (B) Bullous pemphigoid-dyshidrosiform: Multiple vesicles and bullae on the sides of the hand. *Images courtesy*: Dr Raghavendra Rao and Dr Vinay Keshavamurthy.

TABLE 1: Clinical variants of bullous pemphigoid.

Based on morphology	Based on site
Pemphigoid vegetans	Dyshidrosiform (palmoplantar)
Pemphigoid nodularis	Pretibial
Vesicular pemphigoid	Peristomal
Papular pemphigoid	Umbilical
Eczematous pemphigoid	Vulvar
Erythrodermic pemphigoid	Seborrheic
Lichen planus pemphigoides	Distal aspect of amputated limb
Erythema multiforme and toxic epidermal necrolysis-like pemphigoid	Paralyzed limb
	Radiotherapy site
Intertrigo-like pemphigoid	Site of trauma/surgery/burns
Ecthyma gangrenosum-like pemphigoid	
Lymphomatoid papulosis-like pemphigoid	

Infantile and Childhood Pemphigoid

BP rarely occurs in children. The disease has two peaks of onset—first at a median age of 4 months, in the infantile form, and a second peak at 8 years, in the childhood form of BP. The lesions typically occur on the face, palms and soles or may even generalize in infantile BP. Genital involvement, particularly vulvar, is common in the childhood variant (40% vs. 9% in adults). Localized vulvar BP typically occurs in girls 7–12 years of age, and has to be differentiated from sexual abuse, herpes infection, erosive lichen planus, and lichen sclerosus.

Although infections, drugs, and vaccinations (diphtheria, pertussis, tetanus, poliomyelitis, *Haemophilus influenzae* type B, pneumococcus, meningococcus C, and hepatitis B) have been implicated as possible triggers in this age group, most cases likely simply reflect a coincidental temporal association, but immune activation cannot be excluded in some cases. The latency between vaccine administration and the onset of lesions varies from a few hours to 3 weeks, hence a causal relationship is debatable. In affected patients, subsequent vaccines are not contraindicated. The prognosis is generally good, response to treatment is quick, and remission is usually observed. The average duration of disease is about 14 months.

Topical steroids can be used for the localized vulvar disease. Oral corticosteroids (1–2 mg/kg/day) with or without dapsone are the mainstay of therapy. Steroid-sparing options include cyclosporine, azathioprine, doxycycline with niacinamide (in children older than 8 years), erythromycin, mycophenolate mofetil, intravenous immunoglobulin, and rituximab. Relapses are uncommon.

DRUG-INDUCED BULLOUS PEMPHIGOID

Case control studies and a meta-analysis suggest that use of diuretics in particular aldosterone antagonists, anticholinergics, and dopaminergic medications is epidemiologically significantly associated with BP, implying a causal link. Several other drugs, the association of which remains uncertain, have been occasionally reported to trigger BP, such as non-steroidal anti-inflammatory drugs (NSAIDs), antibiotics, angiotensin-converting enzyme (ACE) inhibitors, calcium channel blockers, and tumor necrosis factor-alpha (TNF-α) inhibitors. More importantly, dipeptidylpeptidase-4 inhibitors, particularly vildagliptin and linagliptin, and immune checkpoint inhibitors are significantly associated with and may cause BP. In the latter cases, the delay between their initiation and onset of BP may be more than a year. The odds of developing BP with some of these drugs are enlisted in **Table 2**.

Drug-induced cases seem to occur at a younger age compared to classic BP. There is intense pruritus. Unusual features such as erythema multiforme-like lesions, lesions occurring on the palms and soles and face and a positive Nikolsky sign, have been anecdotally described. Marked peripheral eosinophilia may be present.

Histological findings include necrotic keratinocytes and a subepidermal blister, with the blister cavity containing numerous eosinophils and neutrophils. The dermis shows a dense infiltrate of eosinophils along with neutrophils and lymphocytes.

It is yet unclear whether withdrawal of the culprit drug has a positive impact on the disease course. In BP cases triggered by immune check point inhibitors, the decision to stop immunotherapy critically depends on the tumor response, BP activity and the ability to control skin lesions with the use of topical corticosteroids or low doses of oral corticosteroids.

TABLE 2: Odds of developing bullous pemphigoid with various drugs.

Drug class	Odds ratio
Neuroleptics	3.7
Antibiotics	3.4
Anticholinergics	3.2
Aldosterone antagonist (spironolactone)	2.3–3.1
Dipeptidyl peptidyl peptidase-4 inhibitors	2.13
Loop diuretics (furosemide)	2.0–3.8
Beta blockers	1.7
Angiotensin-converting enzyme inhibitors	1.1
Calcium channel blockers	1.1

Source: Adapted from Lloyd-Lavery A, *et al*. The associations between bullous pemphigoid and drug use: a UK case-control study. *JAMA Dermatol.* 2013;149: 58-62.

Dipeptidyl Peptidase-4 Inhibitor-induced Bullous Pemphigoid

DPP-4i are incretin-based oral drugs, approved in 2006 for the treatment of T2DM. There is more than threefold increased risk of developing BP with DDP-4i **(Fig. 10)**. The number of DPP-4i-associated BP cases is rising, because of increasing use of this drug class. DPP-4 is expressed on the surface of many cell types including keratinocytes and T cells. The inhibition of this peptidase may result in an increase of pro-inflammatory cytokines with eosinophilic stimulation, and an impact on plasminogen activation and plasmin formation. The latter is a serine protease which can proteolytically cleave BP180 and produce epitopes with increased antigenicity. The time to onset of lesions after the introduction of DPP-4i is highly variable, ranging from 8 days to 37 months, with a median of 10 months. This long delay suggests that BP in these patients is drug-aggravated rather than drug-induced. Among the DPP-4i, vildagliptin is associated with the maximum risk, followed by teneligliptin and linagliptin. Vildagliptin is less selective for DPP-4 and in addition, causes inhibition of DPP-8 and DPP-9 compared to other DPP-4i. **Table 3** shows the odds of developing BP with various DPP-4i. Prevalence of human leukocyte antigen (HLA)-DQB1*03:01 is higher in Japanese patients with DPP-4i-associated BP. In one Japanese study, the authors reported that patients with gliptin-triggered BP show less inflammatory features with less erythema, urticarial lesions, and blistering and solitary erosions compared to classical BP, while European studies were unable to confirm these findings.

Some studies have shown the upper extremities and trunk to be more commonly affected. Mucosal involvement is more frequent and severe. The absolute eosinophil count is either normal or slightly raised, and on histopathology, eosinophilic spongiosis is less frequent and dermal eosinophilic infiltrate is scant. These results are concordant with the non-inflammatory clinical phenotype. The circulating antibody titers against NC16A are lower compared to the idiopathic cases. A few Japanese studies have also shown that antibodies in DPP-4i-associated disease target antigenic regions of the extracellular domain of BP180, distinct from the NC16A domain. Hence, enzyme-linked immunosorbent assay (ELISA) using the BP180 NC16A may be negative and use of full length recombinant BP180 substrate is recommended. Some studies have detected antibodies to NC16A if drug exposure is continued in cases who had tested negative earlier. A lower incidence of anti-BP230 reactivity has also been reported. However, European studies have found no significant difference in the clinical and immunological features between the idiopathic/classical and DPP-4i-induced BP.

Few studies have shown the mean prednisolone dose required for treatment to be significantly lower, and remission rates to be higher in DPP-4i-associated cases, both on and off therapy. Median time to improvement after drug withdrawal was 35 days. However, other studies could not confirm these observations, and found no difference in disease evolution and management requirement.

To summarize, it is as yet unclear whether gliptin-triggered BP has a distinct immunological profile based on conflicting results reported. Prospective comprehensive immunological studies with systematic adequate controls are required to gain better insights into this debated question. Based on the scant knowledge and contradictory results from various studies, no clear recommendations to either stop or continue the culprit drug can be made. Nonetheless, switching to a different anti-diabetic class of the drug may be considered.

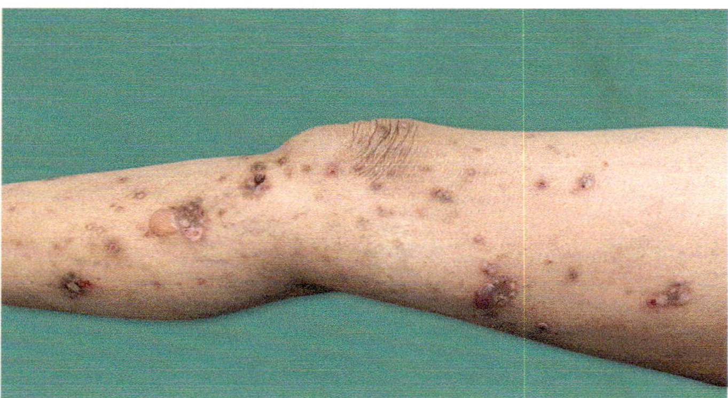

Fig. 10: DPP-4i-induced bullous pemphigoid: Tense blisters overlying normal skin and crusted erosions healing with hypopigmentation on the lower limb in a patient with vildagliptin-induced bullous pemphigoid.

Drug	Adjusted odds ratio
Vildagliptin	5.08
Saxagliptin	2.9
Linagliptin	2.87
Sitagliptin	1.29
Others	1.25

Source: Adapted from Phan K, *et al.* Dipeptidyl peptidase-4 inhibitors and bullous pemphigoid: A systematic review and adjusted meta-analysis. *Australas J Dermatol.* 2020;6:e15-e21.

DIFFERENTIAL DIAGNOSES AND OTHER SUBEPIDERMAL AUTOIMMUNE BULLOUS DISEASES

Based on the wide spectrum of clinical presentations, BP may closely mimic a variety of conditions including contact dermatitis, prurigo, urticarial dermatoses, drug reactions, arthropod reactions, and scabies. In the presence of frank skin blistering, bullous arthropod bites, allergic contact dermatitis, Stevens–Johnson syndrome, bullous drug eruptions, dyshidrotic eczema, pseudoporphyria, or porphyria cutanea tarda should be excluded. In children, bullous impetigo, inherited epidermolysis bullosa, and bullous mastocytosis are clinical differentials. Sometimes pemphigus and dermatitis herpetiformis are also difficult to be clinically distinguished from BP.

Differentiation of BP from the following sAIBDs may be more challenging and requires specific diagnostic immuno-pathological tools, immunoblotting techniques with different extracts or recombinant proteins, and specific in-house ELISAs which are not commercially available.

Pemphigoid Gestationis

It may be considered a distinct subtype of BP typically linked to and associated with pregnancy. Its incidence is estimated between 1:4,000 and 1:60,000 pregnancies. It may rarely occur in association with hydatidiform mole, trophoblastic tumors, and choriocarcinoma. Flares triggered by either the menstrual cycle or use of oral contraceptives have been described. There is strong association with distinct major histocompatibility complex (MHC) class II antigens such as haplotypes HLA-B8, HLA-DR3, and HLA-DR4. Lesions usually develop in the second or third trimester, and rarely in early postpartum period. In half of the patients, disease occurs in the first pregnancy, with high recurrence rate in subsequent pregnancies. It presents with erythematous papulo-vesicles, tense bullae, and urticarial plaques in the periumbilical region **(Figs. 11A and B)**, chest, back, and palms and soles. The lesions are usually intensely pruritic. In early stages, the features may be identical to those observed in polymorphous eruption of pregnancy. Mucosae are usually spared.

Immunologically, there are complement-binding IgG1 autoantibodies directed against BP180 that predominantly recognize antigenic determinants within the NC16A domain. BP180 is also expressed in the placental tissue and fetal membranes starting from the first trimester of pregnancy. This observation suggests cross-reactivity between BP180 expressed in the placental tissue and epidermal basement membrane. The abnormal expression of distinct MHC class II molecules in the placenta may predispose to development of the disease in susceptible subjects.

The prognosis of pemphigoid gestationis is favorable. The disease usually resolves in the postpartum period. Complications include preterm delivery and fetal growth retardation. Neonatal pemphigoid gestationis develops in <5% of newborns due to transplacental transfer of antibodies.

Potent topical corticosteroids or moderate doses of oral corticosteroids are usually sufficient to control the disease. Azathioprine, dapsone, intravenous immunoglobulin, and plasmapheresis have been used in refractory cases.

- *Linear IgA bullous dermatosis (LABD)*: This is covered in Chapter 12.
- *Mucous membrane pemphigoid*: This is covered in Chapter 11.

Lichen Planus Pemphigoides (LPP)

Recent knowledge supports the idea that LPP represents the co-existence of lichen planus and BP, with both conditions sharing the same immunological targets. In fact, cell-mediated and humoral immune responses directed against components of the BMZ including BP180 (BPAG2), are present in lichen planus and BP. LPP usually occurs in patients much younger than BP, with one study reporting a mean age of onset of 46 years. There are typical lichenoid papules and plaques as well as vesicles and bullae arising on both normal appearing skin and on lichenoid lesions **(Fig. 12)**. The latter frequently affect the extremities. Blisters typically develop after the occurrence of lichenoid lesions. Lichenoid involvement of mucosal sites and nails is sometimes observed. Histopathology shows typical features of both lichen planus and BP.

LPP is thus distinct from bullous lichen planus. Anedoctal cases of drug-induced forms such as by ACE inhibitors and statins, have been described. Viral infections such as hepatitis B and varicella have also been implicated. Most importantly, overlap forms of lichen planus and BP

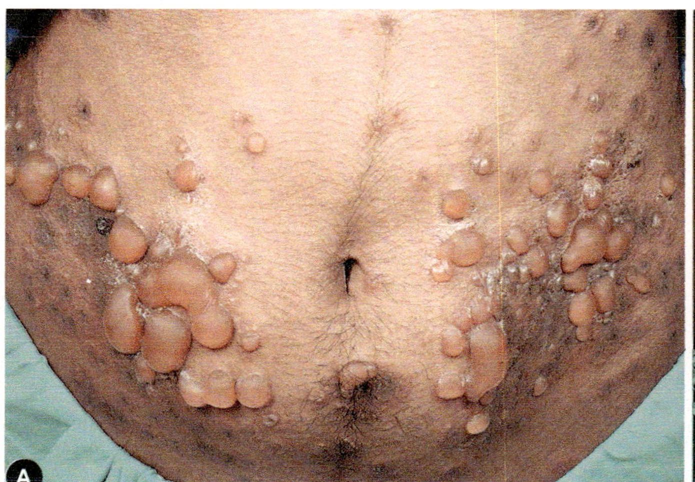

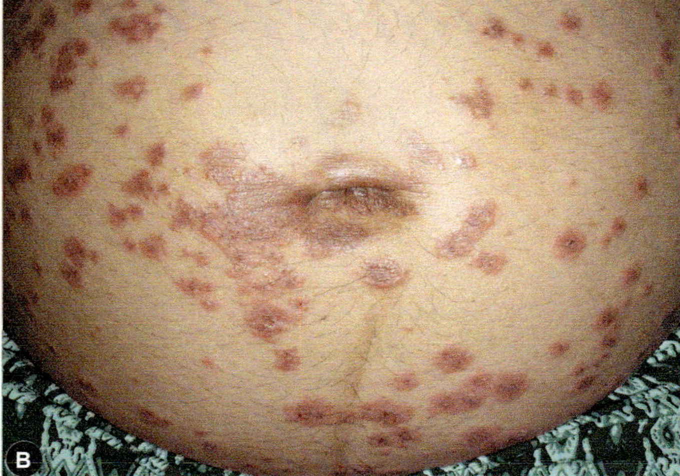

Figs. 11A and B: (A) Pemphigoid gestationis: Tense bullae, crusted erosions, and annular erythematous plaques on the periumbilical area of a 5-month pregnant woman. (B) Pemphigoid gestationis: Multiple annular erythematous plaques with central crusting and vesicles, in periumbilical region and abdomen. *Image courtesy*: Dr. Sujay Khandpur.

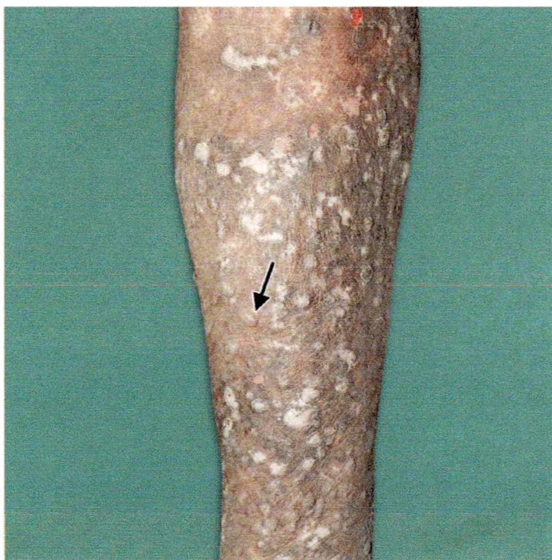

Fig. 12: Lichen planus pemphigoides: Violaceous papules with few having overlying erosions and healing with depigmentation on the upper limb. Tense bullae (arrow) can also be seen arising on normal skin. *Image courtesy*: Dr Raghavendra Rao.

have been increasingly described following therapy with immune check inhibitors such as pembrolizumab and nivolumab, as a result of loss of self-tolerance.

Direct immunofluorescence (DIF) and indirect immunofluorescence (IIF) findings are identical to those found in BP patients. Autoantibodies recognize distinct antigenic regions within the NC16A domain of BP180. Treatment options are similar to those for BP. Oral retinoids such as acitretin have also been tried. The disease course is more favorable than that of BP.

Anti-p200 Pemphigoid

It is a rare subset of pemphigoid, characterized by autoantibodies targeting a 200 kDa (p200) antigen. p200 is an extracellular glycoprotein produced by the keratinocytes and dermal fibroblasts in the epidermal BMZ. In 90% of cases, these antibodies react against laminin γ1, therefore it is also known as anti-laminin γ1 pemphigoid. Experimental studies have also indicated that additional pathophysiologically important antigenic targets exist in anti-p200 pemphigoid.

These patients are younger than BP cases with a mean age of 65.5 years. In a small series of five cases from India, the mean age was even younger—56.6 years (range 42–64 years). Male patients of Asian descent seem to be preferentially affected. The clinical presentation in most cases is similar to BP, inflammatory type of epidermolysis bullosa acquisita (EBA) and LABD **(Figs. 13A and B)**. Annular arrangement of blisters can also be seen. Involvement of the palmoplantar and head and neck regions is observed. Lesions usually heal without scarring and milia formation. Mucosal involvement occurs in up to 40% cases, and seems to be more frequent than in BP. In about 30% of patients, an association with psoriasis has been reported, especially in those of Japanese ethnicity.

On histopathology, subepidermal blister formation is associated with a dense infiltrate of predominantly neutrophils in the papillary dermis. DIF shows linear deposits of IgG and/or C3 along the dermoepidermal junction with an "n-serrated" pattern. On IIF on salt-split normal human skin, the circulating IgG autoantibodies characteristically bind, in contrast to BP, to the floor of the split (floor pattern). Immunoblot assay detects the 200 kDa antigen from human dermal extracts. IB assay and ELISA have shown that

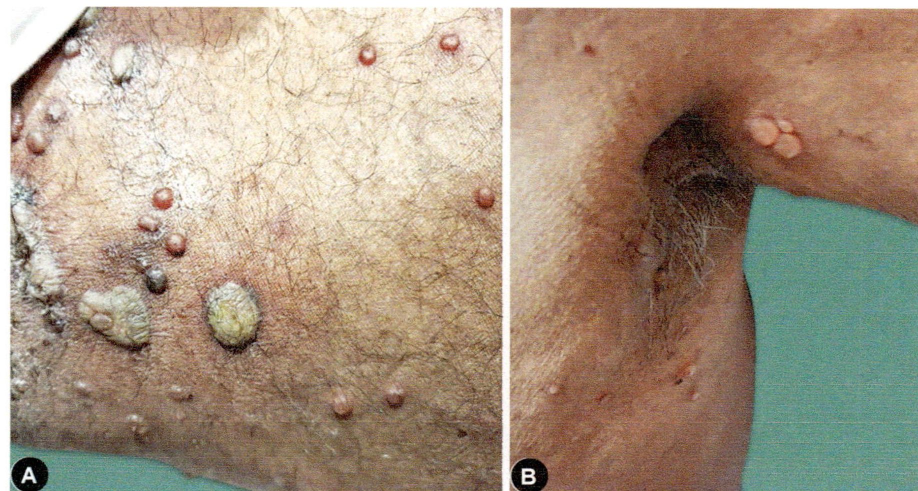

Figs. 13A and B: (A) Anti-p200 pemphigoid: Tense vesicles and bullae, some containing purulent material, arising on normal appearing skin over trunk. (B) Anti-p200 pemphigoid: Tense vesicles and bullae filled with clear fluid, on the lateral and inferior borders of axilla. *Image courtesy*: Dr Raghavendra Rao.

patients' IgG auto-antibodies bind to the C-terminal region of laminin γ1 in 70–90% of cases.

It has been claimed that anti-p200 pemphigoid has a better prognosis than BP. Patients respond well to potent topical steroids or medium dose of oral corticosteroids. Dapsone, tetracyclines, and azathioprine have also been used.

EBA: This is covered in Chapter 11.

Anti-p105 Pemphigoid

The recognition of anti-p105 pemphigoid as a distinct type of sAIBD is controversial. This entity is no longer mentioned in most recent reviews. Early publications claimed that anti-p105 pemphigoid is associated with peculiar clinical and immunopathological features. The latter specifically include the presence of circulating IgG autoantibodies binding to the dermal side of salt-split normal human skin, and immunoblotting a 105 kDa molecular weight protein from the keratinocyte and fibroblast extracts. However, following the first publications, the targeted autoantigens have not been further characterized, and the overall findings have never been confirmed by additional independent groups.

PROGNOSIS AND DISEASE OUTCOME OF BULLOUS PEMPHIGOID

BP runs a chronic course over months to years (average: 3–6 years), with exacerbations and remissions. About 30% of cases relapse in the first year of therapy. Risk factors for relapse include severe disease, dementia, and high serum levels of antibodies against BP180. After discontinuation of treatment, relapses are observed in almost 50% of patients in the first 3 months. Mortality rate varies from 10% to 40%, two- to threefold higher than in age- and sex-matched controls. Risk factors for increased mortality in the first year after diagnosis include advanced age (>80 years), low serum albumin (<3.6 g/dL), raised erythrocyte sedimentation rate (>300 mm/h), extensive disease, requirement of high dose of systemic corticosteroids, Karnofsky score of ≤40, and presence of co-morbidities. Childhood BP has a more favorable prognosis.

PSYCHOLOGICAL MORBIDITY

Pruritus and painful erosions significantly impact the quality of life of BP patients. Validated tools to assess pruritus include the 5-D Itch Scale and Itch Quality of Life questionnaire. Quality of life is measured using Dermatology Life Quality Index and Autoimmune Bullous Quality of Life questionnaire, which assesses the effect on daily activities, social relations, and emotions.

MANAGEMENT OF BULLOUS PEMPHIGOID: OBJECTIVES AND PRINCIPLES

The goals of treatment are to fully control the itch, treat and heal the cutaneous inflammatory lesions, maintain remission either on or off a minimal maintenance therapy, avoid relapses, and minimize therapy-related side-effects. Disease severity (mild disease-BPDAI score <20, moderate disease—BPDAI score ≥20 and <56 and severe disease—BPDAI >56), presence of co-morbidities and patients' age are important factors to consider in managing BP.

The various diagnostic modalities and therapeutic options for BP will be discussed in detail in subsequent chapters. The diagnostic algorithm and therapeutic ladder are summarized in **Flowchart 1 and Figure 14** respectively.

- Clinical features (intense pruritus, classic tense bullae and vesicles or non-bullous/localized lesions, Nikolsky sign negative)
- Assessment of disease extent, quality of life and co-morbidities

↓

- Histopathology: Sub-epidermal bulla with eosinophils and/or neutrophils
- Direct immunofluorescence: Linear deposits of IgG and/or C3 at dermo-epidermal junction, "n-serrated" patten distinguishes BP from EBA

↓

Immunoserological tests:
- Indirect immunofluorescence on salt-split skin (roof pattern of immunoreactant deposition)
- ELISA for anti-BP180 and anti-BP230
- Biochip mosaic to detect 180 kDa antigen
- Immunoblot assay

Flowchart 1: Diagnostic algorithm for bullous pemphigoid.

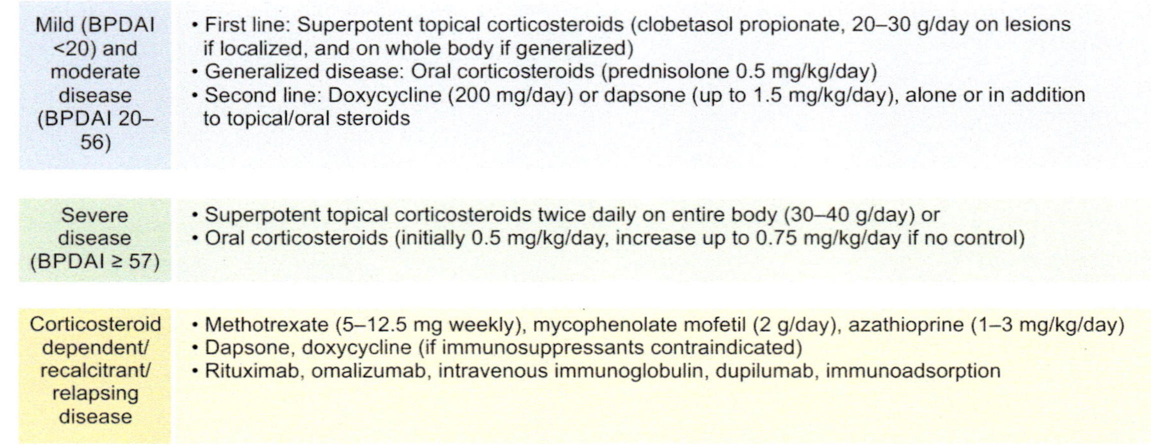

Fig. 14: Therapeutic ladder for bullous pemphigoid.

CONCLUSION

BP is the most frequent sAIBD and affects predominantly old patients. The clinical spectrum of BP is extremely broad, and atypical variants without obvious blistering are not so rare. Strong itch in combination with excoriations, eczematous, vesicular, and/or urticarial lesions may constitute the only manifestations of the disease. Affected patients often have multiple co-morbidities. Its diagnosis critically relies on direct immunofluorescence microscopy and immuno-serological studies.

TAKE HOME MESSAGE

- BP affects younger population in India than in the West and is frequently associated with neurological disorders, diabetes mellitus, and hypertension.
- Classical disease presents with urticarial or eczematous lesions in the prodromal stage accompanied with significant pruritus. This is followed by tense bullae predominantly in the flexures.
- Histologically, it shows a subepidermal split with eosinophil-rich infiltrate in the blister cavity and upper dermis.
- DIF demonstrates linear deposits of IgG and/or C3 along the basement membrane zone.
- Using IIF, circulating antibodies binds to the epidermal side of salt-split normal human skin.
- Childhood BP is rare and shows predilection for the acral and genital sites.
- Anti-p200 pemphigoid is characterized by neutrophilic infiltrate on histopathology and circulating antibodies that bind to the dermal side of salt split skin.
- Pemphigoid gestationis occurs usually in the second or third trimester of pregnancy as urticarial plaques and tense blisters typically in the periumbilical region.
- Distinct drugs have been epidemiologically associated with BP. Therefore, drug triggering should always be considered. Specifically, immune check point inhibitors and DPP-4i have been increasingly reported to potentially cause BP.
- Mild and moderate cases of BP are treated with super-potent topical corticosteroids, while severe disease requires oral steroids with or without steroid-sparing agents and biologicals.

MULTIPLE CHOICE QUESTIONS

1. **Which of these is a feature of childhood pemphigoid?**
   - (a) Peak age of onset is 4 years
   - (b) Lesions commonly occur in flexures
   - (c) Vaccines are implicated as triggering factor
   - (d) It is associated with poor prognosis

2. **Which statement is true regarding anti-p200 pemphigoid?**
   - (a) The age of onset is similar to bullous pemphigoid
   - (b) Psoriasis is associated in 90% of cases
   - (c) Autoantibodies label the floor by IIF on salt-split skin
   - (d) DIF shows u-serrated pattern

3. **All are correct regarding pemphigoid gestationis, *except*:**
   - (a) Periumbilical area is characteristically involved
   - (b) DIF shows IgG deposits at dermoepidermal junction in all cases while C3 is absent
   - (c) The disease in subsequent pregnancies is more severe
   - (d) Mild self-limiting skin lesions may occur in newborns

4. **Starting dose of oral corticosteroid in severe bullous pemphigoid is:**
   (a) 0.5 mg/kg/ day
   (b) 0.25 mg/kg/day
   (c) 1 mg/kg/day
   (d) 1.5 mg/kg/day

5. **Which of these is a poor prognostic factor in bullous pemphigoid?**
   (a) Age >60 years
   (b) Requirement of high doses of oral corticosteroids
   (c) Absence of neurological disease
   (d) High serum albumin levels

6. **Dipeptidyl peptidase-4 inhibitor-induced bullous pemphigoid is characterized by:**
   (a) More inflammatory cutaneous lesions than idiopathic type
   (b) Scanty eosinophilic infiltrate on biopsy
   (c) Higher antibody titers against NC16A BP180 than classic bullous pemphigoid
   (d) Severe and refractory disease course

7. **Which of these morphological types of lesions are not seen in prodromal/non-bullous phase of bullous pemphigoid?**
   (a) Urticarial
   (b) Excoriations
   (c) Lichenoid
   (d) Eczematous

8. **Oral mucosal involvement in bullous pemphigoid is observed in what proportion of cases?**
   (a) 50–60%
   (b) 10–30%
   (c) 1–5%
   (d) 80–90%

9. **Which of these dermatoses is associated with bullous pemphigoid?**
   (a) Psoriasis
   (b) Pityriasis rubra pilaris
   (c) Pityriasis lichenoides chronica
   (d) Seborrheic dermatitis

10. **Which statement is true regarding lichen planus pemphigoides?**
    (a) It affects older patients as compared to bullous pemphigoid
    (b) Head and neck region is commonly involved
    (c) It has less severe course than bullous pemphigoid
    (d) Blisters do not develop outside the lesions of lichen planus

Answers

1. (c)   2. (c)   3. (b)   4. (a)   5. (b)   6. (b)   7. (c)   8. (b)   9. (a)   10. (c)

SUGGESTED READING

1. Khandpur S, Verma P. Bullous pemphigoid. *Indian J Dermatol Venereol Leprol*. 2011;77:450-5.
2. De D, Kaushik A, Handa S, Mahajan R, Chatterjee D, Saikia B, *et al.* Bullous pemphigoid in India: Review of cases registered in an autoimmune bullous disease clinic. *Indian J Dermatol Venereol Leprol*. 2022:1-5
3. Waisbourd-Zinman O, Ben-Amitai D, Cohen AD, Feinmesser M, Mimouni D, Adir-Shani A, *et al.* Bullous pemphigoid in infancy: Clinical and epidemiologic characteristics. *J Am Acad Dermatol*. 2008;58:41-8.
4. Langan M, Groves RW, West J. The relationship between neurological disease and bullous pemphigoid: A population-based case–control study. *J Invest Dermatol*. 2011;131:631-6.
5. Amber KT, Murrell DF, Schmidt E, Joly P, Borradori L. Autoimmune subepidermal bullous diseases of the skin and mucosae: clinical features, diagnosis, and management. *Clinic Rev Allerg Immunol*. 2018;54:26-51.
6. Zenzo GD, della Torre R, Zambruno G, Borradori L. Bullous pemphigoid: From the clinic to the bench. *Clin Dermatol*. 2012;30:3-16.
7. Lamberts A, Meijer JM, Jonkman MF. Nonbullous pemphigoid: A systematic review. *J Am Acad Dermatol*. 2018;78:989-95.
8. Nemeth AJ, Klein AD, Gould EW, Schachner LA. Childhood bullous pemphigoid—Clinical and immunologic features, treatment and prognosis. *Arch Dermatol*. 1991;127:378-86.
9. Lloyd-Lavery A, Chi CC, Wojnarowska F, Taghipour K. The associations between bullous pemphigoid and drug use: a UK case-control study. *JAMA Dermatol*. 2013;149:58-62.
10. Phan K, Charlton O, Smith SD. Dipeptidyl peptidase-4 inhibitors and bullous pemphigoid: A systematic review and adjusted meta-analysis. *Australas J Dermatol*. 2020;6:e15-e21.
11. Lipozencic J, Ljubojevic S, Bukvic-Mokos Z. Pemphigoid gestationis. *Clin Dermatol*. 2012;30:51-5.
12. Goletz S, Hashimoto T, Zillikens D, Schmidt E. Anti-p200 pemphigoid. *J Am Acad Dermatol*. 2014;71:185-91.
13. Chan LS, Fine JD, Briggaman RA, Woodley DT, Hammerberg C, Drugge RJ, *et al.* Identification and partial characterization of a novel 105-kDalton lower lamina lucida autoantigen associated with a novel immune-mediated subepidermal blistering disease. *J Invest Dermatol*. 1993;101:262-7.
14. Borradori L, Van Beek N, Feliciani C, Tedbirt B, Antiga E, Bergman R, *et al.* Updated S2 K guidelines for the management of bullous pemphigoid initiated by the European Academy of Dermatology and Venereology (EADV). *J Eur Acad Dermatol Venereol*. 2022;36:1689-704.

CHAPTER 11

Mucous Membrane Pemphigoid, Anti-laminin 332 Pemphigoid, Epidermolysis Bullosa Acquisita, Bullous Systemic Lupus Erythematosus

Neirita Hazarika, Riti Bhatia

- Mucous membrane pemphigoid
- Anti-laminin 332 mucous membrane pemphigoid
- Epidermolysis bullosa acquisita
- Bullous systemic lupus erythematosus
  - Epidemiology
  - Associated diseases/co-morbidities
- Clinical manifestations
- Prognosis and disease outcome
- Psychological morbidity
- Diagnostic modalities
- Treatment

MUCOUS MEMBRANE PEMPHIGOID

Introduction

Mucous membrane pemphigoid (MMP) is a chronic progressive autoimmune bullous disease (AIBD) occurring most commonly in the older age group, characterized by the development of bullae and erosions in the mucosa that show a tendency for scarring. Scarring can be severe and debilitating, leading to loss of function and significant psychological distress. The term "cicatricial pemphigoid" was used synonymously with MMP until 2002. It is now a separate disease entity with predominant cutaneous involvement in the form of erosions and blisters that heal with scarring and milia formation. Unlike MMP, mucosal involvement is not predominant.

The antigenic targets in MMP are heterogeneous and include various components of the basement membrane zone (BMZ), including bullous pemphigoid 180 (BP 180), BP230, laminin 332, beta-4 peptide of $\alpha6\beta4$ integrin, laminin 311 (shares the $\alpha3$-chain with laminin 332 and is co-targeted), collagen VII, and unspecified 168 kDa and 45 kDa antigens. Exclusive ocular and oral disease is characterized by antibodies targeting the $\beta4$ and $\alpha6$ integrins, respectively. The variant with both mucosal and cutaneous lesions in MMP occurs as a result of autoantibodies against the BP180 antigen.

Epidemiology

MMP is an uncommon disease. The incidence was estimated to be two cases per million population per year in a German study. The incidence of ocular MMP was much higher, 1 in 8,000–46,000 among patients attending ophthalmology outpatients. It occurs in older individuals aged 60–80 years. Young adults and children are rarely affected. There is a predilection for females, with a female to male ratio of 1.5–3:1. There is no geographical or racial predilection.

Associated Diseases/Co-morbidities

MMP has not been clearly associated with malignancy, except for the anti-laminin 332 pemphigoid variant. Some patients may have an association with other autoimmune diseases such as systemic lupus erythematosus (SLE), rheumatoid arthritis, and polyarteritis nodosa.

Clinical Manifestations including Disease on Special Sites

MMP primarily affects the mucosae. Cutaneous involvement is seen in around 10–25% of cases. Among the mucosal sites, the oral cavity is most frequently involved in 85% cases, followed by ocular conjunctiva (64%), pharyngeal mucosa (19%), external genitalia (17%), nasal mucosa (15%), larynx (8%), rectum, anus, and esophagus (4% each). It has a relapsing and remitting course.

Oral MMP commonly involves the gingival and buccal mucosae in the form of desquamative or erosive gingivitis **(Fig. 1)**. The tongue, alveolar ridge, palate, and lips are less frequently affected. Clinical features include edema, intact vesicles, bullae, erythematous patches, and pseudomembranous lesions. Patients who have the disease limited to only the oral mucosa usually have a good prognosis, with mild-to-moderate disease associated with minimal scarring. Oral MMP lesions can closely mimic

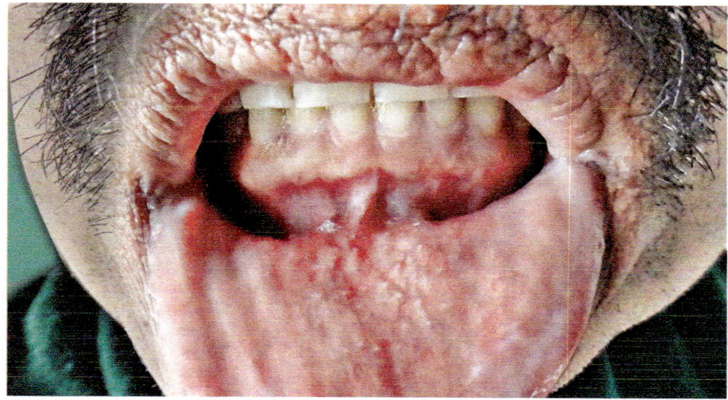

Fig. 1: Oral mucous membrane pemphigoid: Desquamative gingivitis with adhesions in the lower gingiva. *Image courtesy*: Dr Vinay Keshavamurthy.

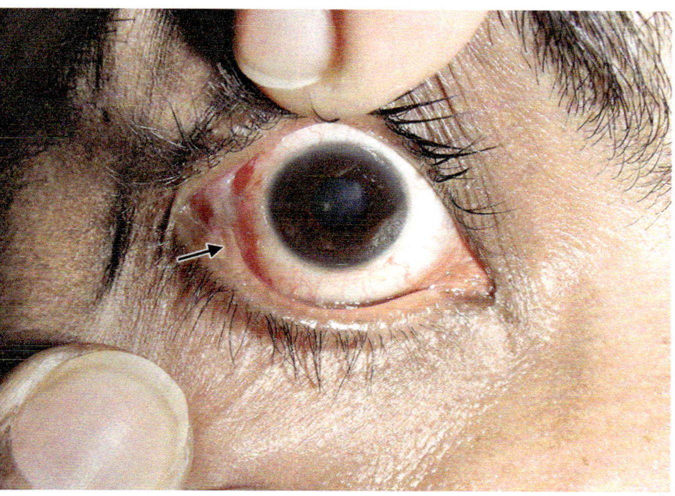

Fig. 2: Ocular mucous membrane pemphigoid: Adhesion formation (arrow) between the bulbar and palpebral conjunctiva (symblepharon formation). *Image courtesy*: Dr Sujay Khandpur.

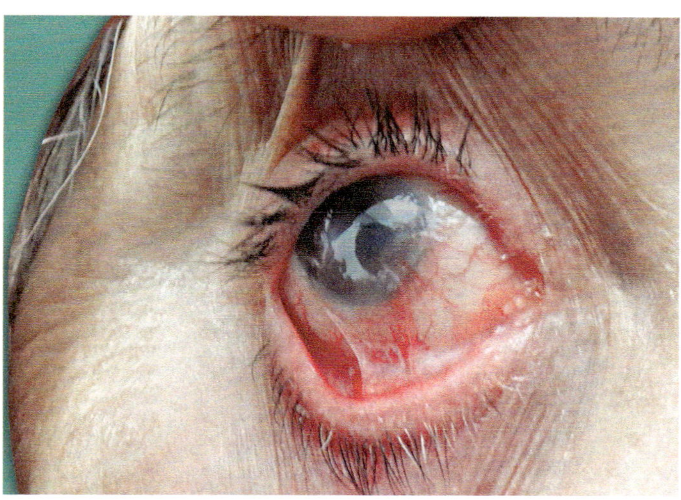

Fig. 3: Ocular mucous membrane pemphigoid: Hyperemia of the conjunctiva with adhesion formation between the bulbar and palpebral conjunctiva (symblepharon formation). *Image courtesy*: Dr Vinay Keshavamurthy.

pemphigus vulgaris (PV), oral erosive lichen planus, and bullous pemphigoid (BP). The lesions are less painful than the mucosal lesions of PV. Scarring is a common consequence of MMP that distinguishes this variant from mucosal involvement in BP, which typically does not scar. Reticulated, white striations representing mucosal fibrosis are often present at sites of healed lesions, and functional limitations secondary to scarring may occur.

Involvement of the laryngeal and tracheal mucosae in MMP can result in hoarseness, stridor, and asphyxiation.

Ocular MMP occurs due to immunoglobulin G (IgG) antibodies against the β4 integrin subunit. It usually involves the conjunctiva, progressing from unilateral to bilateral involvement over 2–3 years. The initial symptoms include irritation, burning, and mucus discharge. Staging of conjunctival inflammation in ocular MMP was described by Foster, *et al* in 1986:

Stage 1: Subepithelial fibrosis

Stage 2: Shortening of fornices

Stage 3: Symblepharon (adhesions between bulbar and palpebral conjunctiva) **(Figs. 2 and 3)**

Stage 4: Ankyloblepharon (fusion of upper and lower lid margins), keratinization of the whole ocular surface

Later in the course of the disease, trichiasis (inward growth of eyelashes), distichiasis (a duplicate row of eyelashes in which one or both grow inward against the eye), entropion, lagophthalmos, limbal stem cell deficiency, and absent tear formation are observed. Corneal ulcers and perforation, and loss of visual acuity are other complications that may occur despite systemic treatment. Ocular MMP should be distinguished from scarring resulting from toxic epidermal necrolysis, trauma, paraneoplastic pemphigus, other subepidermal blistering diseases such as linear IgA bullous disease, epidermolysis bullosa acquisita (EBA), and chronic use of topical ophthalmic medications.

Cutaneous manifestations include tense bullae typically involving the head and neck and upper trunk that heal with scarring. Urticarial plaques surrounding the bullae are seen in variable number of cases.

The clinical scoring systems for MMP include the Mucous Membrane Pemphigoid Disease Area Index (MMPDAI) for milder forms of disease, Autoimmune Bullous Skin Disorder Intensity Score (ABSIS) based on the amount of body surface area (BSA) involved and the degree of activity/healing observed, and the Oral Disease Severity Score (ODSS).

Bedside test: False Nikolsky sign is seen in all subepidermal AIBDs. It is elicited by pulling the peripheral remnant roof of a ruptured blister, thus extending the erosion on the surrounding normal skin. The subepidermal cleft is limited in size, does not show a tendency for spontaneous extension, and heals rapidly.

Prognosis and Disease Outcome

MMP is a slowly progressive chronic disease with a relapsing and remitting course. The outcome is poor compared to the other subepidermal AIBDs. Oral disease usually has a benign outcome, while ocular MMP is associated with treatment resistance. Ocular MMP progresses from initial conjunctival inflammation to blindness in about 10–30 years. Some patients progress more quickly, with intermittent periods of worsening and rapid scarring. MMP can lead to severe irreversible complications such as esophageal and anal stenosis and urethral strictures. Early diagnosis and prompt treatment are key factors in the prevention of adverse disease sequelae. Long-term remission (average 36 months) is possible in approximately one-third of cases.

Psychological Morbidity

MMP is associated with significant psychological distress due to functionally detrimental sequelae of scarring that include blindness, dysphagia, urethral and anal strictures, and airway compromise. Patient-reported outcome measurements including Dermatology Life Quality Index (DLQI), Autoimmune Bullous Disease Quality of Life (ABQOL), and Treatment of Bullous Disease Quality of Life (TABQOL), can be used for assessment of quality of life pre- and post-treatment.

Diagnostic Modalities

Histopathology: Biopsy is preferably obtained from a recent and intact blister from the oral mucosa. Histopathology reveals a subepidermal cleft with lymphocytes and occasional eosinophils. At a later stage, dermal fibrosis is distinctly noted. Histopathology is, however, a non-specific diagnostic modality and does not help to distinguish MMP from other pemphigoid disorders.

Direct immunofluorescence (DIF): It shows linear IgG and/or IgA and C3 deposits in n-serrated pattern at the basement membrane, on a perilesional buccal mucosal biopsy. Ocular biopsy is not usually preferred. It is taken in case the buccal mucosa biopsy is negative. Conjunctival biopsy is obtained from the upper fornix or limbus after a week's course of topical steroid and antibiotic.

Indirect immunofluorescence (IIF): IIF using 1 M NaCl split human skin shows IgG/IgA antibody binding to the blister roof or floor, depending upon the antigen involved. Epidermal/roof binding is due to involvement of $\alpha6\beta4$integrin, BP180 or BP230, and dermal/floor binding is due to antigens laminin 332 and collagen VII. IgG autoantibodies are more frequently detected in MMP than IgA, which are found in around 60% of cases. The occurrence of IgA autoantibodies, alone or in combination with IgG autoantibodies, may indicate more severe disease and progression. The sensitivity of IIF with human split skin and monkey esophagus is 36–84% and 10%, respectively in MMP, thus monkey esophagus can serve as a useful substrate when pemphigus is a close differential diagnosis due to much higher sensitivity in pemphigus. Autoantibodies on IIF using human skin are less often detected in MMP than in BP, and with lower dilutions (1:10–1:40).

Enzyme-linked immunosorbent assay (ELISA)/immunoblot (IB) assay/immunoprecipitation: For cases with epidermal staining on IIF split skin, further testing can be done with ELISA or IB assay with recombinant or cell-derived BP180, BP230, and $\alpha6\beta4$ integrin for IgG autoantibodies. For cases with dermal staining pattern, further testing with recombinant or cell-derived laminin 332 and type VII collagen is recommended. These tests are available only in specialized diagnostic centers.

Treatment

Various modalities include potent topical steroids, tetracycline and nicotinamide combination, or dapsone 50–100 mg/day, in low-risk patients (disease limited to oral mucosa, with or without skin involvement). In non-responsive cases, oral steroid 0.5 mg/kg/day, with or without azathioprine 100–150 mg per day are initiated. High-risk patients, with any other mucosal site affected, are treated with oral steroid (1–1.5 mg/kg/day) along with azathioprine (100–150 mg/day), mycophenolate mofetil (2 g/day), cyclophosphamide (1–2 mg/kg/day orally or 500–1,000 mg intravenously every 4 weeks), dexamethasone pulse (DP) or dexamethasone-cyclophosphamide pulse (DCP). Additional supportive measures include oral hygiene, ocular lubricants, lid hygiene, and breakage of scars with glass rod. For mild ocular disease (hyperemia and edema), low-potency topical steroid or topical cyclosporine are recommended. For moderate disease (hyperemia and intense infiltration), dapsone/methotrexate/mycophenolate mofetil or azathioprine are administered. Severe disease (hyperemia, conjunctival ulceration, limbitis) is managed with oral prednisolone (1 mg/kg/day) and cyclophosphamide (1 mg/kg/day). Recalcitrant disease is managed with intravenous immunoglobulin (IVIg), rituximab, or anti-tumor necrosis factor alpha (TNF-α) agents. Surgical interventions for ocular MMP include amniotic membrane transplantation, tectonic keratoplasty, keratoprosthesis, entropion surgery, tarsorrhaphy, and mucous membrane grafting.

ANTI-LAMININ 332 MUCOUS MEMBRANE PEMPHIGOID

Introduction

Anti-laminin 332 MMP is a rare variant of MMP with laminin 332 autoantigen (i.e., laminin-5, epiligrin, BM600, ladsin, nicein, kalinin, and GB3 antigen), a heterotrimeric glycoprotein consisting of $\alpha3$, $\beta3$, and $\gamma2$ subunits, found at the interface of lamina lucida and lamina densa, tightly bound to the anchoring filament complex of the BMZ. It is associated with a risk of solid organ malignancy. Clinically, it cannot be distinguished from the other variants of MMP.

Epidemiology

Anti-laminin 332 pemphigoid most commonly affects the elderly, of median age 60–65 years. It comprises about 25% cases of MMP.

Associated Diseases/Co-morbidities

It is associated with an increased risk of malignancy, which occurs in about 30% cases. The malignancy is usually diagnosed within a year of diagnosis of MMP. Solid organ malignancies such as visceral adenocarcinoma of various tissues are the most common, though Hodgkin lymphoma, acute myelocytic leukemia, and cutaneous T cell lymphoma have also been reported.

Clinical Manifestations Including Disease on Special Sites

Anti-laminin 332 pemphigoid is clinically and histopathologically indistinguishable from MMP. Involvement of the laryngeal mucosa is commonly seen, specifically the supraglottis. It manifests as hoarseness of voice, stridor, and in extreme cases, laryngeal stenosis requiring tracheostomy. Similar to MMP, erosions that heal with scarring involve the oral, ocular, pharyngeal, laryngeal, esophageal, anal, and genital mucosa. Cutaneous bullae are seen on trauma-prone sites, head and neck, and trunk. These heal with scarring and milia formation.

Prognosis and Disease Outcome

This subset of MMP is associated with a poorer outcome owing to severe disease with frequent recurrences and a high risk of concurrent neoplasms.

Psychological Morbidity

Anti-laminin 332 pemphigoid is associated with high psychosocial morbidity due to functionally debilitating scarring.

Diagnostic Modalities

- *Histopathology and DIF* are similar to MMP. On DIF, n-serrated pattern is seen.
- *IIF* using 1 M NaCl split skin demonstrates dermal localization (floor pattern) of antibodies.
- *ELISA* is used for detection of circulating anti-laminin 332 IgG antibodies, and less frequently IgA and IgE antibodies. This test has both diagnostic and prognostic significance, as antibody titers correlate with disease severity. ELISA is performed with native, recombinant laminin 332 and laminin 332-rich keratinocyte extracellular matrix antigens. None of the serological tests are commercially available yet.
- *Immunoblot assay and immunoprecipitation*: It is undertaken using extracellular matrix of cultured human keratinocytes. IB assay using bovine gingival lysate is helpful in the detection of $\alpha6\beta4$ integrin-specific antibodies.

MMP cases in whom the antibodies bind to the dermal side of BMZ on salt-split skin, should undergo age- and sex-appropriate cancer screening. Additional evaluation for malignancy is recommended based on clinical features.

Treatment

Ocular disease in anti-laminin 332 MMP is particularly resistant to treatment. Treatment options are similar to MMP, including potent topical steroids and topical cyclosporine, lubricants, breakage of scars with glass rod, systemic corticosteroids (1–1.5 mg/kg/day), dapsone, immunosuppressive drugs such as azathioprine (100–150 mg/day), mycophenolate mofetil (2 g/day), cyclophosphamide (50 mg/day), DP or DCP, rituximab, and IVIg. Immunopheresis along with rituximab was successfully used in a case that was refractory to DCP and oral cyclophosphamide.

EPIDERMOLYSIS BULLOSA ACQUISITA

Introduction

EBA is a rare mechanobullous disorder characterized by fragility of the skin, tense bullae formation, milia and scarring. The term "epidermolysis bullosa acquisita" was coined by Hundley and Smith. Roenigk, *et al* proposed the first diagnostic criteria for the classical/mechanobullous EBA.

Pathogenesis

It is due to autoantibodies against type VII collagen, a major component of anchoring fibrils in the BMZ of skin and mucosa. Autoantibodies are commonly seen against non-collagenous (NC) 1 domain and rarely against NC2 domain. These antibodies interfere with antiparallel dimer formation of type VII collagen, inhibiting anchoring fibril assembly, and also disrupt interactions of type VII collagen with the other BMZ or upper dermal components such as type IV collagen, laminin 5 (laminin 332), and fibronectin. In inflammatory EBA, antibody-induced complement fixation also leads to inflammation and damage at the dermo-epidermal junction (DEJ), with subsequent blister formation. The role of resident microbial communities such as firmicutes, proteobacteria, actinobacteria, and bacteroidetes, has also been suggested.

Epidemiology

The incidence of EBA is <0.5/million population. Two age peaks in the second and seventh decades are described. Pediatric cases are rare, with 40 cases reported so far, with age ranging from 2 days (due to placental transfer of autoantibodies) to 16 years.

Clinical Features

There are two clinical variants:
1. *Classical (non-inflammatory/mechanobullous form) EBA*: It is characterized by skin fragility, non-inflammatory tense vesicles, bullae, and erosions. Bullae

appear immediately/few hours after minimal trauma and are commonly seen on the hands, feet, elbows, knees, and lower back **(Figs. 4 to 6)**. Erosions heal with scarring and milia formation **(Fig. 5C)**. Oral **(Figs. 7A and B)**, nasal, ocular, pharyngeal, laryngeal, esophageal, and anogenital mucosae may be involved. Alopecia, nail loss, fibrosis of the hands and fingers (leading to mitten-like deformity), esophageal stenosis, and webbing occur in severe cases.

2. *Inflammatory (non-classical/non-mechanobullous form) EBA*:

   a. *BP-like EBA* meets the clinical criteria of both EBA and BP. Patients have pruritus, tense bullae, and erosions on erythematous/urticated skin, along with trauma-induced bullae on normal skin, involving the trunk, extremities, and flexures. Mucosal involvement is not predominant. Lesions heal with scarring and milia formation.

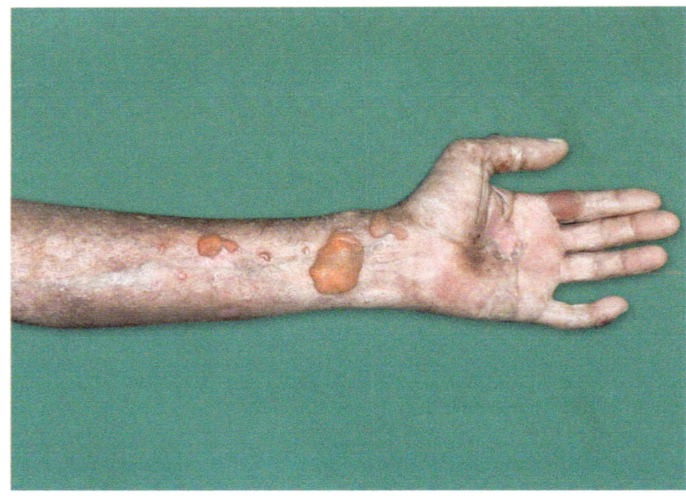

Fig. 4: Non-inflammatory epidermolysis bullosa acquisita: Tense, non-inflammatory vesicles and bullae on the left hand and forearm. *Image courtesy*: Dr Raghavendra Rao.

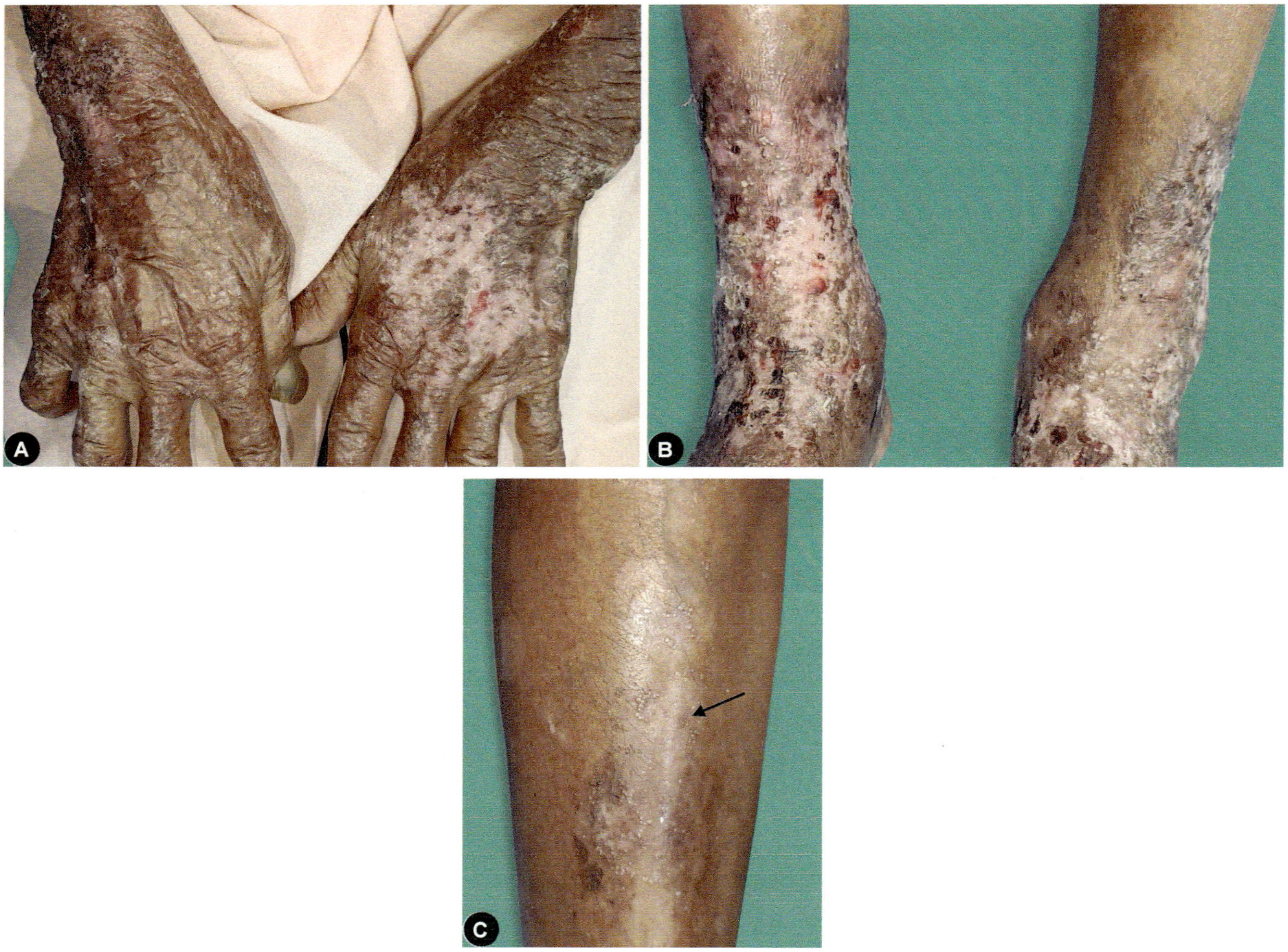

Figs. 5A to C: (A) Epidermolysis bullosa acquisita: Depigmentation, few erosions, atrophy and milia formation over dorsa of both hands. (B) Epidermolysis bullosa acquisita: Hemorrhagic vesicles, crusted plaques, depigmentation, atrophy and milia formation over both ankles. (C) Epidermolysis bullosa acquisita: Multiple milia (arrow) over right shin. *Image courtesy*: Dr. Neetu Bhari.

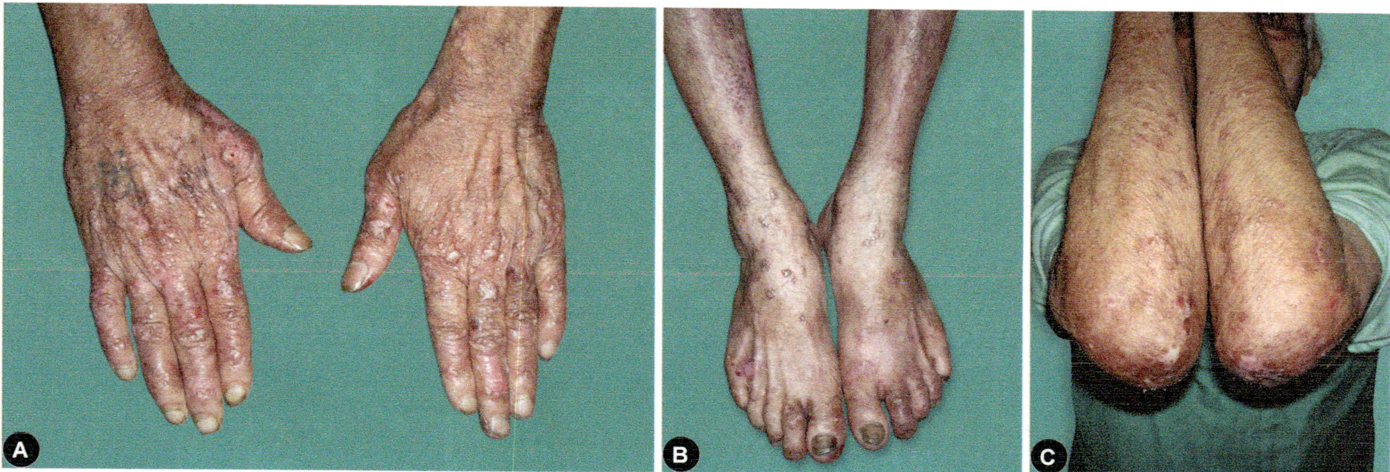

Figs. 6A to C: (A) Epidermolysis bullosa acquisita: Healing erosions and milia on dorsa of hands. (B) Epidermolysis bullosa acquisita: Healing erosions and milia on dorsa of feet with anonychia in few toe nails. (C) Epidermolysis bullosa acquisita: Healing erosions and milia on elbows. *Image courtesy*: Dr. Sujay Khandpur.

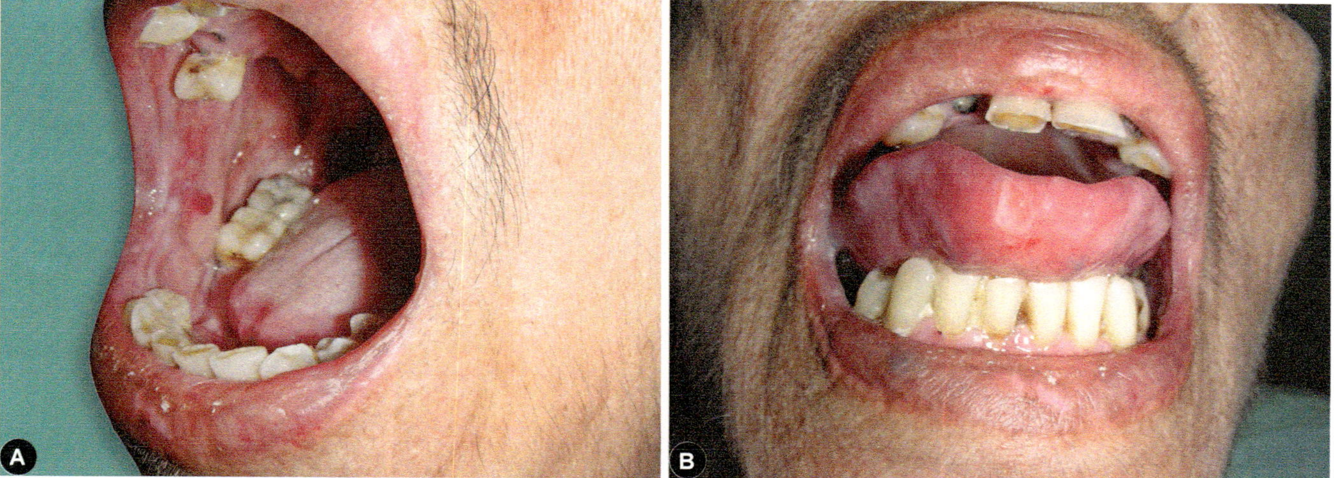

Figs. 7A and B: (A) Epidermolysis bullosa acquisita: multiple erosions in right buccal mucosa. (B) Epidermolysis bullosa acquisita: erosions present on tongue. *Image courtesy*: Dr. Sujay Khandpur.

b. *MMP-like EBA*: This mainly affects the mucosae lined by squamous epithelium—oral mucosa, pharynx, esophagus, epiglottis, conjunctiva, genitalia, anus, trachea, and bronchi. Intact mucosal blisters are seen, unlike in MMP. The mucosal lesions are asymptomatic in up to one-third of cases. Cicatricial lesions (atrophic scars, synechiae, stenosis) are identical in MMP–EBA and MMP. They have mild consequences in the mouth and genitalia, but severe impairment in the esophagus, larynx, trachea, bronchi, and conjunctiva.

c. *IgA bullous dermatosis-like EBA* resembles linear IgA disease (LAD) with erythematous arciform lesions and few scars and milia.

d. *Brunsting–Perry pemphigoid-like EBA* manifests as cutaneous lesions without erythematous or urticarial plaques occurring in the head and neck area, leaving behind atrophic scars. There is no mucosal involvement.

Recent reports suggest that inflammatory phenotype is more common (2/3rd of cases) than classical phenotype.

The clinical presentation may change over time, i.e., patients may switch from a BP-like EBA to classical EBA.

Childhood EBA: As described above, EBA rarely occurs in children, with varied presentation. A literature review identified 40 childhood EBA cases (21 females and 19 males). These included inflammatory EBA ($n = 31$), classical mechanobullous EBA ($n = 7$), and a mix of both phenotypes ($n = 2$). There was cutaneous involvement in 39 of 40 cases, mucosal involvement in 29, and nail dystrophy in 8 of 40 cases.

Severe EBA: It is defined as the occurrence of ≥10 cutaneous bullae and/or ≥3 mucosal sites and/or conjunctival, laryngotracheal or esophageal involvement.

Associated Disorders

EBA may be associated with inflammatory bowel disease (IBD) in up to 25% cases, SLE, amyloidosis, thyroiditis, multiple endocrinopathy syndrome, rheumatoid arthritis, pulmonary fibrosis, chronic lymphocytic leukemia, thymoma, and diabetes.

Diagnostic Modalities

The first diagnostic criteria for EBA was given by Roenigk, *et al* in the early 1970s. These were: (1) spontaneous or trauma-induced blisters resembling hereditary dystrophic EB; (2) adult onset; (3) a negative family history for EB; and (4) exclusion of all other bullous diseases.

- *Histopathology*: It reveals a subepidermal blister with varied inflammatory infiltrate. Classic EBA is pauci-inflammatory. Inflammatory EBA is associated with a neutrophil-rich infiltrate admixed with eosinophils and lymphocytes, and sometimes a mild infiltrate with predominant fibrin deposition. Small epidermal cysts (milia) and dermal fibrosis may be seen. Routine histopathology does not distinguish EBA from other sub-epidermal AIBDs.
- *DIF*: Shows broad, linear deposits of IgG (± C3, IgA, IgM) along the DEJ in a linear u-serrated pattern with 'grass-like' appearance of Ig deposition. In some cases, the serration pattern may not be discernible, especially in mucosal biopsies. In these cases, further thin sections of the biopsy can be helpful.
- *IIF*: Anti-collagen VII IgG antibodies (less commonly IgA) on salt-split skin bind to the dermal side (floor pattern). A commercially available IIF-based assay of NC1-expressing human cells (Euroimmun, Lübeck, Germany) for the detection of IgG autoantibodies against type VII collagen can be done. Its sensitivity is about 92%. The antibody titers correlate with disease activity. However, half of the EBA patients may be seronegative. IIF on hereditary EB skin deficient of type VII collagen is available at selected research centers.
- *ELISA*: Commercially available ELISA based on both the NC1 and NC2 domains (MBL, Nagoya, Japan; Euroimmun, Lubeck) can be used. Its sensitivity is 94%. Similar to IIF, antibody titers correlate with disease activity.
- *IB* assay using dermal extract, human amnion, or cultured A431 cells to detect type VII collagen antibodies, has been undertaken.
- *Fluorescent overlay antigen mapping (FOAM)*: It is a technique based on the possibility of visualizing a target antigen relative to a topographic marker. In EBA, it shows antibody deposits localized below the lamina densa.
- *Immune electron microscopy (IEM)*: It shows autoantibodies specifically binding to the anchoring fibrils and lamina densa where anchoring fibrils originate and terminate. It is considered the diagnostic gold standard.
- Transmission electron microscopy also identifies reduction in anchoring fibrils. Amorphous material beneath the lamina densa represents Ig deposits on anchoring fibrils.

Treatment

General and local measures include:
- Avoidance of trauma
- Gentle cleansing of skin
- Hydrogel or semiocclusive hydrocolloid dressings on clean wounds; silver impregnated dressings or topical antibiotics for infected wounds.

Systemic treatment includes systemic corticosteroids with or without dapsone, colchicine, and immunosuppressive adjuvants including azathioprine, cyclosporine, mycophenolate mofetil, methotrexate, and cyclophosphamide. Rituximab in combination with immunosuppressants, IVIg, or immunoadsorption have been used for refractory EBA. A retrospective analysis of 30 EBA cases showed median time to remission of 9 months, and observed in 33%, 33%, and 45% of the patients at 1, 3, and 6 years follow-up, respectively. In a review on the treatment of EBA published between 1971 and 2016, IVIg and rituximab were found to be associated with complete remission.

Emerging treatments include etanercept, daclizumab, sulfasalazine, anti-granulocyte–macrophage colony-stimulating factor (anti-GM-CSF), 5-lipoxygenase inhibitor (zileuton), recombinant IL-6, roflumilast, therapies targeting complement factors C3, C5 or C5R, cell-derived nanoparticles, and highly galactosylated immune complex treatment.

Prognosis

Overall prognosis of EBA is guarded. Minimal skin fragility without bullous lesions persists for many years. Cicatricial lesions increase morbidity and may be life-threatening.

BULLOUS SYSTEMIC LUPUS ERYTHEMATOSUS

Bullous systemic lupus erythematosus (BSLE) is a rare, acute, transient, vesiculobullous eruption occurring in the setting of SLE and is caused by autoantibodies directed against type VII collagen (anchoring fibrils) at the DEJ. Differentiation of BSLE from EBA presents a diagnostic challenge.

Epidemiology

It affects mainly females in the second to fourth decades, with predominance among the darker phototypes (skin types V–VI).

Clinical Features

BSLE is characterized by acute onset, mildly pruritic, tense bullae (like BP) or small, grouped vesicles [like dermatitis herpetiformis (DH)], appearing on normal/erythematous/urticated skin on the trunk **(Fig. 8)**, upper extremities, face and neck **(Fig. 9)**. Photo-distribution of lesions or history of photosensitivity may be present. The lesions heal with pigmentary changes, without scarring or milia formation. Mucosal involvement is seen in half the cases. Blisters along the vermilion border of lips are characteristic. Patients can exhibit associated symptoms of SLE such as fever, arthritis, renal, and hematologic manifestations. Whether blistering correlates with systemic activity of SLE remains debatable, but it is said to parallel the activity of lupus nephritis.

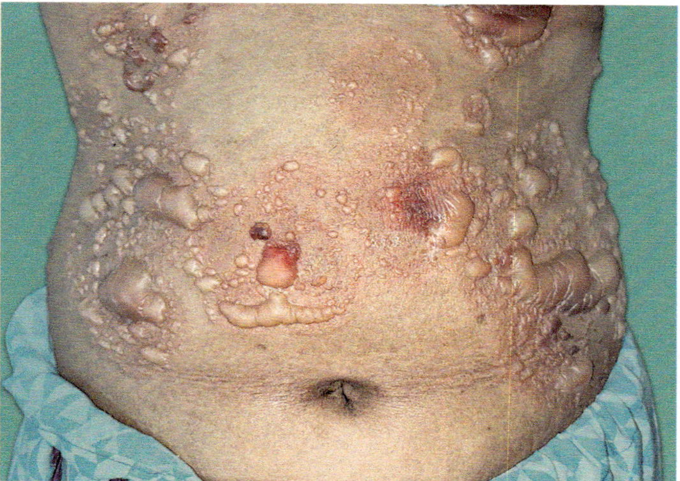

Fig. 8: Bullous systemic lupus erythematosus: Multiple tense vesicles and bullae, some containing hemorrhagic fluid over the abdomen. *Image courtesy*: Dr Manoj Nayak.

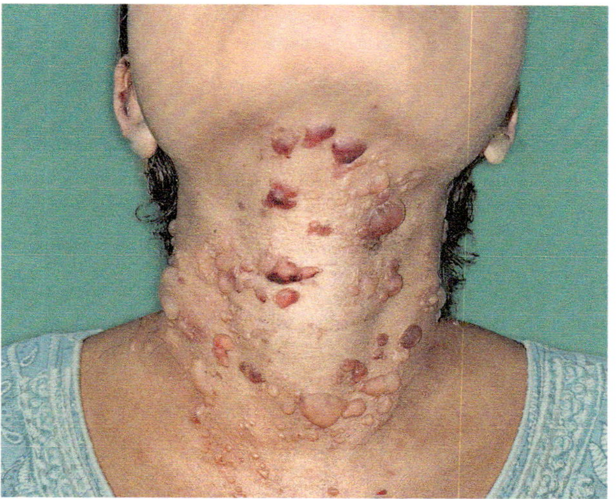

Fig. 9: Bullous systemic lupus erythematosus: Multiple tense vesicles and bullae, some containing hemorrhagic fluid over the neck. *Image courtesy: Dr Manoj Nayak.*

BSLE is classified into two types based on the target antigen:

1. *Type I BSLE*: Most common type; autoantibody is targeted against the 145-kDa amino-terminal NC1 domain and 34-kDa carboxyl-terminal NC2 domain of type VII collagen.
2. *Type II BSLE*: Autoantibodies are targeted against BP180, BP230, and laminin 5 or 6.

However, no clinical differences exist between the two types.

Diagnostic Criteria

These include:

- A pre-existing or new diagnosis of SLE
- Acute vesiculobullous eruption arising on but not limited to sun-exposed skin
- *Histopathology*: Subepidermal blistering, neutrophil-predominant infiltrate in the superficial dermis
- *DIF*: Linear IgG, IgM, C3 ± IgA deposition at the BMZ
- Evidence of antibodies to type VII collagen via DIF or IIF on salt-split skin, IB assay, immunoprecipitation, ELISA, or IEM

All five criteria should be fulfilled to diagnose type I BSLE, whereas only the first four criteria are needed for type II BSLE.

Diagnostic Modalities

- *Histopathology*: Subepidermal spilt with neutrophil-predominant inflammatory infiltrate, either in the dermal papillae (dermatitis herpetiformis-like) or distributed in a continuous band beneath the BMZ (linear IgA dermatosis-like). Leukocytoclasis is common, papillary tip "microabscesses" may be present. Mucin deposition in the dermis is present but basal cell vacuolization is absent.
- *DIF*: Linear continuous deposition of IgG and C3 at the DEJ, sometimes the fluorescence may be granular. IgM and IgA deposits are often seen. A "u-serrated" staining pattern is seen.
- *ELISA*: Serum autoantibodies detected by ELISA are against type VII collagen in type I BSLE and against BP 230, BP 180, or laminin 5 or 6 in type II BSLE.
- IB assay on dermal skin extract shows reactivity against the 290 kDa or 145 kDa antigens of type VII collagen.
- *Direct IEM*: Ig deposits are co-distributed with anchoring fibrils within and below the lamina densa.
- ANA positivity is usually seen and anti-dsDNA, anti-Sm, anti-Ro/SS-A, anti-La/SS-B, anticardiolipin antibodies may also be detected.
- Low levels of complement (C3, C4, CH50), anemia, leukopenia, thrombocytopenia, proteinuria or cellular casts (upon urinalysis), and elevated erythrocyte sedimentation rate (ESR) are usually detected.

Treatment

Dapsone at doses of 50–100 mg/day alone or in combination with prednisolone is the treatment of choice. For refractory disease, hydroxychloroquine, methotrexate, mycophenolate mofetil, colchicine or rituximab, with systemic glucocorticoids are given. Anakinra, an interleukin-1 receptor antagonist, has shown satisfactory results in some studies.

Prognosis

BSLE usually remits in about a year, irrespective of the activity of systemic disease.

The salient features of MMP, EBA and BSLE are summarized in **Table 1**.

CONCLUSION

MMP, anti-laminin 332 pemphigoid, EBA and BSLE are subepidermal AIBDs with varying degrees of mucocutaneous involvement, often healing with scarring and milia formation (except BSLE). A combination of histology, immunopathology and immunoblot assay help in diagnostic confirmation and differentiation of these entities. There is variable response to treatment in these dermatoses.

TAKE HOME MESSAGE

- MMP is a chronic, progressive, subepithelial immunobullous disease primarily involving the oral and ocular mucosae and less often other mucosae and skin. It is associated with functionally and psychologically debilitating scarring.
- Anti-laminin 332 pemphigoid is a rare variant of MMP characterized by a high-risk of predominantly solid organ malignancies.
- EBA is a rare, chronic disorder characterized by skin fragility and non-inflammatory/inflammatory tense bullae that heal with milia and scarring. Colchicine or dapsone is the first line of treatment.
- BSLE is a transient, vesiculobullous eruption occurring in the setting of SLE that heals with pigmentation but without milia or scarring. BSLE shows drastic improvement with dapsone.

TABLE 1: Clinical and diagnostic features in MMP, EBA, and bullous SLE.

Disease	Target antigens	Clinical features	HPE	DIF	Salt-split IIF	DIF pattern analysis
Mucous membrane pemphigoid (MMP)	• BP180 • Laminin 332 • BP230 • α6β4 integrin • Laminin 311 • Type VII collagen	• Tense blisters and erosions with scarring • *Predilection sites:* Mucosa of the mouth, eyes, nose, larynx, esophagus or anogenital region • *Anti-laminin 332 MMP:* Risk of malignancy	Subepidermal bulla with lymphocytes, histiocytes ± eosinophils, neutrophils in upper dermis	Linear IgG ± C3, occasionally IgA, IgM, fibrin at the dermo-epidermal junction	• *Anti-BP180 MMP:* Epidermal/roof pattern • *Anti-laminin 332 MMP:* Dermal/floor pattern	n-serrated
Epidermolysis bullosa acquisita (EBA)	Type VII collagen	• *Classical EBA:* Skin fragility, trauma-induced blisters and erosions *Predilection sites:* Extensors of extremities ± mucosa • *Inflammatory EBA:* Tense blisters on erythematous or normal appearing skin *Predilection sites:* Usually trunk, extremities ± mucosa	Subepidermal blister with a varied inflammatory infiltrate (non-/pauci-inflammatory in classic EBA, neutrophil-rich infiltrate with eosinophils or lymphocytes in inflammatory EBA)	Linear IgG and C3 (± IgA, IgM, properdin), at the dermo-epidermal junction	Dermal or floor pattern	u-serrated
Bullous SLE	• Type VII collagen • Others- BP180, BP230, laminin 5 or 6	Tense blisters on normal or erythematous skin, herpetiform arrangement in patients of SLE; frequently, oral lesions; pruritus severe; Predilection sites: Trunk, upper extremities, face and neck, and flexures	Subepidermal bulla with neutrophilic infiltrate	Linear or granular deposition of IgG (± IgM, IgA, C3) at the dermo-epidermal junction	Dermal (rarely epidermal or combined binding)	u-serrated

(EBA: epidermolysis bullosa acquisita; DIF: direct immunofluorescence; HPE: histopathological examination; IgG: immunoglobulin G; IIF: indirect immunofluorescence; SLE: systemic lupus erythematosus)

MULTIPLE CHOICE QUESTIONS

1. A 56-year-old caucasian man with anti-laminin 332 pemphigoid and extensive oral and nasal erosions as well as severe conjunctival involvement did not respond to intravenous dexamethasone-cyclophosphamide pulses combined with oral cyclophosphamide. Which of the following should be the next logical treatment option?
   (a) Mycophenolate mofetil
   (b) Rituximab
   (c) Dapsone
   (d) Oral prednisolone (1.5–2 mg/kg/day)

2. A 61-year-old man presents with burning and redness in the eyes since last 1 year. The patient also complains of occasional dysphagia and difficulty in micturition. On examination, there is a shortening of fornices of conjunctiva along with redness in bilateral eyes. Oral cavity revealed desquamative gingivitis. There is scarring in the genital mucosa. Histopathological evaluation of lesional skin reveals subepidermal bulla with lymphocytes and eosinophils. A direct immunofluorescence of the perilesional skin reveals linear deposits of IgG and C3 along the DEJ. A further pattern analysis of the DIF reveals an n-serrated pattern. Which of the following is the likely implicated antigen?
   (a) $\alpha6\beta4$ integrin
   (b) Laminin 332
   (c) BP180
   (d) Any of these

3. Consider the following options in the two columns and select the best match.

p. beta-4 integrin	(i) Bullous pemphigoid
q. alpha-6 integrin	(ii) MMP
r. C-terminus of BP180	(iii) Oral MMP
s. N-terminus of BP180	(iv) Ocular MMP

   (a) p (iii), q (iv), r (i), s (ii)
   (b) p (iv), q (iii), r (ii), s (i)
   (c) p (iii), q (iv), r (ii), s (i)
   (d) p (ii), q (iv), r (i), s (iii)

4. A 20-year-old female presents with tense bullae over her face, trunk, and upper extremities. She also has history of photosensitivity and joint pains in the past. Workup revealed ESR of 94 mm/h, antinuclear antibody titer of 1:1280, homogenous pattern. A biopsy of bullae is taken. Which is the most confirmatory histopathology finding?
   (a) Micropapillary neutrophilic abscesses in the upper dermis
   (b) Subepidermal blistering, neutrophilic infiltrate, mucin in the reticular dermis
   (c) Subepidermal blistering with lymphocytic infiltration
   (d) Epidermal blistering with eosinophilic infiltrate

5. Given the likely diagnosis in the above question, what is the most appropriate next step in evaluation?
   (a) Urine toxicology for illicit drug use
   (b) Serum transglutaminase-2/3 antibody testing
   (c) Urinalysis with 24-hour urinary protein estimation
   (d) Serially monitor antinuclear antibody titer

6. A 50-year-old female patient presents to the hospital with multiple tense bullae on her bilateral feet. DIF reveals IgG deposits distributed in a continuous, broad, linear pattern along the basement membrane zone. IIF salt-split skin shows circulating antibodies binding to the dermal side of the artificial blister. Which of the following is to be started?
   (a) Plasmapheresis
   (b) Colchicine
   (c) Rituximab
   (d) IV immunoglobulins

7. In salt-split skin preparations of perilesional skin, the immune deposits are typically located on the epidermal side of the cleavage in all, *except*:
   (a) Bullous pemphigoid
   (b) Cicatricial pemphigoid
   (c) Linear IgA bullous dermatosis
   (d) Epidermolysis bullosa acquisita

8. A u-serrated immune deposition pattern on direct immunofluorescence is seen in:
   (a) Bullous pemphigoid
   (b) Cicatricial pemphigoid
   (c) Linear IgA bullous dermatosis
   (d) Epidermolysis bullosa acquisita

9. Which is true regarding the anatomy of the basement membrane zone?
   (a) Anchoring fibrils are comprised of collagen VII
   (b) Lamina densa is composed of collagen XVII arranged in a lattice-like configuration
   (c) Laminin-332 is superficial to $\alpha6\beta4$ integrin
   (d) Anchoring plaques are present in the lamina lucida

10. Which of the following diagnostic modalities is available in most reference laboratories and can reliably distinguish bullous pemphigoid from epidermolysis bullosa acquisita?
   (a) Direct immunofluorescence
   (b) Indirect immunofluorescence with salt-split skin testing
   (c) Laser scanning confocal microscopy
   (d) Direct immunoelectron microscopy

Answers

1. (b)   2. (d)   3. (b)   4. (b)   5. (c)   6. (b)   7. (d)   8. (d)   9. (a)   10. (b)

SUGGESTED READING

1. Chan LS, Ahmed AR, Anhalt GJ, Bernauer W, Cooper KD, Elder MJ, *et al.* The first international consensus on mucous membrane pemphigoid: definition, diagnostic criteria, pathogenic factors, medical treatment, and prognostic indicators. *Arch Dermatol.* 2002;138:370-9.

2. Bruch-Gerharz D, Hertl M, Ruzicka T. Mucous membrane pemphigoid: clinical aspects, immunopathological features and therapy. *Eur J Dermatol.* 2007;17:191-200.

3. Li X, Qian H, Natsuaki Y, Koga H, Kawakami T, Tateishi C, *et al.* Clinical and immunological findings in 55 patients with anti-laminin 332-type mucous membrane pemphigoid. *Br J Dermatol.* 2021;185:449-51.

4. Lehman JS, Camilleri MJ, Gibson LE. Epidermolysis bullosa acquisita: concise review and practical considerations. *Int J Dermatol.* 2009;48:227-35.

5. Schmidt E, Zillikens D. Pemphigoid diseases. *Lancet.* 2013;381:320-32.

6. Kim JH, Kim YH, Kim SC. Epidermolysis bullosa acquisita: a retrospective clinical analysis of 30 cases. *Acta Derm Venereol.* 2011;91:307-12.

7. Iwata H, Vorobyev A, Koga H, Recke A, Zillikens D, Prost-Squarcioni C, *et al.* Meta-analysis of the clinical and immunopathological characteristics and treatment outcomes in epidermolysis bullosa acquisita patients. *Orphanet J Rare Dis.* 2018;13:153.

8. Yell JA, Allen J, Wojnarowska F, Kirtschig G, Burge SM. Bullous systemic lupus erythematosus: revised criteria for diagnosis. *Br J Dermatol.* 1995;132:921-8.

9. Grover C, Khurana A, Sharma S, Singal A. Bullous systemic lupus erythematosus. *Indian J Dermatol.* 2013;58:492.

10. Contestable JJ, Edhegard KD, Meyerle JH. Bullous systemic lupus erythematosus: a review and update to diagnosis and treatment. *Am J Clin Dermatol.* 2014;15:517-24.

Linear Immunoglobulin A Disease, Chronic Bullous Disease of Childhood, Dermatitis Herpetiformis

Chandana Shajil, Dharshini Sathishkumar, Minu Jose Chiramel

- Linear immunoglobulin A disease
- Chronic bullous disease of childhood
- Dermatitis herpetiformis
  - Epidemiology
  - Etiology and associated diseases
  - Pathophysiology
- Clinical features
- Investigations
- Differential diagnoses
- Treatment
- Complications and prognosis

INTRODUCTION

Linear immunoglobulin A (IgA) disease (LAD), chronic bullous disease of childhood (CBDC), and dermatitis herpetiformis (DH) are rare subepidermal autoimmune bullous diseases (sAIBDs) that exhibit dermal neutrophilic infiltration, show characteristic IgA reactivity on immunofluorescence studies and respond to treatment with dapsone. Due to their distinct co-morbidities and prognosis, it is important to differentiate these conditions and make a precise diagnosis. This chapter reviews their clinico-pathological features and management strategies.

LINEAR IMMUNOGLOBULIN A (IgA) DISEASE

LAD is a mildly pruritic vesiculobullous disorder with or without mucosal involvement, characterized by linear IgA deposits along the dermoepidermal junction (DEJ). Though the ectodomain of bullous pemphigoid 180 (BP180) is considered the primary target antigen, autoantibodies against other antigens of the DEJ are also reported. A similar condition, barring few clinical attributes, seen in infancy and childhood, designated CBDC, is discussed later in this chapter. Mixed immunobullous disease is a subset of LAD cases, characterized by equal IgA and IgG immunofluorescence at the DEJ.

Epidemiology

The incidence of LAD is 0.2–2.3 cases per million/year, and there is no racial or ethnic predilection. It usually affects adults, with a peak age of onset above 60 years, and with a marginally higher female preponderance in some studies.

Etiology and Associated Diseases

Various disease susceptibility loci including *human leukocyte antigen (HLA)-B8, Cw7, DR3, DR2*, and *tumor necrosis factor 2 (TNF2)* have been identified in adults.

Most cases of LAD are idiopathic. Several drugs, particularly antibiotics and non-steroidal anti-inflammatory drugs, are known to trigger LAD within a month of their initiation. Vancomycin is the most common offending agent, the others being penicillins, cephalosporins, sulfonamides, captopril, diclofenac, naproxen and phenytoin. Infections, trauma, vaccinations, and UV radiation have also been cited as inciting factors.

Lymphoproliferative disorders, solid organ malignancies, and inflammatory bowel disease (IBD) are systemic co-morbidities reported in conjunction with LAD. These along with the other lesser-known and unverified associations are enlisted in **Table 1**.

TABLE 1: Co-morbidities associated with linear immunoglobulin A (IgA) disease.

Classification of co-morbidities	Diseases
Gastrointestinal diseases	Ulcerative colitis, Crohn's disease
Malignancies	B-cell lymphoma, chronic lymphocytic leukemia, renal, bladder, esophagus, colon, breast, uterus, and thyroid cancer
Connective tissue disorders	Systemic lupus erythematosus, dermatomyositis, rheumatoid arthritis
Autoimmune diseases	Thyrotoxicosis, autoimmune hemolytic anemia, alopecia areata, autoimmune hepatitis, multiple sclerosis

Pathophysiology

An aberrant humoral and cellular immune response is central to the pathogenesis of LAD. Circulating IgA autoantibodies, specifically the IgA1 subclass, are directed against the components of DEJ. It is proposed that drugs act as haptens, modifying the native proteins of the DEJ or dermis, leading to disruption of immune tolerance and production of autoantibodies. In LAD patients who also suffer from IBD, the inflamed bowel is hypothesized to produce IgA1 autoantibodies.

The two main antigens are the 97kDa (LABD97) and 120kDa proteins (LAD-1), located on the ectodomain of BP180, the key transmembrane protein maintaining DEJ integrity. Over the years, IgA autoantibodies targeting BP180 non-collagenous 16A (NC16A) domain, BP230, type VII collagen, a 285kDa protein (LAD 285), laminin 332, and p200 have been recognized. Identification of more than one target antigen in a patient may be explained by epitope spreading. Depending on the location of autoantibodies on immune electron microscopy or indirect immunofluorescence (IIF), LAD can either be of lamina lucida-type, sublamina densa-type, or both. The binding of circulating antibodies along the DEJ is postulated to trigger an inflammatory cascade leading to neutrophil chemotaxis and dermal-epidermal split due to the proteolytic enzymes released by inflammatory cells.

Clinical Features

The classical presentation includes tense bullae and vesicles, with variable pruritus, arising on normal-appearing or inflamed skin, and urticated plaques, developing on the trunk and extremities **(Fig. 1)**. Their arrangement in an

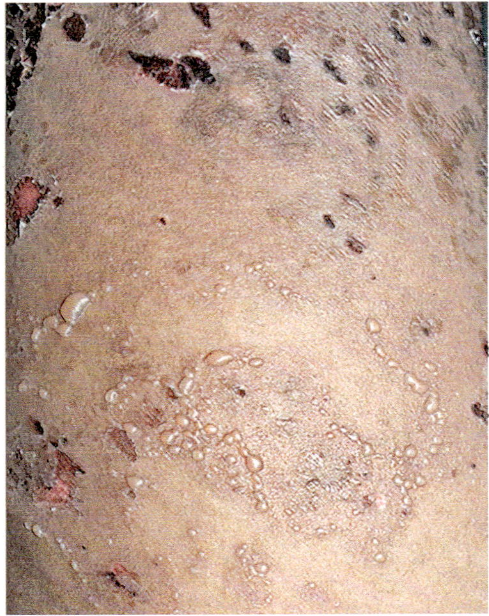

Fig. 1: Linear immunoglobulin A (IgA) disease: Multiple vesicles in an annular configuration and erosions on the trunk. *Image courtesy:* Dr Sujay Khandpur.

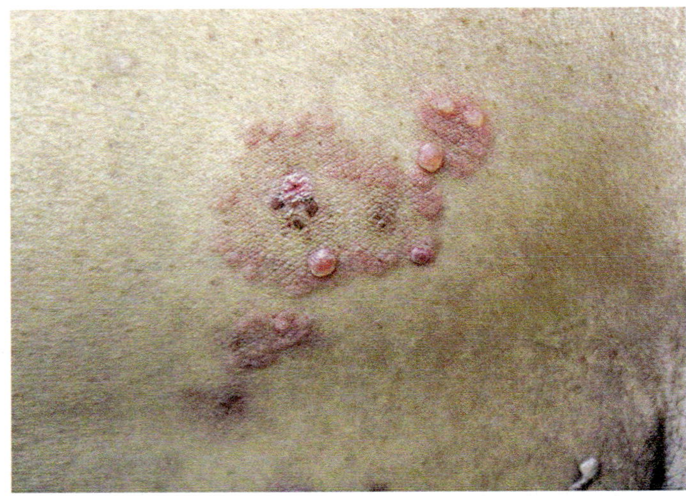

Fig. 2: Linear immunoglobulin A (IgA) disease: Vesicles located along the periphery of a resolving lesion with annular configuration, giving a "string of pearls" appearance.

annular configuration is a striking feature of LAD, termed the "string of pearls", "crown of jewels", or "cluster of jewels" sign **(Fig. 2)**. They subsequently form erosions that usually heal without scarring. Unlike BP, mucosal erosions/ulcers are commonly seen in 70% of cases. Oral cavity is often affected, with rare involvement of the ocular, nasal, genital, pharyngeal, laryngeal, esophageal, and anal mucosa. Within the oral cavity, palatal and buccal mucosal erosions are more frequent, and erosive gingivitis and cheilitis may also occur. Redness of the eyes, discharge, pain, and foreign body sensation are the common complaints with eye involvement.

Morphological variants of LAD include toxic epidermal necrolysis (TEN)-like, prurigo-like, urticarial or erythema multiforme-like presentation. TEN-like presentation is a severe form of the disease, often triggered by vancomycin. Extensive disease, large skin erosions, atypical presentation, a positive Nikolsky sign, focal necrotic keratinocytes and dermal eosinophilic infiltrate on histopathology, and C3 deposits at the DEJ on direct immunofluorescence (DIF) are largely encountered in drug-induced LAD. Mucosal involvement and detectable circulating autoantibodies are comparatively uncommon in the drug-induced variant.

Investigations

- *Tzanck smear*: Predominantly neutrophils are seen.
- *Histopathology*: In biopsy obtained from an intact vesicle, subepidermal blister with predominant neutrophilic infiltrate in the blister cavity, papillary dermis and in perivascular location is seen. The dermal neutrophilic collections may form papillary microabscesses, resembling DH. Additional dermal infiltration of eosinophils may present a BP-like picture. However, the "line up" of neutrophils at the basement membrane is a histopathological pointer in favor of LAD.
- *DIF*: Linear IgA deposit along DEJ is the characteristic feature. Though weak positivity for IgG, IgM, and C3 is common in LAD, the occasional co-existence, in

equal strength of both IgA and IgG, can complicate an otherwise straightforward diagnosis. These cases of linear IgA/IgG bullous dermatosis or mixed immuno-bullous disease likely represent an overlap between LAD and BP. There are conflicting opinions about its categorization under LAD or BP. Drug-induced LAD may give a false negative DIF.

- *Detection of serum autoantibodies*: IIF using monkey esophagus or 1 M NaCl-split human skin can be employed to screen for autoantibodies, both from serum and blister fluid. IIF using salt-split skin has greater sensitivity, and the binding pattern, i.e., autoantibody binding to the epidermal (roof pattern) or dermal side (floor pattern), forms the basis of its classification into the lamina lucida-type and sublamina densa-type of LAD. The autoantibodies are directed against LAD-1, LABD97, BP180 NC16A domain, and BP230 in the lamina lucida-type (roof pattern), whereas type VII collagen, laminin 332, and p200 are the target antigens in sublamina densa-type (floor pattern). Both epidermal and dermal binding pattern is exhibited by autoantibodies against LAD285. Most of the positive cases are of lamina-lucida type, with a mixed pattern also known to occur.
- Assays such as IgA enzyme-linked immunosorbent assay (ELISA) and immunoblot are rarely used as diagnostic adjuncts, especially when histology and DIF yield ambiguous results. However, positive results are more common in CBDC than in LAD.

Differential Diagnoses

LAD cases with overlapping features of BP, epidermolysis bullosa acquisita (EBA), or mucous membrane pemphigoid (MMP) may be encountered. Stevens–Johnson syndrome (SJS), TEN, acute generalized exanthematous pustulosis (AGEP), bullous fixed drug eruption (FDE), and erythema multiforme are other differentials that may be considered in the context of a drug etiology.

Treatment

LAD usually responds well to standard treatment. Pharmacotherapy of LAD is as follows:
- Dapsone (0.5–3 mg/kg) is regarded as the first-line treatment. It is used alone or combined with other topical or systemic agents, based on the clinical response.
- Prednisolone at a low dose of 0.25–0.5 mg/kg can be administered initially for rapid control.
- Sulfapyridine (15–60 mg/kg/day) and sulfamethoxypyridazine (1,000–1,500 mg/day) are alternatives to dapsone that are less toxic and do not require strict monitoring.
- Antibiotics such as tetracycline, doxycycline, dicloxacillin, erythromycin and trimethoprim–sulfamethoxazole, and anti-inflammatory agents such as colchicine and nicotinamide have been found useful in patients intolerant to dapsone or sulfa drugs.
- Superpotent topical corticosteroids are combined with systemic agents or used as monotherapy for localized or limited disease. Similarly, topical tacrolimus is a therapeutic adjunct that may reduce the requirement for systemic treatment.
- Other modalities such as cyclosporine, methotrexate, azathioprine, mycophenolate mofetil, cyclophosphamide, IVIg, immunoadsorption, rituximab, or etanercept are reserved for refractory cases.

Drug-induced LAD is known to improve as early as 4–8 weeks after stopping the inciting drug. Remission following colectomy was noted in a case with ulcerative colitis.

Complications and Prognosis

Skin lesions heal with pigmentary changes; but scarring and milia formation due to secondary infection may occur. Mucosal disease, particularly of the eyes, is prone to scarring with disastrous outcomes such as adhesions, symblepharon, and sometimes blindness. Rarely, pharyngeal, laryngeal, or esophageal strictures add to the morbidity. IgA nephropathy is an extremely rare but serious complication. Complete recovery of nephropathy following withdrawal of the culprit drug may occur in drug-induced cases.

The disease has an unpredictable course that may last for months to years. *TNF2* allele is associated with a longer disease duration and poor prognosis. Gottlieb, *et al*, have suggested age <70 years and mucosal involvement as indicators of chronic disease. After achieving clinical remission, maintenance treatment is necessary for several weeks as the disease may relapse. Symptomatic improvement or disease remission observed during pregnancy may be followed by relapses in the postpartum period. Drug-induced LAD carries a better prognosis, with complete recovery upon drug withdrawal.

CHRONIC BULLOUS DISEASE OF CHILDHOOD

CBDC or LAD of childhood is the most common AIBD in children. CBDC is similar to LAD in terms of its broad clinical picture, pathogenesis, immunogenetics, immunopathology, and management. Linear IgA deposition at the DEJ is the diagnostic feature; however, "mixed immunobullous disease of childhood", characterized by mixed IgA and IgG positivity, represents a discrete immunopathological group.

Epidemiology

CBDC is typically seen among preschool children, with an average age of onset between 4 and 5 years. Neonatal cases are rare, with blistering seen even at birth. There is no definite gender or ethnic predilection.

Etiology and Associated Diseases

Genetic susceptibility in CBDC is linked to *HLA-B8, DR3, DQ2, Cw7,* and *TNF2* alleles. Though largely idiopathic, bacterial and viral infections, vaccinations, antibiotics, and non-steroidal anti-inflammatory drugs were thought to trigger the disease in some reports. Unlike LAD, drug-induced CBDC is rare. We have encountered a case of neonatal CBDC following vancomycin use in our center.

CBDC, like LAD, is associated with IBD and autoimmune lymphoproliferative syndrome. The lack of substantial evidence of its association with lymphoproliferative disorders or malignancies could be attributed to the young age of disease onset.

Pathophysiology

The pathogenesis of CBDC is similar to LAD.

Clinical Features

Since CBDC is the childhood variant of adult-onset LAD, overall presentation remains the same. The disease has an abrupt onset of tense polymorphic blisters and erosions, with or without pruritus, occurring on normal to erythematous skin, with lesions initially appearing on the perianal region, perineum and lower abdomen, and later spreading to the buttocks **(Fig. 3)**, thighs **(Figs. 4 and 5)**, and other parts of the body including the trunk **(Fig. 6)** and extremities **(Fig. 7)**. Facial, particularly perioral involvement, and annular or polycyclic blistering showing the "string of pearls" or "cluster of jewels" sign, is more frequent and prominent in CBDC **(Figs. 8 to 11)**. CBDC has a variable incidence of mucosal disease; neonatal cases usually have mucosal involvement.

Investigations

The findings in CBDC are similar to LAD.

Differential Diagnoses

CBDC may be occasionally confused with herpes infection, epidermolysis bullosa, and infection-induced erythema multiforme.

Treatment

Treatment is similar to LAD. Dapsone (0.5–2 mg/kg/day) with or without systemic steroids, is most frequently used. Tetracycline and doxycycline cannot be administered to children <8 years of age as they produce permanent teeth discoloration. In a survey conducted by Farrant, *et al*, erythromycin combined with other systemic agents was found to be beneficial, though as monotherapy, it failed to sustain the clinical response. Rituximab administered as 375 mg/m^2/dose, two doses 2 weeks apart, has been found effective in refractory cases.

Complications and Prognosis

The complications discussed under LAD are rarely encountered in CBDC. In neonatal cases, mucosal disease is common, often leading to serious complications such as airway compromise, feeding difficulties, and blindness.

Spontaneous remission often occurs by 2 years from disease onset or by 6–8 years of age, with the majority recovering by adolescence. However, it may rarely persist into adulthood. *TNF2* allele is associated with longer disease duration and poorer prognosis.

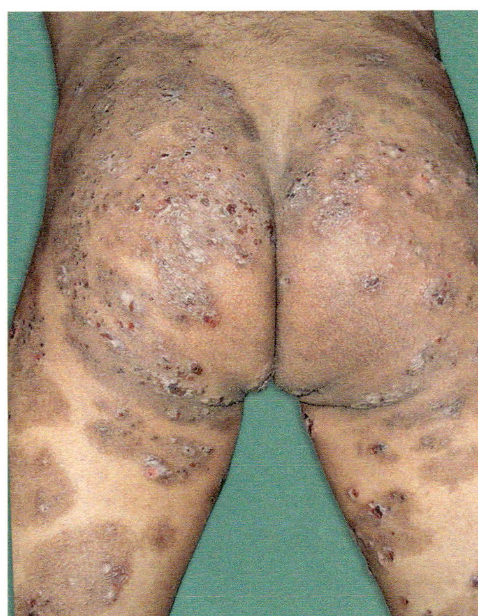

Fig. 3: Chronic bullous disease of childhood: Blisters in annular configuration in perianal area, buttocks, and upper thighs. *Image courtesy*: Dr Sujay Khandpur.

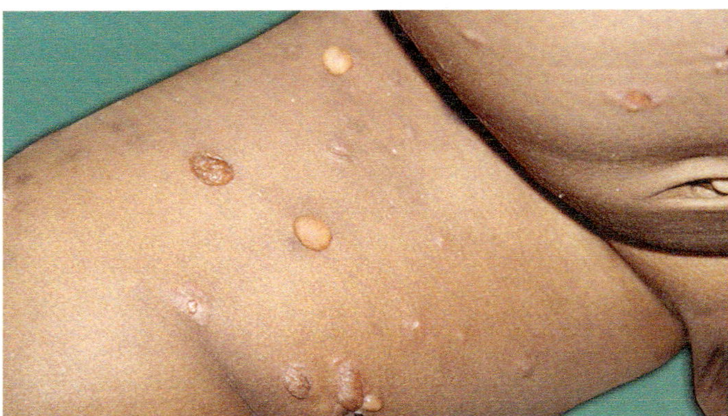

Fig. 4: Chronic bullous disease of childhood: Multiple tense and ruptured bullae on the thigh.

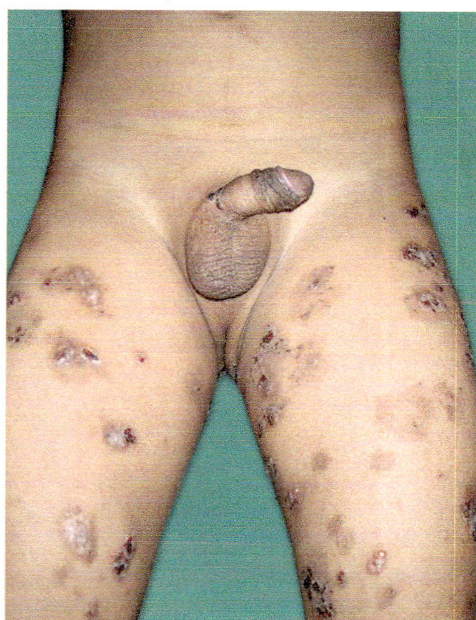

Fig. 5: Chronic bullous disease of childhood: Multiple crusted plaques and vesicles on both thighs and penis. *Image courtesy*: Dr Sujay Khandpur.

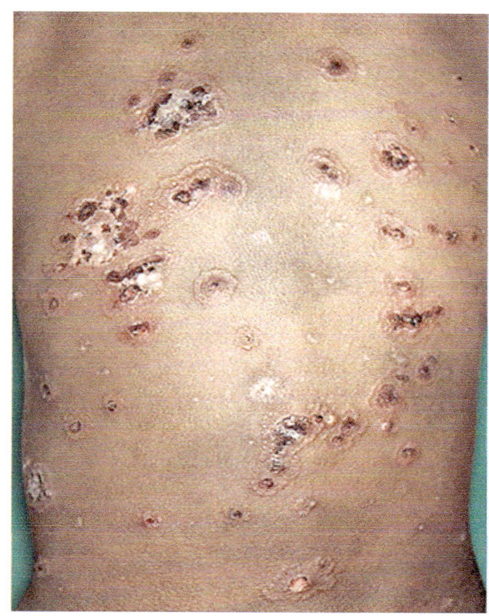

Fig. 6: Chronic bullous disease of childhood: Vesicles arranged in an annular pattern on the trunk.

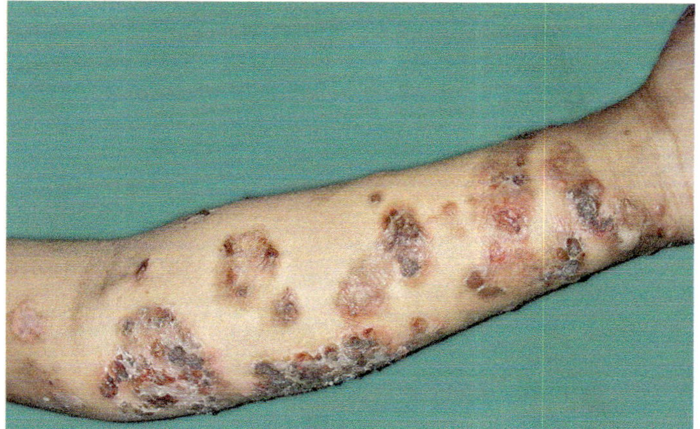

Fig. 7: Chronic bullous disease of childhood: Multiple annular plaques with peripheral vesiculation on left forearm. *Image courtesy*: Dr Sujay Khandpur.

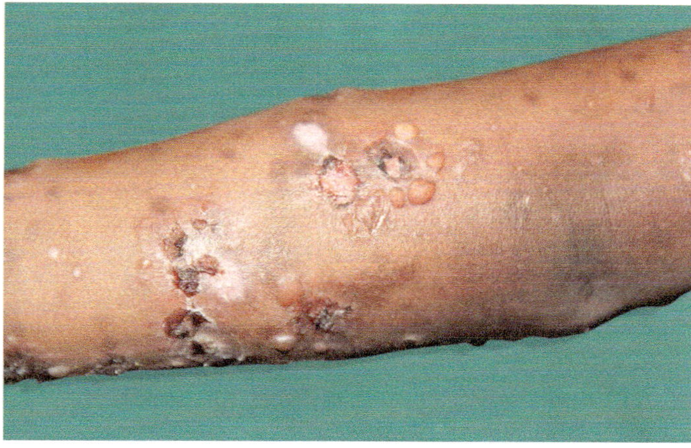

Fig. 8: Chronic bullous disease of childhood: Vesicles on forearm showing "string of pearls" arrangement.

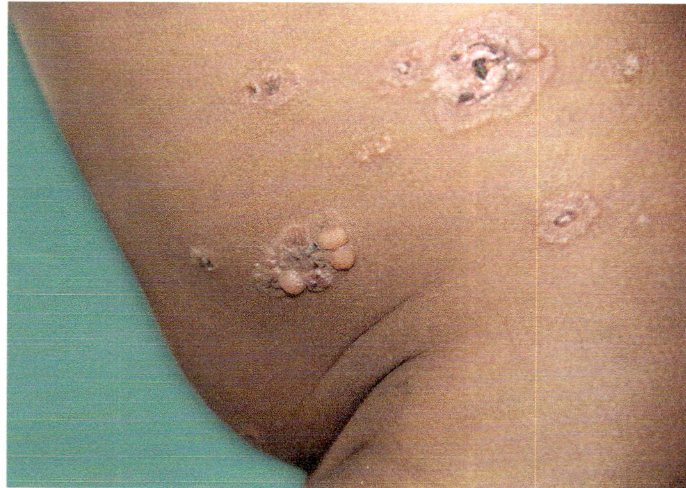

Fig. 9: Chronic bullous disease of childhood: Vesicles on lower abdomen showing "string of pearls" arrangement.

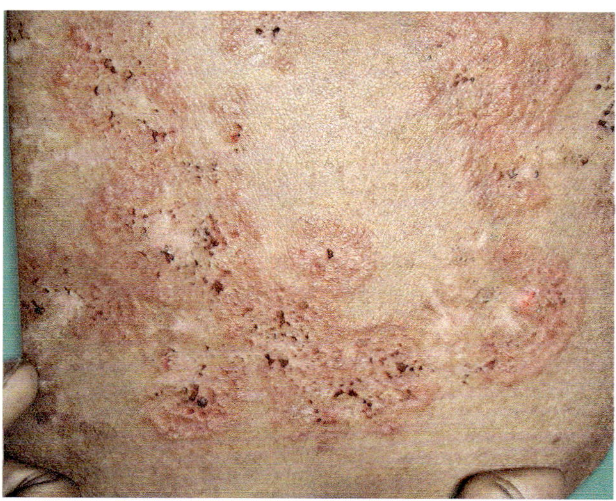

Fig. 10: Chronic bullous disease of childhood: Multiple annular and polycyclic lesions with peripheral vesiculation. *Image courtesy*: Dr Sujay Khandpur.

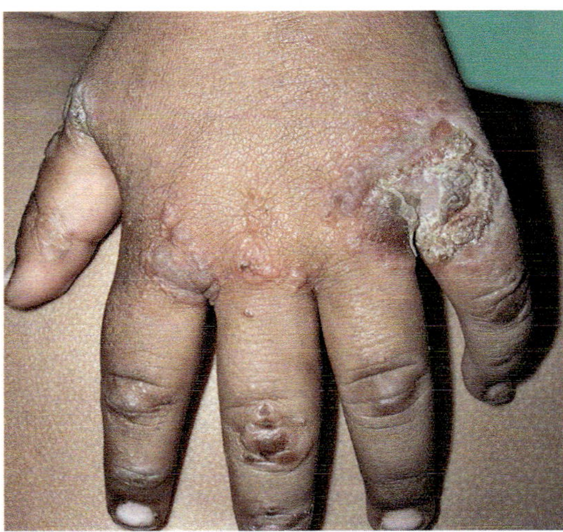

Fig. 11: Chronic bullous disease of childhood: Vesicles in an annular configuration on the dorsum of hand. *Image courtesy*: Dr Sujay Khandpur.

DERMATITIS HERPETIFORMIS

DH or Duhring–Brocq disease is a chronic, pruritic condition often accompanied by gluten-sensitive enteropathy (GSE) or celiac disease of variable severity. The characteristic granular IgA deposits in the papillary dermis target epidermal transglutaminase.

Epidemiology

The disease usually occurs during the fourth decade of life, though any age group can be affected. Pediatric and elderly cases are seldom encountered. Unlike GSE, which is more common in women, DH shows a male predilection with male to female ratio of 1.5:1 to 2:1. It is common among Caucasians, with incidence ranging from 0.4 to 3.5 per 1,00,000 people/year. It is rare in Africans and Asians, who lack the predisposing genes. Recent studies from Europe have noted a decrease in the incidence of DH as opposed to GSE. The highest prevalence of DH, reported in a 40-year prospective study from Finland was 75 per 1,00,000 population. In a retrospective study from north India by Handa, *et al*, DH constituted 9.47% of immunobullous diseases. The mean age of onset was 40.9 ± 16.39 years, with a male to female ratio of 1.4:1.

Etiology and Associated Diseases

HLA-DQ2 and *HLA-DQ8* alleles predispose to both DH and GSE.

DH has a strong association with GSE, with almost 90% of cases having some degree of enteropathy. However, this association appears to be weaker in Asians. Autoimmune disorders such as autoimmune thyroid disease (4.3%) and type 1 diabetes mellitus (T1DM) (2.3%) are more commonly associated compared to pernicious anemia, vitiligo, Addison's disease, myasthenia gravis, and connective tissue disorders. In the study by Handa, *et al*, only 24% of DH patients had endoscopic biopsy-proven GSE and 23% had

associated autoimmune co-morbidities. DH was also found to increase the risk of developing BP; hence, BP should be considered in a DH patient who develops large bullae and becomes unresponsive to a gluten-free diet (GFD).

Pathophysiology

Dietary gluten intolerance is an important aspect of both DH and GSE pathogenesis. Epidermal transglutaminase (TG3), the major target antigen of DH synthesized by the keratinocytes and found in both epidermis and dermis, is homologous to tissue transglutaminase (TG2), the target antigen of GSE. Gliadin, the key antigenic component of gluten, is deaminated by TG2 in the intestinal mucosa, contributing to its immunogenicity. Deaminated gliadin binds to HLA-DQ2 and HLA-DQ8 on antigen-presenting cells. T- and B-cell mediated immune response against the altered gliadin leads to inflammation, with subsequent tissue damage and production of autoantibodies, respectively. As a result of epitope spreading, autoantibodies against multiple antigens including gliadin, TG2, TG3, and endomysium (tissue covering the smooth muscle of the digestive tract) can be found in blood. It is theorized that circulating IgA anti-TG3 autoantibodies or the antigen-antibody complex get deposited in the dermis, resulting in inflammation, neutrophil migration, and proteolytic cleavage at the DEJ. However, this requires further clarification.

Clinical Features

Typically, intensely pruritic, erythematous, grouped or herpetiform papules, vesicles, erosions, and excoriations are symmetrically distributed over the extensor aspect of elbows **(Figs. 12A and B)**, knees **(Figs. 13A and B)**, scalp, back especially the sacral area, and buttocks. A generalized, extensive rash may be seen in severe cases. The paucity of intact vesicles on examination can be attributed to the severe pruritus experienced by these patients. Hence, DH must be considered in an undiagnosed or treatment-refractory pruritic rash. Lesions may heal with dyspigmentation, rarely producing scarring.

Oral mucosal burning, erythema, vesiculation, and erosions and palmoplantar purpura are rare presentations. Acral purpuric lesions and petechiae, especially digital purpura, are sometimes the early manifestation of DH that may be detected only by dermoscopy. Other uncommon cutaneous manifestations include isolated facial lesions, extensive macular lesions, leukocytoclastic vasculitis-like, urticaria-like, or prurigo-like lesions, and palmoplantar keratosis. Dental enamel defects such as pits, horizontal grooves, and discoloration are shared features of GSE and DH.

Gastrointestinal involvement: Approximately one-third of the patients may complain of abdominal symptoms such as bloating, nausea, abdominal pain, diarrhea, constipation, and weight loss due to associated GSE. In 75–90% of the patients, small bowel mucosal biopsy may show normal villous architecture with just intraepithelial lymphocytes to

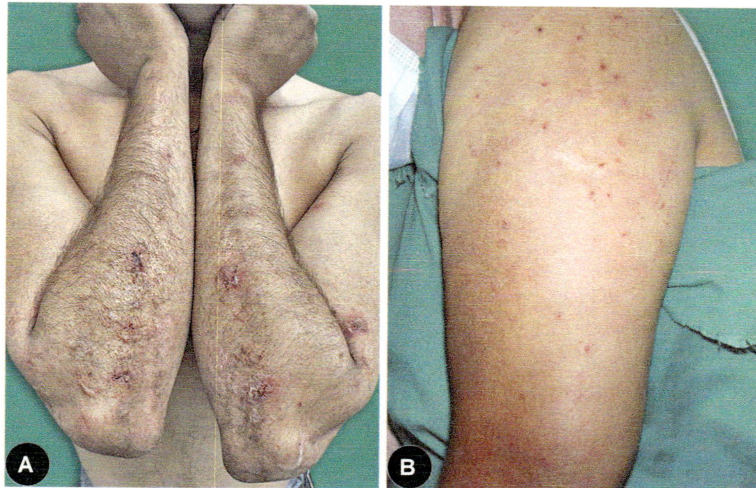

Figs. 12A and B: (A) Dermatitis herpetiformis: Grouped vesicles and erosions on erythematous base around elbows. *Image courtesy*: Dr Vinay Keshavamurthy. (B) Dermatitis herpetiformis: Multiple excoriations and crusted papules on erythematous base on left arm in a patient with celiac disease. *Image courtesy*: Dr Sujay Khandpur.

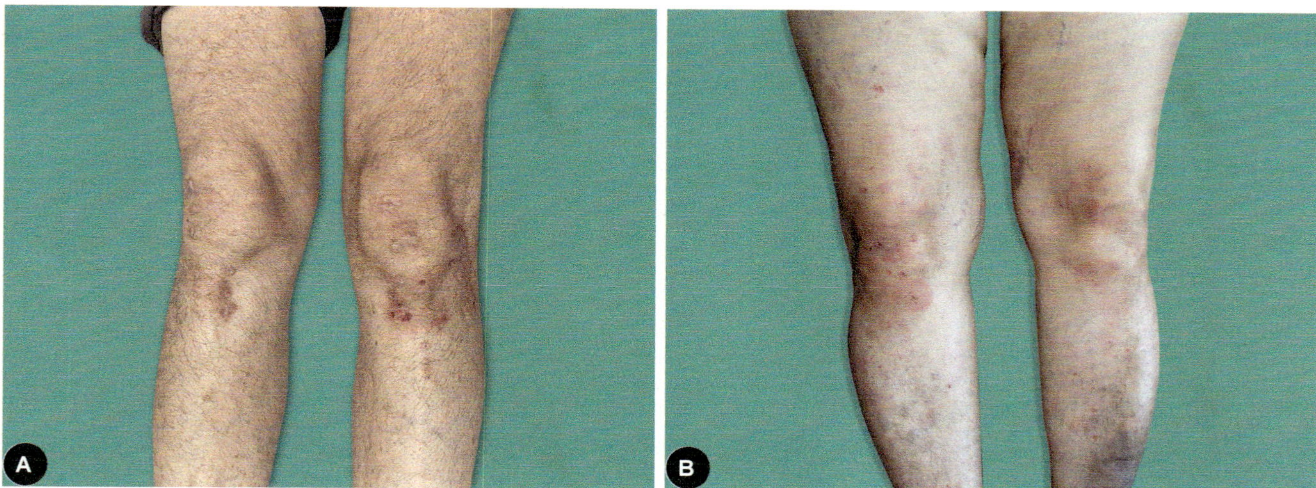

Figs. 13A and B: (A) Dermatitis herpetiformis: Grouped erosions and post-inflammatory hypopigmentation on knees. Image courtesy: Dr Vinay Keshavamurthy. (B) Dermatitis herpetiformis: Multiple vesicles and excoriations on erythematous base on both knees in a patient with celiac disease. *Image courtesy*: Dr Sujay Khandpur.

crypt hyperplasia, and villous atrophy. However, it is neither mandatory for diagnosis nor routinely done in DH.

Iodide exposure due to ingestion of certain foods, medications, or topical application can cause worsening of disease; whereas, smoking tobacco may improve the symptoms.

Investigations

- On Tzanck smear, predominantly neutrophils are seen.
- *Histopathology*: It shows small, focal, subepidermal blister or collection of fibrin, with neutrophilic infiltrate at the tips of dermal papillae forming papillary microabscesses. Early lesions show only neutrophils ± eosinophils in the dermal papilla and older lesions reveal subepidermal vesiculation coalescing into multiloculated bulla-containing inflammatory cells and fibrin.

- *DIF*: It demonstrates granular or fibrillar (particularly in Asians) IgA deposits in the dermal papillae and/or granular IgA deposits at the DEJ. Besides IgA, other immunoreactants such as IgM, C3, and IgG may also be detected. DIF may yield negative result in patients following a strict gluten-free diet (GFD), whereas pharmacotherapy does not affect DIF result.

- *Serology*: It is done to detect IgA antibodies against TG2, TG3, and endomysium in the patient's serum. Given its high sensitivity, ELISA for anti-TG2 IgA antibody is the commonly performed screening test for both DH and GSE. ELISA for anti-TG3 IgA antibody has comparable sensitivity; but like the aforementioned test, it is not

119

specific for DH and also not easily available. Although immunofluorescence-based antiendomysial antibody test has high specificity, it is tedious, expensive, and not commonly done. Though selective IgA deficiency is not as common in DH as in celiac disease, it should be ruled out when serology is negative. IgG-based assays are useful in such patients. At least one serological test should be performed in suspected cases. It is an important diagnostic tool when DIF cannot be performed or is repeatedly negative, and to monitor response to dietary restriction. However, DH cannot be excluded purely based on negative serology results.

- *Iodide sensitivity*: Iodine exposure leads to DH flare by an unknown mechanism. Detection of iodine intolerance by the iodine patch test or iodine oral challenge test was a diagnostic tool used by clinicians before the advent of DIF. Patch testing with 50% potassium iodide in petrolatum for 24 hours provokes erythema and blistering, with histological features of DH.

The diagnostic criteria published in the consensus statement by European Academy of Dermatology and Venereology (EADV) are as follows: major criteria include clinical features compatible with DH, and DIF positivity. Minor criteria include histology compatible with DH, at least one positive serology test, evidence of celiac disease on duodenal biopsy, HLA testing compatible with DH, positive iodine patch test or oral iodine challenge, rapid response to dapsone and response to long-term gluten-free diet. Two major criteria, or typical clinical features with combination of minor criteria suggests DH.

Given its close association with GSE, a gastroenterologist's opinion should be sought. Patients should be tested for diabetes mellitus, thyroid, and other autoimmune disorders as appropriate.

Differential Diagnoses

Other itchy dermatoses such as scabies, insect bite hypersensitivity, and eczema may be indistinguishable from DH.

Treatment

A lifelong GFD is an integral part of the management of DH and associated GSE. Alone, it brings about only gradual improvement of both skin and gastrointestinal disease. Nevertheless, dietary restriction is the long-term treatment option, which not only maintains disease remission after withdrawal of pharmacotherapy, but also reduces the risk of lymphoma. Its impact on associated autoimmune diseases however is unclear. Wheat, barley, and rye contain gluten. Wheat products such as breads, pastas, and baked products, cereals, soups, sauces, and processed food should be avoided. Fresh fruits and vegetables, poultry, meat, seafood, dairy, legumes, and nuts are naturally gluten-free.

Grains such as rice, millet, corn, sorghum, certified gluten-free oats, and starchy foods such as potato and tapioca can be consumed. Due to high lipid, sugar, and salt content, GFD increases cardiometabolic risk. Hence, a dietician's consultation is essential to plan a strict GFD.

The addition of the following therapeutics to GFD ensures faster recovery:

- Dapsone is considered the treatment of choice (started at 25–50 mg/day and gradually increased to a maximum of 300 mg/day) as it produces remarkable improvement, with pruritus subsiding in 72 hours and skin lesions clearing within days.
- Other sulfonamide drugs such as sulfamethoxy-pyridazine (0.25–1.5 g daily), sulfapyridine (1–2 g/day), and sulfasalazine (1–4 g/day) are alternate treatment options.
- When sulfa drugs are contraindicated, ineffective or not tolerated, anti-inflammatory agents such as colchicine (0.5–2.5 mg/day) or tetracycline (500 mg four times a day) with nicotinamide (500 mg thrice a day), can be administered.
- Immunosuppressive agents such as azathioprine, methotrexate, mycophenolate mofetil, and rituximab have also been found useful in some reports. Cyclosporine is not recommended because of the requirement of a dangerously high dose.

Potent topical steroids may be used to ameliorate pruritus, but systemic steroids are ineffective in DH. Following improvement, medication can be slowly tapered to a minimum maintenance dose and eventually withdrawn, while continuing on GFD.

Complications and Prognosis

DH is a chronic disease with lifelong relapses and remissions; spontaneous remission is rare. A GFD is paramount to sustain remission off all systemic therapy, improve the quality of life and protect against lymphoma. Patients unresponsive to several years of GFD, known as refractory DH, constitute 2% of the cases and carry a poor prognosis.

Complications due to associated GSE include malabsorption leading to anemia, osteoporosis, weight loss, short stature, and rarely extraintestinal co-morbidities such as liver disease, nephropathy, ataxia, neuropathy, and infertility. DH patients are at a greater risk of gastrointestinal malignancies, including non-Hodgkin lymphoma during the first 5 years following diagnosis. Owing to a common genetic background of DH and GSE, the first-degree relatives of patients suffering from either of the two conditions are prone to both these diseases and must be screened.

The clinico-pathological characteristics and management of LAD, CBDC and DH are summarized in **Table 2**.

TABLE 2: Clinico-pathological characteristics and management of LAD, CBDC, and DH.

	Linear IgA disease (LAD)	Chronic bullous disease of childhood (CBDC)	Dermatitis herpetiformis (DH)
Age	Above 60 years	4–5 years	30–40 years
Gender (Male:Female)	Slight female preponderance	No gender predilection	1.5:1 to 2:1
Autoantigen(s)	• *Major*: LABD97 and LAD-1 • *Others*: BP180 NC16A domain, BP230, type VII collagen, LAD 285, laminin 332, p200	Same as LAD	TG3
Clinical features	• *Lesions*: Tense bullae, vesicles, urticated plaques, erosions • *Common sites*: Trunk, extremities, oral mucosa • *Pruritus*: +/–	• *Lesions*: Tense bullae, vesicles, urticated plaques, erosions • *Common sites*: Periorificial, perineum, lower trunk, face, limbs • *Pruritus*: +/–	• *Lesions*: Grouped papulo-vesicles, erosions, excoriations • *Common sites*: Extensor aspect of elbows, knees, back, and buttocks Oral mucosa involvement rare • *Pruritus*: Severe
Triggers/exacerbating factors	Drugs (especially vancomycin), infections, trauma, vaccinations, UV radiation	Drugs, infections, vaccinations	Gluten-containing diet, iodide exposure through food, medications, or topical application
Common associations	Lymphoproliferative disorders, solid organ malignancies, IBD	IBD	Celiac disease, autoimmune thyroid disease, type 1 diabetes mellitus (T1DM)
Histopathology	Subepidermal blister with neutrophils ± eosinophils in papillary dermis	Same as LAD	Subepidermal blister, dermal neutrophilic infiltrate forming papillary-tip microabscesses
DIF	Linear IgA along DEJ	Same as LAD	Granular IgA in dermal papillae and/or DEJ
Serology	Serum IgA autoantibodies bind to DEJ on IIF using monkey esophagus or 1 M NaCl-split human skin	Same as LAD	ELISA for IgA anti-TG2 antibody, IgA anti-TG3 antibody (when available)
First-line treatment	Dapsone ± systemic steroid	Same as LAD	Gluten-free diet + dapsone
Alternate treatment	Sulfapyridine, sulfamethoxypyridazine, colchicine, doxycycline, erythromycin, nicotinamide, immunosuppressants	Same as in LAD, tetracycline and doxycycline are avoided	Sulfamethoxypyridazine, sulfapyridine, sulfasalazine
Prognosis	Chronic course when age <70 years and mucosal involvement; usually requires prolonged treatment for months to years except in drug-induced LAD	Spontaneous remission in 2 years	Chronic disease with relapses and remissions; strict gluten-free diet improves prognosis
Major complications	Conjunctival scarring and adhesions, blindness; pharyngeal, laryngeal, esophageal strictures	Complications as in LAD, frequent in neonatal cases	Small bowel lymphoma, complications linked to malabsorption

(DEJ: dermoepidermal junction; DIF: direct immunofluorescence; ELISA: enzyme-linked immunosorbent assay; IBD: inflammatory bowel disease; IgA: immunoglobulin A; IIF: indirect immunofluorescence; TG2: tissue transglutaminase; TG3: epidermal transglutaminase; UV: ultraviolet)

CONCLUSION

LAD, CBDC, and DH are subepidermal immunobullous diseases characterized by papillary dermal neutrophilic infiltration with dermo-epidermal split on histopathology, and IgA positivity on DIF. Dapsone is considered the treatment of choice in all three conditions. Besides pharmacotherapy, a lifelong GFD is a crucial part of DH management.

TAKE HOME MESSAGE

- LAD, CBDC, and DH are sAIBDs with autoantibodies directed against proteins located at the DEJ or dermis, leading to papillary dermal neutrophilic infiltration and dermoepidermal split.
- Exclusive or predominant linear IgA deposits are seen along the DEJ in LAD and CBDC, whereas, granular or fibrillar papillary dermal deposits of IgA are characteristic of DH.

- LAD and CBDC are now considered a single entity due to their similar clinicopathological features, lacking any major differences.
- A subset of LAD cases having equally mixed linear deposits of IgA and IgG at the DEJ are labeled as linear IgA/IgG bullous dermatosis or mixed immunobullous disease. LAD cases with overlapping clinical and immunopathological features of BP, EBA or MMP may be encountered, making a precise diagnosis difficult.
- Dapsone produces remarkable improvement and is the preferred treatment in all the three conditions.
- Owing to the strong association of DH with GSE, GFD forms a crucial part of its treatment.

MULTIPLE CHOICE QUESTIONS

1. Which of the following drugs commonly triggers LAD?
 (a) Co-amoxiclav
 (b) Penicillin
 (c) Phenytoin
 (d) Vancomycin

2. Which is the major target antigen of LAD?
 (a) BP180 NC16A domain
 (b) 120 kDa protein on the ectodomain of BP180
 (c) BP230
 (d) Type VII collagen

3. Which is true regarding CBDC?
 (a) The 'string of pearls' sign is rarely seen
 (b) Perineum and perioral involvement are prominent features
 (c) It is frequently associated with lymphoproliferative disorders
 (d) It has a long disease duration

4. Which medication is not used in the treatment of CBDC?
 (a) Colchicine
 (b) Dapsone
 (c) Doxycycline
 (d) Erythromycin

5. Which MHC gene is strongly associated with DH?
 (a) *HLA-B8*
 (b) *HLA-Cw7*
 (c) *HLA-DQ2*
 (d) *HLA-DR3*

6. Which of the following is considered a long-term treatment option for DH?
 (a) Colchicine
 (b) Dapsone
 (c) Gluten-free diet
 (d) Systemic steroids

7. Which statement is false regarding drug-induced LAD?
 (a) Usually seen within a month of starting the drug
 (b) Extensive disease and atypical presentations are reported
 (c) Mucosal involvement is a common feature
 (d) Has a better prognosis

8. Which statement accurately describes mixed immuno-bullous disease?
 (a) Cases exhibiting overlapping clinical features of LAD and BP
 (b) Cases exhibiting intraepidermal and subepidermal cleft
 (c) Cases exhibiting mixed linear deposits of IgA and IgG at the DEJ
 (d) Cases exhibiting IgA binding to the epidermal and dermal side of salt-split skin

9. What is true regarding clinical features of DH?
 (a) Disease onset is in childhood
 (b) One-third of the patients have gastrointestinal symptoms
 (c) Lesions develop initially over the flexural aspect of extremities
 (d) Oral erosions are common in DH

10. Which statement is true regarding diagnosis of DH?
 (a) Eosinophils are seen on Tzanck smear
 (b) In addition to IgA, DIF may be positive for IgM, C3, and IgG
 (c) ELISA for antiendomysial antibody is commonly performed as screening test
 (d) Small bowel mucosal biopsy is routinely done for diagnosing DH

Answers

1. (d)   2. (b)   3. (b)   4. (c)   5. (c)   6. (c)   7. (c)   8. (c)   9. (b)   10. (b)

SUGGESTED READING

1. Guide SV, Marinkovich MP. Linear IgA bullous dermatosis. *Clin Dermatol*. 2001;19:719-27.

2. Genovese G, Venegoni L, Fanoni D, Muratori S, Berti E, Marzano AV. Linear IgA bullous dermatosis in adults and children: a clinical and immunopathological study of 38 patients. *Orphanet J Rare Dis*. 2019;14:115.

3. Collier PM, Wojnarowska F, Welsh K, Mcguire W, Black MM. Adult linear IgA disease and chronic bullous disease of childhood: the association with human lymphocyte antigens Cw7, B8, DR3 and tumour necrosis factor influences disease expression. *Br J Dermatol*. 1999;141:867-75.

4. Lammer J, Hein R, Roenneberg S, Biedermann T, Volz T. Drug-induced linear IgA bullous dermatosis: a case report and review of the literature. *Acta Derm Venereol*. 2019;99:508-15.

5. Gottlieb J, Ingen-Housz-Oro S, Alexandre M, Grootenboer-Mignot S, Aucouturier F, Sbidian E, *et al*. Idiopathic linear IgA bullous dermatosis: prognostic factors based on a case series of 72 adults. *Br J Dermatol*. 2017;177:212-22.

6. Görög A, Antiga E, Caproni M, Cianchini G, De D, Dmochowski M, *et al*. S2k guidelines (consensus statement) for diagnosis and therapy of dermatitis herpetiformis initiated by the European Academy of Dermatology and Venereology (EADV). *J Eur Acad Dermatol Venereol*. 2021;35:1251-77.

7. Nguyen CN, Kim SJ. Dermatitis Herpetiformis: An update on diagnosis, disease monitoring, and management. *Medicina (Kaunas)*. 2021;57:843.

8. Handa S, Dabas G, De D, Mahajan R, Chatterjee D, Saika UN, *et al*. A retrospective study of dermatitis herpetiformis from an immunobullous disease clinic in north India. *Int J Dermatol*. 2018;57:959-64.

9. Shin L, Gardner JT 2nd, Dao H Jr. Updates in the diagnosis and management of linear IgA disease: a systematic review. *Medicina (Kaunas)*. 2021;57:818.

10. Farrant P, Darley C, Carmichael A. Is erythromycin an effective treatment for chronic bullous disease of childhood? A national survey of members of the British Society for Paediatric Dermatology. *Pediatr Dermatol*. 2008;25:479-82.

Scoring Systems and Clinical Approach to Pemphigus and other Autoimmune Bullous Diseases

CHAPTER 13

Scoring Systems and Quality of Life Indices

Abir Saraswat, Swastika Suvirya, Sonal Sachan

- Disease outcome measures for autoimmune bullous diseases
  - Disease outcome measures for pemphigus
    - Pemphigus Disease Area Index (PDAI)
    - Autoimmune Bullous Skin Disorder Intensity Score (ABSIS)
    - Pemphigus Vulgaris Activity Score (PVAS)
  - Other disease outcome measures for pemphigus
  - Disease outcome measures for bullous pemphigoid
    - Autoimmune Bullous Skin Disorder Intensity Score (ABSIS)
    - Bullous Pemphigoid Disease Area Index (BPDAI)
  - Disease outcome measure for mucous membrane pemphigoid
    - Mucous Membrane Pemphigoid Disease Area Index (MMPDAI)
  - Disease outcome measure for epidermolysis bullosa acquisita
    - Epidermolysis Bullosa Acquisita Disease Area Index (EBADAI)
- Quality of life indices
  - Autoimmune bullous disease-specific quality of life instrument
    - Autoimmune Bullous Disease Quality of Life (ABQOL)
    - Treatment Autoimmune Bullous Disease Quality of Life (TABQOL)
  - Other quality of life instruments used widely in various medical specialties including dermatology
    - Dermatology Life Quality Index (DLQI)
    - 36-Item Short Form Survey (SF-36)
    - Skindex
    - General Health Questionnaire

INTRODUCTION

The incorporation of validated scoring systems in assessing disease severity and treatment response in dermatology has significant value. This is because unlike other medical branches where objective parameters such as laboratory values and radiological investigations are good proxies, assessments in dermatology mostly depend upon the patients' clinical features. Standardized disease severity measurement instruments like Psoriasis Area and Severity Index (PASI) for psoriasis have been used for many years in dermatological diseases. Similarly, such tools are also required to measure disease severity in autoimmune bullous diseases (AIBDs). This chapter discusses disease scoring systems and quality of life (QoL) indices used in the context of AIBDs.

DISEASE OUTCOME MEASURES FOR AUTOIMMUNE BULLOUS DISEASES

AIBDs are rare, chronic, and potentially fatal cutaneous disorders which have significant deleterious effects on patients' health. The activity of AIBD alters according to disease evolution and management, making it essential to develop a standardized and validated scoring system that can objectively measure these changes. Such disease outcome measures not only help in evaluating patient's well-being and titrating drug dosage, but are also extremely important in standardizing the way disease severity, treatment response, relapse, etc. are defined and communicated in literature. Obviously, this is the key to our ability to determine the best treatment strategies for our patients, based on data from clinical trials.

Disease Outcome Measures for Pemphigus

Pemphigus Disease Area Index (PDAI)

Pemphigus Disease Area Index (PDAI) was formulated in 2008 by a panel of dermatologists named the International Pemphigus Definitions Group **(Table 1)**.

The total PDAI score varies from 0 to 263, and evaluates the involvement of skin and mucosa by assessing the number and size of vesiculobullous lesions, erosions or newly developed erythema, visible within each anatomical site. This includes a total of 12 body sites with scalp as a separate site, and 12 sites in the oral cavity. Individual score for both the cutaneous and mucosal components varying from 0 to 10, is assigned to each anatomical site.

For damage scores, individual anatomic sites are evaluated. The damage (post-inflammatory hyperpigmentation or erythema from resolving lesions) is evaluated and scored as 1 and 0 for presence and absence of these damage features, respectively. A total damage score of 13 is calculated by adding individual points as per the anatomic distribution (12 points and 1 point assigned for skin and scalp damage, respectively). Thus, the highest scores for skin, scalp, and mucous membrane are 120, 10, and 120 each. A score of 250 amounts to disease activity, and 13 represents damage caused by the disease.

TABLE 1: Pemphigus Disease Area Index (PDAI) scoring sheet.

Body area	Anatomical sites	Activity	Damage
Skin		(Erosions/blisters/new erythema)	(Post-inflammatory hyperpigmentation/ erythema from resolving lesion)
	Ears	0—Absent	0—Absent
	Nose	1—1–3 lesions, 1 up to diameter >2 cm, none >6 cm	1—Present
	Rest of the face	2—2–3 lesions, at least 2 >2 cm diameter, none >6 cm	
	Neck	3—>3 lesions, none >6 cm diameter	
	Chest	5—>3 lesions and/or at least 1 >6 cm diameter	
	Abdomen	10—>3 lesions and/or at least 1 >16 cm diameter or entire area	
	Back, buttocks		
	Arms		
	Hands		
	Legs		
	Feet		
	Genitals		
	Total score	(0–120)	(0–12)
Scalp		(Erosions/blisters/new erythema)	(Post-inflammatory hyperpigmentation/ erythema from resolving lesions)
		0—Absent	0—Absent
		1—In 1 quadrant	1—Present
		2—2 quadrants	
		3—3 quadrants	
		4—Affects whole scalp	
		10—At least 1 lesion >6 cm	
	Total score	(0–10)	(0–1)
Mucous membrane		(Erosions/blisters)	
	Eyes	0—Absent	
	Nose	1—1 lesion	
	Buccal mucosa	2—2–3 lesions	
	Hard palate	3—>3 lesions or 2 lesions >2 cm	
	Soft palate	10—Entire area	
	Upper gingival		
	Lower gingival		
	Tongue		
	Floor of mouth		
	Labial mucosa		
	Posterior pharynx		
	Anogenital		
	Total score	(0–120)	–

Total activity score: Total skin activity score + total scalp activity score + total mucosal activity score. Maximum score: 250

Total damage score: Total skin damage score + total scalp damage score. Maximum score: 13

Sources: Grover S. Scoring systems in pemphigus. *Indian J Dermatol.* 2011;56:145-9. Adapted from Murrell DF, *et al.* Consensus statement on definitions of disease, end points, and therapeutic response for pemphigus. *J Am Acad Dermatol.* 2008;58:1043-6. PDAI scoring sheet developed by the International Pemphigus Definitions Group with support of the International Pemphigus and Pemphigoid Foundation.

Autoimmune Bullous Skin Disorder Intensity Score (ABSIS)

Pfütze, *et al* (2007) established Autoimmune Bullous Skin Disorder Intensity Score (ABSIS) for the purpose of objective and subjective assessment of pemphigus severity **(Fig. 1)**. The scores before ABSIS were either subjective or physician-dependent. However, due to the markedly variable manifestations of pemphigus, multiple parameters were required which could precisely reflect the phenotypic variability of pemphigus and were sensitive enough to measure the slightest therapeutic response. Considering this, ABSIS, a standardized scoring system for pemphigus, was devised.

ABSIS score ranges from 0 to 206 and separately measures cutaneous and oral involvement. A higher ABSIS score indicates more significant disease activity. The skin score uses two forms of measurement: affected body surface area (BSA) and quality of lesions. BSA is calculated using the

Date:
Patient's weight (kg):

	Legend for weighting factor (most dominant appearance of skin lesions):	
1.5	Erosive, exudative lesions	
1	Erosive, dry lesions	
0.5	Re-epithelialized lesions (including post-inflammation) erythema and/or hyperpigmentation	

Skin involvement (Max BSA):	Patient's BSA	Weighting factor
Head and neck (9%):		
L Arm including hand (9%):		
R Arm including hand (9%):		
Trunk (front and back) (36%):		
L Leg (18%):		
R Leg (18%):		
Genitals (1%):		

(Skin involvement total score: %BSA × weighing factor = 0–150 points) — calculated by the program.

Oral involvement:

I. Extent (enter 1 for presence of lesions, 0 for absence of any lesion):

Upper gingival mucosa		Tongue	
Lower gingival mucosa		Floor of the mouth	
Upper lip mucosa		Hard palate	
Lower lip mucosa		Soft palate	
Left buccal mucosa		Pharynx	
Right buccal mucosa			

(Total score ranges from 0 to 11)

Severity (discomfort during eating/drinking)

Food	Level	Factor of discomfort	Severity score
Water	1		
Soup	2		
Yogurt	3		
Custard	4		
Mashed potatoes/scrambled egg	5		
Baked fish	6		
White bread	7		
Apple/raw carrot	8		
Fried steak/whole grain bread	9		

(Severity score = Level multiplied by the factor of discomfort = 0–45 points)

	Legend for factor of discomfort	
1	Pain/bleeding occurred always	
0.5	Pain/bleeding occurred sometimes	
0	Never experienced problems	

Fig. 1: Autoimmune Bullous Skin Disorder Intensity Score (ABSIS) scoring sheet.
(BSA: body surface area; L: left; R: right)

Sources: Grover S. Scoring systems in pemphigus. *Indian J Dermatol*. 2011;56:145-9. Adapted from Pfütze M, *et al*. Introducing a novel Autoimmune Bullous Skin Disorder Intensity Score (ABSIS) in pemphigus. *Eur J Dermatol*. 2007;17:4-11.

Wallace's rule of nines, conventionally designed for burn patients. As per this rule, each anatomical site is assumed to be 9%, such that in an adult body, the head and neck is 9%, trunk is 36% (18% each for anterior and posterior aspects), upper and lower limbs comprise 9% and 18%, respectively, and the genitals are scored as 1%. Lesion quality is evaluated by multiplying assigned weighting factor with the estimated BSA percentage.

A weighting factor of 1.5 is taken for exudative, erosive lesions, and positive Nikolsky sign. On the other hand, a weighting factor of 1.0 is assigned for dry, erosive lesions, and 0.5 for lesions which have re-epithelialized. The weighting factor is determined according to the predominant lesion type at a particular anatomical site. A maximum score of 150 is obtained with this scale.

The score for oral involvement has been incorporated from a severity score originally devised by Saraswat and Kumar in 2003. It takes into account both the anatomical location (maximum score 11) and symptom severity (maximum score 45) of oral lesions. For extent of lesions present on each of 11 different anatomical areas in the oral cavity, a score of 0 is assigned for absence and 1 for presence of lesions. These 11 areas include upper and lower lip mucosae, right and left buccal mucosae, upper and lower gingival mucosae, floor of the oral cavity, tongue, hard and soft palate, and pharynx. The severity is determined by pain/bleeding associated with a specific type of food. The factor discomfort is given a score of 1 for persistent pain/bleeding, 0.5 when pain/bleeding occurs occasionally, and 0 when no symptoms are experienced. The final severity score is calculated by adding the factor discomfort value with the food-specific score.

Pemphigus Vulgaris Activity Score (PVAS)

The Pemphigus Vulgaris Activity Score (PVAS) was formulated to overcome the flaws in previous scoring systems, such as complexity in PDAI, and non-inclusion of other mucosal sites apart from oral mucosa in ABSIS. PVAS is based on three crucial components:

1. Extent of the lesions, incorporating the number of lesions (N) and different anatomical regions (D) in the skin(s) and all mucosal sites (m).
2. Elicitation of Nikolsky sign (S).
3. Weightage of morphological type of cutaneous lesions (T) as per the healing phase. The coefficients for skin lesion type are 1, 0.5, and 0 for bulla or erosions, crusts, and pigmentation, respectively. This depicts the different healing stages of cutaneous lesion from active bullae with erosions converted to crusted lesions which later progressively re-epithelize into post-inflammatory hyperpigmentation. The coefficient for bulla, or erosion and ulceration in the mucosa is 1 and 0.5 respectively.

In the mucosa, the healing process is slightly different from cutaneous lesions. As the mucosal erosions heal, they become more well-defined and transform into ulcers, that might be more painful than the preceding erosion. However, this pain does not indicate more significant disease activity. Therefore, symptoms may not be good indicators for defining disease activity.

The cutaneous score is calculated by multiplying the skin lesion type coefficient (T_s) with the sum of skin lesions number (N_s), distribution of these cutaneous lesions in different body regions (D_s), and manifestation of Nikolsky sign (S_s). Likewise, the mucosal score is evaluated by multiplying the mucosal lesion type coefficient (T_m) with the sum of mucosal lesions number (N_m) and the distribution of mucosal lesions at different anatomic sites (D_m). The total score for each cutaneous and mucosa score is 11 and 7, respectively. Thus, PVAS has a score range of 0–18, measured by using the formula:

$$PVAS = [T_s(N_s + D_s + S_s)] + [T_m(N_m + D_m)]$$

The advantages and drawbacks of these scoring systems are mentioned in **Table 2**.

TABLE 2: Comparison between major pemphigus disease scoring systems.

Scoring system with year of introduction	Mean calculation time (minutes)	Advantages	Disadvantages
ABSIS (2007)	3.9 ± 0.18	• A comprehensive score incorporating both quantitative (skin score) and qualitative (oral mucosa score) parameters; hence a better guide for therapeutic titration • Simple and less time-consuming • Can be additionally used for measuring disease severity of other AIBDs such as bullous pemphigoid and epidermolysis bullosa acquisita	• Lesser reliability and validity • Specifically designed for pemphigus, and its implementation in other AIBDs is less accurate because it lacks few disease-specific parameters of those diseases like pruritus in bullous pemphigoid • It does not take into account other mucosal sites except for oral mucosa • It does not include damage caused by the disease • ABSIS uses the rule of nines and BSA, which is impractical in the initial phase of disease where disease activity is high but BSA is less

Continued

Continued

Scoring system with year of introduction	Mean calculation time (minutes)	Advantages	Disadvantages
PDAI (2008)	4.7 ± 0.18	• Highest reliability and validity • Objective measurement of pemphigus activity, especially in mild-to-moderate cases, unlike ABSIS • Takes into consideration residual changes like PIH, unlike ABSIS • A valuable tool for determining the therapeutic efficacy of novel therapeutics for pemphigus in clinical trials	• More time-consuming • It is not easy to comprehend and implement • Contrary to the ABSIS scoring system, PDAI cannot be used in other AIBDs
PVAS (2013)	3.1 ± 0.2	• Simple and less time-taking • The anatomical distribution of pemphigus lesions is known to correlate with expression of pemphigus antigens, which are more concentrated in the head and neck region. Therefore, initial involvement of these areas signifies milder disease activity. In view of this, the appearance of lesions in the lower body parts indicates more severe disease activity, which could be measured more accurately by PVAS • PVAS clarifies that symptoms such as painful ulcerative mucosal lesions are part of the healing process, and they may not necessarily reflect more severe disease activity • PVAS differentiates between active lesion types, crusted lesions, and post-inflammatory changes, unlike others	Reliability and validity better than ABSIS but lower than PDAI (inter-observer variation depends on elicitation of Nikolsky sign, which could vary)

(ABSIS: Autoimmune Bullous Skin Disorder Intensity Score; AIBD: autoimmune bullous disease; BSA: body surface area; PDAI: Pemphigus Disease Area Index; PIH: post-inflammatory hyperpigmentation; PVAS: Pemphigus Vulgaris Activity Score)

Other Disease Outcome Measures for Pemphigus

Besides the three major scoring systems, ABSIS, PDAI, and PVAS, several (>100) other disease outcome measures exist for assessing pemphigus disease severity, but most lack proper validation. Therefore, they are not widely accepted. Few such outcome measures are described in **Table 3**.

TABLE 3: Concise description of lesser-known pemphigus disease scoring systems.

Type of outcome measure	Parameters affecting the score	Advantages	Disadvantages
Serum markers	Anti-desmoglein antibody (anti-Dsg Ab) levels by ELISA: • Anti-Dsg 1 Ab • Anti-Dsg 3 Ab	Establishes relation between anti-Dsg levels and disease severity	• Low sensitivity and not enough validation • Laboratory-dependent

Pemphigus Area and Activity Score (PAAS)	Skin and mucosal scores are included:
	• Skin involvement (0–18):
	  ○ The body is divided into four parts: Head, upper limbs, trunk, and lower limbs
	  ○ Each body part includes activity (for example, new blisters each day) and the percentage of area involved
	• Mucosal involvement (0–6):
	  ○ Area
	  ○ Severity
		Easy and rapid	• PAAS is dependent on BSA, so a significant change in surface area involvement might drastically change the severity score
			• Daily count of blisters is a poor manifestation of disease activity as it does not precisely reflect the stage or size of the lesions

Ikeda Index	Four items have been suggested for evaluation (0–12): 1. Skin lesions: Percentage area affected (0–3) 2. Nikolsky sign (0–3) 3. Number of new blisters each day (0–3) 4. Oral lesions: Percentage area affected (0–3)	• Simple assessment • Less time-consuming	• It does not include other mucosal regions except for oral mucosa • It does not take into account the anatomic distribution and morphology of lesions • The use of Nikolsky sign creates chances of inter-observer variability

Continued

Continued

Type of outcome measure	Parameters affecting the score	Advantages	Disadvantages
Level of corticosteroid and/or adjuvant medication use	Two items are evaluated (0–10): 1. The extent of disease (0–4) 2. Level of corticosteroid and/or adjuvant drug given (0–6)	Simple and rapid	• Unreliable because corticosteroid and/or immunosuppressive drug use depends on extrinsic factors such as physician's experience and patient's co-morbid illness • It does not include mucosal involvement, and no individual score has been provided for erosions
Pemphigus Activity Score (PAS)	It is based on (0–12): • Number of erosions in oral mucosa • Number of skin erosions • Number of daily blisters • Anti-Dsg1 and 3 antibody ELISA titers	Good accuracy: correlates antibody titers to disease activity	• Poor sensitivity due to assessment of body surface area (BSA) • No scores are given to size and site of erosions • Laboratory-dependent
BSA involvement	• Both cutaneous and mucosal involvement are included. • It is based on two factors: 1. The extent of BSA involvement 2. Functional impairment • Categorization is done as per the above parameters as mild, moderate, severe or extensive	Easy and quick	• Low sensitivity: fails to depict gradual improvement as disease condition is classified into four broad categories • BSA does not provide information on the number and distribution of lesions; which are of paramount importance for assessing disease activity • Major changes in BSA and functional status are required; thus slight changes go unnoticed • Not appropriate for use in clinical trials
Commitment Index of Skin and Mucous in Pemphigus Vulgaris (ISMPIV)	It depends on several parameters (0–100): • Number of blisters and erosions (0–25) • Size of blisters and erosions (0–25) • Nikolsky sign (0–20) • Mucous membrane involvement and sepsis (0–30)	• High inter-rater reliability • Standardized management by correlating the treatment provided with disease severity • Helps in the determination of disease prognosis	The incorporation of Nikolsky sign makes it observer-dependent
Measure for oral pemphigus	It measures two factors: 1. The extent of oral mucosa involvement (0–11) 2. Functional impairment (pain and bleeding assessed for nine food items)	• Does not rely on measurement of size/count of lesions • Includes patient-reported parameters • Better sensitivity for measuring the activity of oral disease, thus later included in ABSIS	• Other mucosal sites are ignored • It can only be used for oral pemphigus
Oral Disease Severity Score (ODSS)	It is based on the following parameters: • The extent of oral mucosa involvement (divided into 17 anatomical sites) • Type of lesions	• High inter-observer reliability • Quick and straightforward to perform • It is accurate as it incorporates 17 oral mucosal sites, which is more than any other scoring system	It was devised for use in oral lichen planus (OLP). However, later utilized for other oral diseases that caused confusion because the erosion in pemphigus extends to the epithelial level, but in OLP, they are deeper. Thus, the terminologies used cannot accurately reflect oral pemphigus disease activity
Pemphigus Oral Lesions Intensity Score (POLIS)	It includes the following factors: • Extent, number, and type of oral lesions • Functional impairment	• A more sensitive and accurate tool as it is formulated specifically for oral pemphigus • High inter-observer reliability	• Complex to evaluate • More time-consuming

 (ABSIS: Autoimmune Bullous Skin Disorder Intensity Score; ELISA: enzyme-linked immunosorbent assay)

Disease Outcome Measures for Bullous Pemphigoid

Autoimmune Bullous Skin Disorder Intensity Score (ABSIS)

Detailed description is given in **Figure 1**.

Bullous Pemphigoid Disease Area Index (BPDAI)

It was formulated by the International Pemphigoid Committee in 2012. It incorporates both objective and subjective components **(Table 4)**. The clinical assessment based on disease activity score, damage score for skin lesions, and activity score for mucosa, reflects the objective nature of BPDAI. Pruritus was part of the subjective BPDAI scoring system, with scores varying from 0 to 360 for disease activity. The total damage score range is 0–12. It is crucial to note that damage is separately scored in this severity scoring system. The reason is that it guides the observers/raters to be aware of the fact that not every lesion depicts active disease.

BPDAI divides the cutaneous and mucosal factors into 12 anatomical regions, with each region being assigned

TABLE 4: Bullous Pemphigoid Disease Area Index (BPDAI).

Skin	Activity		Activity		Damage
Anatomical location	Erosions/blisters	Number of lesions if <3	Urticarial/erythema/other	Number of lesions if <3	Pigmentation/other
	0—Absent		0—Absent		0—Absent 1—Present
	1—1–3 lesions, none >1 cm diameter		1—1–3 lesions, none >6 cm diameter		
	2—1–3 lesions, at least 1 lesion >1 cm diameter		2—1–3 lesions, at least 1 lesion >6 cm diameter		
	3—>3 lesions, none >2 cm diameter		3—>3 lesions, or at least 1 lesion >10 cm		
	5—>3 lesions, and at least 1 lesion >2 cm		5—>3 lesions and at least 1 lesion >25 cm		
	10—>3 lesions, and at least 1 lesion >5 cm diameter or entire area		10—>3 lesions and at least 1 lesion >50 cm diameter or entire area		
Head					
Neck					
Chest					
Left arm					
Right arm					
Hands					
Abdomen					
Genitals					
Back/buttocks					
Left leg					
Right leg					
Feet					
Total skin	/120		/120		
Mucosa	Erosions/blisters				
	1—1 lesion				
	2—2–3 lesions				
	5—>3 lesions, or 2 lesions >2 cm				
	10—Entire area				
Eyes					
Nose					
Buccal mucosa					

Continued

Continued

Skin	Activity		Activity		Damage
Hard palate					
Soft palate					
Upper gingiva					
Lower gingiva					
Tongue					
Floor of mouth					
Labial mucosa					
Posterior pharynx					
Anogenital					
Total mucosa	/120				

Source: Adapted from Murrell DF, *et al*. Definitions and outcome measures for bullous pemphigoid: recommendations by an international panel of experts. *J Am Acad Dermatol*. 2012;66:479-85.

individual scores. The final BPDAI activity score is the summation of points for activity related to the phenotype of skin lesions, which are blisters and erosions (0–120 points); elicitation of erythema and urticaria (0–120 points); and mucosal erosions and blisters (0–120 points). Based on the post-inflammatory hyperpigmentation or scarring noticed over each cutaneous anatomical site, damage is calculated wherein, 1 point is given for their presence and 0 if found absent. The BPDAI damage score is the sum of these above mentioned scores and directly correlates with disease severity. The patient-reported pruritus incorporated here is known as BPDAI pruritus. The component of pruritus could signify the initial phase of disease or recurrence, and also its effect on patient's daily routine activity. Hence, to assess the affected QoL, several questions related to patient's pruritus are asked, like "how severe has your itching been in the last 24 hours/last week/last month?" These are answered on a visual analog scale (VAS), with each question scored between 0 (no itch) and 10 (maximum itch). The total BPDAI pruritus score is measured out of 30 by adding these individual scores. However, if the patient fails to interpret or provide an answer to these questions, such as in cases of mental instability or cognitive distortions, an alternate method is adopted to determine the severity of pruritus. This procedure is physician-dependent, wherein the degree of pruritus is assigned a score depending on the severity of visible cutaneous excoriations. The pruritus scores are assigned as follows: for no excoriations (0), for isolated excoriations at up to two body sites (10), excoriations on three body sites or disruption of activities of daily living (20), and generalized excoriations or sleep disturbance (30).

Advantages of BPDAI:
- BPDAI has good accuracy, validity, and sensitivity.
- The inter-rater reliability of BPDAI is better than ABSIS.
- The inclusion of BPDAI pruritus adds the additional benefit of assessing disease recurrence and quality of patient's life.

Disadvantages of BPDAI: BPDAI damage score does not reveal disease activity.

Disease Outcome Measure for Mucous Membrane Pemphigoid

Mucous Membrane Pemphigoid Disease Area Index (MMPDAI)

The disease activity and damage are measured separately for scalp, eyes and mucosal sites, and other body areas **(Table 5)**. The skin and mucosa are divided into 12 anatomic regions, where activity scoring is performed, ranging from 0 to10 points. The presence of damage scores 1 point, and absence scores 0. Scalp activity scoring is performed depending upon the number of affected quadrants, with a score of 0 for absence of lesion and a score of 10 if at least a single lesion of size >6 cm is present. The damage score of scalp is measured and assigned 1 point for presence and 0 for absence of any damage. Likewise, each quadrant of the eye (upper, lower, medial, and lateral) is scored separately based on the degree of erythema, varying from 0 to 4 (no erythema to bright red). The activity score for each eye quadrant sums up to subtotal 0–16 points, which is then incorporated into the formula to obtain activity scores (0–10 points) for the individual eye. For damage score, 1 point is assigned for presence and 0 for absence of the damage caused and is calculated for left and right eyes separately. Similarly, scores for other mucosal and cutaneous (forehead, shoulders, lower limbs) sites are also recorded and measured.

Advantages of MMPDAI:
- MMPDAI is highly sensitive and detects more minor changes in clinical response.
- It includes all mucosal sites, unlike other scoring systems.
- A higher score weightage is given to mucosa because they are commonly involved in this dermatosis.
- Incorporation of scarring in the damage score reflects more accuracy specific to mucous membrane pemphigoid.

Disadvantage of MMPDAI: Proper validation of this scoring tool is still lacking.

TABLE 5: **Mucous Membrane Pemphigoid Disease Area Index (MMPDAI).**

Skin	Activity		Damage
Anatomic location	Erosion/blisters or new erythema		Post-inflammatory hyperpigmentation or erythema from resolving lesion or scarring
	0—Absent 1—1–3 lesions, up to 1 lesion >2 cm in any diameter, none >6 cm 2—2–3 lesions, at least 2 lesions >2 cm diameter, none >6 cm 3—>3 lesions, none >6 cm diameter 5—>3 lesions, and/or at least 1 lesion >6 cm 10—>3 lesions, and/or at least 1 lesion >16 cm diameter or entire area	No. of lesions if ≤3	0—Absent 1—Present
Ears			
Forehead			
Rest of the face			
Neck			
Chest			
Abdomen			
Shoulders, back			
Buttocks			
Arms and hands			
Legs and feet			
Anal			
Genitals			
Total skin	/120		/12
Scalp	Erosions/blisters or new erythema	No. of lesions if ≤3	Post-inflammatory hyperpigmentation or erythema from resolving lesion/scarring
	0—Absent 1—1 quadrant 2—2 quadrants 3—3 quadrants 4—Affects whole scalp 10—At least 1 lesion >6 cm		0—Absent 1—Present
Total scalp (0–10)	/10		/1
Mucous membrane	Damage		
Anatomic location	Erosions/blisters		Post-inflammatory hyperpigmentation or erythema from resolving lesion/scarring
Eyes (quadrants upper, lower, medial, and lateral)	0—No erythema 1—Light pink 2—Moderate pink 3—Dark pink 4—Bright pink Add up quadrants	Subtotal	0—Absent 1—Present
Left eye (0–16) × 0.625	/10	/16	
Right eye (0–16) × 0.625	/10	/16	
	0—Absent 1—lesion 2—3 lesions 5—>3 lesions or 2 lesions >2 cm 10—Entire area	Number of lesions if ≤3	0—Absent 1—Present

Continued

Continued

Skin	Activity		Damage
Nasal			
Buccal mucosa			
Palate			
Upper gingiva			
Lower gingiva			
Tongue/floor of mouth			
Labial			
Posterior pharynx			
Anal			
Genital			
Total mucosa	/120		/12

Total activity score: [ ]   Total activity score: [ ]

Source: Adapted from Murrell DF, *et al.* Definitions and outcome measures for mucous membrane pemphigoid: recommendations of an international panel of experts. *J Am Acad Dermatol.* 2015;72:168-74.

Disease Outcome Measure for Epidermolysis Bullosa Acquisita

Epidermolysis Bullosa Acquisita Disease Area Index (EBADAI)

Epidermolysis Bullosa Acquisita Disease Area Index (EBADAI) has been suggested for better measurement of disease severity specific to epidermolysis bullosa acquisita (EBA). However, the final consensus-based instrument is yet to be published.

QUALITY OF LIFE INDICES

The QoL indices have been designed for chronic diseases wherein treatment is more important than cure. In AIBDs, cure is often an impossible goal to achieve, pertaining to their relapsing and remitting course, which could hamper the patient's physical and mental well-being, thereby altering his QoL. Hence, multiple QoL tools have been formulated, including AIBD-specific QoL instruments (use limited to AIBD), skin-specific QoL tools (use limited to cutaneous diseases), and generic QoL tools (applied widely in the field of medicine, including dermatology). QoL instruments direct the physicians to tailor their management according to individual patients' needs.

Autoimmune Bullous Disease-specific Quality of Life Instrument

Autoimmune Bullous Disease Quality of Life (ABQOL)

The Autoimmune Bullous Disease Quality of Life (ABQOL) question-sheet based items address the patient's obligations or limitations to daily activities, physical difficulties or impairment, and psychiatric effects. Individual items are given scores ranging from 0 to 3, wherein higher the score, worse is the QoL. The final ABQOL score varies from 0 to 51 on adding up all the item scores. On comparing the convergent validity of ABQOL with the two more common instruments, the 36-item short form (SF-36) survey and Dermatology Life Quality Index (DLQI), the results were found to be moderate, showing correlation coefficients of 0.69 and 0.63 each. The explanation for this dissimilarity could be the fact that ABQOL precisely measures the impairment in QoL for patients with AIBD, unlike DLQI and SF-36, which are used in dermatological disorders in general. Thus, ABQOL is a sensitive and specific tool for estimating changes in QoL in AIBD.

Treatment Autoimmune Bullous Disease Quality of Life (TABQOL)

AIBDs are chronic cutaneous diseases, therefore immuno-suppressive medications are given for longer duration, leading to adverse effects. This has a deleterious impact on the patient's health and also adds to the financial burden. Treatment Autoimmune Bullous Disease Quality of Life (TABQOL) questionnaire is designated to measure therapy-related impact on QOL. It consists of 17 items related to the plausible physical, functional, psychological, and financial burden on patient's QoL because of the treatment prescribed in AIBDs. Like ABQOL, each item scores between 0 and 3, denoting worse QoL with each additional point in the total score. On adding up these scores, a maximum TABQOL score of 51 is obtained.

TABQOL has high validity, internal consistency, and reliability, which depicts its usefulness in the measurement of treatment burden, and evaluation of disease remission in research.

The combined implementation of these disease-specific QoL indices (ABQOL and TABQOL) with the validated clinical outcome measures, such as ABSIS and PDAI, help in better monitoring of the disease. The physicians are able to detect the exact difficulties faced by AIBD patients, such as physical impairment, psychosocial factors, and financial burden. The items most applicable to a particular patient are identified, and management of each patient is customized accordingly.

Other Quality of Life Instruments Used Widely in Various Medical Specialties Including Dermatology

These are of two types: generic and skin-specific. The generic ones can be applied to a wide range of diseases and over a large population. Skin-specific QoL tools are more detailed and utilized explicitly for cutaneous ailments.

Dermatology Life Quality Index (DLQI)

DLQI, a commonly applied skin-specific QOL tool, comprises 10 sets of questions used to assess the effects of cutaneous disorders on QoL. Questions 1 and 2 are prepared to measure the symptoms and feelings of patients; questions 3 and 4 reflect the impact on patients' daily activities; questions 5 and 6 denote leisure-time affected, questions 7 and 8 reflect problems experienced at work and school; question 9 shows the effects on sexual activity due to skin disease; and question 10 gives information on treatment response. Responses for each question include "not at all/not relevant", "a little", "a lot", or "very much", which are scored as 0, 1, 2, or 3 respectively. Each of these scores are summed up to get the total DLQI score, where high scores indicate worse QoL.

36-Item Short Form Survey (SF-36)

The SF-36 survey is a common generic QoL instrument utilized widely in the medical field. It consists of 36 items on a Likert scale format that covers eight individual health-related points: (1) physical limitations caused by health conditions; (2) disrupted social life due to physical or emotional issues; (3) decrease in daily activities/roles due to impaired physical health; (4) disruption in daily activities/roles related to emotional issues/stress; (5) mental well-being; (6) bodily pain; (7) levels of energy and fatigue; and (8) general health perceptions. The individual domain scores 0–100, with a greater score reflecting better health status.

Skindex

Skindex is another questionnaire-based skin-specific QoL tool designed to gauge the effects of cutaneous disorders on QoL. Initially, it was developed as a 61-item questionnaire. However to improve the discriminative and evaluative ability of the skindex tool and reduce the burden on the respondent, it was revised to make more concise sets of questions, comprising 29, 17, and 16 items, namely Skindex-29, Skindex-17, and Skindex-16, respectively.

Skindex assesses three essential areas that address QoL: symptoms, emotions, and functioning. In Skindex-29, individual items evaluate the patients' experience of one of these areas in the last 4 weeks, with the responses "never",

"rarely", "sometimes", "often", and "all the time" arranged on a scale ranging from 0 ("never") to 100 ("all the time"). The points individually for these three areas are measured by taking out an average of scores (0–100). A greater score reflects worse QoL. In Skindex-16, four items measure symptoms, seven measure emotions, and five items measure functioning. It is a shorter and more straightforward system, which is scored similar to the previous versions but with more emphasis on how frequently the patients are affected by the particular symptoms of their cutaneous disorder rather than how frequently the symptoms are perceived or experienced.

General Health Questionnaire

Due to the visible nature of dermatological diseases, patients suffer from psychological problems due to social insecurities, which could negatively affect their personal, professional, and social life. These psychological problems must be ascertained for evaluating QoL in AIBDs. The General Health Questionnaire (GHQ-12) with a total score ranging from 0 to 12, was introduced for measuring psychological distress. It contains 12 items that enquire about the degree of psychological burden experienced by the patient in the past few weeks. The binary method (0-0-1-1) is utilized for recording the patient's answers on a four-point scale. GHQ-12 is a simple QoL instrument that aids in screening non-psychotic psychiatric disorders such as depression and anxiety, which are experienced in cutaneous disorders.

CONCLUSION

There are multiple scoring systems to capture disease severity and impact on life of patients suffering from AIBDs. Due to the dynamic nature of diseases and the extraordinary variability of clinical symptoms, no single scoring system can capture the full spectrum of their physical and psychological impact. This brief overview can help the clinician and researcher to decide which score(s) to use in a particular patient or study to best fulfill their requirements. A better understanding of these scoring systems will hopefully lead to more widespread use and further refinements. This can only mean better care to the patients who suffer from these debilitating and sometimes life-threatening diseases.

TAKE HOME MESSAGE

- Disease outcome measures and QoL indices when applied in amalgamation shift our focus from providing only medical care to holistic patient-oriented care in AIBDs. Sometimes, clinical improvement may not correlate well with the psychological well-being of AIBD patients, which necessitates the requirement of such scoring systems and QoL indices.
- Though ABSIS was formulated keeping pemphigus in mind, this scoring system is widely accepted and can be implemented in all AIBDs.
- Among the various pemphigus severity scoring systems, PDAI is the most comprehensive one.

- The best scoring tool for bullous pemphigoid is BPDAI, as the inclusion of pruritus enables us to additionally measure the patient's QoL.
- Separate scoring systems for MMP and EBA can provide a better severity picture of these illnesses, which was not possible with ABSIS. However, these scores still require more validation data.
- AIBD-specific QoL instruments, namely ABQOL and TABQOL, when used in amalgamation with disease-specific scoring systems for assessing severity, can guide physicians in tailoring treatment to individual patients.
- Various studies have validated the outcome measures, but are yet awaiting routine application in day-to-day medical practice.
- In future, with frequent utilization of these scoring systems and indices, we await revision and refinement of these valuable tools.

MULTIPLE CHOICE QUESTIONS

1. **Which of the following are the three major disease outcome measures for pemphigus?**
   - (a) PDAI, PAS, and ODIS
   - (b) ABSIS, PDAI, and ISMPIV
   - (c) PDAI, PVAS, and ABSIS
   - (d) ABSIS, BPDAI, and PVAS

2. **Which disease outcome measure incorporates Nikolsky sign in its calculation?**
   - (a) PVAS
   - (b) ABSIS
   - (c) Both (a) and (b)
   - (d) PDAI

3. **Rule of nines to measure body surface area of involvement is used in which scoring system?**
   - (a) BPDAI
   - (b) PVAS
   - (c) MMPDAI
   - (d) ABSIS

4. **What are the main anatomical sites in PDAI for evaluating pemphigus disease activity?**
   - (a) Skin (body and scalp) and mucous membranes
   - (b) Skin (body, scalp, and nails) and mucous membranes
   - (c) Skin (body and scalp) and oral mucosa
   - (d) Skin (body, scalp, nails) and oral mucosa

5. **What are the drawbacks of serum markers like anti-desmoglein antibody levels for assessing disease severity in pemphigus?**
   - (a) Serial anti-Dsg Ab titers are poorly correlated with disease severity while monitoring treatment response in clinical research
   - (b) Lack enough validation studies
   - (c) Both (a) and (b)
   - (d) It correlates well with disease severity, and there are no drawbacks

6. **The maximum disease activity score of BPDAI is:**
   - (a) 360
   - (b) 206
   - (c) 263
   - (d) 150

7. **Incorporation of which feature in damage score makes MMPDAI better than other AIBD scoring systems for measuring MMP disease severity?**
   - (a) Erythema
   - (b) Erosions
   - (c) Ulceration
   - (d) Scarring

8. **What are the disease-specific QoL tools used for measuring QoL in AIBD patients?**
   - (a) Autoimmune Bullous Disease Quality of Life (ABQOL) and Treatment Autoimmune Bullous Disease Quality of Life (TABQOL)
   - (b) Dermatology Life Quality Index (DLQI) and SF-36 survey
   - (c) Skindex and Global Health Questionnaire (GHQ)
   - (d) Physician Global Assessment (PGA)

9. **How many items are included in Treatment Autoimmune Bullous Disease Quality of Life (TABQOL)?**
   - (a) 21
   - (b) 60
   - (c) 15
   - (d) 17

10. **What are the advantages of utilizing the disease outcome measures in amalgamation with disease-specific QoL in AIBD patients?**
    - (a) Shifts the goal from disease-oriented care to disease plus patient-oriented care
    - (b) Better practice of evidence-based medicine
    - (c) Helpful in evaluating the efficacy and safety of newer drugs in clinical trials
    - (d) All of the above

Answers

136 1. (c)   2. (c)   3. (d)   4. (a)   5. (c)   6. (a)   7. (d)   8. (a)   9. (d)   10. (d)

SUGGESTED READING

1. Bak GG, Murrell DF. Autoimmune blistering disease: Outcome measures. In: Maibach H, Osman N (Eds). Cutaneous Biometrics, 1st edition. Switzerland: Springer, Cham; 2019. pp. 1-30.

2. Daniel BS, Hertl M, Werth VP, Eming R, Murrell DF. Severity score indexes for blistering diseases. *Clin Dermatol.* 2012;30:108-13.

3. Saraswat A, Kumar B. A new grading system for oral pemphigus. *Int J Dermatol.* 2003;42:413-4.

4. Wijayanti A, Zhao CY, Boettiger D, Chiang YZ, Ishii N, Hashimoto T, *et al.* The Reliability, Validity and Responsiveness of Two Disease Scores (BPDAI and ABSIS) for Bullous Pemphigoid: Which One to Use? *Acta Derm Venereol.* 2017;97:24-31.

5. Hanna S, Kim M, Murrell DF. Validation studies of outcome measures in pemphigus. *Int J Womens Dermatol.* 2016;2:128-39.

6. Ormond M, McParland H, Donaldson ANA, Andiappan M, Cook RJ, Escudier M, *et al.* An Oral Disease Severity Score validated for use in oral pemphigus vulgaris. *Br J Dermatol.* 2018;179:872-81.

7. Murrell DF, Daniel BS, Joly P, Borradori L, Amagai M, Hashimoto T, *et al.* Definitions and outcome measures for bullous pemphigoid: recommendations by an international panel of experts. *J Am Acad Dermatol.* 2012;66:479-85.

8. Murrell DF, Marinovic B, Caux F, Prost C, Ahmed R, Wozniak K, *et al.* Definitions and outcome measures for mucous membrane pemphigoid: recommendations of an international panel of experts. *J Am Acad Dermatol.* 2015;72:168-74.

9. Sebaratnam DF, Hanna AM, Chee SN, Frew JW, Venugopal SS, Daniel BS, *et al.* Development of a quality-of-life instrument for autoimmune bullous disease: the autoimmune bullous disease quality of life questionnaire. *JAMA Dermatol.* 2013;149:1186-91.

10. Tjokrowidjaja A, Daniel BS, Frew JW, Sebaratnam DF, Hanna AM, Chee S, *et al.* The development and validation of the treatment of autoimmune bullous disease quality of life questionnaire, a tool to measure the quality of life impacts of treatments used in patients with autoimmune blistering disease. *Br J Dermatol.* 2013;169:1000-6.

11. Pfütze M, Niedermeier A, Hertl M, Eming R. Introducing a novel Autoimmune Bullous Skin Disorder Intensity Score (ABSIS) in pemphigus. *Eur J Dermatol.* 2007;17:4-11.

CHAPTER 14

Clinical Approach to Autoimmune Bullous Diseases

Vignesh Narayan R, Rashmi Sarkar

- History taking in a patient of autoimmune bullous disease
- Examination
- Assessment for complications
- Special signs
- Scoring systems for disease severity
- Algorithm for diagnosis

INTRODUCTION

From previous chapters we have learnt that autoimmune bullous diseases (AIBDs) can be intraepidermal or subepidermal. Each subtype has its unique clinical presentation, including morphology and distribution of lesions, natural course, treatment response, and prognosis. Hence, delineating a particular subtype, assessing disease extent and severity, associated co-morbidities and the effect of disease on patient's quality of life besides obtaining information on previous treatment taken and response to treatment, are an integral part of the clinical approach which helps to individualize management.

HISTORY TAKING

A detailed history in a patient suspected of AIBD must include:

Demographic Details

Age of the Patient

Certain AIBDs are more likely to present at a particular age. In the pemphigoid group, both bullous pemphigoid (BP) and mucous membrane pemphigoid (MMP) occur in patients older than 60 years of age. The risk of developing these diseases increases with age, with the relative risk being 300 times higher in patients >90 years of age compared to those <60 years. Pemphigus vulgaris (PV) and pemphigus foliaceus (PF) occur in middle-aged patients, typically around 40–60 years of age. In India, most patients are younger, with disease onset <40 years of age. Endemic pemphigus also preferentially affects younger population, with up to one-third of the cases being <20 years of age.

The patients' age also has a bearing on disease course and prognosis, e.g., childhood BP and PV usually have a better prognosis than the adult forms.

The distribution of lesions too varies with age, e.g., childhood form of linear immunoglobulin A (IgA) disease (LAD) [chronic bullous dermatosis of childhood (CBDC)] tends to involve periorificial areas. Childhood BP has a predilection for palms and soles, and genitalia (vulvar BP). A summary of the age at presentation of various AIBDs is given in **Table 1**.

TABLE 1: Common age at presentation of various autoimmune bullous diseases.

Disease	Age in years
Pemphigus vulgaris (PV)/ pemphigus foliaceus (PF)	40–60 In India, <40
Paraneoplastic pemphigus (PNP)	45–70 Children (mean age of 11 years, when associated with Castleman disease)
Bullous pemphigoid (BP)	69–83 In India, slightly younger age (around 60 years)
Drug-induced pemphigoid	40–60
Anti-p200 pemphigoid	42–64
Mucous membrane pemphigoid (MMP)	60–80
Pemphigoid gestationis	Pregnant women (second or third trimester)
Linear immunoglobulin A (IgA) disease (LAD)	>60 <5 [chronic bullous dermatosis of childhood (CBDC)]
Dermatitis herpetiformis (DH)	30–40
Epidermolysis bullosa acquisita (EBA)	44–55 (two peaks, in second and seventh decade)
Bullous systemic lupus erythematosus (SLE)	20–40
Lichen planus pemphigoides	35–44

Gender

Hormonal, immunological, epigenetic, and microbiotic variations may explain the gender-based differences in AIBDs **(Table 2)**. BP, PNP (few studies), DH, anti-p200 pemphigoid, and drug-induced pemphigoid are more common in males, while MMP, PV, and PF (few studies) are more common in females.

Female PV patients tend to have more severe mucosal involvement, younger age of disease onset and a personal and family history of other autoimmune diseases.

TABLE 2: Gender predilection of autoimmune bullous diseases.

Gender	Autoimmune bullous disease more prevalent
Males	BP, PNP, DH, anti-p200 pemphigoid, drug-induced pemphigoid
Females	Other AIBDs

(BP: bullous pemphigoid; DH: dermatitis herpetiformis; PNP: paraneoplastic pemphigus)

Geographic Location of the Patient

Environmental and genetic constitution varies with geography, and this manifests as a difference in disease phenotype. Indian pemphigus patients tend to have a younger age of onset (third to fourth decade of life compared to third to sixth decade elsewhere), Brazilian patients living in rural areas close to rivers suffer from endemic PF or fogo selvagem, EBA is more common in black people of African descent, and DH is more common in individuals of North European descent.

Socioeconomic Status

This helps to navigate and counsel regarding the various treatment options that may be afforded by the patient.

Onset/Triggering Factors

Most of the AIBDs have an insidious onset and a chronic course. However, there may be some variations, e.g., CBDC tends to have an abrupt onset, compared to its adult counterpart (LAD).

Certain triggering factors **(Table 3)** such as infection, drugs **(Tables 4 and 5)**, vaccination, and ultraviolet (UV) exposure are associated with the onset of these diseases.

TABLE 3: Important triggers for autoimmune bullous diseases.

PV	

Infections	• *Viral*:
	  ○ Herpes simplex
	  ○ EBV
	  ○ CMV
	  ○ HHV-8
	• *Bacterial*:
	  ○ *Staphylococcus aureus*
	  ○ *Proteus vulgaris*
	  ○ *Pseudomonas aeruginosa*

Continued

Continued

Drugs	Refer to **Table 4**
Other agents	Pesticides
Pemphigus erythematosus	
	Ultraviolet (UV) exposure
Endemic PF (fogo selvagem)	
	Simulium (Black fly)
PNP	
	Lymphoproliferative malignancies: Non-Hodgkin's lymphoma, CLL, Castleman disease
BP	
Physical agents	• UV radiation • X-ray therapy • Trauma • Post-surgery • Vaccines
Drugs	Refer to **Table 5**
DH	
	Gluten-containing diet: • Wheat • Barley • Rye *Iodine-rich food*: • Kelp and marine oil • Iodine supplements
LAD	
	Drugs, infection, trauma, vaccination, UV radiation
Bullous SLE	
	Sun exposure
EBA	
	Trauma, contact allergy to metals

(BP: bullous pemphigoid; CLL: chronic lymphocytic leukemia; CMV: cytomegalovirus; DH: dermatitis herpetiformis; EBA: epidermolysis bullosa acquisita; EBV: Epstein–Barr virus; HHV-8: human herpesvirus-8; LAD: linear immunoglobulin A disease; PF: pemphigus foliaceus; PNP: paraneoplastic pemphigus; PV: pemphigus vulgaris; SLE: systemic lupus erythematosus)

TABLE 4: Various drugs associated with drug-induced pemphigus.

Thiol (induce PF > PV, and 39–53% remit on drug withdrawal)	Penicillamine, captopril, penicillin, piroxicam, lisinopril, thiopronine, bucillamine
Phenol (induce PV > PF, and only 15% remit on drug withdrawal)	Rifampicin, cefadroxil, levodopa, aspirin, heroin, phenobarbital
Non-thiol non-phenol	Glibenclamide, calcium channel blockers, progesterone, NSAIDs, secukinumab, tocilizumab
Topical agents (contact pemphigus)	Imiquimod, phenol, tincture of benzoin

(NSAID: non-steroidal anti-inflammatory drug; PF: pemphigus foliaceus; PV: pemphigus vulgaris)

TABLE 5: Autoimmune bullous diseases that can be drug-induced.

PV	• 7% patients develop pemphigus after taking penicillamine for at least 6 months • Penicillamine (33.1%), captopril (7.7%), and bucillamine (6.5%) are commonly reported drugs • Mean latency after drug intake is 154.27 ± 277.5 days (median of 60 days)
BP	• Dipeptidyl peptidase-4 inhibitor (DPP-4i)—gliptins • PD-1/PD-L1 inhibitors (immune checkpoint inhibitors) • Furosemide • Spironolactone • Sulfasalazine • Ibuprofen • Captopril • Penicillamine • Antibiotics • Neuroleptics • Anticholinergic agents *Topical agents*: • Benzyl benzoate • 5-fluorouracil • Chemical peels
LAD	Vancomycin (most common), NSAIDs (diclofenac, naproxen), penicillin, cephalosporins, sulfonamides, captopril, phenytoin
Bullous SLE	Hydralazine

(BP: bullous pemphigoid; LAD: linear immunoglobulin A disease; NSAID: non-steroidal anti-inflammatory drug; PD-1: programmed cell death 1; PD-L1: programmed cell death ligand 1; PV: pemphigus vulgaris; SLE: systemic lupus erythematosus)

Initial Site of Involvement and Distribution of Lesions

The disease may preferentially involve a particular site initially, e.g., oral mucosa is often the first site of involvement in 50–70% of PV cases. In PNP too, the presenting sign is stomatitis, usually involving the vermilion border of lips. The mechanobullous variant of EBA occurs at sites of trauma and extremities. Pemphigoid gestationis occurs around the periumbilical region, and MMP involves the oral mucosa in 85% cases followed by the conjunctiva **(Table 6)**.

The distribution of lesions is easy to discern and gives a rapid way of ruling in or disregarding a diagnosis **(Table 6)**. PF lesions are distributed along the seborrheic sites, pemphigoid gestationis occurs on the abdomen and extremities, BP involves the flexors, DH occurs on the extensors, and the localized form of BP, on pretibial region.

Mucosal Involvement

The mucosa is unique with its differential expression of antigens, and the pattern of involvement gives a clue to the diagnosis. Mucosal involvement is almost universal in PV,

TABLE 6: Sites of onset and distribution of lesions in various autoimmune bullous diseases.

Sites of onset in various AIBDs	
Disease	*Initial site of involvement*
PV	Oral mucosa (50–70%)
PF	Scalp, face, trunk
PNP	Oral mucosa
MMP	Oral mucosa >conjunctiva
Pemphigoid gestationis	Periumbilical region
LAD	Lower abdomen, limbs
CBDC	Periorificial areas, limbs
EBA	Extremities, trunk
DH	Elbows/knees, lower back
Distribution of lesions in AIBDs	
Disease	*Distribution*
PV	Pure mucosal (16.5%), mucocutaneous (64.7%), pure cutaneous (10.7%) (scalp/face/flexures/trunk)
PF	Seborrheic sites
IgA pemphigus	Flexures, trunk, extremities
Pemphigus vegetans	Flexures, angles of mouth, dorsa of hands and feet
PNP	Mucosae, upper body, palmoplantar
BP	Trunk, limbs, flexures
MMP	Oral (85%) and ocular (65%) mucosa, head, neck, upper trunk (25–30%)
Pemphigoid gestationis	Abdomen, extremities
DH	Extensors of limbs, lower back
LAD	Perineum, face, trunk, limbs
EBA	Mechanobullous variant (sites of trauma-extensors) Inflammatory variant (generalized)
Bullous SLE	Photo-exposed sites, neck, trunk

(BP: bullous pemphigoid; CBDC: chronic bullous disease of childhood; DH: dermatitis herpetiformis; EBA: epidermolysis bullosa acquisita; IgA: immunoglobulin A; LAD: linear IgA disease; MMP: mucous membrane pemphigoid; PF: pemphigus foliaceus; PNP: paraneoplastic pemphigus; PV: pemphigus vulgaris; SLE: systemic lupus erythematosus)

PNP, and MMP. It is almost always spared in PF and DH **(Table 7)**.

Patients with oral mucosa involvement complain of pain, burning in the mouth, difficulty in swallowing solid and semisolid food, and sometimes drooling of saliva. Lesions involving the conjunctival mucosa present with grittiness and foreign body sensation and may at times form adhesions. Involvement of the nasal mucosa may present as nasal stuffiness, crusting, epistaxis, and nasal discharge. Laryngeal involvement manifests as hoarseness of voice, and esophageal involvement causes heartburn, odynophagia, and dysphagia. Vulvar involvement, as in localized BP in children, may be mistaken for sexual abuse or infection.

TABLE 7: Frequency of mucosal involvement in various autoimmune bullous diseases.

Disease	Mucosal involvement
PV	Almost all cases (85%)
PF	Almost never
PNP	• Severe and recalcitrant mucositis • Oral (93%), ocular (41%), genital (35%), bronchial (30%)
BP	10–25%, mild
MMP	• Almost all, full-thickness, desquamative gingivitis • Oral (85%), ocular (64%), genital (17%)
LAD	70%
EBA	50%
Pemphigoid gestationis	Rare
DH	Rare

(BP: bullous pemphigoid; DH: dermatitis herpetiformis; EBA: epidermolysis bullosa acquisita; LAD: linear immunoglobulin A disease; MMP: mucous membrane pemphigoid; PF: pemphigus foliaceus; PNP: paraneoplastic pemphigus; PV: pemphigus vulgaris)

Course of Disease

Some AIBDs have a self-limiting course, with multiple relapses and remissions; some rarely go into remission spontaneously except in cases of localized disease; some diseases responds well to therapy, improve with pregnancy, and subsequent episodes tend to be milder; few diseases completely regress with treatment and usually do not flare up again; few are difficult to treat and respond poorly to therapy, while others like DH require diet modification (DH patients with gluten-sensitive enteropathy who respond well to a gluten-free diet fare better than those who do not respond well to this diet) **(Table 8)**.

Other Important Symptoms

Other additional features may give a clue toward the diagnosis, e.g., pruritus prior to lesions is seen in BP and DH, the latter may also have associated gastrointestinal symptoms; PNP may be associated with significant weight loss; pemphigus erythematosus (PE) is often accompanied by photosensitivity, joint pains, and oral ulcers; patients of cicatricial pemphigoid may complain of deafness when it involves the ears, and EBA cases may give history of loss of hair and nails.

Drug History

Drugs may cause biochemical interaction and an aberrant immune stimulation, leading to AIBD **(Tables 4 and 5)**.

Past History/Co-morbidities

History of co-morbidities is important as it may influence treatment decision and prevent unwanted drug interactions **(Table 9)**. This is especially important for diseases that present in the elderly.

TABLE 9: Important co-morbidities associated with autoimmune bullous diseases.

Disease	Co-morbidities
PV	Graves' disease, autoimmune thyroiditis, lupus erythematosus, rheumatoid arthritis, thymoma, myasthenia gravis, hypertension (37.5%), psoriasis, inflammatory bowel disease, malignancies—both solid organ (esophageal and laryngeal cancers) and hematological (chronic lymphocytic leukemia, multiple myeloma, non-Hodgkin's lymphoma)
PE	Lupus erythematosus
PNP	Hematological neoplasms (70–80%), non-hematological neoplasms (16–25%)
IgA pemphigus	IgA gammopathy, inflammatory bowel disease, HIV infection
BP	Parkinsonism, schizophrenia, bipolar disorder, dementia, ischemic stroke, epilepsy, diabetes (29.8%), hypertension (41%)
Anti-p200 pemphigoid	Psoriasis
DH	Celiac disease, gluten-sensitive enteropathy, autoimmune thyroiditis, type 1 diabetes mellitus
LAD	Lymphoproliferative disorders, solid organ malignancies, inflammatory bowel disease
MMP	SLE, rheumatoid arthritis, polyarteritis nodosa
Anti-laminin 332 pemphigoid	Solid organ malignancy—lung, gastric, colon
EBA	Multiple myeloma, inflammatory bowel disease (25% cases), SLE, amyloidosis, thyroiditis, multiple endocrinopathy syndrome, rheumatoid arthritis, pulmonary fibrosis, chronic lymphocytic leukemia, thymoma, diabetes
Bullous lupus erythematosus	SLE

(BP: bullous pemphigoid; DH: dermatitis herpetiformis; EBA: epidermolysis bullosa acquisita; HIV: human immunodeficiency virus; IgA: immunoglobulin A; LAD: linear immunoglobulin A disease; MMP: mucous membrane pemphigoid; PE: pemphigus erythematosus; PNP: paraneoplastic pemphigus; PV: pemphigus vulgaris; SLE: systemic lupus erythematosus)

TABLE 8: Course of various autoimmune bullous diseases.

Course	Disease
Self-limiting course with multiple relapses and remissions	BP, LAD, pemphigoid gestationis
Good response to therapy with multiple relapses	PV
Complete remission with therapy, with rare recurrence	Bullous SLE
Fluttering course without complete resolution	PF
Poor response to therapy	EBA
Fulminant disease course	PNP

(BP: bullous pemphigoid; EBA: epidermolysis bullosa acquisita; LAD: linear immunoglobulin A disease; PF: pemphigus foliaceus; PNP: paraneoplastic pemphigus; PV: pemphigus vulgaris; SLE: systemic lupus erythematosus)

Personal History

Smoking decreases the severity of PV and DH, while tannins present in red wine may worsen PV. Diseases involving the oral mucosa may cause pain and difficulty in eating, resulting in malnutrition. Bowel habits may be altered due to poor food intake or associated diseases. Bladder habits may be altered due to ongoing fluid loss or involvement of the urethral mucosa.

Dietary History

Certain food items have a possible role in disease causation or triggering of the disease by biochemical or immunological mechanisms **(Table 10)**.

TABLE 10: Role of food in autoimmune bullous diseases.

Food	Disease
• *Thiols*: Onion, garlic, leek, chive • *Phenols*: Mango, cashew, pistachio, black pepper • *Tannins*: Raspberry, cranberry, blackberry, red chillies, cassava, wine • *Isothiocyanates*: Mustard, radish, turnip, cabbage, cauliflower	PV
Nickel	BP
Gluten	DH, LAD
Iodides (seafood)	DH

(BP: bullous pemphigoid; DH: dermatitis herpetiformis; LAD: linear immunoglobulin A disease; PV: pemphigus vulgaris)

EXAMINATION

A thorough examination is a pivotal step in the diagnosis of AIBDs. Finding a single blister may provide immense information about the diagnosis; whereas its absence does not rule out an AIBD. Patients may sometimes present only with wheals, erythema, papules, nodules, or secondary lesions such as erosions and crusting. Blisters may be missed especially in the mucosae or flexures.

General Examination

A detailed general physical and systemic examination including measurement of vital parameters is important to assess baseline status of the patient, monitor for complications that may occur with extensive disease due to loss of barrier function, temperature dysregulation, protein and electrolyte imbalance, secondary infection or sepsis causing multiorgan involvement, and to detect associated co-morbidities. It is also important for patient management with various anti-inflammatory and immunosuppressive agents.

Cutaneous Examination

Morphology

The morphology of lesions may vary across spectrum **(Table 11)**. The characteristic of the blister is determined

TABLE 11: Morphologies of important autoimmune bullous diseases.

Disease	Morphology
PF	Frank blistering rare, superficial erosions with cornflake-like crust
PV	Flaccid bullae, large superficial erosions
IgA pemphigus	Vesicopustules, pustules
PNP	Polymorphic lesions—EM-like, TEN-like, LP-like, BP-like
Pemphigus herpetiformis	Grouped vesicles on erythematous base, annular lesions
BP	Urticarial plaques, tense bullae on erythematous base
Pemphigoid gestationis	Annular urticarial plaques, targetoid lesions, tense vesicles
LAD/CBDC	Smaller vesicles in annular "crown of jewel" or "string of pearls" configuration
DH	Excoriated papules/papulovesicles; frank vesicles rarely seen
EBA	• Tense blisters on non-inflamed skin (non-inflammatory) • Tense blisters and urticarial plaques (inflammatory) • Lesions with angular contour (indicate skin fragility)
Lichen planus pemphigoides	Tense vesicles on both pre-existing LP lesions and uninvolved skin

(BP: bullous pemphigoid; CBDC: chronic bullous disease of childhood; DH: dermatitis herpetiformis; EBA: epidermolysis bullosa acquisita; EM: erythema multiforme; IgA: immunoglobulin A; LAD: linear immunoglobulin A disease; LP: lichen planus; PF: pemphigus foliaceus; PNP: paraneoplastic pemphigus; PV: pemphigus vulgaris; TEN: toxic epidermal necrolysis)

by the level of split. Intraepidermal bullous diseases present with flaccid blisters, whereas the subepidermal ones have tense blisters. The former rupture easily leaving behind erosions that usually have ill-defined-to-jagged margins with peripheral extension. They have little tendency to heal and are usually covered with serosanguinous crust. Subepidermal blisters do not rupture easily and often have hemorrhagic fluid within them. They show a tendency to settle on their own without rupturing (known as autografting). The erosions/ulcers are discrete, well-defined, and do not show peripheral extension.

Ongoing inflammation and activity may manifest with underlying erythema with associated pruritus.

The morphology of residual lesions may also provide clues to a particular disease subtype, e.g., diffuse hyperpigmentation occurs in PV, while hypopigmentation with perifollicular repigmentation is a feature of BP. Milia and scarring indicate disruption of the basement membrane, as seen in EBA. Mucosal scarring is a sequelae of MMP.

Arrangement/Configuration of Lesions

This may give important pointers to the diagnosis **(Table 12)**.

TABLE 12: Arrangement/configuration of lesions in various autoimmune bullous diseases.

Disease	Arrangement of lesions
IgA pemphigus	Vesicopustules/pustules coalesce in an annular or circinate pattern with central crusting, in a "sunflower-like" centrifugation
Pemphigus herpetiformis	Closely grouped vesicles (herpetiform arrangement)
LAD/CBDC	New lesions often arising around resolving lesions leading to an annular "string of pearls" or "crown of jewels" appearance
DH	Closely grouped papulo-vesicles (herpetiform arrangement)

(CBDC: chronic bullous disease of childhood; DH: dermatitis herpetiformis; IgA: immunoglobulin A; LAD: linear immunoglobulin A disease)

Sites of Predilection of Lesions

This aspect has been discussed in the history section **(Table 6)**.

Examination of the Oral Cavity

Some findings in the oral cavity may indicate a particular AIBD **(Table 13)**.

TABLE 13: Oral cavity involvement in autoimmune bullous diseases.

Disease	Morphology
PV	Irregular erosions with jagged margins that extend peripherally with shedding of epithelium, desquamative gingivitis
Pemphigus vegetans	Cerebriform tongue, vegetative lesions over angles of mouth
PNP	Severe mucosal involvement with recalcitrant oral stomatitis, involvement of vermilion border of lips and hemorrhagic crusting, desquamative gingivitis
MMP	Desquamative gingivitis that heals with whitish reticulate scarring; sequelae like adhesions between tongue and floor of mouth or between gingiva and labial mucosa, shortening of frenulum and deviation of uvula may occur. Tongue, alveolar ridges, palate, and lips are less frequently affected
DH	Dental enamel pits
Lichen planus pemphigoides	Lichenoid lesions in buccal mucosa

(DH: dermatitis herpetiformis; MMP: mucous membrane pemphigoid; PNP: paraneoplastic pemphigus; PV: pemphigus vulgaris)

Genital Examination

Genital involvement in MMP presents with erosions, scarring, introital shrinkage, and labial fusion. Anogenital involvement can occur in severe variants of pemphigus. Vulvar lesions occur in childhood BP. Peri-genital involvement is seen in CBDC.

Examination of the Nails

Nails may be affected due to involvement of the nail folds, matrix, and nail bed. Nail changes including hemorrhagic changes are associated with severe disease. Nail lesions can sometimes relapse before cutaneous recurrences.

PV may present with subungual hematoma, acute paronychia, Beau's lines, and onychomadesis. Nail folds may be the site of predilection in PNP. Nail dystrophy, pterygium formation and anonychia can be seen in EBA. BP may also present with nail scarring and pterygium formation.

Examination of the Eyes

During ocular examination, eyelashes are examined for inversion; eyelids for presence of erosions (PV and ocular pemphigoid); bulbar and palpebral conjunctiva for erythema, erosions (PV, PNP, LAD, ocular pemphigoid), scarring and synechiae formation (ocular pemphigoid); and cornea for opacities and vascularization (ocular pemphigoid).

Examination of the Palms and Soles

Due to a thick stratum corneum on the palms and soles, intraepidermal blisters may falsely appear to be tense.

Palmoplantar involvement is more often seen in PNP than PV (dyshidrosiform type). It occurs in dyshidrosiform BP. Infantile BP tends to be located on the palms and soles. Punctate purpura on palms and soles is seen in DH.

Examination of the Scalp and Hair

Different portions of the hair follicle express antigens leading to scalp involvement. PV and PF present with easy extractability of anagen hair. This anagen effluvium is regarded as equivalent of Nikolsky sign. PF may just present with scalp scaling and crusting while tufting of hair follicles may be noted in PV. Scarring alopecia occurs in those AIBDs where the disease targets lamina lucida and below.

Examination to Look for Complications

Careful examination must be undertaken to look for local and systemic complications. These may be due to secondary viral, bacterial, or fungal infection, a consequence of extensive and severe disease, or a side effect of treatment **(Table 14)**. A long-standing and non-healing lesion may be due to infection like herpes (eczema herpeticum). Patients with mucosal involvement may manifest signs and symptoms of nutritional deficiency. Extensive involvement may lead to dehydration, hypothermia, and sepsis. Pulmonary embolism has frequently been seen in BP patients.

TABLE 14: **Complications seen in various autoimmune bullous diseases.**

Complication	Condition
Infections: Eczema herpeticum, oral candidiasis, secondary bacterial infection—in extensive mucocutaneous AIBD	
Malnutrition, weight loss	Mucosal PV, PNP, other paraneoplastic AIBDs
Hypoproteinemia	Extensive AIBD
Dehydration, hypothermia	Extensive AIBD
Evidence of sepsis	Extensive AIBD
Pulmonary	
Bronchiolitis obliterans	PNP
Interstitial lung disease	PV, BP, LAD
Pulmonary embolism	BP > PV
Medication-related side effects	

(BP: bullous pemphigoid; LAD: linear immunoglobulin A disease; PF: pemphigus foliaceus; PNP: paraneoplastic pemphigus; PV: pemphigus vulgaris)

SPECIAL SIGNS

Nikolsky Sign

Procedure: Apply lateral pressure with thumb/finger pad on a bony prominence. This shearing force dislodges upper epidermis from lower epidermis, creating an erosion.

Interpretation:
- Positive in intraepidermal bullous disease.
- In patients on immunosuppression, a negative sign indicates end of acute disease.
- Reappearance indicates flare-up of disease and may need an increase in immunosuppression.

Some key terminologies related to Nikolsky sign are given in **Table 15**.

Lutz Sign (Bulla Spread Sign)

Procedure:
- Mark the margin of bulla with a pen.
- Apply slow, careful unidirectional pressure causing peripheral extension.
- *For small intact/tense bulla, apply vertical pressure*: Asboe–Hansen sign.

Interpretation:
- *Pointed*: PV
- *Rounded*: Pemphigoid
- *Negative due to roof fragility*: Hailey–Hailey disease and staphylococcal scalded skin syndrome

A list of the common signs seen in AIBDs are summarized in **Table 16**.

TABLE 15: **Various terminologies related to the Nikolsky sign.**

Marginal Nikolsky/ indirect Nikolsky	Nikolsky sign may be elicited over normal looking skin of a pemphigus patient close to existing lesions
Direct Nikolsky	<ul><li>Nikolsky sign over normal skin at a distant site from existing lesions</li><li>Positive means severe disease activity</li><li>First sign to disappear as disease responds to therapy</li></ul>
Pseudo-Nikolsky	<ul><li>Positive in erythematous areas</li><li>Cause is necrosis</li><li>Positive in SJS/TEN/burns</li></ul>
Nikolsky phenomenon	The superficial layer of the epidermis is felt to move over the deeper layer, and instead of immediately forming an erosion as in Nikolsky sign, a blister develops after some time
Modified Nikolsky	Peripheral extension of blister on applying pressure to its surface; helpful in those without fresh bulla
False Nikolsky/ Sheklakov sign	<ul><li>Positive in subepidermal bullous disorders</li><li>Pulling the peripheral remnant roof of a ruptured blister and extending to surrounding normal skin</li><li>Plane of cleavage is subepidermal</li></ul>
Microscopic Nikolsky	Pathological changes that are induced at the subclinical level after applying tangential pressure to skin/mucosa
Dry Nikolsky	Eroded base dry
Wet Nikolsky	Eroded base wet

(SJS: Stevens–Johnson syndrome; TEN: toxic epidermal necrolysis)

TABLE 16: **Common signs seen in autoimmune bullous diseases.**

Nikolsky sign	Application of lateral shearing pressure with thumb/ finger pad on a bony prominence dislodges upper epidermis from lower epidermis creating erosion
Lutz sign	Unidirectional lateral pressure causing spread of bulla
Asboe–Hansen sign	Vertical pressure on a vesicle causes it to spread
Premlatha sign	Cerebriform tongue seen in pemphigus vegetans
String of pearls sign	Annular arrangement of blisters and erythema seen in LAD, CBDC, and BP
Hypopyon sign/ half-half blister	Presence of small, discrete, flaccid vesicles that rapidly turn pustular, with pus characteristically accumulating in the lower half, seen in PV and IgA pemphigus
Fried egg sign	Dermoscopic feature of scalp pemphigus, showing multiple yellowish dots surrounded by a white halo

(BP: bullous pemphigoid; CBDC: chronic bullous disease of childhood; LAD: linear immunoglobulin A disease)

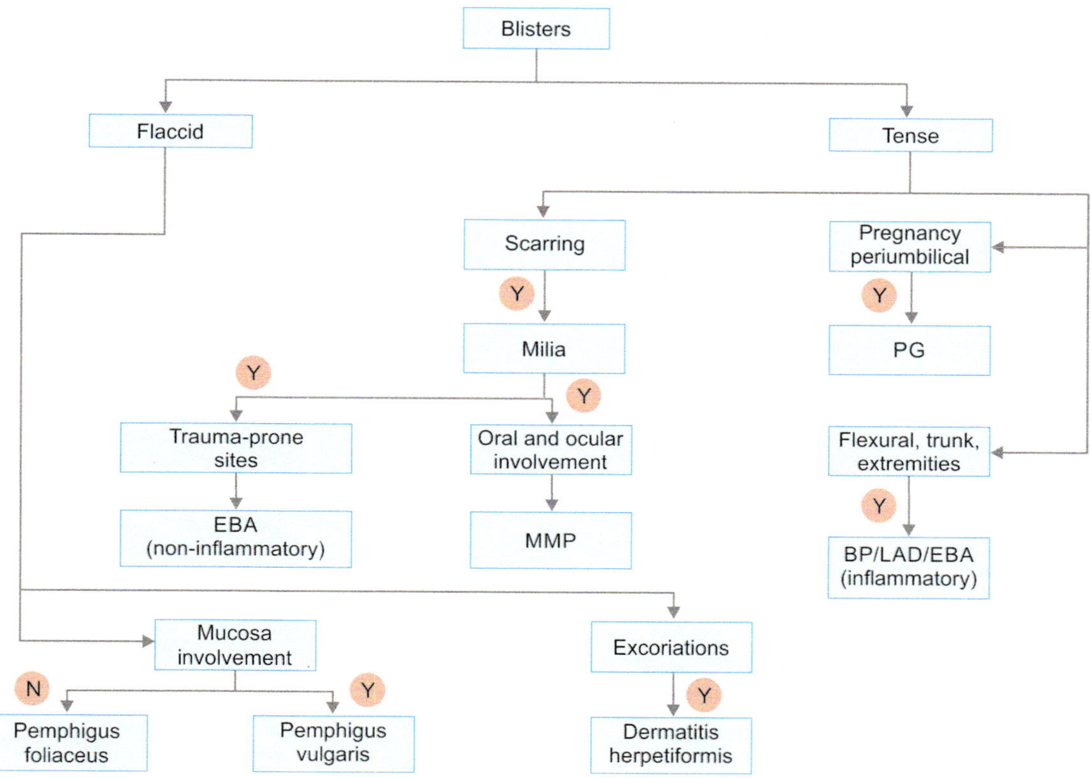

Flowchart 1: The algorithmic clinical approach in a patient with autoimmune bullous disease.
(BP: bullous pemphigoid; EBA: epidermolysis bullosa acquisita; LAD: linear immunoglobulin A disease; MMP: mucous membrane pemphigoid; PG: pemphigoid gestationis; Y: yes; N: no)

SCORING SYSTEMS FOR DISEASE SEVERITY

These have been developed to evaluate baseline disease severity and response to therapy. The various scoring systems have been discussed in Chapter 13.

ALGORITHM FOR DIAGNOSIS

Now that we have learnt the various aspects of history taking and clinical examination of AIBDs, we can apply the following algorithm to arrive at a diagnosis **(Flowchart 1)**.

CONCLUSION

A well planned clinical approach can help in early and accurate diagnosis of AIBDs. This would be crucial for effective management and prevention of long-term morbidity and mortality.

TAKE HOME MESSAGE

- A detailed history followed by thorough general physical, systemic, and dermatological examination is important to make a diagnosis of AIBD.
- History taking should include demographic details (name, age, sex, residence, socioeconomic status) and disease characteristics (onset/triggering factors, initial site of lesions, their distribution, course of disease, and mucosal involvement). Other relevant history including drug history, past history, history of associated co-morbidities, personal, family, and dietary history should be taken.
- Examination should include general physical, systemic, and mucocutaneous examination (morphology, arrangement, distribution of lesions, examination of the oral cavity, genitalia, nails, eyes, palms and soles, and scalp).
- Assessment for complications should be undertaken.
- Special signs should be elicited.
- The disease should be scored using a validated score at baseline and during follow-up periods.

MULTIPLE CHOICE QUESTIONS

1. **In which disease, blisters can occur on erythematous skin?**
   - (a) Dermatitis herpetiformis
   - (b) Pemphigus vulgaris
   - (c) Bullous pemphigoid
   - (d) All of the above

2. **Dermatitis herpetiformis is associated with which of the following diseases?**
   - (a) Autoimmune thyroiditis
   - (b) IgA monoclonal gammopathy
   - (c) Alzheimer's disease
   - (d) Rheumatoid arthritis

3. **False Nikolsky sign is seen in:**
   - (a) SJS–TEN
   - (b) Remitting pemphigus vulgaris
   - (c) Bullous pemphigoid
   - (d) Herpes simplex

4. **Which of the following food contains tannins?**
   - (a) Onion
   - (b) Pistachio
   - (c) Red chilly
   - (d) Radish

5. **Which of the following is most likely to have mucosal involvement?**
   - (a) Dermatitis herpetiformis
   - (b) Bullous pemphigoid
   - (c) Pemphigus foliaceous
   - (d) Linear IgA disease

6. **Which of the following is true about penicillamine and pemphigus?**
   - (a) Pemphigus foliaceous is more likely
   - (b) 35–50% cases resolve on drug withdrawal
   - (c) It belongs to phenol group of drug
   - (d) Both (a) and (b)

7. **Lichen planus pemphigoides is likely to occur in which age group?**
   - (a) 35–45
   - (b) 25–35
   - (c) 85–90
   - (d) <5 years

8. **Which of the following diseases shows 'string of pearls' sign?**
   - (a) Pemphigus vulgaris
   - (b) Dermatitis herpetiformis
   - (c) EBA
   - (d) Chronic bullous dermatosis of childhood

9. **In which of the following disease, the initial lesion is a pustule?**
   - (a) Pemphigus foliaceous
   - (b) Pemphigus vegetans
   - (c) Dermatitis herpetiformis
   - (d) Cicatricial pemphigoid

10. **An important infectious complication seen in pemphigus is:**
    - (a) Gianotti–Crosti disease
    - (b) Eczema herpeticum
    - (c) Scabies
    - (d) Miliary tuberculosis

Answers

1. (d) 2. (a) 3. (c) 4. (c) 5. (d) 6. (d) 7. (a) 8. (d) 9. (b) 10. (b)

SUGGESTED READING

1. Tosti A, André M, Murrell DF. Nail involvement in autoimmune bullous disorders. *Dermatol Clin*. 2011;29:511-3.
2. Elchahal S, Kavosh ER, Chu DS. Ocular manifestations of blistering diseases. *Immunol Allergy Clin North Am*. 2008;28:119-36.
3. Miteva M, Murrell DF, Tosti A. Hair loss in autoimmune cutaneous bullous disorders. *Dermatol Clin*. 2011;29:503-9.
4. Tull TJ, Benton E. Immunobullous disease. *Clin Med (Lond)*. 2021;21: 162-5.
5. Maity S, Banerjee I, Sinha R, Jha H, Ghosh P, Mustafi S. Nikolsky's sign: A pathognomic boon. *J Family Med Prim Care*. 2020;9: 526-30.
6. Kaimal S, Thappa DM. Diet in dermatology: revisited. *Indian J Dermatol Venereol Leprol*. 2010;76:103-15.
7. Juratli HA, Avci P, Horváth B. Clinicians' pearls and myths in pemphigus. *Ital J Dermatol Venereol*. 2021;156:142-6.

Diagnostic Aspects of Pemphigus and other Autoimmune Bullous Diseases

CHAPTER 15

Histopathological Aspects

Neha Taneja, Rhea Ahuja, M Ramam

- Histopathological features of autoimmune bullous disorders (epidermal and subepidermal bullous disorders)
- Epidermal vesiculo-bullous disorders include pemphigus group of disorders
- Subepidermal bullous disorders include bullous pemphigoid, anti-p200 pemphigoid, mucous membrane pemphigoid, linear IgA disease, chronic bullous dermatosis of childhood and dermatitis herpetiformis

INTRODUCTION

Autoimmune bullous diseases (AIBDs) usually show a 'vesiculo-bullous' reaction pattern on histopathology. These can be categorized on the basis of the anatomical level of split, as intraepidermal, which occurs due to keratinocyte acantholysis (pemphigus group of disorders), or subepidermal, due to damage to the components of basement membrane zone (pemphigoid group of disorders) **(Table 1)**. Though this distinction is usually straightforward, re-epithelizing subepidermal blisters may look like intraepidermal blisters because of the regenerating epithelium at the base of blister. Similarly, regenerating pemphigus might show an intraepidermal split at a higher level than expected.

Besides the level of split, other ancillary features which help in making a diagnosis include other epidermal changes, presence of dyskeratotic keratinocytes, interface dermatitis, and type and intensity of the dermal infiltrate.

CHOOSING THE APPROPRIATE BIOPSY SITE

Skin biopsies for routine histopathological evaluation in blistering disorders should be taken from lesional skin, ideally an intact bulla <24 hours old. In case of a small vesicle, the entire vesicle can be removed using a 4-mm punch, while in a larger bulla, biopsy should be taken from the edge, including two-thirds blister and one-third perilesional skin. In the absence of an intact vesicle, biopsy may be taken from the edge of an erosion. Taking a biopsy from the oral mucosa is more challenging as one rarely sees an intact bulla, the affected mucosa is friable and easily erodes and is not always easily accessible. In patients who only have oral lesions, a carefully taken mucosal punch biopsy is of great diagnostic value.

PEMPHIGUS GROUP OF DISORDERS

Pemphigus group of disorders are clinically characterized by flaccid blisters and erosions of the skin and mucous membranes and histologically by acantholysis that leads to formation of intraepidermal blisters. These intraepidermal blisters can occur at subcorneal, intraspinous or suprabasal levels, along with different types of inflammatory infiltrates, resulting in the following subtypes:

- Pemphigus vulgaris, with its variant, pemphigus vegetans (P. vegetans)

TABLE 1: Vesiculo-bullous reaction pattern in autoimmune bullous diseases according to the anatomical level of split.

Intraepidermal	
Subcorneal	• Pemphigus foliaceus and variants • Immunoglobulin A (IgA) pemphigus (subcorneal pustular dermatosis variant)
Intraspinous	IgA pemphigus (intraepidermal variant)
Suprabasal	• Pemphigus vulgaris and variants • Paraneoplastic pemphigus
Subepidermal	
Epidermal basement membrane zone destruction or disruption	• Bullous pemphigoid • Mucous membrane pemphigoid • Pemphigoid gestationis • Dermatitis herpetiformis • Linear IgA bullous dermatosis and its childhood variant chronic bullous dermatosis of childhood • Bullous systemic lupus erythematosus • Epidermolysis bullosa acquisita

- Pemphigus foliaceus (PF), with its lupus erythematosus-like variant, pemphigus erythematosus, and its endemic variant, fogo selvagem
- Pemphigus herpetiformis
- Paraneoplastic pemphigus (PNP)
- Immunoglobulin A (IgA) pemphigus

Pemphigus Vulgaris

Pemphigus vulgaris (PV) presents with oral erosions along with variably-sized, flaccid vesicles and bullae which rupture easily and leave behind erosions with overlying crusts.

Histopathologically, it is characterized by acantholysis of basal keratinocytes leading to formation of a suprabasal cleft in the epidermis. The basal keratinocytes, although separated from each other, remain attached to the basement membrane, giving a "row of tombstones" appearance (**Fig. 1**). Acantholytic keratinocytes are larger, round cells with large central nuclei, a perinuclear halo, and basophilic cytoplasm at the periphery (**Fig. 2**). These cells are present in the cleft or on the roof and floor of the blister. In addition, the cleft contains a few inflammatory cells such as lymphocytes, neutrophils and eosinophils, fibrin and red blood cells. The dermal infiltrate is usually sparse but may be of variable density, being particularly intense in mucosal lesions. It is composed of lymphocytes and histiocytes, with occasional eosinophils and neutrophils and is accompanied by some dermal edema. It is not uncommon to note that only a small portion of the intraepidermal cleft is suprabasal while the remainder of the cleft is intraspinous (**Fig. 3**). This should be reported as PV. In some biopsies, the suprabasal cleft extends into the epithelium of the hair follicle (**Fig. 4**) and eccrine duct. However, it is not clear if adnexal involvement on biopsy has any clinical significance.

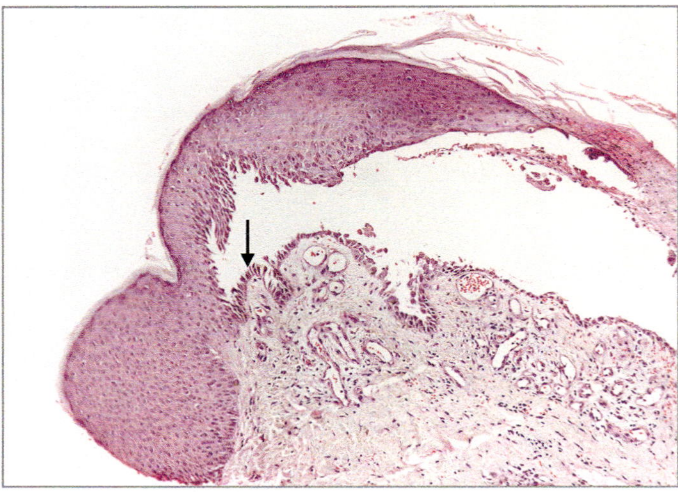

Fig. 1: Pemphigus vulgaris: Suprabasal cleft with a 'row of tombstones' appearance (arrow) (H&E; ×100).

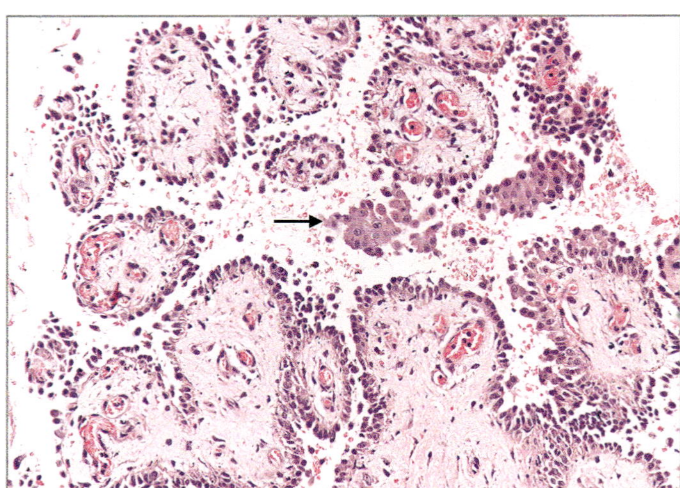

Fig. 2: Pemphigus vulgaris: Large rounded acantholytic keratinocytes (arrow) are seen in the center of the image. Note the dermal papillae lined by basal cells in a "row of tombstones" appearance (H&E; ×200).

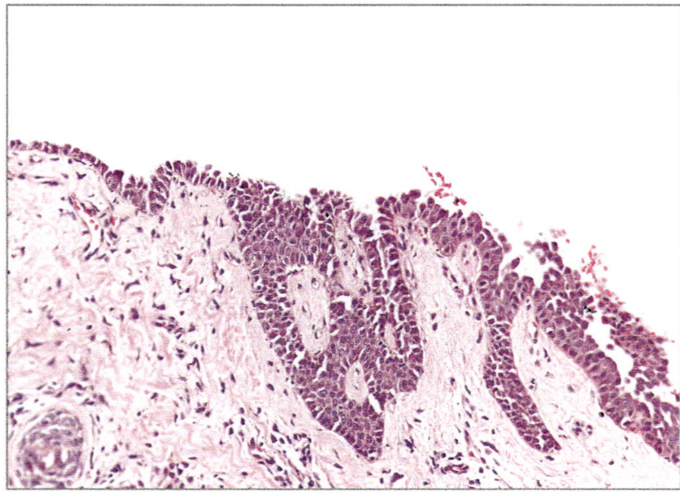

Fig. 3: Pemphigus vulgaris: On the left, the floor is composed of a single row of basal cells while it is two to three layers thick over the rest of the blister (H&E; ×200).

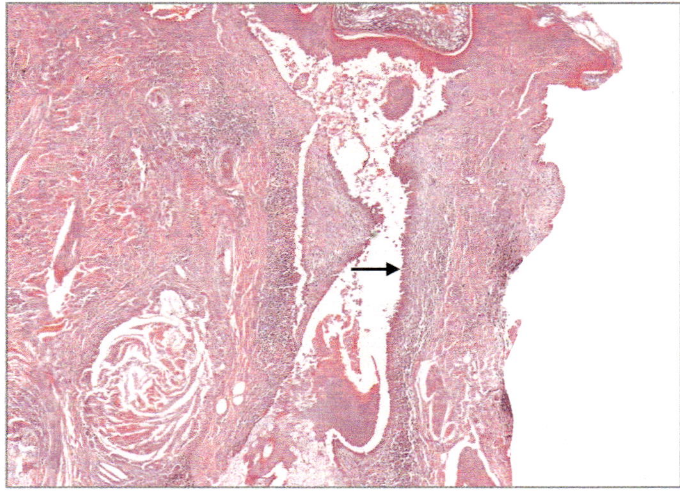

Fig. 4: Pemphigus vulgaris: Suprabasal clefting extends down the entire length of the hair follicle (arrow) (H&E; ×40).

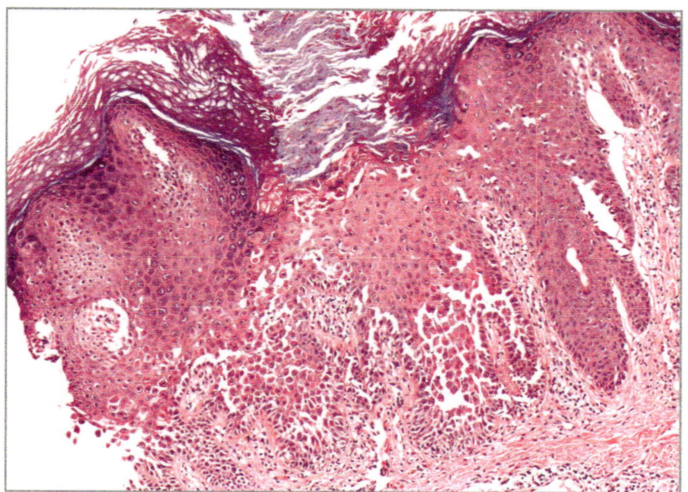

Fig. 5: Hailey–Hailey disease: Many acantholytic cells in the spinous layers accompanied by overlying hyperkeratosis and parakeratosis (H&E; ×200).

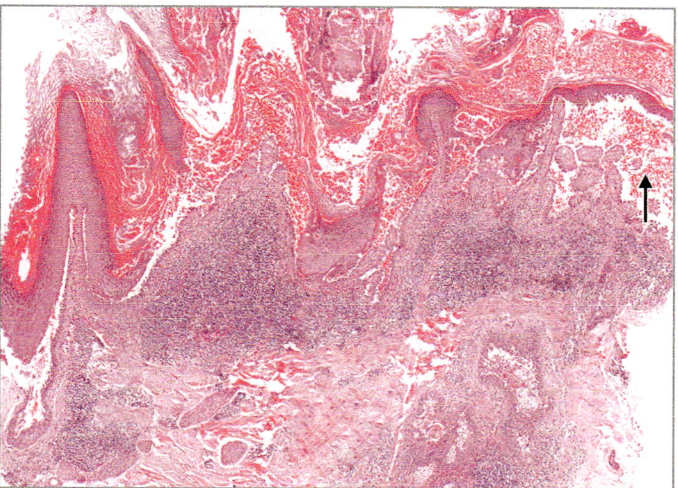

Fig. 6: Pemphigus vegetans: Marked hyperkeratosis, papillomatosis, and acanthosis of the epidermis with a suprabasal cleft most prominent at the right margin of the section (arrow). There is a dense infiltrate in the upper dermis and around a hair follicle (H&E; ×40).

If a biopsy obtained from a small vesicle does not show a cleft, step sections should be requested as diagnostic changes may be found deeper in the block. When a biopsy is taken from the edge of a blister, the cleft may be confined to the edge of the section and may have to be carefully looked for. Biopsy taken at the pre-vesicular stage or from the erythematous edge of a blister shows eosinophilic spongiosis (exocytosis of eosinophils in the epidermis along with spongiosis). In the appropriate clinical context, this finding is consistent with a diagnosis of PV. However, eosinophilic spongiosis is not specific to PV and can also be seen in other AIBDs, such as bullous pemphigoid (BP), PF, P. vegetans, and pemphigus herpetiformis.

Acantholytic cells are a characteristic finding in pemphigus but may also be seen in some other intraepidermal blistering conditions such as bullous impetigo and viral blisters, and in the group of acantholytic dyskeratotic disorders. In other intraepidermal blisters, acantholytic cells are infrequent and other findings specific for the disease help to differentiate them. In our experience, acantholytic cells in pemphigus are frequently dyskeratotic and this is not useful as a finding in differentiating it from acantholytic dyskeratotic disorders (Hailey–Hailey disease, transient acantholytic dermatosis, and Darier's disease). The presence of hyperkeratosis and parakeratosis in acantholytic dyskeratotic disorders is a more reliable clue **(Fig. 5)**.

Pemphigus Vegetans

P. vegetans is an uncommon variant of PV, mostly localized to the intertriginous areas and characterized by malodorous, moist vegetative plaques preceded by vesico-pustules.

Histopathologically, it is characterized by pseudoepitheliomatous hyperplasia of the epidermis with hyperkeratosis and irregular acanthosis. Numerous eosinophils are usually present within the epidermis and dermis, producing both eosinophilic spongiosis and eosinophilic pustules and microabscesses. Suprabasal split and acantholysis may be focal, and not as prominent as in PV,

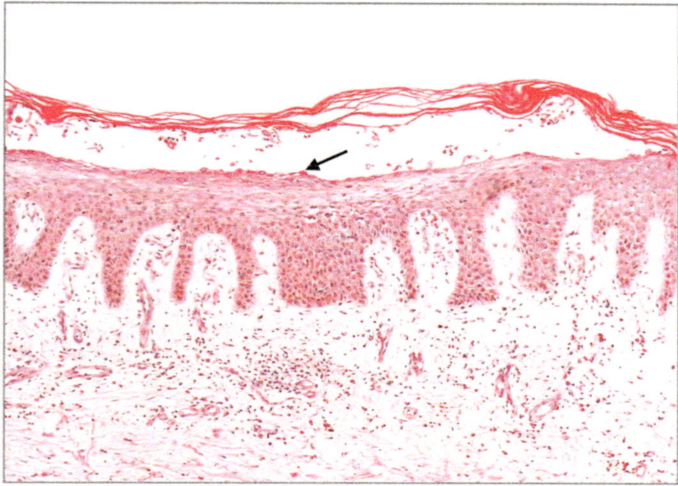

Fig. 7: Pemphigus foliaceus: Subcorneal split with a few neutrophils in the blister cavity and an occasional acantholytic keratinocyte (arrow) in the floor (H&E; ×100).

but should be carefully looked for as it helps to clinch the diagnosis **(Fig. 6)**.

Pemphigus Foliaceus

The cutaneous blisters in PF are more superficial and flaccid than in PV. So, patients with PF usually present with scaly, crusted erosions especially in a seborrheic distribution rather than intact blisters. Mucosal involvement is quite rare.

Histopathology reveals relatively subtle findings and low power examination of some biopsies may appear nearly normal because the subcorneal split resembles the common artifact of a separated stratum corneum. In these cases, the bumpy appearance of the underlying granular layer, because of occasional acantholytic cells, is a clue to the diagnosis **(Fig. 7)**. There is a subcorneal cleft containing fibrin, some neutrophils and eosinophils, and few scattered acantholytic keratinocytes. Acantholytic granular cells are a characteristic finding **(Fig. 8)** and are often seen more prominently in the follicular infundibulum. These acantholytic cells are flatter, somewhat diamond shaped and more basophilic, as compared to PV. Rarely, there may be prominent eosinophilic spongiosis with intraepidermal eosinophilic pustules and microabscesses.

Pemphigus erythematosus also known as Senear–Usher syndrome is a localized form of PF which encompasses the clinical and immunological features of both PF and lupus erythematosus. Skin lesions are present in a malar distribution, typical of lupus erythematosus, in addition to the usual seborrheic sites. Histopathology shows features similar to those of PF. Direct immunofluorescence (DIF) shows intercellular IgG and C3 deposits as in pemphigus, and also along the dermoepidermal junction as in lupus. Antinuclear antibodies (ANA) are observed in 30–80% of cases along with circulating antibodies to desmoglein 1 (Dsg1).

Pemphigus Herpetiformis

Pemphigus herpetiformis is a rare variant of pemphigus which clinically presents as itchy, grouped, erythematous papules and tense vesicles, resembling dermatitis herpetiformis (DH). Sometimes, there may be annular to arcuate, erythematous or urticarial plaques with central healing and peripheral papulo-vesicles. These lesions may later evolve into a more classical PF or rarely PV.

The characteristic histopathological finding is eosinophilic spongiosis **(Fig. 9)** or neutrophilic spongiosis that may or may not be accompanied by focal, mild acantholysis. However, a wide range of histopathological changes may be seen in pemphigus herpetiformis including eosinophilic/neutrophilic spongiosis alone, to typical suprabasal or intraspinous acantholysis. Immunofluorescence studies are helpful in making a diagnosis given the variable histological features, and show intercellular deposition of IgG and C3 in the epidermis, as in pemphigus.

Paraneoplastic Pemphigus

PNP, now known as paraneoplastic autoimmune multi-organ syndrome (PAMS), is an AIBD occurring in the presence of an underlying neoplasm such as non-Hodgkin's lymphoma, chronic lymphocytic leukemia, Castleman's disease, thymoma, retroperitoneal sarcoma and Waldenström's macroglobulinemia. It is characterized by recalcitrant and extensive oral stomatitis along with polymorphic cutaneous lesions: flaccid vesicles like in pemphigus, erythema multiforme-like lesions, lichenoid lesions, or tense blisters as in pemphigoid.

Depending on the clinical morphology of skin lesions, the histological features may vary. Skin biopsy may show intraepidermal acantholysis with suprabasal cleft (pemphigus-like), vacuolar interface dermatitis with necrotic keratinocytes (erythema multiforme-like) **(Fig. 10)**, a lichenoid lymphocyte-rich infiltrate with overlying basal cell damage [lichen planus (LP)-like] or rarely subepidermal blistering. Sometimes, a combination of these findings may

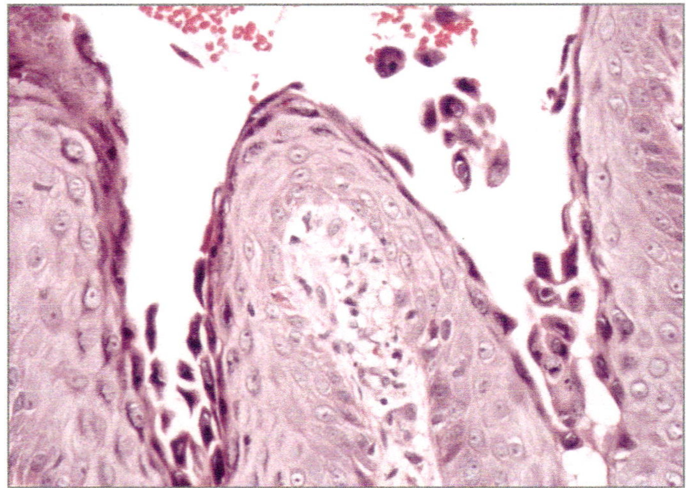

Fig. 8: Pemphigus foliaceus: Acantholytic cells of the granular layer (H&E; ×400).

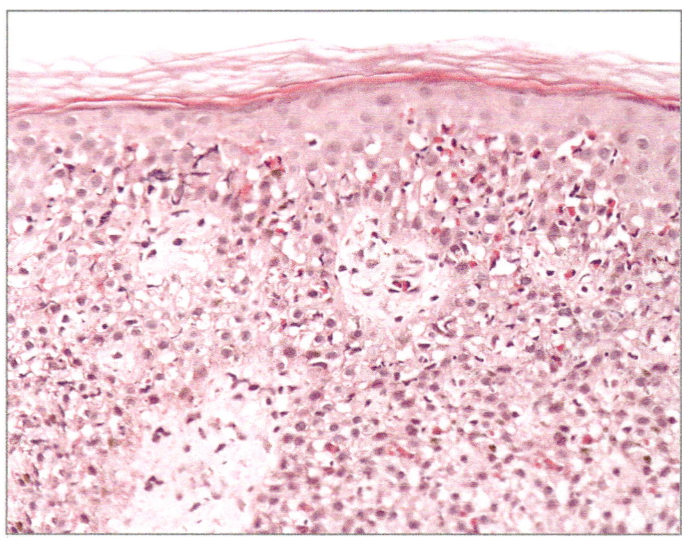

Fig. 9: Pemphigus herpetiformis: Multiple eosinophils in the epidermis accompanied by spongiosis (H&E; ×200).

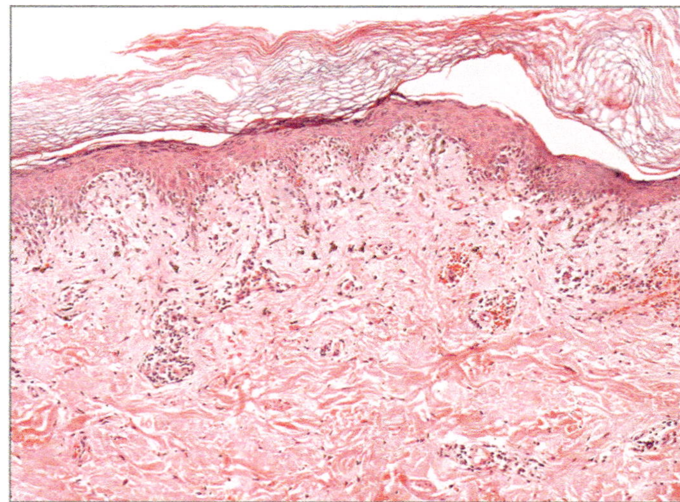

Fig. 10: Paraneoplastic pemphigus: Vacuolar basal cell damage with an occasional necrotic keratinocyte and a mild papillary dermal infiltrate of lymphocytes with several melanophages (H&E; ×40).

be present in the same section. Usually, the histological features are those of a lichenoid tissue reaction with overlying necrotic keratinocytes, with or without acantholysis.

Immunoglobulin A pemphigus

IgA pemphigus is characterized by circulating and bound IgA autoantibodies against desmosomal and non-desmosomal proteins. It is divided into two major forms based on histopathology and autoantigens involved—(1) the subcorneal pustular dermatosis (SPD) type and (2) intraepidermal neutrophilic (IEN) type. Desmocollin 1 (Dsc1) has been identified as the autoantigen in SPD type, whereas desmogleins (Dsgs) and desmocollins (Dscs) are the target autoantigens in the IEN variant. Patients present with small flaccid vesicles that soon transform to pustules with a predilection for intertriginous areas. These form annular plaques with superficial circinate pustules at the periphery.

The histopathology of the SPD subtype of IgA pemphigus reveals a subcorneal cleft containing neutrophils. The classic description is that of a pustule sitting on top of the epidermis, without underlying spongiosis. In contrast, the IEN type displays intraepidermal pustules with small to moderate numbers of neutrophils. Acantholysis is not a prominent finding in either subtype of IgA pemphigus. As the name suggests, DIF shows intercellular deposition of IgA in the epidermis with increased staining in the upper layers of the epidermis in the SPD type, while the IEN type has IgA staining throughout the epidermis. Although similar to Sneddon–Wilkinson disease and pustular psoriasis histopathologically, the SPD type of IgA pemphigus is distinguishable from both conditions by its positive DIF results. The presence of parakeratosis and neutrophils in the stratum corneum and spongiosis adjacent to or beneath the subcorneal blister may favor a diagnosis of pustular psoriasis over IgA pemphigus, but these are not reliable distinguishing features.

SUBEPIDERMAL BULLOUS DISEASES

Subepidermal bullous diseases are characterized by blisters below the basal layer. Histologically, these can be classified on the basis of the predominant composition of the inflammatory infiltrate in the cleft and underlying dermis **(Table 2)**. To further delineate a particular subepidermal disorder, immunofluorescence (see Chapter 16 for more details), salt-split assay and serological studies (Chapters 16 and 17) are required.

When dealing with subepidermal bullous diseases, it is important to differentiate a true cleft from an artifactual split. Dermo-epidermal junction is the weakest link in the skin, hence, any shearing force during tissue handling and biopsy processing may result in an artifactual cleft at this level. The presence of a subepidermal split extending throughout the section, with dermal papillae projecting into the overlying cleft and an infiltrate present both within the cleft and in the dermis are pointers toward a true split.

TABLE 2: Classification of subepidermal bullous disorders based on composition of the inflammatory infiltrate.

Subepidermal blister with little inflammation (pauci-inflammatory)	• Cell-poor variant of bullous pemphigoid • Epidermolysis bullosa acquisita (mechano-bullous variant)
Subepidermal blister with eosinophils	• Bullous pemphigoid • Pemphigoid gestationis
Subepidermal blister with neutrophils	• Linear IgA bullous dermatosis • Dermatitis herpetiformis • Anti-p200 pemphigoid • Bullous systemic lupus erythematosus • Mucous membrane pemphigoid (along with eosinophils) • Epidermolysis bullosa acquisita, inflammatory variant

Bullous Pemphigoid and Pemphigoid Gestationis

BP is a subepidermal AIBD that affects primarily the elderly, and presents with large, tense bullae on an urticarial base, commonly involving the lower trunk, extremities and flexures. It may start with a pre-bullous phase of itching and urticarial eruptions that can persist for several weeks to months. Blisters heal spontaneously in a few days leaving behind post-inflammatory changes such as hypo- or depigmentation with follicular pigmentation. Less commonly, scarring and milia formation may be seen. Pemphigoid gestationis also shows similar lesions, however, a periumbilical involvement in the form of annular urticarial plaques, targetoid lesions and tense blisters is characteristic of this disease.

Biopsy from a developed bullous lesion shows a subepidermal cleft. The intensity of the infiltrate is proportional to the erythema surrounding the blister. Blisters that clinically show erythema and edema have moderately dense, eosinophil-rich infiltrates within the cleft and in the underlying dermis **(Figs. 11 and 12)**. Neutrophils are often admixed with eosinophils in variable proportions. If neutrophils are prominent, anti-p200 pemphigoid should be suspected (see below). When blisters develop on non-inflammatory skin, the biopsy shows a pauci-inflammatory or cell-poor subepidermal blister with minimal to mild infiltrates in the cleft and underlying dermis **(Fig. 13)**.

In early non-bullous urticarial lesions, a subepidermal cleft is usually absent. There is an infiltrate of eosinophils in the papillary dermis with eosinophils tagging along the basal layer. Eosinophilic spongiosis may be noted in the epidermis. In most instances, the eosinophilic infiltrates of BP are confined to or are most prominent in the upper dermis and this is a differentiating feature from other causes of dermal eosinophilic infiltrates.

Pemphigoid gestationis shows histopathological features similar to cell-rich BP.

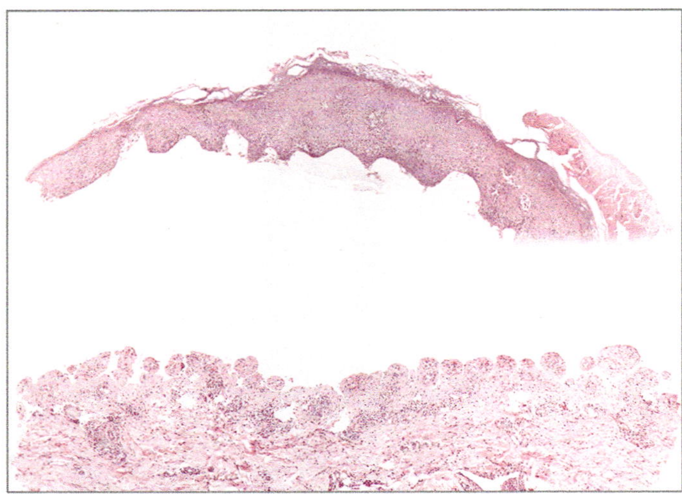

Fig. 11: Bullous pemphigoid: Subepidermal cleft with festooning of dermal papillae and a moderately dense upper dermal infiltrate (H&E; ×40).

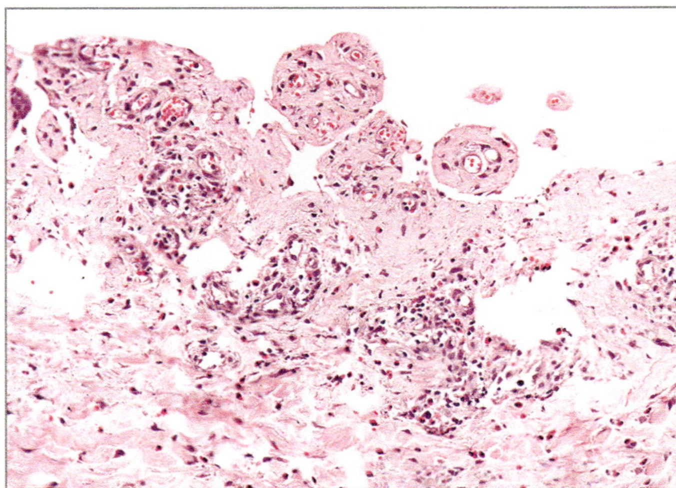

Fig. 12: Bullous pemphigoid: The dermal infiltrate shows many eosinophils (H&E; ×200).

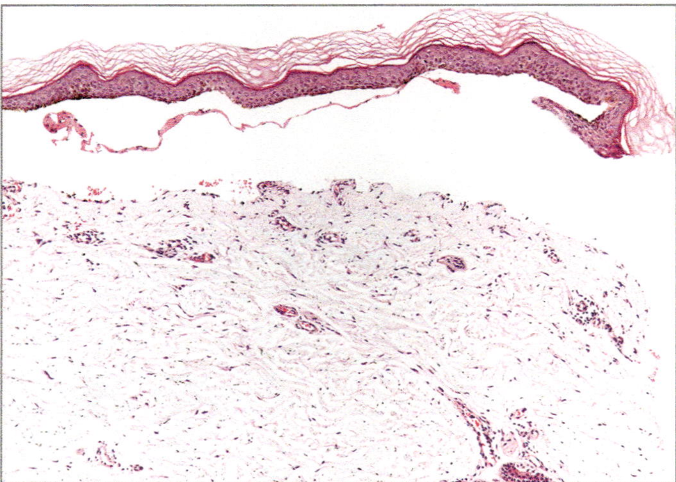

Fig. 13: Bullous pemphigoid: Subepidermal blister with no significant inflammatory infiltrate within and below the cleft (H&E; ×100).

Mucous Membrane Pemphigoid

Mucous membrane pemphigoid (MMP) is a subepidermal bullous disorder affecting the elderly, with preferential involvement of the mucosae and a tendency to heal with scarring. The term "cicatricial pemphigoid" is often used synonymously with MMP, but is better reserved for cases with prominent skin involvement.

Oral erosions are present in almost all cases, often in the form of full-thickness desquamative gingivitis and erosions on the buccal mucosa, which may heal with whitish reticulated scarring. Other affected mucosae include the ocular and anogenital mucosa and uncommonly, nasal,

pharyngeal and laryngeal mucosa. Skin may be involved in about a quarter of the cases.

Histopathology from the blister reveals a subepithelial or subepidermal cleft with the lamina propria showing an infiltrate of lymphocytes, histiocytes, some plasma cells, some eosinophils and occasional neutrophils. Eosinophils are usually fewer than in BP. At later stages, dermal fibrosis may be noted, consistent with scarring seen clinically, which can help in distinguishing it from other subepidermal bullous diseases. However, it is inconsistently seen, and has been reported in only around one-fourth of specimens.

Linear IgA Disease and Chronic Bullous Dermatosis of Childhood

Linear IgA disease (LAD) and chronic bullous dermatosis of childhood (CBDC) are adult and childhood counterparts of the same subepidermal bullous disorder where the predominant immunoreactant is IgA directed against LABD antigen 1 (LABD97 and ladinin-1 (LAD-1). These disorders are characterized by vesicles and bullae on normal or erythematous skin, commonly arranged in an annular pattern (crown of jewels sign). Oral involvement is seen in 50–80% of cases and is more common than in BP. A predilection for periorificial sites such as perioral and perineal areas is noted, especially in CBDC.

Histopathological examination shows a subepidermal cleft with a neutrophil-rich infiltrate in the blister cavity and upper dermis **(Figs. 14 and 15)**. The infiltrate often contains eosinophils, which are seen in >50% cases. Papillary microabscesses similar to those seen in DH are found in 8% of cases.

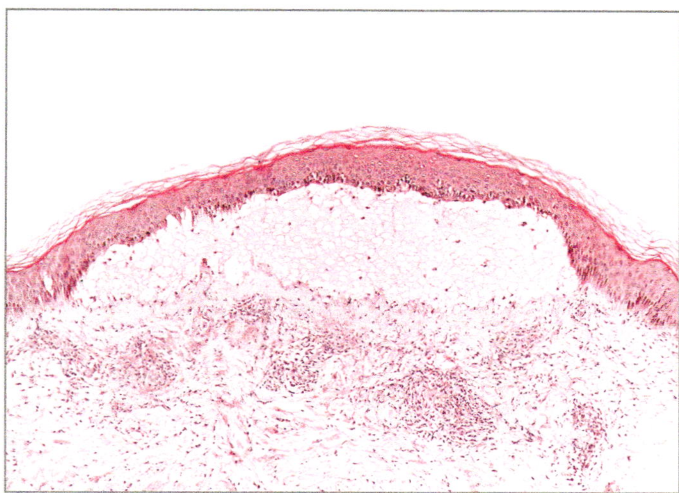

Fig. 14: Neutrophil-rich subepidermal blister: Subepidermal cleft with neutrophils within the blister cavity and in the upper dermis (H&E; ×100).

Fig. 15: Neutrophil-rich subepidermal blister: A few neutrophils in the cleft and many in the underlying dermis (H&E; ×200).

Dermatitis Herpetiformis

DH is an extremely pruritic, subepidermal AIBD with IgA autoantibodies directed against epidermal transglutaminase (eTG) or tissue transglutaminase 3 (tTG3). Patients are usually young to middle-aged adults who present with grouped, itchy, erythematous papulo-vesicles, crusted erosions and excoriated papules, symmetrically distributed on the elbows, knees, buttocks and back. It is associated with an underlying gluten-sensitive enteropathy in 90% of cases.

Papillary tip microabscesses, i.e., accumulation of neutrophils at the tips of dermal papillae, are an early histopathological finding **(Fig. 16)**. A crescentic cleft is seen between the neutrophilic microabscess and the overlying epidermis. Initially, there may be multiple small subepidermal clefts which may fuse to form a larger unilocular bulla.

Identical histopathological findings are seen in bullous systemic lupus erythematosus (SLE), which also shows a similar clinical presentation and rapid response to dapsone therapy. The co-existence of SLE helps to differentiate the two diseases. Neutrophilic microabscesses may also be seen in LAD, MMP, and anti-p200 pemphigoid.

Epidermolysis Bullosa Acquisita

This is a mechano-bullous disorder with antibodies targeted against NC1 domain of type VII collagen. It can present as non-inflammatory tense bullae on trauma-prone sites (hands, feet, elbows and knees) which heal with milia formation and scarring. Sometimes, it presents as an inflammatory bullous eruption on the trunk and extremities similar to BP. MMP-like and LAD-like presentations have also been described.

Histopathological findings largely depend on the clinical presentation. In the classic mechano-bullous variant, a pauci-inflammatory subepidermal cleft is noted. In the inflammatory subtypes, there is a subepidermal cleft with a fairly dense infiltrate both within the cleft and in the underlying dermis. The dermal infiltrate may be neutrophil-rich or has a mixed composition with lymphocytes, histiocytes and eosinophils. Papillary dermal fibrosis is present in late-stage lesions, consistent with the clinical finding of scarring. An epidermal cyst representing a milium may be seen, if biopsied with the blister **(Fig. 17)**.

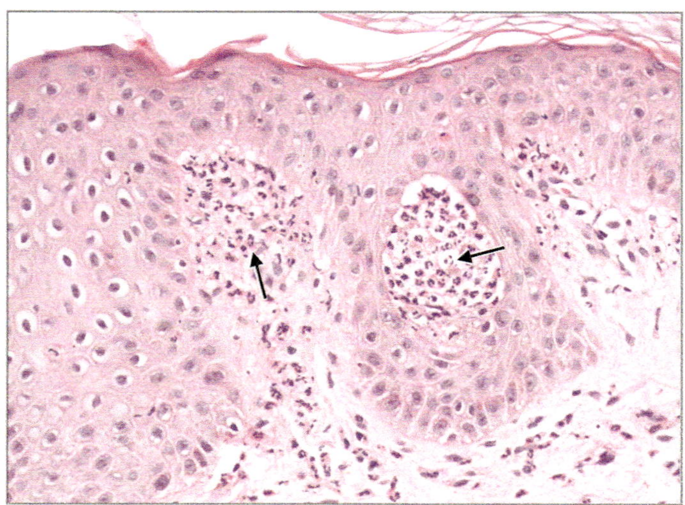

Fig. 16: Dermatitis herpetiformis: Focal collections of neutrophils at the tips of dermal papillae (papillary microabscesses) (arrows) (H&E; ×100). *Image courtesy*: Dr Sudheer Arava.

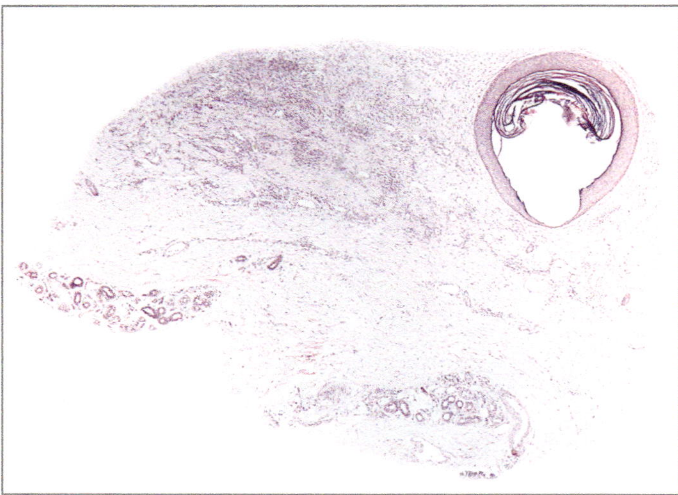

Fig. 17: Epidermolysis bullosa acquisita: Subepidermal cleft with dermis containing neutrophils, and associated dermal fibrosis and a milium (epidermal cyst) (H&E; ×40)

Lichen Planus Pemphigoides

This is a rare variant of BP characterized by co-existence of lesions of both LP and BP. Bullae are noted on papules and plaques of LP (as in bullous LP) and also on erythematous or normal skin (as in BP).

Biopsy from a blister on normal/urticated skin shows features similar to BP, with a subepidermal cleft rich in eosinophils. Neutrophilic predominance has also been described, so has a cell-poor variant with minimal dermal inflammation. DIF and indirect immunofluorescence (IIF) studies yield results similar to that seen in BP. Histopathology from a lichenoid lesion shows features of LP, with a dense band-like inflammatory infiltrate in the papillary dermis and marked basal cell damage. In bullous lesions overlying lichenoid papules and plaques, there is in addition, a prominent cleft at the dermoepidermal junction.

Anti-p200 Pemphigoid

Anti-p200 pemphigoid is a rare immunobullous disorder with autoantibodies against a 200 kDa protein, the C-terminus of laminin-γ1. It has a polymorphic clinical presentation that mimics BP and less commonly, MMP and other subepidermal bullous disorders. Co-existing psoriasis is noted in up to one-third of cases. It runs a self-limiting course and rapidly resolves without scarring, with treatment.

Histopathology reveals a subepidermal blister with an inflammatory infiltrate that is commonly neutrophil-rich (41%), composed of both eosinophils and neutrophils (40%), or rarely eosinophil-rich (11%).

CONCLUSION

Histopathological examination is an important tool in the diagnosis of autoimmune bullous diseases. Skin biopsies are usually taken either from a small intact vesicle or the edge of a larger bulla. Based on the level of split, the disease can be classified as subcorneal, suprabasal, or subepidermal. Additional features that help to make a specific diagnosis include the presence or absence of dermal inflammation, composition of the infiltrate, and other findings such as fibrosis and milia formation.

TAKE HOME MESSAGE

- Skin biopsies for routine histopathological evaluation in blistering disorders should be taken from lesional skin, either from a small intact vesicle or edge of a larger bulla.
- Vesiculo-bullous disorders can histologically be classified based on the level of split—intraepidermal (subcorneal or suprabasal) and subepidermal. The subepidermal group can further be characterized based on the predominant composition of the inflammatory infiltrate in the cleft and underlying dermis.
- Histology of PV shows acantholysis of basal keratinocytes leading to formation of a suprabasal cleft in the epidermis. The basal keratinocytes, although separated from each other, remain attached to the basement membrane giving a "row of tombstones" appearance.
- PF shows a subcorneal cleft containing fibrin, some neutrophils and eosinophils, and a few scattered acantholytic keratinocytes. Subcorneal pustular dermatosis-type of IgA pemphigus also shows a subcorneal cleft containing neutrophils, classically described as a pustule sitting on top of the epidermis.
- A subepidermal blister with an eosinophil-rich dermal infiltrate is seen in BP and pemphigoid gestationis. In early non-bullous lesions, the histological features are variable and include eosinophilic spongiosis and papillary dermal edema, with or without a subepidermal cleft.
- LAD, DH, anti-p200 pemphigoid and bullous SLE are characterized by a subepidermal blister with neutrophilic predominance in the dermal infiltrate.
- An interface dermatitis along with a suprabasal cleft is present in PNP while lichenoid inflammation with a subepidermal blister is seen in LP pemphigoides.
- Histopathological findings in EBA depend on the clinical presentation of the disease. In the classic mechano-bullous variant, a pauci-inflammatory subepidermal cleft is noted, while in the inflammatory subtypes, the dermal infiltrate may be neutrophil-rich or has a mixed composition with mononuclear cells and eosinophils.

MULTIPLE CHOICE QUESTIONS

1. **Biopsy in a vesiculo-bullous disorder should be taken:**
   (a) Preferably from oral mucosa
   (b) From the edge of large bulla
   (c) From a blister > 24 hours old
   (d) From a fresh erosion compared to an intact bulla

2. **Histopathology of pemphigus vulgaris:**
   (a) May show dyskeratotic acantholytic cells
   (b) Shows hyperkeratosis and parakeratosis
   (c) Does not involve follicular epithelium
   (d) May show neutrophilic spongiosis in pre-vesicular stage

3. **Dense eosinophilic spongiosis forming microabscesses is a feature of:**
   (a) Pemphigus vulgaris
   (b) Pemphigus foliaceus
   (c) Pemphigus vegetans
   (d) Paraneoplastic pemphigus

4. **Histopathological differentials of subcorneal pustular dermatosis-type of IgA pemphigus include all, *except*:**
   (a) Pustular psoriasis
   (b) Pemphigus foliaceus
   (c) Subcorneal pustular dermatosis
   (d) Intraepidermal neutrophilic IgA pemphigus

5. **Which of the following is not true?**
   (a) Biopsy of paraneoplastic pemphigus shows a lichenoid tissue reaction with overlying necrotic keratinocytes with or without acantholysis
   (b) In IgA pemphigus, acantholysis is usually not a prominent feature
   (c) Pemphigus herpetiformis shows eosinophilic or neutrophilic spongiosis with prominent acantholysis
   (d) Acantholytic granular cells are a characteristic finding of pemphigus foliaceus

6. **Pemphigus erythematosus shows:**
   (a) Suprabasal clefting
   (b) Vacuolar interface change
   (c) Multiple necrotic keratinocytes
   (d) Histopathology identical to pemphigus foliaceus

7. **Which of the following does not favor a true subepidermal cleft over an artifactual split?**
   (a) Infiltrate in the cleft
   (b) Festooning of dermal papillae
   (c) Infiltrate in the dermis
   (d) Focal clefting limited to a part of the section

8. **Which of the following is not a neutrophil-rich subepidermal blistering disease?**
   (a) Chronic bullous dermatosis of childhood
   (b) Dermatitis herpetiformis
   (c) Anti-p200 pemphigoid
   (d) Pemphigoid gestationis

9. **Mechano-bullous variant of epidermolysis bullosa acquisita shows a:**
   (a) Pauci-inflammatory subepidermal cleft
   (b) Neutrophil-rich subepidermal cleft
   (c) Eosinophil-rich subepidermal cleft
   (d) Interface dermatitis

10. **Which of the following is not true?**
    (a) Small subepidermal crescentic clefts are seen in dermatitis herpetiformis
    (b) Pre-bullous phase of bullous pemphigoid may show eosinophils tagging along the basal layer
    (c) Pemphigoid gestationis can be reliably distinguished from bullous pemphigoid on H&E alone
    (d) Dermal fibrosis may be appreciated in late stages of mucous membrane pemphigoid

Answers

1. (b) 2. (a) 3. (c) 4. (d) 5. (c) 6. (d) 7. (d) 8. (d) 9. (a) 10. (c)

SUGGESTED READING

1. Manocha A, Tirumalae R. Histopathology of pemphigus vulgaris revisited. *Am J Dermatopathol*. 2021;43:429-37.
2. Hodge BD, Roach J, Reserva JL, Patel T, Googe A, Schulmeier J, *et al*. The spectrum of histopathologic findings in pemphigoid: Avoiding diagnostic pitfalls. *J Cutan Pathol*. 2018;45:831-8.
3. Junkins-Hopkins JM, Busam KJ. Blistering skin diseases. In: Busam KJ (Ed). Dermatopathology, 2nd edition. Philadelphia: Elsevier Saunders; 2016. pp. 207-48.
4. Wu H, Bennett HAB, Harrist TJ. Noninfectious vesiculobullous and vesiculopustular diseases. In: Elder DE (Ed). Lever's Histopathology of the Skin, 10th edition. Philadelphia: Lippincott; 2010. pp. 235-78.
5. Tintle SJ, Cruse AR, Brodell RT, Duong B. Classic findings, mimickers, and distinguishing features in primary blistering skin disease. *Arch Pathol Lab Med*. 2020;144:136-47.
6. Verdolini R, Cerio R. Autoimmune subepidermal bullous skin diseases: the impact of recent findings for the dermatopathologist. *Virchows Arch*. 2003;443:184-93.
7. Yeh SW, Ahmed B, Sami N, Razzaque Ahmed A. Blistering disorders: Diagnosis and treatment. *Dermatol Ther*. 2003;16:214-23.

CHAPTER 16

Immunofluorescence and Immune Electron Microscopy

Raghavendra Rao, Pallavi Hegde

- Types and technique of immunofluorescence
- Indications and site of biopsy
- Transportation of specimen
- Interpretation of results
- Modifications of technique
- Immune electron microscopy

INTRODUCTION

Immunofluorescence (IMF) is an immunohistochemical technique to identify the antibodies bound to antigens in the tissue or present in the serum. It is considered the gold standard test to demonstrate tissue-bound antibodies in autoimmune bullous diseases (AIBDs). IMF not only helps to confirm the diagnosis but is also a useful tool in prognostication, assessing disease activity and predicting disease relapse. There are various techniques and variations of IMF that can be employed depending on the provisional clinical diagnosis.

TYPES OF IMMUNOFLUORESCENCE

Direct immunofluorescence (DIF) and indirect immuno-fluorescence (IIF) are the two main and commonly practiced techniques of IMF. DIF is a technique of detecting tissue-bound immunoreactants in the skin and/or mucosae or from plucked hair, while IIF detects the circulating autoantibodies in patient's serum. A modification of IIF, known as *complement fixation technique* is specifically used to demonstrate circulating antibodies in patients with pemphigoid gestationis.

TECHNIQUES OF IMMUNOFLUORESCENCE

Direct Immunofluorescence (DIF) Technique

The timing and site of biopsy, transportation, staining procedure, and storage conditions such as temperature, moisture, and pH are crucial for the proper interpretation of results. Punch biopsy (size of 3–3.5 mm) is considered superior to scalpel biopsy in suspected AIBD.

Selection of Biopsy Site

Selection of the optimal site for biopsy is crucial as the diagnostic ability of DIF depends on the presence of intact epidermis/epithelium along all or most of the specimen. The ideal site of biopsy in a suspected case of AIBD is perilesional skin, i.e., within 1–2 cm from the blister/erosion. The lesional skin must be avoided as the immunoreactants would have been consumed or undergone degradation during the inflammation, rendering a negative DIF test.

Mucosal biopsies can be tricky due to complex anatomical structure, difficulty in accessing the perilesional site and fragility of the mucosa. As immune deposits are likely to be present throughout the mucosa, punch biopsies may be taken from normal appearing buccal mucosa. The buccal mucosa can be exposed by everting the cheek, placing the thumb at the commissure and reflecting the corner of the mouth, and applying external pressure on the cheek with the index finger to present the buccal mucosa. Labial mucosa may be preferred alternatively as it is more convenient to obtain a biopsy from the lip. In conditions where the pathology is confined to the gingiva as in cases of desquamative gingivitis, the reflected alveolar mucosa is considered as the optimal site. A modified punch biopsy technique, "*stab-and-roll*" method, has been recommended to obtain gingival tissue as there might be inadvertent loss of epithelium by the lateral forces exerted during the traditional punch biopsy procedure. In this technique, all the cutting forces are directed internally to the bone. Gentle pressure is applied on the gingiva with the tip of a no. 15 blade until the bone surface is reached, and then the blade is rolled from the tip along the entire cutting edge. The sample is then gently removed from the bone using a small non-serrated tissue forceps to avoid tissue damage.

Some experts have advocated to take two biopsies in patients with mucosal-dominant disease; one from the perilesional site and the other from the normal mucosa away from the lesion. In patients with a strong clinical suspicion of AIBD, if DIF is unrewarding, a repeat biopsy should be undertaken. A study has shown that the sensitivity of DIF in mucous membrane pemphigoid (MMP) increased from 69% to 85% after processing repeat biopsy specimens. Immune deposits along the basement membrane zone (BMZ) have been demonstrated in the oral mucosa in patients with ocular MMP; hence, an oral biopsy may be considered in patients with ocular MMP.

Another technical consideration while performing the biopsy for DIF is to avoid formalin contamination of the biopsy specimen. A common scenario where formalin contamination occurs is using the same forceps (that was used to obtain the first biopsy for hematoxylin and eosin sections); a touch of formalin will render the specimen unsuitable for DIF microscopy. Formalin contamination of biopsy specimens causes certain artifactual changes. Formalin exposure up to 2 minutes causes complete loss of immunoreactants especially in pemphigus; prolonged exposure up to 10 minutes or more stains the nucleus of keratinocytes, mimicking in vivo antinuclear antibody (ANA) pattern seen in connective tissue diseases. To avoid this, when two biopsies are planned, the first biopsy should always be taken for DIF followed by the histopathology sample.

Processing of Biopsy Samples

The principle and steps involved in DIF are enumerated in **Figure 1 and Flowchart 1**.

Unlike histopathological slides, IMF slides cannot be preserved for long period as the stains degrade rapidly on exposure to a light source. Though a previous study has shown that IMF slides could be preserved at room temperature for 5 years, this may not be possible in a tropical climate like India. However, they can be preserved in deep freezer for a few months.

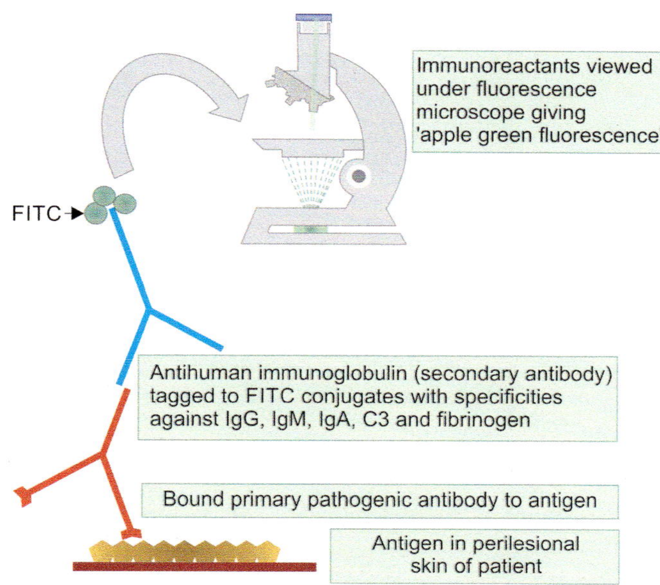

Fig. 1: Principle of direct immunofluorescence.
(DIF: direct immunofluorescence; FITC: fluorescein isothiocyanate)

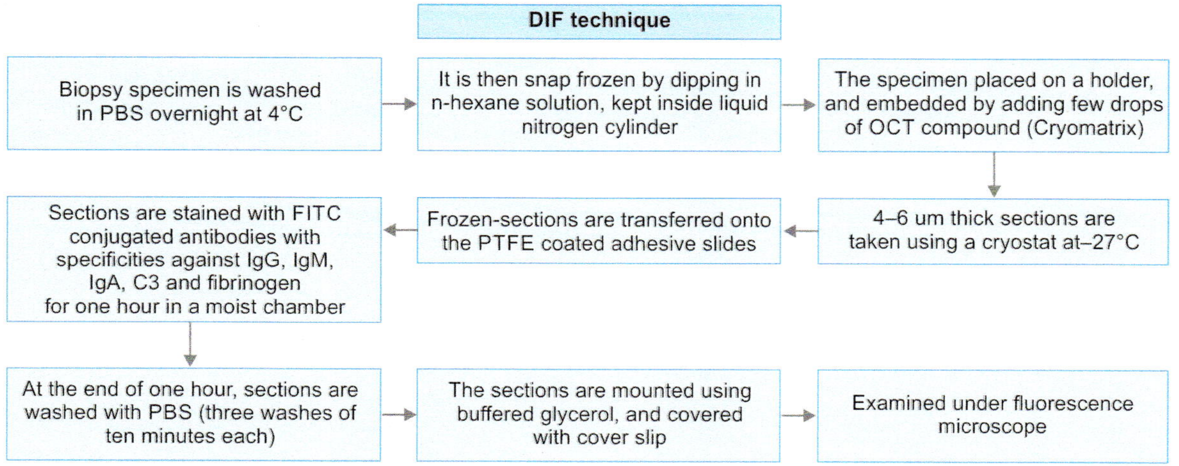

Flowchart 1: Steps involved in the technique of direct immunofluorescence.
(DIF: direct immunofluorescence; FITC: fluorescein isothiocyanate; OCT: optimum cutting temperature; PBS: phosphate buffered saline; PTFE: polytetrafluoroethylene)

Transport Media for DIF Biopsy Samples

Michel's medium (MM) has traditionally been considered as the ideal transport medium for skin biopsy specimens. Immunoreactants are preserved for up to 28 days at room temperature when biopsy specimens are stored in MM; a previous study has shown long-term reliability (up to 6 months) of MM. Besides this, normal saline or phosphate buffered saline (PBS) can be used to transport the skin biopsy specimen to the IMF laboratory, provided it can be shipped within 24 hours; this is suitable in places where IMF facility is available in-house. We have shown the utility of honey as a transport medium of skin biopsy specimens; immunoreactants are preserved for up to 2 weeks, making it a suitable medium for clinicians who do not have MM in their clinic. Honey can be easily procured in any departmental store making it an easily accessible transport medium.

Indirect Immunofluorescence (IIF) Technique

IIF is a two-step procedure performed on the patient's serum **(Fig. 2)**. About 3 mL of blood without anticoagulants is collected, and serum is separated by centrifugation. In the first step, serial dilutions of the patient's serum are incubated with frozen sections of a suitable substrate to allow circulating autoantibodies to bind to the respective antigens in the substrate. These antibodies are detected in the second step using fluorescein conjugated immunoglobulin G (IgG) and IgA. The second step is similar to DIF.

IIF helps in assessing disease severity, prognostication, and monitor treatment response. IIF shows positivity in about 80–90% of patients with active pemphigus vulgaris (PV); negative results are seen in the very early stage of the disease and in patients during remission. The sensitivity of IIF highly depends on the substrate used; the ideal substrates are monkey esophagus for PV, normal human skin for pemphigus foliaceus (PF) and rat bladder epithelium for paraneoplastic pemphigus (PNP). It also depends on technical factors like storage of sera. All sera should be deep frozen until the tests are performed. The antibody levels decline gradually over many months or years and this is further accelerated by repeated freezing and thawing. In general, five or more freeze-thaw cycles can cause almost complete loss of activity.

Salt-split Skin Technique (SST)

This technique is extremely useful to distinguish the various subepidermal AIBDs (sAIBDs) which reveals BMZ staining with identical immunoreactants. Normal human skin is incubated in 1 M solution of sodium chloride for 12–24 hours; then it is gently teased with forceps to separate the epidermis from the dermis [indirect salt-split technique]. An artificial split is induced within the BMZ at the level of lamina lucida, so that the upper lamina lucida remains on the epidermal side (roof-pattern) and lower lamina lucida and lamina densa on the dermal side (floor-pattern). This is followed by the IIF technique, i.e., incubating split skin substrate with the patient's serum for 60 minutes and subsequently staining with fluorochrome-tagged IgG/IgA conjugates. Alternatively, the patient's skin may be incubated and studied (direct SST), but being a pathological substrate, the split may not always occur at the level of lamina lucida; hence, indirect SST is preferred over direct SST.

Dermo-epidermal separation may also be induced rapidly (within few hours) by using suction apparatus such as a handheld vacuum pump. Alternatively, enzyme digestion using trypsin may be used to induce a split. This is achieved by incubating the sample in 0.5% trypsin in balanced salt solution at 37°C for about 90 minutes. The process slows down at lower temperatures. Since the process is quicker, it also allows large areas of the skin to be separated easily.

INTERPRETATION

Interpretation of DIF findings in AIBDs **(Table 1)** are based on the following parameters:
- The primary site of immune deposits
- Any additional site of deposit
- Extent of deposit—focal or diffuse
- The type of immunoreactants deposited
- Pattern of deposit—granular, linear or ragged
- Serration pattern analysis—"n" or "u" serration pattern
- Most intense deposits, in case of multiple deposits

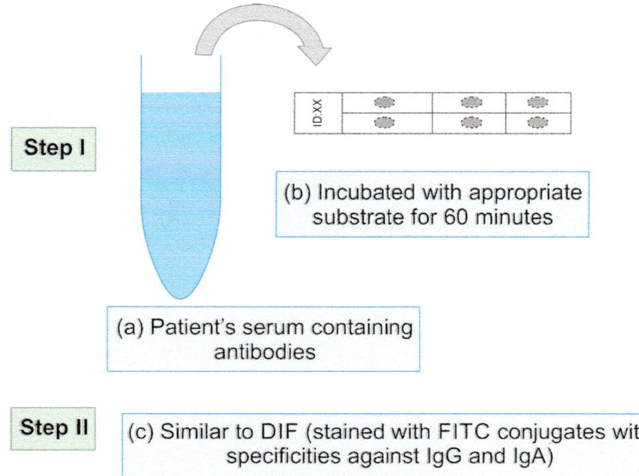

Fig. 2: Principle of indirect immunofluorescence.

TABLE 1: Interpretation of direct immunofluorescence findings in autoimmune bullous diseases.

Condition	Pattern	Type of immunoreactants	Additional comments
Pemphigus (except IgA pemphigus, PE, and PNP)	ICS **(Fig. 3)**	IgG, C3	• The staining pattern is identical in pemphigus vulgaris (PV) and pemphigus foliaceus (PF) • Gives a "chicken-wire"/"fish-net" appearance • Localization/difference in intensity of staining might differentiate the two in few cases • C3 deposition usually indicates active disease • The sensitivity of DIF in active disease is 90–100% • DIF on Tzanck smear samples has been evaluated and the results were comparable with respective skin biopsies
IgA pemphigus	ICS	IgA	• Subcorneal pustular dermatoses (SPD) type—intensity of staining is more at the upper epidermal layers/subcorneal layer • Intraepidermal neutrophilic (IEN) type—uniform intensity of ICS throughout the epidermis
PE	ICS and BMZ	IgG > C3	Fish-net pattern in the epidermis; in addition, granular staining of BMZ similar to lupus erythematosus
PNP	ICS and BMZ	IgG, C3	• ICS and linear BMZ staining with IgG and C3 • ICS—weak and non-specific as compared to classic PV • BMZ staining resembles BP • IIF on transitional epithelium (rat bladder) is diagnostic
Pemphigoid group	Linear BMZ staining **(Fig. 4)**	C3, IgG occasionally with other immunoreactants	• Pemphigoid group includes BP, MMP, PG, LP pemphigoides and anti-p200 pemphigoid • Intensity of staining is more with C3 compared with other immunoreactants • "n" serration pattern of immunoreactant deposit seen at BMZ
LAD	Linear BMZ staining	IgA only or predominantly IgA	• Sharp and thin band compared to other sAIBDs • "n" serration pattern of immunoreactant deposit seen at BMZ
DH	Granular staining at the tips of papillary dermis	IgA **(Fig. 5)**	• Fibrillar pattern of IgA is the other pattern. It has been reported especially from Japan and recently from Indian patients **(Fig. 6)** • Fibrillar pattern may be associated with atypical clinical picture
EBA	Linear BMZ staining	IgG, C3, occasionally with other immunoreactants	• BMZ staining is more intense with IgG compared to C3 • Frequently, BMZ staining is seen with multiple immunoreactants • "u" serration pattern of immunoreactant deposit seen at BMZ
b-SLE	Linear BMZ staining	IgG, IgM, IgA, C3	"u" serration pattern of immunoreactant deposit seen at BMZ

(BMZ: basement membrane zone; BP: bullous pemphigoid; b-SLE: bullous systemic lupus erythematosus; DH: dermatitis herpetiformis; EBA: epidermolysis bullosa acquisita; ICS: intercellular staining; LAD: linear IgA disease; LP: lichen planus; MMP: mucous membrane pemphigoid; PE: pemphigus erythematosus; PG: pemphigoid gestationis; PNP: paraneoplastic pemphigus)

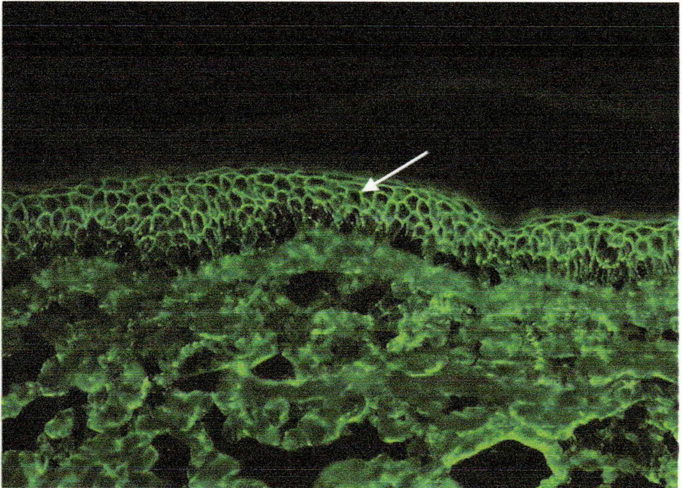

Fig. 3: DIF pattern in pemphigus: Intercellular staining with IgG giving a "fish-net" appearance (arrow) (FITC; ×200).

(DIF: direct immunofluorescence; FITC: fluorescein isothiocyanate; IgG: immunoglobulin G)

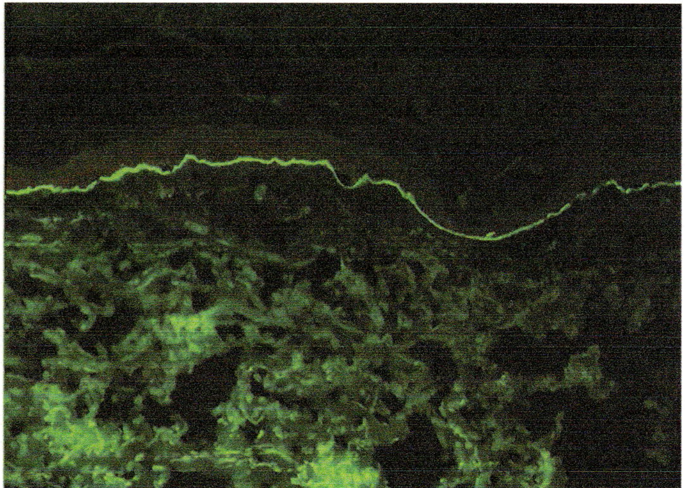

Fig. 4: DIF pattern in bullous pemphigoid: Linear staining of BMZ with C3 (FITC; ×200).

(BMZ: basement membrane zone; DIF: direct immunofluorescence; FITC: fluorescein isothiocyanate)

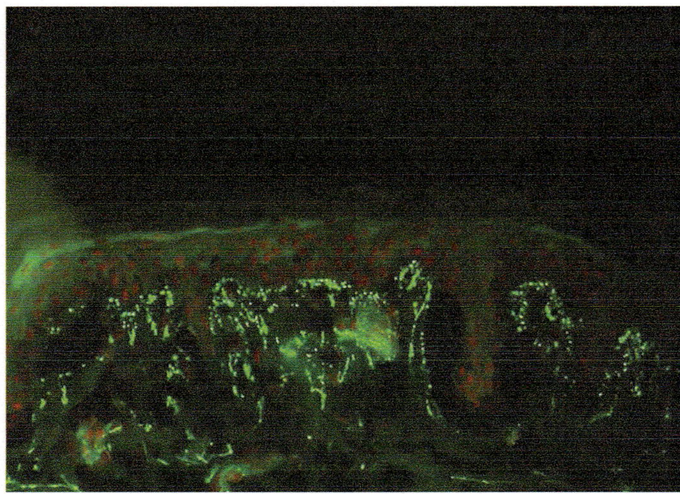

Fig. 5: DIF pattern in dermatitis herpetiformis: Granular staining at the tips of dermal papillae with IgA (FITC; ×200).

(DIF: direct immunofluorescence; FITC: fluorescein isothiocyanate; IgA: immunoglobulin A)

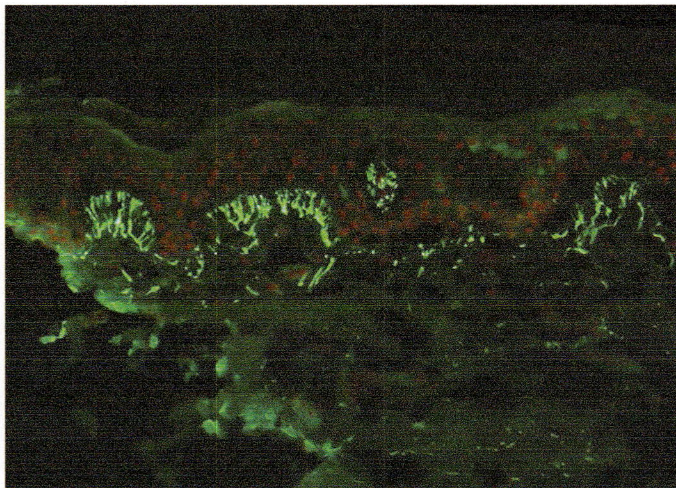

Fig. 6: DIF pattern in dermatitis herpetiformis: Fibrillar staining at the tips of dermal papillae with IgA (FITC; ×200).

(DIF: direct immunofluorescence; FITC: fluorescein isothiocyanate; IgA: immunoglobulin A)

Interpretation of IIF findings and SST in AIBDs are shown in **Table 2**.

TABLE 2: Interpretation of indirect immunofluorescence findings and salt-split technique in autoimmune bullous diseases.

Pattern	Conditions
BMZ staining on epidermal side of the split (roof-pattern) **(Fig. 7)**	BP (70% of cases), PG, MMP, LAD
BMZ staining on dermal side of the split (floor-pattern) **(Fig. 8)**	<ul><li>EBA</li><li>MMP (anti-laminin 332)</li><li>b-SLE</li><li>Anti-p200 pemphigoid</li></ul>
Combined	BP (30% of cases), LAD

(BMZ: basement membrane zone; BP: bullous pemphigoid; b-SLE: bullous systemic lupus erythematosus; EBA: epidermolysis bullosa acquisita; LAD: linear IgA disease; MMP: mucous membrane pemphigoid; PG: pemphigoid gestationis)

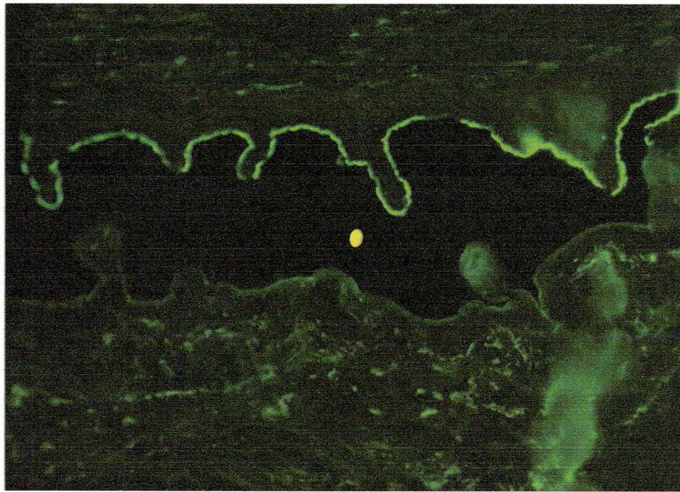

Fig. 7: IIF of salt-split skin (yellow circle indicates the level of split) in bullous pemphigoid: It shows staining with IgG on the epidermal side of the split (roof-pattern) (FITC; ×400).

(FITC: fluorescein isothiocyanate; IgG: immunoglobulin G; IIF: indirect immunofluorescence)

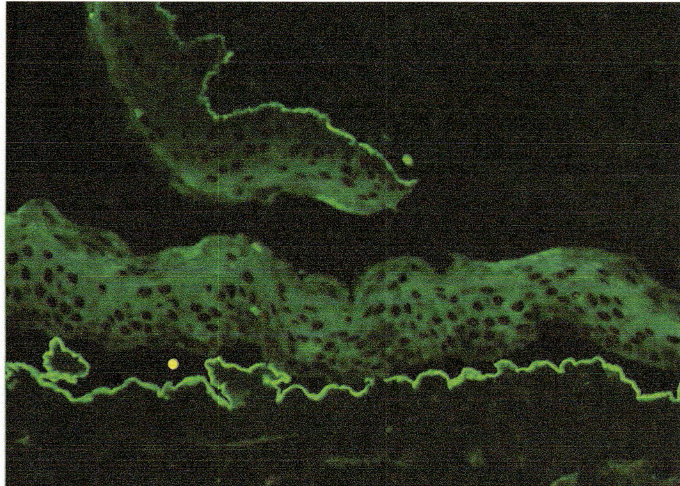

Fig. 8: IIF of salt-split skin (yellow circle indicates the level of split) in epidermolysis bullosa acquisita: It shows staining with IgG on the dermal side (floor-pattern) (FITC; ×200).

(FITC: fluorescein isothiocyanate; IgG: immunoglobulin G; IIF: indirect immunofluorescence)

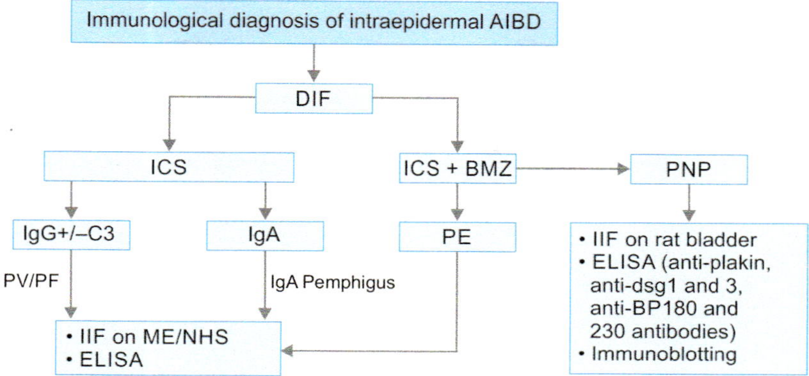

Flowchart 2: Interpretation of immunological diagnosis of intraepidermal autoimmune bullous diseases.

(AIBD: autoimmune bullous disease; BMZ: basement membrane zone; BP: bullous pemphigoid; DIF: direct immunofluorescence; Dsg: desmoglein; ELISA: enzyme-linked immunosorbent assay; FITC: fluorescein isothiocyanate; ICS: intercellular staining; IgA: immunoglobulin A; IgG: immunoglobulin G; IIF: indirect immunofluorescence; ME: monkey esophagus; NHS: normal human skin; PE: pemphigus erythematosus; PF: pemphigus foliaceus; PNP: paraneoplastic pemphigus; PV: pemphigus vulgaris)

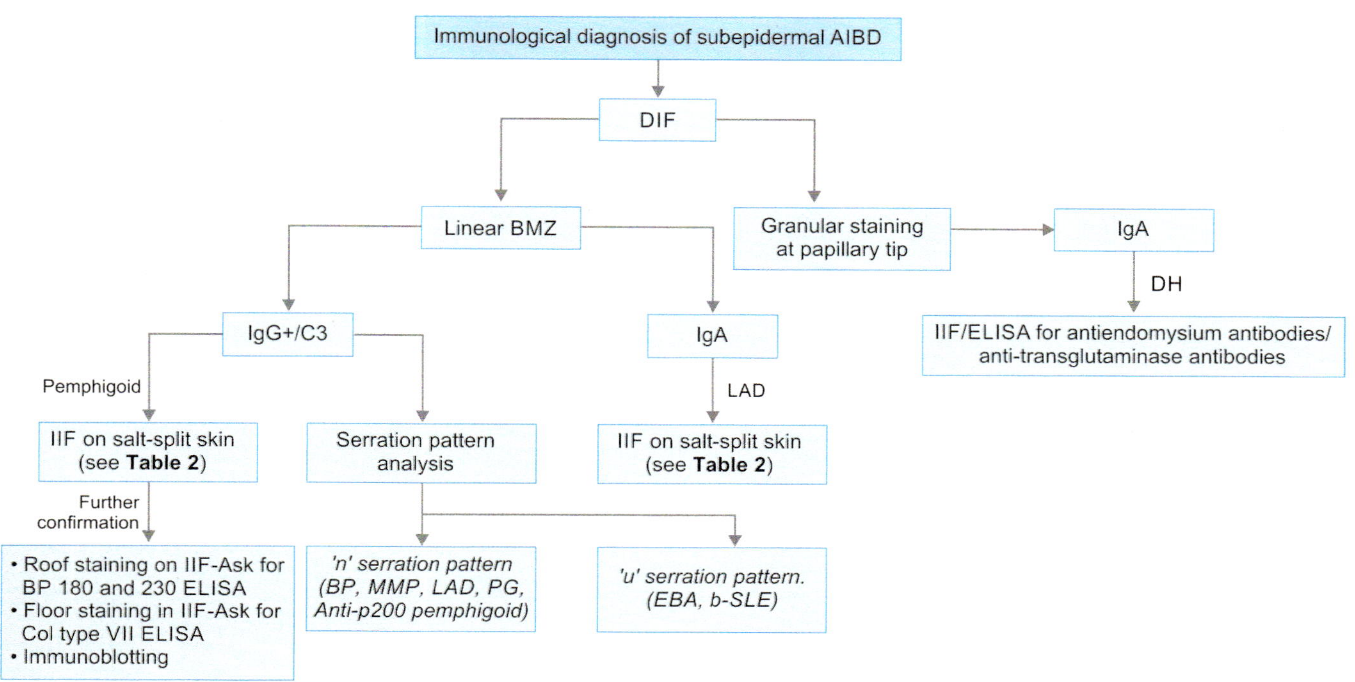

Flowchart 3: Interpretation of immunological diagnosis of subepidermal autoimmune bullous diseases.

(AIBD: autoimmune bullous disease; BMZ: basement membrane zone; BP: bullous pemphigoid; b-SLE: bullous systemic lupus erythematosus; DH: dermatitis herpetiformis; DIF: direct immunofluorescence; EBA: epidermolysis bullosa acquisita; ELISA: enzyme-linked immunosorbent assay; IgA: immunoglobulin A; IgG: immunoglobulin G; IIF: indirect immunofluorescence; LAD: linear IgA disease; MMP: mucous membrane pemphigoid; PF: pemphigus foliaceus; PG: pemphigoid gestationis; PV: pemphigus vulgaris)

Step-wise approach to immunological diagnosis of intraepidermal and subepidermal AIBDs are depicted in **Flowcharts 2 and 3**.

MODIFICATIONS OF DIRECT AND INDIRECT IMMUNOFLUORESCENCE

- ***DIF of plucked hair in pemphigus:*** It has been found to be a useful diagnostic test especially in patients who do not give consent for a skin biopsy. The outer root sheath (ORS) of anagen hair is structurally analogous to the epidermal keratinocytes; hence, pemphigus-specific fluorescence pattern can be appreciated. In this technique, hair are plucked using a rubber-tipped artery forceps and approximately five anagen hair are chosen. The plucked hair are examined under a light microscope to ascertain the presence of ORS. They are then washed in PBS and placed on a glass slide. They are stained with fluorescein isothiocyanate (FITC)-conjugated IgG for 60 minutes at room temperature in a moist chamber. Subsequently, the slides are washed in PBS (three times each, lasting for 10 minutes) and air dried. The slides are mounted with buffered glycerol and examined under fluorescence microscope. DIF of plucked hair was found to be positive in 80–100% of patients with pemphigus.

- ***Formalin-fixed paraffin embedding (FFPE) for DIF specimen:*** A biopsy specimen preserved in formalin cannot be processed for DIF microscopy as formalin destroys the immune reactants deposited in the skin. A previous study elucidated the utility of DIF on formalin-fixed paraffin-embedded skin biopsy specimens (DIF-P). The 5-μm thick sections were taken on glass slides; the slides were then deparaffinized and rehydrated and placed in PBS for 10 minutes at 37°C. Then the sections were digested with 0.05% proteinase in PBS for 30 minutes at 37°C. After washing with PBS, the slides were fixed with 95% ethanol for 10 minutes and then rinsed with PBS before staining. The slides were then processed for DIF. It was found to be less sensitive than conventional DIF on frozen sections (DIF-F). The characteristic immunopathological findings on DIF-P were identified in 20–100% of cases depending upon the underlying condition. It showed good diagnostic value in pemphigoid group such as bullous pemphigoid (BP) and pemphigoid gestationis.

- ***Automated DIF analysis of skin biopsies:*** A study conducted in Lubeck, Germany compared DIF performed using the manual method with the automated technique. Though the sensitivity of both techniques were comparable, the slides stained by the automated method displayed more intense specific IMF signals and less background staining. This improves the diagnostic accuracy and saves reagents. However, larger comparative studies are required to further explore the utility of these methods over manual staining techniques.

- ***IIF of other fluids:*** Studies comparing antibody titers of blister fluid and serum in patients with subepidermal AIBDs have concluded that IIF sensitivity on blister fluid is similar to that in serum. The blister fluid can be used as an alternative to serum especially in the pediatric or geriatric population and in those with extensive skin involvement and poor IV access. Using IIF, autoantibodies have also been detected in other body fluids such as saliva and urine.

- ***Mosaic BIOCHIP method:*** The BIOCHIP is a novel multiplex IIF technique used in the serological diagnosis of AIBDs. The BIOCHIP method combines the screening of autoantibodies and target antigen-specific substrates in a single miniature incubation field. The conventional BIOCHIP slide has 10 incubation fields each having 6 different substrates (Mosaic 7) including (1) frozen tissue section of monkey esophagus, (2) 1M NaCl-split skin, (3) human embryonic kidney (HEK293) cells transfected with desmoglein 1 (Dsg1) protein ectodomain, (4) HEK293 cells transfected with Dsg3 protein ectodomain, (5) microdrops of BP180 free antigen, and (6) HEK293 cells transfected with C-terminal globular domain of the BP230 domain, thus enabling testing 10 serum samples

in a single slide. It showed better specificity than sensitivity in the diagnosis of BP, PV, or PF. Hence, it not only detects antibodies in the tissues (monkey esophagus/salt-split skin), but also helps in the detection of target antigens in pemphigus and BP.

Further details on this method are available in Chapter 17.

ARTIFACTS IN IMMUNOFLUORESCENCE MICROSCOPY

Interpretation of IMF results depends to a great extent on technical factors; artifacts are often observed in DIF microscopy and are a potential source of diagnostic confusion. The recognition of IMF artifact patterns and their differentiation from specific IMF patterns is essential for accurate interpretation of the results. Proper controls and expertise in the field are required to interpret specific reactions and distinguish these from non-specific artifacts and other patterns which cause diagnostic confusion.

Artifact Patterns Resembling AIBD Pattern

Pemphigus-like pattern can be produced by cytoplasmic fluorescence, freezing artifact, and forceps-induced crushing artifact. It results in focal discontinuous intercellular epidermal fluorescence with almost all conjugates. There are also reports of incidental detection of a pemphigus-like pattern in the lesional and non-lesional skin of vasculitis patients, the clinical significance of which is yet to be elucidated. It is proposed that blisters observed in cutaneous small vessel vasculitis might be attributed to these antibodies. Linear and granular basement-membrane zone patterns resembling sAIBD may be present in the sun-exposed skin in normal individuals, though the intensity of staining is often weak. To avoid such confusion, the biopsy site must be chosen carefully. Collagen fibers in thin skin sections curl up and produce linear fluorescence along the dermal side of BMZ. It appears as a narrow pencil line. Basal cell cytoplasmic fluorescence is sometimes found in IIF with low dilutions of sera that might appear as BMZ staining.

ADVANTAGES AND LIMITATIONS OF IMMUNOFLUORESCENCE TECHNIQUES IN AIBDs

Advantages

- DIF is the gold standard test to demonstrate tissue-bound antibodies in patients with AIBDs and is virtually positive in all patients with active disease.
- It not only confirms the diagnosis but also directs the clinician regarding further testing, e.g., if DIF shows the presence of intercellular staining in the epidermis, the clinician will order for Dsg enzyme-linked immuno-sorbent assay (ELISA) or perform immunoblotting using epidermal extracts. On the other hand, if there is BMZ

staining, ELISA should be performed with BP180/230 kits ("roof staining pattern" on salt-split skin) or using other kits containing BMZ antigens such as type VII collagen or laminin 332 ("floor staining" pattern on salt-split skin). Immunoblotting in patients showing BMZ staining should be performed with dermal extracts.

Limitations

- It is relatively expensive and not widely available.
- Due to photodegradation, DIF slides cannot be preserved for long periods making retrieval of slides difficult.
- There can be overlapping IMF patterns in pemphigus and pemphigoid group of diseases.
- Artifacts are common and may mimic the specific staining pattern leading to diagnostic dilemma especially to the inexperienced observer.

IMMUNE ELECTRON MICROSCOPY (IEM)

The ultrastructural localization of antibodies can be detected by electron microscopy using electron dense material such as horseradish peroxidase or colloidal gold. IEM combines the specificity and sensitivity of immunological methods with the high structural resolution of electron microscopy, providing an in situ correlation and visualization of the antigen-binding sites. Direct IEM allows the detection of in vivo bound IgA, IgG, IgM, and/or C3. This is of value in differentiating various sAIBDs showing the floor-staining pattern. The indirect IEM allows localization of the target antigens of circulating autoantibodies by testing the serum of patient on normal skin. With the availability of advanced techniques for serological diagnosis such as ELISA, IEM has rarely been used even in research laboratories around the globe.

CONCLUSION

Immunofluorescence techniques are of immense importance in the management of AIBDs. Thorough knowledge of various immunofluorescence techniques, their variations and interpretations are essential for optimum utilization of these facilities for the better management of patients.

TAKE HOME MESSAGE

- Immunofluorescence is the gold standard test to demonstrate pathological antibodies in patients with AIBDs.
- DIF and IIF are used to detect tissue—bound and circulating antibodies, respectively. IIF using salt-split technique helps to sub-categorize subepidermal AIBDs into "epidermal or roof" staining pattern and "dermal or floor" staining pattern.
- Other modifications of IMF techniques, serration pattern analysis on DIF, or IIF using knock-out skin, are also useful in the diagnosis of subepidermal AIBDs.
- The timing and site of biopsy, transportation, staining procedure, and storage condition such as temperature, moisture, and pH are crucial for proper interpretation of the results. It is very important to avoid formalin contamination of the biopsied specimen posted for DIF.

MULTIPLE CHOICE QUESTIONS

1. **All the following can be used to induce dermo-epidermal separation in salt-split technique,** *except*:
   - (a) 1 molar sodium chloride
   - (b) Trypsin
   - (c) Suction apparatus
   - (d) Formalin

2. **Rat bladder is used as a substrate for indirect immunofluorescence in the serodiagnosis of:**
   - (a) Pemphigus vulgaris
   - (b) Mucous membrane pemphigoid
   - (c) Paraneoplastic pemphigus
   - (d) Dermatitis herpetiformis

3. **Honey can be used safely to preserve the immunoreactants in biopsy samples for up to:**
   - (a) 2 weeks
   - (b) 4 weeks
   - (c) 6 weeks
   - (d) 8 weeks

4. **'Stab and roll' method of obtaining biopsy is indicated in the following site:**
   - (a) Conjunctiva
   - (b) Gingiva
   - (c) Tongue
   - (d) Cervix

5. **Dermal staining pattern (floor-pattern) on salt-split IIF is seen in all the following conditions,** *except*:
   - (a) Anti-laminin 332 MMP
   - (b) Epidermolysis bullosa acquisita
   - (c) Lichen planus pemphigoides
   - (d) Anti-p200 pemphigoid

6. **Mosaic 7 biochip slides have the following substrates,** *except*:
   - (a) BP180
   - (b) BP230
   - (c) Desmocollin 1
   - (d) Salt-split skin

7. **Which chemical is deleterious to the specimen to be used for DIF studies?**
   (a) Saline
   (b) Distilled water
   (c) Formalin
   (d) Gluteraldehyde

8. **IIF has been performed using the following body fluids, *except*:**
   (a) Saliva
   (b) Blister fluid
   (c) Tear
   (d) Urine

9. **Fibrillar pattern of IgA along the BMZ has been associated with:**
   (a) Lichen planus
   (b) Dermatitis herpetiformis
   (c) Paraneoplastic pemphigus
   (d) Linear IgA disease

10. **A combination of ICS and BMZ staining is seen in the following condition:**
   (a) IgA pemphigus
   (b) Bullous pemphigoid
   (c) Pemphigus erythematosus
   (d) Pemphigus herpetiformis

Answers

1. (d)   2. (c)   3. (a)   4. (b)   5. (c)   6. (c)   7. (c)   8. (c)   9. (b)   10. (c)

SUGGESTED READING

1. Chhabra S, Minz RW, Saikia B. Immunofluorescence in dermatology. *Indian J Dermatol Venereol Leprol.* 2012;78:677-91.
2. Shetty VM, Subramaniam K, Rao R. Utility of immunofluorescence in dermatology. *Indian Dermatol Online J.* 2017;8:1-8.
3. Margo C, Barnes JR, Crowson AN. Direct immunofluorescence testing in the diagnosis of immunobullous disease, collagen vascular disease, and vascular injury syndromes *Dermatol Clin.* 2012;4:763-98.
4. Mohan KH, Pai S, Rao R. Sripathi H, Prabhu S. Techniques of immunofluorescence and their significance. *Indian J Dermatol Venereol Leprol.* 2008;74:415-9.
5. Kamaguchi M, Iwata H. The diagnosis and blistering mechanisms of mucous membrane pemphigoid. *Front Immunol.* 2019;10:1-8.
6. Arbesman J, Grover R, Helm TN, Beutner EH. Can direct immuno-fluorescence testing still be accurate if performed on biopsy specimens after brief inadvertent immersion in formalin? *J Am Acad Dermatol.* 2019;65:106-11.
7. Valencia-Guerrero A, Deng A, Dresser K, Bouliane G, Cornejo KM. The value of direct immunofluorescence on proteinase-digested formalin-fixed paraffin-embedded skin biopsies. *Am J Dermatopathol.* 2018;40:111-7.
8. Jenkins RE, Bhogal BS, Willsteed E, Black MM. Artefacts in immunofluorescence microscopy: a potential source of diagnostic confusion. *J Eur Acad Dermatol Venereol.* 1992;1:171-7.
9. Carey B, Joshi S, Abdelghani A, Mee J, Andiappan M, Setterfield J. The optimal oral biopsy site for diagnosis of mucous membrane pemphigoid and pemphigus vulgaris. *Br J Dermatol.* 2020;182:747-5.
10. Pavlović MD, Zecević RD. Cutaneous small-vessel vasculitis with unexpected circulating and in situ bound pemphigus autoantibodies. *Dermatol Online J.* 2005;11:19.
11. Lemcke S, Sokolowski S, Rieckhoff N, Buschtez M, Kaffka C, Winter-Keil A, *et al.* Automated direct immunofluorescence analyses of skin biopsies. *J Cutan Pathol.* 2016;43:227-35.

CHAPTER 17

Newer Diagnostic Techniques

Ananya Sharma, Sujay Khandpur

- Introduction to various newer diagnostic techniques in autoimmune bullous diseases, including enzyme-linked immunosorbent assay (ELISA), Biochip mosaic, immuno-histochemistry on paraffin embedded sections, optical coherence tomography (OCT) and reflectance confocal microscopy (RCM)
- Principle and procedure of various techniques
- Utility in diagnosis and prognosis
- Advantages and limitations
- Current availability and cost

INTRODUCTION

Autoimmune bullous diseases (AIBDs) are reliably diagnosed on the basis of clinical presentation, histopathology, and immunofluorescence. Direct immunofluorescence (DIF) is often considered the diagnostic gold standard in this group of disorders by detecting patterns of deposition of immunoreactants in tissue samples. Indirect immuno-fluorescence (IIF) detects circulating antibodies in the serum against specific antigens, using animal/human tissue substrates. IIF is a time-consuming, operator-dependent process with limited availability of the substrate. These techniques have limited ability to distinguish between the various AIBDs. Newer techniques have emerged that offer the advantage of being non-invasive (require a serum sample rather than tissue), with some tests, like the ELISA (enzyme-linked immunosorbent assay), providing additional information regarding prognosis. They may also be of benefit when a patient does not have active disease. However, the sensitivity, specificity, and reliability of some of these tests is yet to be firmly established. Newer imaging modalities such as reflectance confocal microscopy (RCM) and optical coherence tomography (OCT) have recently been used as a rapid tool for visualizing both intraepidermal and subepidermal clefts akin to an "optical biopsy", but the cost and availability has been prohibitory for widespread usage.

ENZYME-LINKED IMMUNOSORBENT ASSAY (ELISA)

The ELISA test, a labeled immunoassay for the detection of circulating antibodies, was first attempted in AIBDs by Ishii K, *et al* in 1997 using recombinant extracellular domains of the desmoglein (Dsg) 1 and 3 antigens produced by baculovirus expression. The antigens can also be developed in insect or human embryonic kidney 293 (HEK293) cell lines. The ELISA test is typically performed in 48 or 96-well polystyrene plates coated with the antigens (or antibodies) of interest, the counterpart of which is to be detected in the patient's serum. It is a semi-quantitative/quantitative method reflecting the antibody load and reported in relative units/milliliter (RU/mL).

Principle

ELISA is based on the interaction of antigen and antibody to form the antigen-antibody complex, and measures qualitatively or semi-quantitatively their amount in blood or tissues with the help of an enzyme-substrate reaction to develop a visible color or fluorescence. The color developed is quantified using a photometer.

ELISA is performed in broadly four steps: coating, blocking, detection, and final reading **(Fig. 1)**. Commercially available ELISA kits are pre-coated with the antigen of interest. In AIBDs, the indirect ELISA method is used in which antigen-coated plates (48 or 96 microwells on each plate) and two sets of antibodies are used **(Fig. 2)**. Diluted patient sera (1:100) containing the primary antibody to be detected is pipetted on to polystyrene plate wells, along with positive and negative controls and calibrators that have a pre-defined concentration of antibodies (200 RU/mL, 20 RU/mL, 2 RU/mL) **(Fig. 3)**. This is incubated at room temperature for 30 minutes to allow the antibodies to bind. Following this, excess fluid is decanted, the wells are washed using a buffer and a secondary, synthetic enzyme-linked antibody complementary to the primary antibody is added with another period of incubation. These secondary enzyme-linked antibodies would only bind to those wells in which the primary antibody from

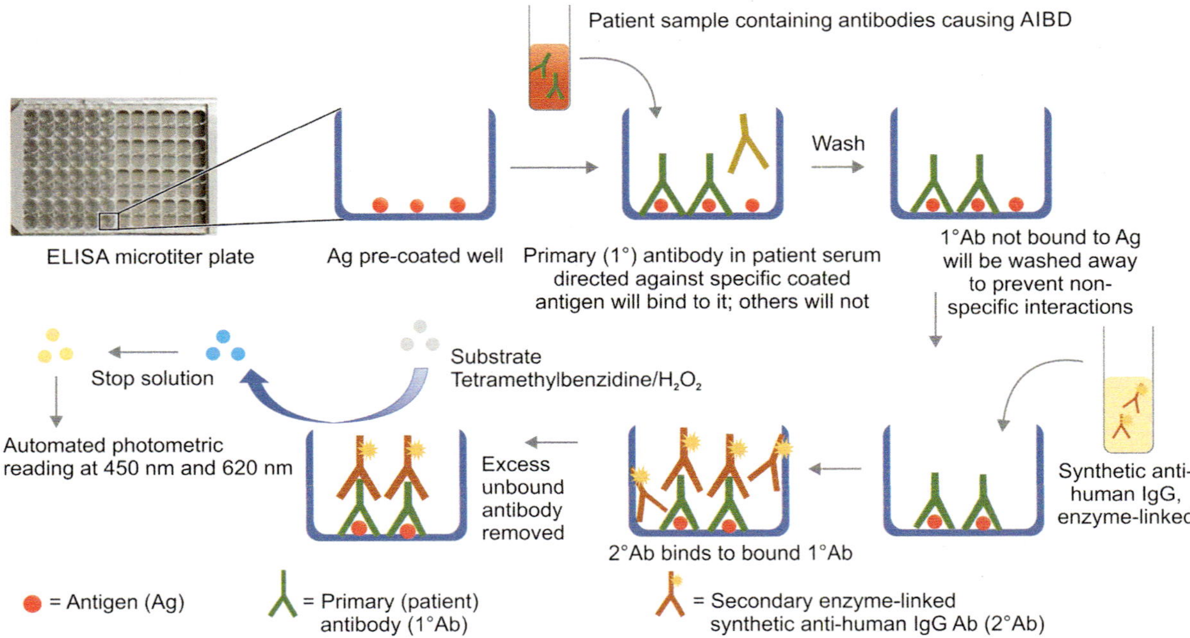

Fig. 1: Indirect ELISA test: Flow diagram to show the principle of indirect ELISA.
(AIBD: autoimmune bullous disease; ELISA: enzyme-linked immunosorbent assay; H₂O₂: hydrogen peroxide; IgG: immunoglobulin G)

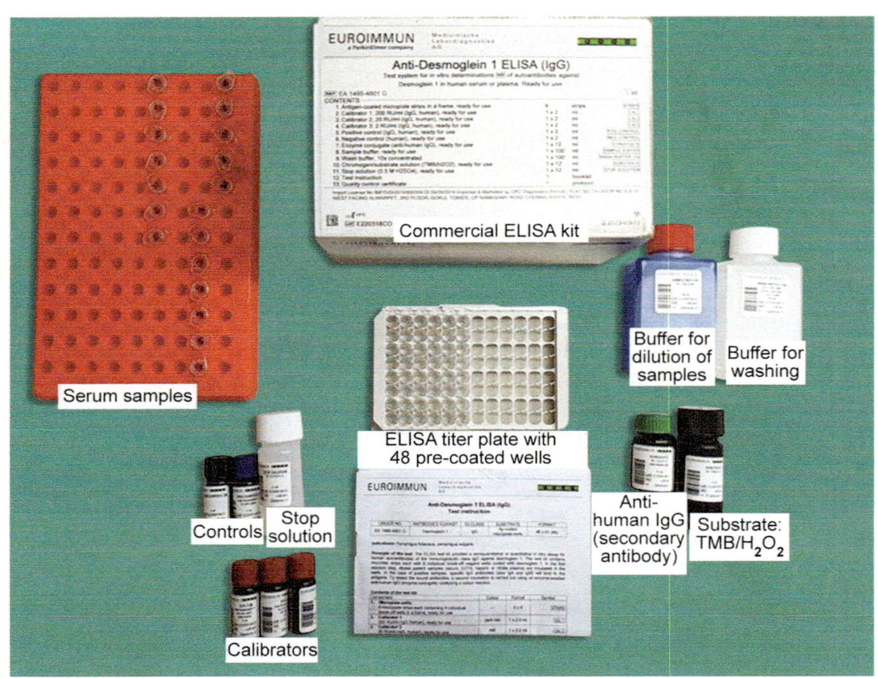

Fig. 2: ELISA test: Components of a commercial ELISA kit (anti-Dsg1, Euroimmun®, Germany).
(Dsg: desmoglein; ELISA: enzyme-linked immunosorbent assay; IgG: immunoglobulin G; TMB/H₂O₂: tetramethylbenzidine/hydrogen peroxide)

the patient sera were already bound. The addition of a substrate/chromogen in the presence of these enzymes is then used to elicit a color change. Common enzymes and their substrates used include horseradish peroxidase which oxidizes 3,3′,5,5′-tetramethylbenzidine/hydrogen peroxide resulting in a deep blue color change **(Fig. 4A)**; and alkaline phosphatase which dephosphorylates para-nitrophenyl phosphate to result in the yellow color of nitrophenol A.

A stop solution is added to halt and stabilize the enzymatic process **(Fig. 4B)** followed by automated photometric reading at 450 nm and 620 nm **(Fig. 4C)**. The test can be used qualitatively, semi-quantitatively or quantitatively, depending on the calibrators used. A cutoff is provided by the manufacturer for interpretation, e.g., <20 RU/mL is taken as negative and ≥20 RU/mL is taken as positive.

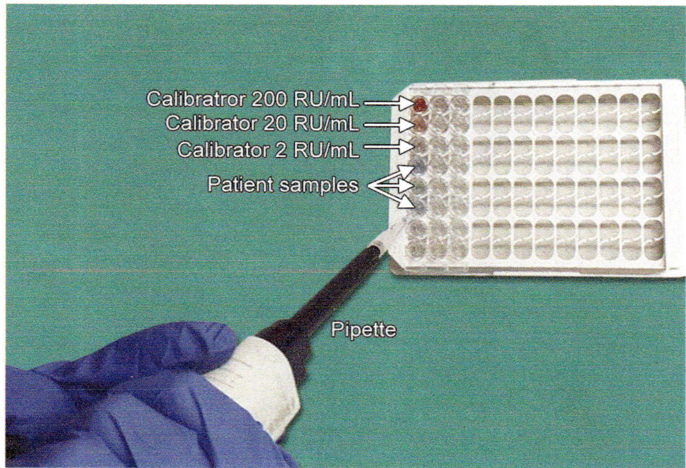

Fig. 3: Enzyme-linked immunosorbent assay (ELISA): Calibrator controls and patient samples pipetted on to ELISA plate.

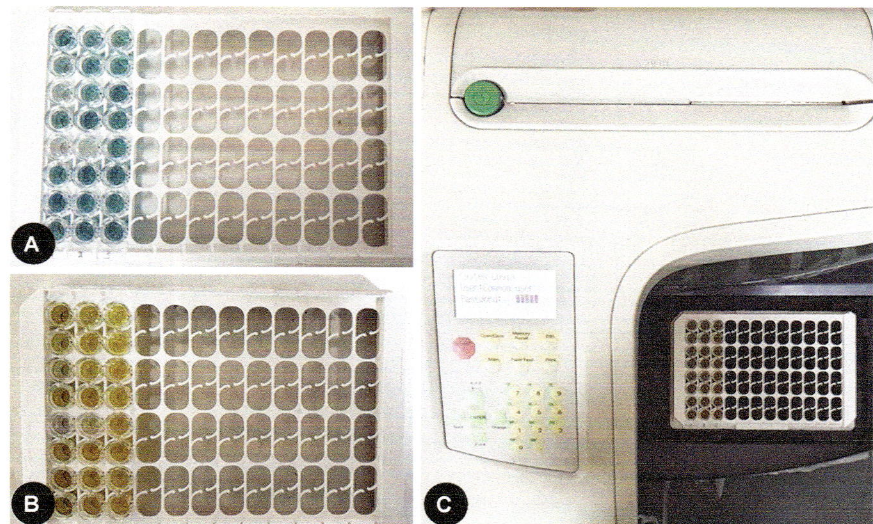

Figs. 4A to C: Enzyme-linked immunosorbent assay (ELISA) test in pemphigus: (A) Addition of substrate (tetramethylbenzidine/hydrogen peroxide) to all wells containing sample showing blue color change indicating presence of anti-Dsg antibody; (B) yellow color of solution after addition of stop solution; (C) automated photometric reading of color intensity in various wells. (Dsg: desmoglein)

Utility

Recombinant and cell-derived forms of various target antigens have been developed in order to utilize the ELISA test for diagnostic and prognostic use in AIBDs.

For Diagnosis

A patient is considered to have a diagnosis of pemphigus vulgaris (PV), if anti-Dsg3 antibody is detected in their serum, regardless of Dsg1 (though Dsg1 is positive in 60% of PV patients). If the serum tests positive for anti Dsg1 antibody alone, a diagnosis of pemphigus foliaceus (PF) is made. A cutoff value is established using normal and disease controls to formulate definitions for negative and positive test results. This is variable in studies, e.g., in pemphigus, a cutoff of 10 and 11 RU/mL for Dsg3 and Dsg1 respectively was established by Amagai, *et al*, whereas it was 30 RU/mL for Dsg3 and 25 (females) to 40 RU/mL (males) for Dsg1 in a study by Harman, *et al*. When the control sera of healthy individuals were tested by Amagai, *et al*, the positivity for Dsg3 and Dsg1 was seen in 2.2% and 1.1% cases respectively. The ELISA test has shown excellent specificity (85–97%) and moderate-to-good sensitivity (56–94%) in the diagnosis of pemphigus, which is comparable to IIF in head-to-head comparisons. In a cohort of 32 PV patients by Zagorodniuk I, *et al*, sensitivity and specificity of ELISA was 81% and 94% respectively, compared to 81% and 100% with IIF. There was concordance of IIF and ELISA results in 69%, whereas 31% tested positive in only one of the modalities.

ELISA in pemphigus could theoretically also help in differentiating PV from PF. This distinction is not always easily made on DIF, due to overlapping immunofluorescence patterns. Although some studies found anti-Dsg3

TABLE 1: Diagnostic utility of ELISA test in autoimmune bullous diseases and comparison with indirect immunofluorescence.

ELISA (Ab)	Disease	ELISA		IIF	
		Sensitivity	Specificity	Sensitivity	Specificity
Dsg1	PF	57–94%	86–98%	55–93%	87–99.6%
Dsg3	PV	68–94%	88–97%	72–90%	91–98%
Envoplakin	PNP	83%	100%	74%	90–100%
BP230	BP	58–60%	65–99%	62–89%	50–98%
BP180	BP	79–94%	94%		
BP230	MMP	5–21%	83–93%	36–54%	97.5–99%
BP180	MMP	24–41%	85–91%		
Laminin 332	MMP	53–90%	71–93%		
Collagen VII	EBA	30–95%	98.7%	92%	98–99.8%

(Ab: antibody; BP: bullous pemphigoid; Dsg: desmoglein; EBA: epidermolysis bullosa acquisita; ELISA: enzyme-linked immunosorbent assay; IIF: indirect immuno-fluorescence; MMP: mucous membrane pemphigoid; PF: pemphigus foliaceus; PNP: paraneoplastic pemphigus; PV: pemphigus vulgaris)

to be specific for PV and uniformly negative in PF [Huang, *et al* 2007, *n* = 29 (20 PV and 9 PF); Kullkolakarn, *et al* 2008, *n* = 35 (27 PV and 7 PF)], other studies have found it to be raised in more than half of PF cases [Khandpur, *et al* 2010, *n* = 66 (64 PV and 12 PF)]. However, higher values above a cutoff of 184.84 RU/mL would give 100% specificity for PV (Khandpur S, *et al* 2010). Meanwhile, antibodies against Dsg1, considered pathogenic for PF, have been found in a high proportion of PV across studies (60–95%), with no established cutoff used to determine the subtype. Thus, the detection of anti-Dsg3 (above a cutoff) on ELISA could establish a diagnosis of PV over PF.

In a study by Harman, *et al* on 104 patients (80 PV and 24 PF), the titers of anti-Dsg3 antibody could be correlated to mucosal disease severity in PV (10-unit increase in Dsg3 ELISA associated with 25% chance of a higher severity score) and titers of anti-Dsg1 could be correlated to cutaneous disease severity in both PV and PF (10-unit increase in Dsg1 ELISA associated with 34% chance of having a higher severity score). There was no correlation of anti-Dsg1 with mucosal disease severity, thus establishing a phenotypic correlation with the pathogenic antibodies.

In the pemphigoid group, the sensitivity of ELISA for bullous pemphigoid (BP) 180 [BP antigen 2 (BPAG2)/type XVII collagen] (79–94%) is higher than that of BP230 (BPAG1) (58–60%) for diagnosing BP; and also shows a slightly higher specificity. The additional diagnostic value of BP230 over BP180 alone is low (~5%). Within BP180, the non-collagenous (NC) 16a domain (a membrane proximal NC region) is the main antigenic site, but antibodies may be directed against other intra- and extracellular domains too. Sensitivity improves if ELISA is performed with the recombinant antigens that include these domains. However, up to 7.4% of the normal population has been shown to test positive for BP180 and/or BP230 on ELISA.

Antibodies in mucous membrane pemphigoid (MMP) include a wide spectrum, including those against the BP180, BP230, laminin 332, α6β4 and collagen XVII antigens. However, they react with the C-terminus of collagen XVII rather than the NC16a domain targeted in BP, and hence

immunoassays need to include this component; 75% immunoassays of MMP patients showed positivity to full length recombinant human collagen XVII, whereas only 42% showed so to the NC16a domain alone.

The sensitivity of collagen VII ELISA for the diagnosis of epidermolysis bullosa acquisita (EBA) in most studies has been poor, especially in those who were salt-split skin negative.

The diagnostic utility of ELISA test in AIBDs and its comparison with IIF is depicted in **Table 1**.

For Prognosis or as a Predictor of Disease Relapse

In a multicentric study from 13 hospitals in France comprising 26 pemphigus patients (19 PV and 7 PF) who were followed up over a 17-month period, levels of anti-Dsg1 antibody were found to correlate well with cutaneous disease activity (p = 0.03) and could be used to predict relapse in the skin. However, anti-Dsg3 antibody levels were found to be poorly specific (23%) for mucosal relapse (high anti-Dsg3 values observed in all relapse cases and 10/13 patients with ongoing mucosal remission); unless a high cutoff (130 RU/mL) was used. Anand V, *et al* demonstrated that the levels of both antibodies correlated well with remission and relapse; and calculated a cutoff for relapse of 50 RU/mL for Dsg1 (sensitivity 74%, specificity 73%) and 98.6 RU/mL for Dsg3 antibody (sensitivity 83%, specificity 83%) **(Table 2)**. A Chinese study on 20 PV patients also demonstrated similar findings of correlation of anti-Dsg1 and anti-Dsg3 ELISA index as well as IIF titers with disease activity, with the ELISA index values performing superior to IIF. According to a recent study by Ujjie, *et al* in 42 patients, anti-Dsg1 and 3 titers at first relapse are lower than those at disease onset.

A higher baseline or 3 month post-treatment titer of antibodies correlates with an increased rate of relapse. The mean relapse free time was shorter in anti-Dsg3 positive patients compared to anti-Dsg3 negative patients, though the same was not true for anti-Dsg1 antibodies. ELISA values are affected by immunosuppressive agents administered in

TABLE 2: Utility of ELISA test as a predictor of relapse in pemphigus.

ELISA (Ab)	AIBD	Author	*n*	PPV (relapse)	NPV (relapse)	*p* value
Dsg1	PV (cutaneous) or PF	Abasq, *et al.* 2009 Median follow-up: 22 months Cutoff: 20 RU/mL	19 PV 7 PF	79%	84%	0.03
	PV	Anand, *et al.* 2011 Follow-up: 12 months Cutoff: 50 RU/mL	38	61%	83%	0.001
	PV (cutaneous) or PF	Bracke, *et al.* 2013 Follow-up: 24 months Cutoff: 15 RU/mL	7 PV 3 PF	Sensitivity (79%)	Specificity (88%)	
	PV	Danseshpazhooh, *et al.* 2016 Follow-up: 28 months Cutoff: 20 RU/mL	89	50%	64%	
Dsg3	PV (mucosal)	Abasq, *et al.* 2009 Median follow-up: 22 months* Cutoff: 130 RU/mL	5	84%*	81%*	0.13
	PV	Anand, *et al.* 2011 Median follow-up: 12 months Cutoff: 98.57 RU/mL	38	73%	89%	0.004
	PV	Danseshpazhooh, *et al.* 2016 Follow-up: 28 months Cutoff: 20 RU/mL	89	56%	75%	
					Odds ratio for relapse	*p* value
Dsg1 and Dsg3 together (neither are statistically significant indicator of relapse if considered separately)	PV + PF	Genovese, *et al.* 2022 Median follow-up: 74 months	143	2.42		0.013

*With very high cutoff of 130 IU/mL, otherwise poorly specific for mucosal relapse (23%).

(AIBD: autoimmune bullous disease; Dsg: desmoglein; ELISA: enzyme-linked immunosorbent assay; NPV: negative predictive value; PF: pemphigus foliaceus; PPV: positive predictive value; PV: pemphigus vulgaris)

AIBDs. In a study by Harman, *et al* in 2000 on 82 PV and 25 PF patients, the sensitivity of Dsg1 and Dsg3 ELISA for the diagnosis of PF and PV dropped from 100% to 92% and 95% respectively in patients initiated on immunosuppressive treatment.

In BP, the anti-BP180 titer also fluctuates with disease activity and is a good indicator for relapse. A high baseline titer, lower decrease in anti-BP180 titers in the first 60 days of treatment and higher levels of BP180 at day 150 are all associated with increased relapse. However, the same correlation has not been found with anti-BP230 titers. IIF antibody titers in BP do not correlate with disease activity, and it has been found that the total titer of antibodies deposited at the basement membrane are much higher in patients with BP230 positivity on ELISA. Some authors thus speculate that BP230 forms a major component of these deposited antibodies in such patients with high IIF titers that do not correlate with disease activity.

Advantages of Enzyme-linked Immunosorbent Assay

- This test enables evaluation of a large number of samples (48 or 96) at the same time.
- It is minimally invasive as it requires serum sample rather than tissue for analysis.
- It is an objective method unlike immunofluorescence.
- It is a quantitative method (the result is depicted as a numerical value) that is able to quantify antibody titers against specific antigens and thus helps delineate subsets of AIBDs that cannot be easily differentiated on histopathology/DIF, e.g., many subepidermal blistering disorders may show a linear pattern on DIF, but ELISA would delineate the type of antibody (e.g., BP230, BP180, laminin 332, collagen VII, etc.).
- It is simpler, faster and less expensive than immuno-precipitation and immunoblotting.
- Its sensitivity in the diagnosis of pemphigus is 57–94% and specificity is 86–98%. In BP, sensitivity is 79–94% and specificity is 94% to BP180, in various studies.
- ELISA values correlate well with disease activity. In pemphigus, anti-Dsg1 titer correlates well with cutaneous severity while anti-Dsg3 titer correlates with mucosal severity.
- In pemphigus, the anti-Dsg1 titers correlate well with cutaneous relapse. In BP, the anti-BP180 titer correlates with disease activity and a high titer is a good indicator for relapse.

Limitations of the Enzyme-linked Immunosorbent Assay Test

- A negative ELISA result to the specific antigens tested does not rule out a rarer subtype of an AIBD against another antigen, which would be picked up on DIF.
- In Indian pemphigus patients, both anti-Dsg3 and 1 antibodies may be high in PV and PF, requiring high anti-Dsg3 cutoffs to differentiate between them.
- ELISA values may turn negative if patients are on immunosuppressive therapy.
- In PV, anti-Dsg3 titers do not correlate well with mucosal relapse.
- Performance of these assays in the pediatric population has not been established.

Variations of Enzyme-linked Immunosorbent Assay

Multiplex/profile ELISA: For a faster, simultaneous analysis of multiple antibodies implicated in AIBDs, 'profile' immunoassays are available commercially that combine a set of antigens, e.g., MESACUP anti-Skin Profile (MBL) covers five target antigens (Dsg1, Dsg3, BP180, BP230, type VII collagen) (88% concordance with individual ELISA systems).

Dermatology Profile ELISA (Euroimmun) includes the above mentioned five antigens as well as envoplakin. Concordant results with this multivariant ELISA against DIF/multistep diagnostic algorithm were seen in 91–94% of patients with pemphigus and 71–88% of patients with pemphigoid. Half (52.6%) of the incongruent results could be explained by antibodies against other target antigens and immunoglobulin A (IgA) reactivity. Other authors have also mentioned the possibility of IgE antibodies in BP for false negative ELISA results.

Conformational ELISA index: The poor correlation of anti-Dsg3 antibodies to remission and relapse in PV in some studies (i.e., high anti-Dsg3 antibodies in patients despite mucosal remission) has been hypothesized to be due to non-pathogenic antibodies, which have been characterized as antibodies directed against the non-calcium-dependent epitopes of Dsg3 (EC3-5) in animal models. EDTA (ethylenediaminetetraacetic acid)-treated ELISA chelates calcium, and thus modifies the calcium-dependent epitope (EC 1-2), to which the pathogenic antibodies cannot bind. This thus gives the titer of non-pathogenic antibodies alone. Subtracting this value from conventional ELISA would give an estimate of the pathogenic antibodies called conformational ELISA index, which has been shown to correlate better with disease activity.

Restricted ELISA: It is an ELISA developed using a protein extract from trypsin-digested fresh bovine skin to detect antibodies in a new variant of endemic PF from El Bagre, Colombia. This antigen (a conformational 45 kDa fragment of Dsg1 ectodomain) was found to be recognized by antibodies from all PF patients, and about half of PV patients. It was more sensitive than DIF and IIF to diagnose endemic PF.

ELISA test on salivary fluid: Salivary IgG has been found to correlate with serum IgG in inflammatory conditions. Salivary anti-Dsg1 was found to be 52.3% sensitive and 98.9% specific for PV at a cutoff of 7.7 RU/mL, whereas salivary anti-Dsg3 showed 77.9% sensitivity and 97.8% specificity. ELISA on salivary fluid is performed undiluted, in contrast to ELISA on serum which is performed at 1:100 dilution. This could be used as a non-invasive test for the diagnosis of pemphigus when there is difficulty in obtaining blood samples, as in pediatric patients.

IgA ELISA: Conventional ELISA systems detect IgG antibodies. However, in a subset of pemphigoid patients and especially in linear IgA disease, the pathogenic antibodies are IgA subtype and are missed on conventional ELISA. Csorba, *et al* developed a system for the detection of the same using a recombinant BP180 antigen and antihuman IgA antibodies.

Paper-based ELISA for BP: Hsu, *et al* developed a method of using a Whatman no.1 filter paper along with wax printer to create hydrophilic-hydrophobic wells coated with the recombinant NC16a antigen. This has been used as a low-cost and rapid ELISA to diagnose BP with good sensitivity (82%) and specificity (75%) and it requires only 2 µL of sample.

Availability and Cost

- MBL, Japan and Euroimmun, Germany are the two major providers.
- Dsg1/3 IgG ELISA (for single antigen, 48 wells): INR 29,000 + 5% GST.
- Euroimmun Dermatology Profile ELISA (IgG) (profile ELISA): a pack of 12 tests for INR 39,000 + 5% GST.

IMMUNOHISTOCHEMISTRY ON PARAFFIN-EMBEDDED SECTIONS

Diagnosis of AIBDs is often confirmed by immunofluorescence studies on frozen perilesional sections; however, they may not always be available and require special transport media (e.g., Michel's media) and specialized laboratories for processing. The same immunoreactants, IgG or subset IgG4, and stable factors of alternate and classical complement pathway respectively, i.e., C3d and C4d, may be detected on formalin-fixed paraffin embedded tissue through immunoenzymatic methods employing the commercially available mouse monoclonal and rabbit polyclonal antibodies. Immunohistochemistry may be qualitative or semi-quantitative. It is observed as brown intercellular staining in the epidermis in pemphigus group and linear staining at the dermo-epidermal junction in the pemphigoid group.

TABLE 3: Diagnostic utility of immunohistochemistry on paraffin-embedded sections of various immunoreactants in autoimmune bullous diseases.

AIBD	Immunoreactant	Sensitivity
Pemphigus	IgG	24%
	IgG4	77%
	C3d	11%
	C4d	84%
Pemphigoid	IgG	22%
	IgG4	25%
	C3d	86%
	C4d	75%

Note: Specificity with various immunoreactants was reported as 100% with IgG, 98% with IgG4, 99% with C3d, and 99% with C4d.

(AIBD: autoimmune bullous disease; IgG: immunoglobulin G)

Source: Adapted from Kasperkiewicz M, *et al*. Immunoglobulin and complement immunohistochemistry on paraffin sections in autoimmune bullous diseases: A systematic review and meta-analysis. *Am J Dermatopathol*. 2021;43:689-99.

A systematic review and meta-analysis of 124 pemphigus, 321 pemphigoid, and 43 dermatitis herpetiformis cases and 335 controls showed that detection of C3d and/or C4d is a promising modality towards the diagnosis of AIBDs **(Table 3)**. The limitation of this modality is that IgA-mediated AIBDs which show IgA reactivity on DIF, such as granular or linear staining in dermatitis herpetiformis and linear IgA disease, respectively, may not show complement deposition as IgA does not fix complement. Similarly, the predominant antibody deposited in pemphigus and pemphigoid (IgG4) does not activate the classical complement pathway and hence may not show deposition of C4d.

BIOCHIP MOSAIC ASSAY

It is a modified IIF method comprising multiple miniaturized biological substrates arranged on a single solid substrate (usually a glass slide), for faster throughput of samples. It is called a "biochip" in analogy to a computer chip that can perform multiple mathematical operations speedily and simultaneously.

The miniaturized biological substrates (biochips) comprise millimeter-sized fragments of specialized cover slips coated with tissue sections, cultured cells, transfected cells, or antigen dots. These are arranged in an equidistant, precise manner in one reaction field (on a glass slide). There are 10 fields on one biochip slide, each having six miniaturized biological substrates. This "mosaic" can now be used to detect multiple (six) antibodies simultaneously in multiple (ten) samples using a single biochip slide **(Fig. 5)**. The Dermatology Mosaic 7 or Biochip mosaic for AIBDs uses six substrates, including monkey esophagus, monkey 1 M NaCl salt-split skin, BP230gC (C-terminal globular domain of BP230), Dsg1 transfected HEK293 cells, Dsg3 transfected HEK293 cells, and BP180-NC16a purified antigen **(Figs. 6A to C)**. An extended biochip with 12 substrates, including additional NC1 domain of collagen

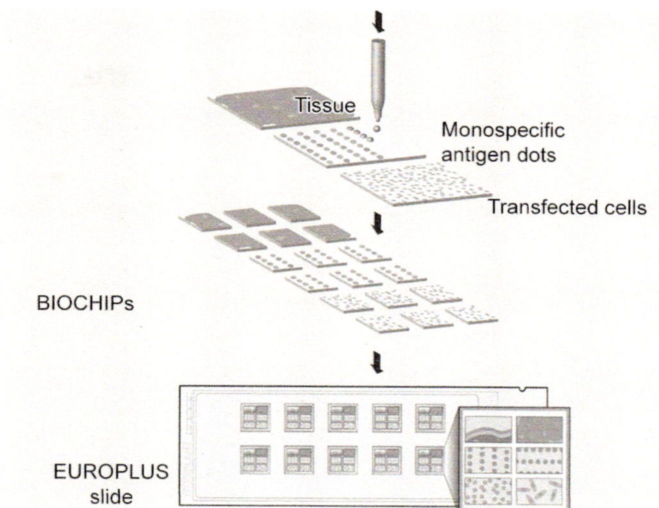

Fig. 5: Biochip mosaic: One slide has 10 fields, each with six miniaturized biological substrates (millimeter-sized fragments of specialized cover slips coated with tissue sections, cultured cells, transfected cells, or antigen dots).

Source: Euroimmun®, Germany.

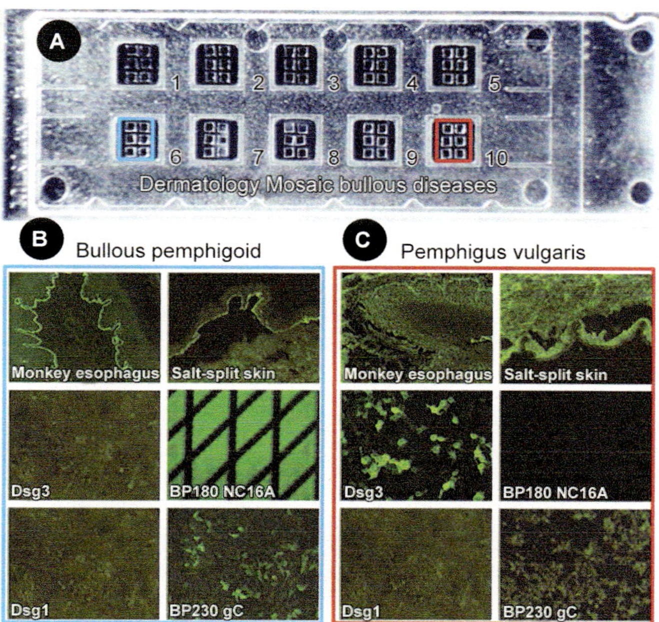

Figs. 6A to C: Biochip mosaic: (A) Dermatology mosaic 7 by Euroimmun (Biochip mosaic for AIBDs); (B) Panel of results in a patient of bullous pemphigoid: linear basement membrane staining on monkey esophagus. roof staining in salt split skin, diamond shaped green fields in front of a dark background signifying positivity to BP180-NC16a, cytoplasmic granular flouroscence in BP230gC, negativity for Dsg1 and Dsg3; (C) Panel of results in a patient of pemphigus vulgaris: intraepidermal intercellular fishnet fluorescence in monkey esophagus and salt-split skin, granular cytoplasmic positivity in Dsg3 and Dsg1 transfected cells, BP180NC16a negativity and ambiguous result for BP230gC.

(AIBD: autoimmune bullous disease; BP: bullous pemphigoid; Dsg: desmoglein; NC: non-collagenous; gC: C-terminal globular domain)

Source: Adapted from van Beek N, *et al*. Serological diagnosis of autoimmune bullous skin diseases: prospective comparison of the BIOCHIP mosaic-based indirect immunofluorescence technique with the conventional multi-step single test strategy. *Orphanet J Rare Dis.* 2012;7:49.

VII, recombinant gliadin for dermatitis herpetiformis, rat bladder, monkey liver, monkey liver with serosa (for paraneoplastic pemphigus) and empty vector, has also been developed.

Principle and Method

The principle is the same as that of IIF. Patients' serum (or plasma) samples to be tested can be stored up to 14 days at 2–8 degree Celsius, and are tested in 1:10 dilution for qualitative evaluation; whereas further dilutions are used for semi-quantitative evaluation. The 'Titerplane' technique has been developed to standardize the method and enable processing of many samples together. In this, a reagent tray containing many reaction fields is utilized, into each of which a fixed volume of sample is pipetted. The biochip slides are fitted corresponding to reagent fields in an inverse fashion from the top and incubated so as to allow antibodies to bind **(Fig. 7)**. A fresh reagent tray is used similarly to bind the secondary fluorescein-labeled antihuman antibody, and the reading is done using a fluorescent microscope at 20× (for tissue sections and transfected cells) or 40× (for cell substrates).

Interpretation of the Biochip mosaic assay is detailed below **(Table 4; Figs. 6B and C)**.

Utility

The positivity of the biochip target antigens Dsg1 and 3 in pemphigus group of disorders has ranged from 12.5–83.3% for Dsg1 (52.3–88.3% for PF), and 63.2–100% for Dsg3 (overall better performance). When evaluated separately for foliaceus and vulgaris groups, Dsg1 shows high sensitivity for PF (90%), which was poor for PV (52.3%), though corroboration with mucosal or cutaneous involvement was not reported. The sensitivity of Dsg3 for PV was 98.5%, with a specificity of 99.6%, showing good diagnostic utility. The monkey esophagus microarray as part of the biochip showed a sensitivity of 60.9% and specificity of 62.2% for PV, whereas it was 87.5% and 61.3% respectively for PF, an overall poorer result than Dsg1/3.

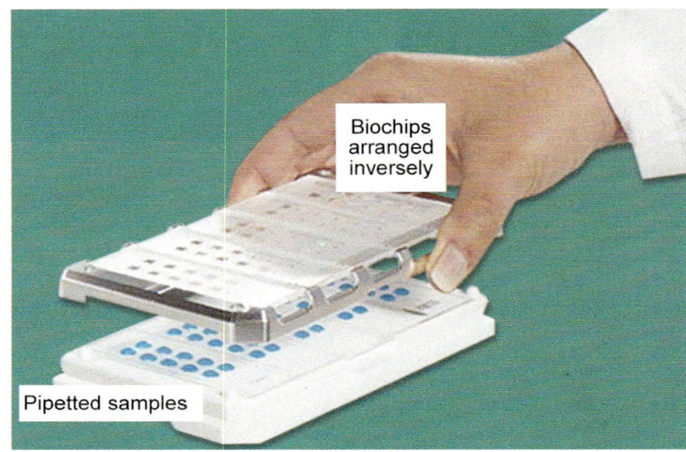

Fig. 7: Biochip mosaic: Titerplane technique to process multiple samples for biochip simultaneously—patient samples pipetted onto a reagent tray with many reaction fields, over which a set of inverted biochips are fitted.
Source: Euroimmun®, Germany.

TABLE 4: Interpretation of Biochip Mosaic Assay for various autoimmune bullous diseases.

Biochip \ AIBD	PV	PF	Bullous pemphigoid	Linear IgA disease	Mucous membrane pemphigoid	Epidermolysis bullosa acquisita
Monkey esophagus	Fine intercellular intraepidermal fluorescence	Fine intercellular intraepidermal fluorescence	Fine linear staining at basement membrane zone	Fine linear staining at basement membrane zone	Fine linear staining at basement membrane zone	Fine linear staining at basement membrane zone
Primate 1 M NaCl salt-split skin	–	–	Fine linear staining at roof	Fine linear staining at roof	Fine linear staining at roof (α6β4) or floor (laminin 332)	Fine linear staining at floor
BP230gC (C-terminal globular domain of BP230)	–	–	Cytoplasmic granular fluorescence	–	–	–
BP180-NC16a purified antigen	–	–	Diamond-shaped green fields in front of a dark background	–	–	–
Dsg1 transfected HEK293 cells	Cytoplasmic granular fluorescence may be seen	Cytoplasmic granular fluorescence	–	–	–	–
Dsg3 transfected HEK293 cells	Cytoplasmic granular fluorescence	–	–	–	–	–

(AIBD: autoimmune bullous disease; BP: bullous pemphigoid; Dsg: desmoglein; HEK: human embryonic kidney; IgA: immunoglobulin A; LABD: linear IgA bullous disease; NC: non-collagenous; PF: pemphigus foliaceus; PV: pemphigus vulgaris)

In the pemphigoid group, positivity for BP180 ranged from 55.3–100%, mostly reporting 80–90% positivity, while that for BP230 was lower at 14–68.3%. The specificity was 96.5–100% for BP180, and lower, i.e., 39–100%. for BP230.

An Indian study by Arunprasath, *et al* (*n* = 18 patients) reported a concordance of 100% of the biochip with DIF in pemphigus. A larger cohort of 108 patients studied by Tirumalae, *et al*, reported a concordance of 89% between the biochip mosaic and biopsy/DIF in pemphigus and 93% in pemphigoid. Good agreement has also been observed with the ELISA test. A recent head-to-head comparison showed an improved overall sensitivity of the six antigen biochip mosaic over the multivariate ELISA for PV (100% with biochip vs. 94% with ELISA) and BP (87.5% for biochip vs. 75% for ELISA).

In EBA, in a pilot study that included 6 cases and 11 controls, the biochip for NC1 domain of collagen VII showed 100% sensitivity and specificity, which was corroborated by ELISA.

Its sensitivity and specificity in various AIBDs is depicted in **Table 5**.

Advantages of Biochip Mosaic Assay

- It is possible to evaluate multiple samples for many diseases simultaneously in a limited time (~100 min), and thus can be used as a screening tool.
- Results are read visually and it does not require photo-metric equipment.

Limitations of Biochip Mosaic Assay

- The results are read visually, so they are subjective and usually qualitative.
- Inter-rater reliability is low and depends on the level of training.
- Sometimes ambiguous staining patterns may occur such as partial or weak staining.
- It may not be possible to distinguish different sub-epidermal disorders beyond that on the basis of salt-split skin, as specific antigen panel is usually only available for BP, or for EBA in the extended panel.
- Cost is high and this equipment is usually procured only at high flow tertiary care centers.

Availability and Cost

It is available in India by the following names:
- *IIFT Mosaic Dsg1/3 by Euroimmun*: Pack size of 50 tests for INR 52,658 + 12% GST
- *IIFT Dermatology Mosaic 7 by Euroimmun*: Pack size of 50 tests for INR 1,27,597+ 12% GST

Kits contain slides with a mosaic of Biochips, fluorescein labeled antihuman IgG (goat), positive control, negative control, cover glasses, PBS-Tween, and embedding medium.

OPTICAL COHERENCE TOMOGRAPHY (OCT)

Histopathology is considered the gold standard of diagnostics in dermatology; however, it is invasive and processing of the tissue requires a few days to a week. Moreover, the yield depends significantly on the chosen lesion and its stage in evolution. "Optical biopsy" techniques attempt to non-invasively visualize tissues at a cellular level across various stages of evolution and offer a potential replacement to conventional histopathology. OCT is one such biomedical imaging modality based on white-light Michelson interferometry **(Fig. 8)**. It has been used in ophthalmology since 1988 and was modified a few years later in 1995 for visualizing skin.

Principle and Method

The skin has high absorption and scattering compared to the eye, and is best visualized using super-luminescent diodes in the 'diagnostic window' of 700–1,300 nm (infrared wavelengths rather than visible light used for ophthalmic OCT) which are able to penetrate deep into the skin. The principle of interferometry is used, wherein the depth of the signal and optical density of the tissue is measured on

TABLE 5: Sensitivity and specificity of autoimmune bullous diseases with the Biochip mosaic assay.

Test	PF	PV	Pemphigoid group	EBA
HEK293 cells transfected with Dsg1	Sensitivity 90%	Sensitivity 52.3%	–	–
HEK293 cells transfected with Dsg3	–	• Sensitivity 98.5% • Specificity 99.6%	–	–
Monkey esophagus microarray	• Sensitivity 87.5% • Specificity 61.3%	• Sensitivity 60.9% • Specificity 62.2%	–	–
HEK293 cells transfected with BP180	–	–	• Sensitivity 80–90% • Specificity 96.5–100%	–
HEK293 cells transfected with BP230	–	–	• Sensitivity 14–68.3% • Specificity 39–100%	–
Extended Biochip-NC1 domain of collagen VII	–	–	–	• Sensitivity 100% • Specificity 100%

(BP: bullous pemphigoid; Dsg: desmoglein; EBA: epidermolysis bullosa acquisita; HEK: human embryonic kidney; NC: non-collagenous; PF: pemphigus foliaceus; PV: pemphigus vulgaris)

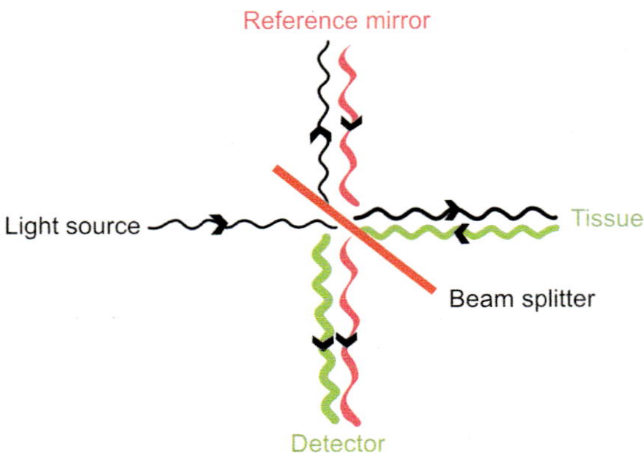

Fig. 8: Optical coherence tomography: Diagrammatic representation of its principle. The principle of interferometry is used, wherein the depth of the signal and optical density of the tissue is measured on the basis of disruption of the coherence of a laser beam passing through the tissue. This disruption is measured against a reference beam of the same coherence that was split-off initially from the same source beam and reflected back from a mirror to combine again with the probe beam backscattered from the tissue.

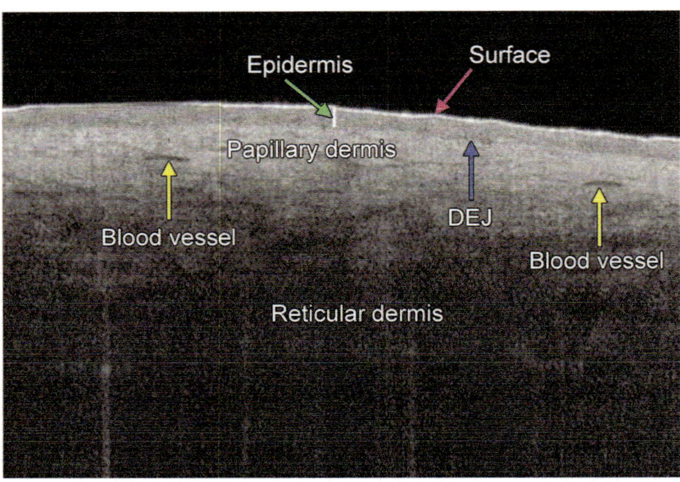

Fig. 9: Optical coherence tomography—Representation of normal skin: It shows stratum corneum as bright white line at the surface (pink arrow), followed by a lesser intensity (darker) zone of epidermis (green arrow), then demarcation with the dermis (dermo-epidermal junction—DEJ) as a second intensity peak (blue arrow), followed by the dermis itself that shows higher intensity (more grey-white shadows) than the epidermis. Thin linear dark structures in dermis (yellow arrows) represent blood vessels.

the basis of disruption of the coherence of a laser beam passing through the tissue. This disruption is measured against a reference beam of the same coherence that was split-off initially from the same source beam and reflected back from a mirror to combine again with the probe beam backscattered from the tissue **(Fig. 8)**.

It provides two-dimensional images with an axial resolution of 3–15 µm, lateral resolution of 20–24 µm and a penetration depth of 0.4–2 mm, thus spanning the epidermis and dermis, sometimes up to the subcutis. There are variations in the parameters as per the technology used: time-domain OCT, spectral-domain OCT, and swept-source or optical-domain OCT, the last two of which are part of 'Fourier-domain OCT' that has enabled speedy real-time scanning (acquisition time 2–4 seconds) and adoption into routine clinical practice (e.g., VivoSight). Dynamic OCT is an angiographic OCT that can detect blood flow. Three-dimensional OCT can reconstruct three-dimensional images of the skin, and artificial intelligence (AI)-enabled OCT utilizes deep learning algorithms for better analysis.

Visualization of Skin on Optical Coherence Tomography

The normal skin is visible as white line on the surface (stratum corneum) due to the reflectivity causing peak signal intensity, followed by a lesser intensity (darker) zone of the epidermis, then demarcation of the dermis (dermo-epidermal junction—DEJ) as a second intensity peak, followed by the dermis itself that shows higher intensity (more gray-white shadows) than the epidermis. Within the dermis, the hair follicles and sweat glands appear as low intensity (darker areas). Blood vessels appear as dark ovoid or elongated structures **(Fig. 9)**.

In AIBDs, the blister cavity is visible as dark, ovoid areas separating the normally continuous layers of the skin, or flatter grayish areas when the blister is not fluid-filled. The location is assessed by delineating whether this cavity is within the epidermis or the epidermis is present as a layer on top of this cavity **(Figs. 10 and 11)**. The inflammatory cells within the blister cavity are seen as gray pinpoint specks, while fibrin is visible as gray homogenous substance within the blister. Dark, thin, and linear structures in the upper dermis represent blood vessels.

Utility

An exploratory pilot study in six patients including three of BP, one of PV and one of subcorneal pustular dermatosis showed that OCT may provide in vivo imaging corresponding to histopathology to classify them as epidermal or subepidermal. In a multicentric study from Europe evaluating 72 lesions (48 lesions of BP and 24 lesions of pemphigus), OCT was able to detect the anatomic level of the blister accurately in all patients. Inflammatory cells within the blister were detected in 62.5% of BP and 25% of pemphigus cases. Fibrin deposition and dilated blood vessels could also be observed in majority of the BP patients. OCT was even able to detect subclinical blistering in 9.4% of BP and 20.8% of pemphigus patients. OCT has also been used to diagnose mucosal lesions of these disorders.

Advantages of Optical Coherence Tomography

- OCT provides cross-sectional/vertical images oriented similar to histopathology.

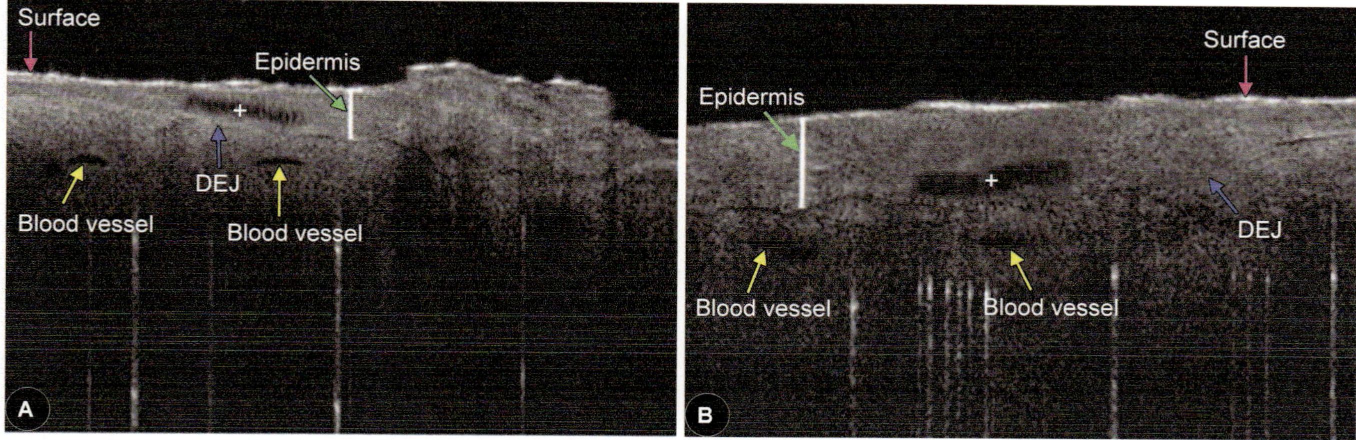

Figs. 10A and B: Optical coherence tomography—Representation of OCT of pemphigus vulgaris: It shows intraepidermal bulla (+), and dilated blood vessels (yellow arrows) in the upper dermis.
(DEJ: dermo-epidermal junction)
Source: Adapted from Mandel VD, *et al*. Reflectance confocal microscopy and optical coherence tomography for the diagnosis of bullous pemphigoid and pemphigus and surrounding subclinical lesions. *J Eur Acad Dermatol Venereol.* 2018;32:1562-9.

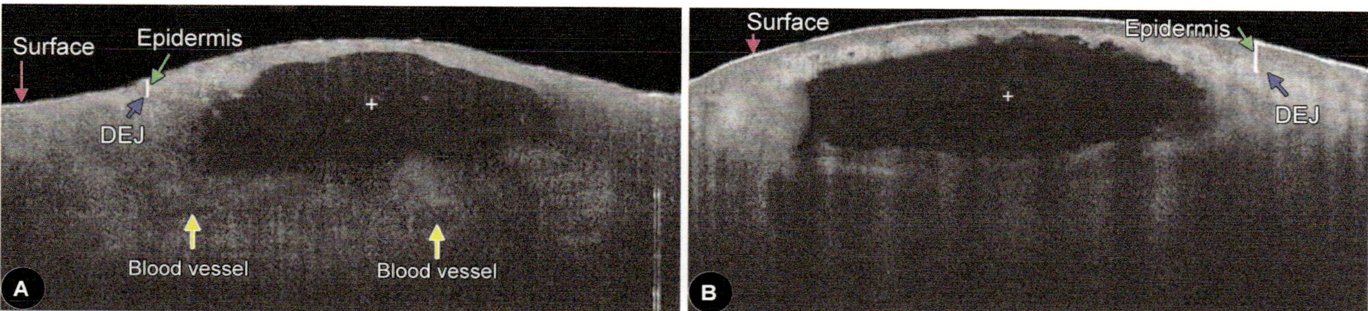

Figs. 11A and B: Optical coherence tomography—Representation of OCT of bullous pemphigoid: It shows subepidermal bulla (+), and dilated blood vessels (yellow arrows) in the upper dermis.
(DEJ: dermo-epidermal junction)
Source: Adapted from Mandel VD, *et al*. Reflectance confocal microscopy and optical coherence tomography for the diagnosis of bullous pemphigoid and pemphigus and surrounding subclinical lesions. *J Eur Acad Dermatol Venereol.* 2018;32:1562-9.

- It provides a compromise between resolution and depth, in between high-frequency ultrasound (low resolution, high penetration) and RCM (high resolution, low penetration).
- Real-time non-invasive imaging makes it possible to visualize multiple areas in one sitting, and on follow-up.
- Subclinical splits may be detected, and it may be used as a screening tool to identify an ideal site for biopsy.

Limitations

- The cellular resolution is poor, so features like acantholytic cells cannot be visualized.
- It is an expensive instrument.

Availability and Cost

- It is not available for dermatological use in India.
- Common commercially available devices include VivoSight and SanTec IVS-300.

REFLECTANCE CONFOCAL MICROSCOPY (RCM)

RCM is a non-invasive imaging technique that uses diode laser to provide high resolution, en face, in vivo images of the skin. It is akin to a virtual biopsy, however, with limited depth of visualization up to the epidermis and superficial dermis. It has been approved by the United States Food and Drug Administration (US FDA) for evaluating the skin and interpreting images in order to decrease the number of unnecessary biopsies for benign cutaneous lesions and inflammatory dermatoses **(Fig. 12)**.

Principle

A near-infrared laser of 830 nm (diode) is the source of light, which passes through collimating optics to an objective lens that focuses the beam on to its focal plane. Only the light reflected back from this focal plane is picked up by the

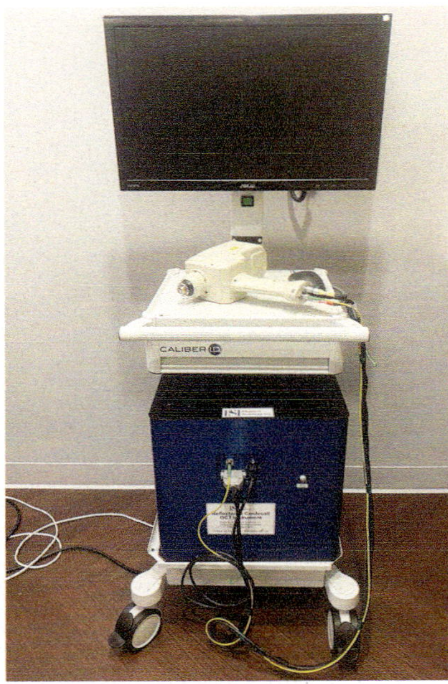

Fig. 12: Equipment used for RCM–OCT. *Image courtesy*: Dr Manu Jain, Associate Attending, Optical Imaging Specialist, Department of Dermatology, Memorial Sloan Kettering Cancer Centre, New York, USA.

(OCT: optical coherence tomography; RCM: reflectance confocal microscopy)

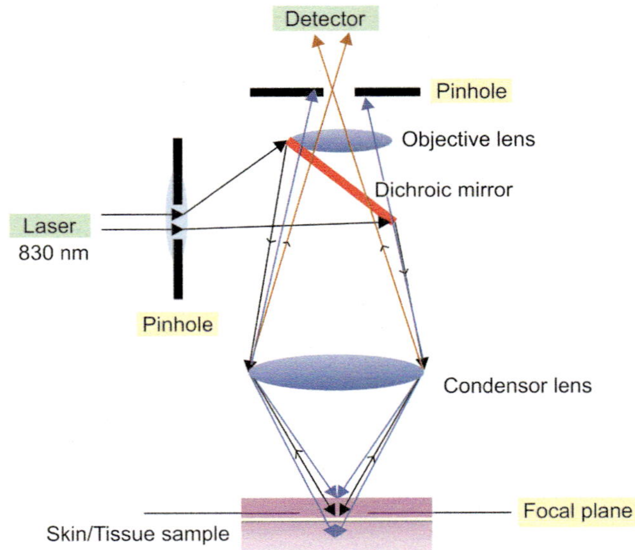

Fig. 13: Reflectance confocal microscopy: Diagrammatic representation of principle of reflectance confocal microscopy. A near-infrared laser of 830 nm (diode) is the source of light, which passes through collimating optics to an objective lens that focuses the beam onto its focal plane. Only the light reflected back from this focal plane is picked up by the detector by virtue of a pinhole, whereas light scattered from adjoining planes is blocked. "Confocal" placement of pinholes (point source of light, illuminated spot in the sample and pinhole aperture all lie in optically conjugated focal planes) allows high resolution images from a single plane within thick tissue.

detector by virtue of a pinhole, whereas light scattered from adjoining planes is blocked, thus decreasing haziness. This "confocal" placement of pinholes allows high-resolution images from a single plane within thick tissue **(Fig. 13)**. A complete image may be generated by adjusting and moving the plane of focus step by step over the entire sample, thus enabling a large field of view. The plane of visualization is like that in dermoscopy, but seen in cellular details.

Images are seen in gray scale, with different tissue elements identifiable by differing brightness determined by their relative refractive indices. The normal stratum corneum (up to 20 μm from skin surface) is a bright and highly reflective surface interspersed by dark skin markings **(Fig. 14A)**. Deeper to this is the stratum granulosum and stratum spinosum (up to 100 μm), that consists of polygonal cells with dark nuclei and grainy cytoplasm (due to organelles and/or keratohyalin granules) that form a regular honeycomb pattern **(Fig. 14B)**. The basal cells appear as bright, round cells forming a cobblestone pattern **(Fig. 14C)**. The bright hue is due to melanin that provides the strongest endogenous contrast in the skin. These surround dark, round areas which are the en face view of projecting dermal papillae **(Figs. 14B and C)**. The papillary (100–150 μm) and reticular dermis (>150 μm) contain bright, long fibrillary collagen and dark, tubular blood vessels.

The horizontal/lateral resolution in RCM is 0.5–1 μm, axial between 3 and 5 μm and penetration depth is 150–200 μm (including entire epidermis and papillary dermis). Optical 'clearance agents' like immersion fluids have been used to increase the depth of RCM imaging.

RCM can identify blister cavities as a dark, homogenous, non-reflective space, the level of which can be discerned by identification of the honeycomb pattern of epidermis below the blister cavity (intraepidermal) **(Fig. 15A)** or solely above it (subepidermal) **(Fig. 15B)**. These may be filled with acantholytic cells (14–17 μm weakly refractive, round-to-ovoid cells with centrally or eccentrically situated nucleus) or inflammatory cells (8–12 μm highly refractive cells).

Utility

Kurzeja, *et al*, in their study of 36 PV and 29 PF lesions, proposed a criteria for the diagnosis of pemphigus, requiring two of the following three features: (1) acantholytic clefts in RCM of a lesion, (2) acantholytic clefts in RCM of healthy-appearing skin adjacent to a lesion, and (3) multiple dilated blood vessels in RCM of the lesion. Mandel, *et al* found that RCM could diagnose 75% of BP patients (n = 16 patients, 48 lesions) and 50% of PV patients (n = 8, 24 lesions). It was also able to discern acantholytic cells in 62.5% of the pemphigus patients. Moreover, subclinical blistering was detected in 9.4% BP and 20.8% pemphigus patients when apparently healthy skin >1 cm away from the lesion was biopsied. In a study by Ardigo, *et al* on nine BP patients, subepidermal split was detected in 100% of the bullae examined but in none of the urticarial lesions.

RCM could identify findings of PV in the oral mucosa in a series of nine patients, and had differing features from recurrent aphthous stomatitis. RCM can also identify cellular details in other blistering conditions such as herpes and Hailey–Hailey disease.

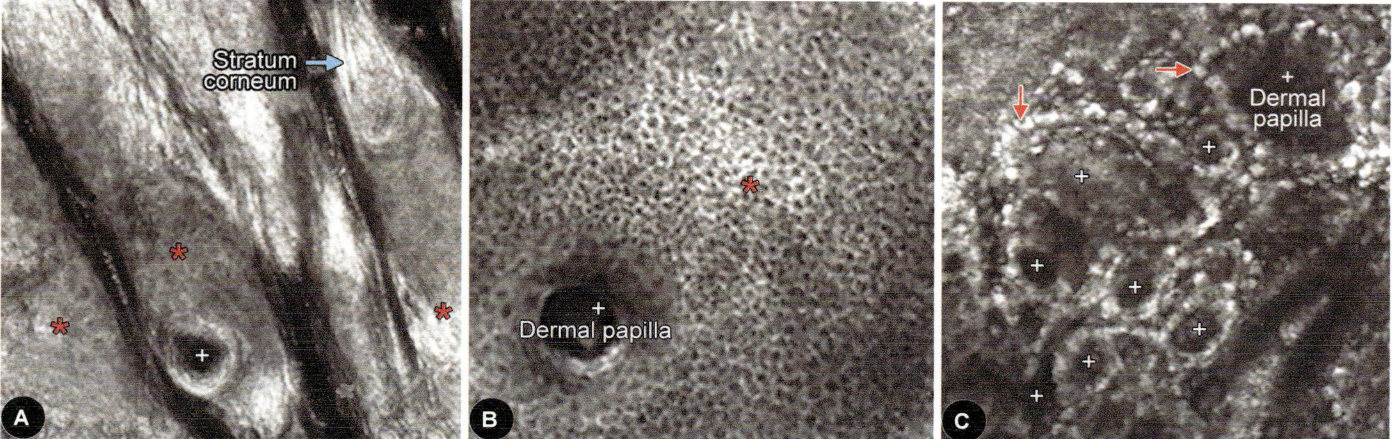

Figs. 14A to C: Reflectance confocal microscopy—Representation of normal skin: (A) It shows stratum corneum as bright and highly reflective surface (blue arrow), with dark linear furrows representing dermatoglyphics (skin folds). There is normal honeycomb pattern of stratum granulosum and stratum spinosum (red asterisk) (B) Stratum granulosum and stratum spinosum showing normal honeycomb pattern (red asterisk) (C) The dermal papillae (+) are encased by bright basal keratinocytes and melanocytes (red arrows) at the dermo-epidermal junction.

Source: Adapted from Levine A, *et al*. Introduction to reflectance confocal microscopy and its use in clinical practice. *JAAD Case Rep*. 2018;4:1014-23.

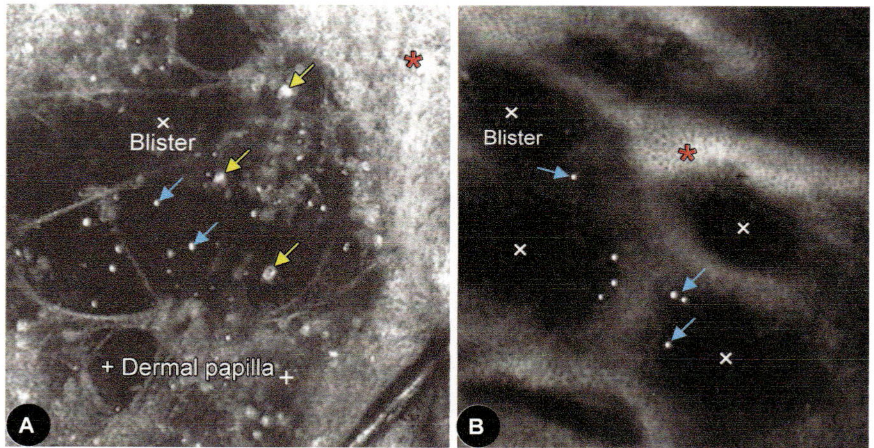

Figs. 15A and B: Reflectance confocal microscopy—(A) Representation of RCM of pemphigus vulgaris: It shows intraepidermal blister (x) containing round to ovoid, mildly refractive acantholytic cells with centrally or eccentrally situated nucleus (yellow arrows) and smaller, round, highly refractive inflammatory cells (blue arrows) (B) Representation of RCM of bullous pemphigoid: It shows presence of sub-epidermal blisters (x) with some inflammatory cells (blue arrows) inside the blisters. Red asterisk denotes normal honeycomb pattern of stratum spinosum.

Sources:

Figure 15A: Adapted from Kurzeja M, *et al*. Criteria for diagnosing pemphigus vulgaris and pemphigus foliaceus by reflectance confocal microscopy. *Skin Research and Technology*. 2011;18:339-46.

Figure 15B: Adapted from Mandel VD, *et al*. Reflectance confocal microscopy and optical coherence tomography for the diagnosis of bullous pemphigoid and pemphigus and surrounding subclinical lesions. *J Eur Acad Dermatol Venereol*. 2018;32:1562-9.

Advantages of Reflectance Confocal Microscopy

- RCM offers rapid, non-invasive, real-time bedside imaging with high cellular resolution.
- It can be used to visualize multiple areas at the same time.

Limitations of Reflectance Confocal Microscopy

- Visualization is limited to en face views which are unfamiliar to most dermatologists and dermatopathologists, thus requiring training to interpret images.
- It has limited depth of visualization.
- It is a costly modality with restricted availability.

Variations

Line-field confocal OCT (LC-OCT): It combines the principles of RCM and OCT to provide cellular resolution of epidermal layers with deeper visualization till the deep dermis. Togentti, *et al* used LC-OCT to assess 30 patients of suspected AIBDs and found 90% accuracy in diagnostic assessment as per confirmatory tests (histology and DIF ± IIF/ELISA).

Availability and Cost

- It can be provided in India through Indian dealers of International companies.
- Commercial systems available in other countries include VivaScope 1500, VivaScope 3000.
- Cost is approximately INR 1 crore.

CONCLUSION

Diagnostics in AIBDs have progressed beyond histopathology and immunofluoroscence. ELISA is able to provide high diagnostic accuracy on serum samples and is able to predict disease activity and relapse. Biochip mosaic assay has made IIF rapid and accessible. Optical biopsy techniques like reflectance confocal microscopy and optical coherence tomography are good non-invasive screening tools, but are limited by their restricted availability and high cost. An understanding of the pathogenesis of disease and principles of these diagnostic modalities is essential for correct interpretation.

TAKE HOME MESSAGE

- ELISA test has excellent specificity (85–97%) and a moderate-to-good sensitivity (56–94%) in the diagnosis of pemphigus group of diseases.
- Levels of anti-Dsg1 and 3 correlate with disease severity, and anti-Dsg1 is a good predictor of cutaneous relapse.

The same is controversial for anti-Dsg3 and mucosal relapse and high cutoff values give improved specificity. For BP, anti-BP180 is a good predictor of relapse.

- Immunohistochemistry on paraffin-embedded sections can be utilized in AIBDs to detect IgG/IgG4 and C3d/C4d deposition (stable components of alternate and classical complement pathway) in paraffin-embedded sections. C4d has good sensitivity for both pemphigus and pemphigoid group of disorders.
- Biochip mosaic is a modified IIF method comprising multiple miniaturized biological substrates arranged on a glass slide that can be used to detect many antibodies simultaneously in multiple (ten) samples using a single biochip slide.
- There is about 90% concordance of biochip with biopsy/DIF, with good sensitivity (98.5%) and specificity (99.6%) of Dsg3 transfected cells in biochip for PV and good sensitivity (90%) of Dsg1 for PF. For pemphigoid group, BP180 performs better than BP230.
- Non-invasive imaging of skin and subcutaneous tissue akin to an "optical biopsy" is now feasible with imaging modalities such as RCM and OCT. While RCM offers cellular resolution, it visualizes limited depth of about 200 μm. Increased depth visualized in OCT of about 0.2–4 mm is at the cost of resolution.
- OCT uses the principle of white light Michelson interferometry with the source of light being 700–1,300 nm infrared laser. The plane of view is coronal, similar to that seen in histopathology. Fourier-domain OCT has enabled real-time scanning of large areas due to the long acquisition time of 2–4 seconds.
- RCM uses diode laser (830 nm) and provides a large field of view but with en face orientation.
- ELISA and Biochip are available and in use in India, However, OCT and RCM are currently not being used in India.

MULTIPLE CHOICE QUESTIONS

1. **What is the usual cutoff for positivity for anti-desmoglein ELISA?**
   - (a) 200 RU/mL
   - (b) 20 RU/mL
   - (c) 100 RU/mL
   - (d) 10 RU/mL

2. **What is conformational ELISA index?**
   - (a) ELISA value (total) – ELISA value (pathogenic antibodies)
   - (b) ELISA value (total) – ELISA value (non-pathogenic antibodies)
   - (c) ELISA value (pathogenic antibodies) × ELISA value (total)
   - (d) ELISA value (pathogenic antibodies)/ELISA value (pathogenic + non-pathogenic antibodies) × 100

3. **Which of the following is false for ELISA in AIBD?**
   - (a) The technique used is direct ELISA
   - (b) Titers of antibodies to Dsg1 can be used to predict relapse in pemphigus vulgaris
   - (c) Anti-BP180 has higher diagnostic utility in bullous pemphigoid than anti-BP230
   - (d) Titers of antibodies to Dsg1 and Dsg3 correlate with disease severity in pemphigus

4. **What is a limitation of ELISA?**
   - (a) Poor specificity compared to DIF
   - (b) Qualitative method
   - (c) Negative result may be obtained if an autoimmune bullous disease is caused by antibodies directed against another, uncommon antigen that was not tested
   - (d) Subjective method

5. **Which of the following antibodies cannot be detected in immunohistochemistry on paraffin embedded sections?**

(a) IgG

(b) C4d

(c) IgA

(d) C3d

6. **Which of the following is not included in the standard biochip for AIBD/Dermatology Mosaic 7?**

(a) BP-230gC (C-terminal globular domain of BP230)

(b) Monkey esophagus

(c) Salt-split primate skin

(d) Rat bladder

7. **What is the term for the technique used in Biochip to process multiple samples together?**

(a) Titerplane technique

(b) Multiplex biochip

(c) Mosaic biochip

(d) Profile technique

8. **What is the penetration depth of OCT?**

(a) Up to 100 μm

(b) Up to 200 μm

(c) Up to 1 mm

(d) Up to 2 mm

9. **Acantholytic cells can be visualized in:**

(a) OCT

(b) RCM

(c) Both (a) and (b)

(d) None of the above

10. **Wavelength of light utilized in RCM is:**

(a) 1,300 nm

(b) 830 nm

(c) 810 nm

(d) 755 nm

Answers

1. (b) 2. (b) 3. (a) 4. (c) 5. (c) 6. (d) 7. (a) 8. (d) 9. (b) 10. (b)

SUGGESTED READING

1. Chan W. The use of ELISA in pemphigus. *Hong Kong Dermatol Venereol Bull.* 2005;13:14-9.

2. Harman KE, Gratian MJ, Seed PT, Bhogal BS, Challacombe SJ, Black MM. Diagnosis of pemphigus by ELISA: a critical evaluation of two ELISAs for the detection of antibodies to the major pemphigus antigens, desmoglein 1 and 3. *Clin Exp Dermatol.* 2000;25:236-40.

3. Schmidt E, Zillikens D. Modern diagnosis of autoimmune blistering skin diseases. *Autoimmun Rev.* 2010;10:84-9.

4. Van de gaer O, de Haes P, Bossuyt X. Detection of circulating anti-skin antibodies by indirect immunofluorescence and by ELISA: a comparative systematic review and meta-analysis. *Clin Chem Lab Med.* 2020;58:1623-33.

5. Anand V, Khandpur S, Sharma VK, Sharma A. Utility of desmoglein ELISA in the clinical correlation and disease monitoring of pemphigus vulgaris. *J Eur Acad Dermatol Venereol.* 2011;26:1377-83.

6. Charneux J, Lorin J, Vitry F, Antonicelli F, Reguiai Z, Barbe C, et al. Usefulness of BP230 and BP180-NC16a enzyme-linked immuno-sorbent assays in the initial diagnosis of bullous pemphigoid: a retrospective study of 138 patients. *Arch Dermatol.* 2011;147:286-91.

7. Saschenbrecker S, Karl I, Komorowski L, Probst C, Dähnrich C, Fechner K, et al. Serological diagnosis of autoimmune bullous skin diseases. *Front Immunol.* 2019;10:1974.

8. Yang A, Xuan R, Melbourne W, Tran K, Murrell DF. Validation of the BIOCHIP test for the diagnosis of bullous pemphigoid, pemphigus vulgaris and pemphigus foliaceus. *J Eur Acad Dermatol Venereol.* 2020;34:153-60.

9. Arunprasath P, Rai R, Venkataswamy C. Comparative analysis of biochip mosaic-based indirect immunofluorescence with direct immunofluorescence in diagnosis of autoimmune bullous diseases: a cross-sectional study. *Indian Dermatol Online J.* 2020;11:915-9.

10. Wan B, Ganier C, Du-Harpur X, Harun N, Watt FM, Patalay R, et al. Applications and future directions for optical coherence tomography in dermatology. *Br J Dermatol.* 2020;184:1014-22.

11. Mandel VD, Cinotti E, Benati E, Labeille B, Ciardo S, Vaschieri C, et al. Reflectance confocal microscopy and optical coherence tomography for the diagnosis of bullous pemphigoid and pemphigus and surrounding subclinical lesions. *J Eur Acad Dermatol Venereol.* 2018;32:1562-9.

12. Levi A, Ophir I, Lemster N, Maly A, Ruzicka T, Ingber A, et al. Noninvasive visualization of intraepidermal and subepidermal blisters in vesiculobullous skin disorders by in vivo reflectance confocal microscopy. *Lasers Med Sci.* 2012;27:261-6.

CHAPTER 18

Immunoblot Assay and Immunoprecipitation

Sujay Khandpur, Xiaoguang Li, Takashi Hashimoto, Vinay Keshavamurthy

- Advantages of immunoblot assay
- Limitations of immunoblot assay
- Substrates for immunoblot and immunoprecipitation assays
- Procedure of immunoblot assay
- Immunoprecipitation
- Some observations in studies on AIBDs using immunoblot and immunoprecipitation assays

INTRODUCTION

Immunoblot (IB) assay and immunoprecipitation (IP) are novel diagnostic strategies that help to identify, quantify, and determine the size of specific proteins. These procedures have revolutionized the field of immunology. They allow immunodetection and quantitation of specific proteins in complex cell homogenates including proteins that are both novel and show flow abundance. Characterization of the epitope specificity of autoantibodies is possible. IB assay can also be used as a semi-quantitative method to determine and compare the expression of specific proteins in various cells and tissues. It can also be used for absolute quantification which requires a linear standard curve of purified target protein.

In autoimmune bullous diseases (AIBDs), IB assay identifies targeted antigen(s) and confirms the diagnosis when there are weak or atypical fluorescence patterns, or when diseases cannot be differentiated on the basis of their serum immunofluorescence binding patterns.

Western blotting was introduced by Towbin, *et al* in 1979. In this process, there is a transfer of proteins from gel to microporous membrane (blotting). Both electrophoretic and non-electrophoretic transfer of proteins to membrane are undertaken. Towbin, *et al* enabled proteins to be electrophoretically separated using polyacrylamide–urea gels and transferred on to a nitrocellulose membrane. Burnette (1981) later employed the more widely used sodium dodecyl sulfate-polyacrylamide gel electrophoresis (SDS-PAGE).

ADVANTAGES OF IMMUNOBLOT ASSAY

IB assay offers several advantages:
- It allows detection of picogram levels of protein in a sample.
- The wet membranes used in the assay are pliable and easy-to-handle compared to gels.
- It allows easy accessibility of the proteins immobilized on the membrane to different ligands.
- Only small amount of reagents are required for transfer analysis.
- It is possible to store transferred proteins prior to use and the same protein transferred can be used for multiple analyses.
- The specificity of the antibody–antigen interaction allows the detection of a target protein in complex mixtures containing >100,000 different proteins.

LIMITATIONS OF IMMUNOBLOT ASSAY

There are several limitations of IB assay:
- It can only be carried out if a primary antibody against the protein/antigen of interest is available.
- The procedure requires significant technical skill, e.g, use of optimum amount of primary antibody, efficiency of protein blotting, retention of antigen during processing, and the final detection/amplification system used.
- The procedure is cumbersome.
- It is expensive including high cost of advanced digital imagers being used.
- The basic IB protocol may be ineffective in detecting a particular protein, and modifications may be required.
- Mechanical, chemical, and thermal separation methods used in epidermal–dermal separation and even sodium dodecyl sulfate may distort the number, structure, conformation, and distribution of some of the antigens.
- Other technical issues may be encountered such as variations in transfer efficiency of proteins. Small proteins (<10 kDa) may not be retained by the membrane after long time transfer, large proteins (>140 kDa) may not all be transferred to the membrane after short time

transfer, and varying gel concentrations may affect transfer efficiency. Other problems include the primary antibody not recognizing the immobilized antigen in its denatured state, the detection signal decaying too quickly, and high background noise.

SUBSTRATES FOR IMMUNOBLOT AND IMMUNOPRECIPITATION ASSAY

Both human and animal substrates have been used. They can be natural skin or cultured skin cells. Human substrate is preferred as it prevents misinterpretation due to species differences.

Antigens/proteins can be obtained from:

- *Normal human epidermis*: such as adult or neonatal foreskin, epidermal grafts such as suction blister or split-skin grafts
- *Cultured keratinocytes*: such as HaCaT keratinocyte cell line monolayers (both on live cells and on fixed and permeabilized cells)
- *Tumor cell lines*: extract of cultured human squamous cell carcinoma cells including KU8 cells derived from penile carcinoma, cell line derived from squamous cell carcinoma of human urinary bladder (SCaBER), or human colorectal adenocarcinoma.
- *Human amniotic membrane*: harvesting proteins from amnion does not require epidermal-dermal separation, and a sufficient yield of desmosomal and hemi-desmosomal antigens can be obtained.
- *Animal substrates*: bovine muzzle desmosome preparation, epithelial bovine tongue extracts, or bovine gingiva

Dermal protein extracts are used in subepidermal disorders.

PROCEDURE OF IMMUNOBLOT ASSAY

In IB assay, the antigens/proteins present in a protein extract are first separated according to molecular weight by electrophoresis over a polyacrylamide slab gel in the presence of SDS-PAGE. The separated proteins are then electrophoretically transferred to an inert membrane filter, which facilitates further incubation and washing steps. Finally the antigen(s) against which the patient's autoantibodies are directed, are visualized.

The apparatus used for IB assay is depicted in **Figure 1**.

Sample Preparation

- The tissue, which is the source of antigens, is rapidly frozen with liquid nitrogen to avoid protease degradation of proteins, or collected and lysed immediately. Repeated freeze/thaw cycles should be avoided as this has an adverse effect on the quality of protein.
- Solid tissue is mechanically broken down using a homogenizer or by sonication in a lysis buffer.
- To obtain epidermal and dermal extracts, different dermo-epidermal separation methods have been used: ethylenediaminetetraacetic acid (EDTA) separation, heat separation, and dispase separation. Studies have shown that heat and EDTA separation methods are superior to dispase method in improving the antigen yield in various AIBDs, and that heat separation is preferred because the preparation time is shorter.

Use of lysis buffers: Lysis buffers used in sample preparation for IB assay should enable efficient protein extraction and maintain antisera recognition of the protein. Various detergents, salts, and buffers have been used to enable lysis of cells and to solubilize proteins. To avoid degradation of protein, protease and phosphatase inhibitors are included in the lysis buffer.

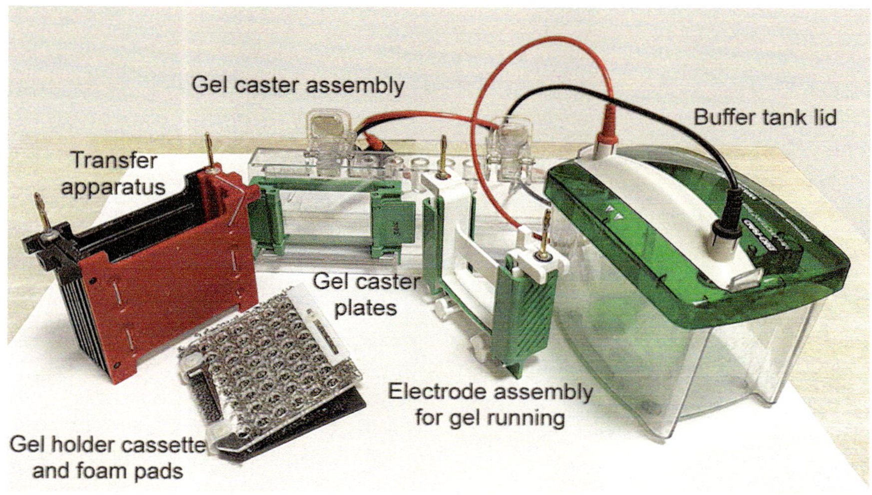

Fig. 1: Apparatus for immunoblot assay. *Image courtesy*: Dr Alpana Sharma.

Determination of Protein Concentration

The protein concentration of the sample to be loaded on the gel needs to be estimated. Quantification is achieved by measuring samples at 280 nm on a spectrophotometer. The Bradford assay (1976) can be used where a standard curve is created to determine unknown sample concentration.

Separation of Proteins/Antigens

- Proteins can be separated on the basis of isoelectric point, molecular weight, electric charge or a combination of these.
- Proteins are separated using gel electrophoresis. The most common type of electrophoresis uses polyacrylamide gels and buffers loaded with SDS (SDS-PAGE). The procedure is based on the principle that SDS is a strongly anionic detergent. Since all proteins do not have the same electrical charge, the mixture is treated with SDS, and the proteins become denatured and negatively charged. This allows separation of proteins on the basis of molecular weight.
- The samples are loaded onto the gel. One lane includes a molecular weight marker that determines the molecular weight of the target protein. Another lane should include an internal control, ideally with a known concentration and molecular weight, to determine if the primary antibody is effective. Since most autoantigens are large molecules with molecular weight >100 kDa, 5% gels are useful in most cases. For antigens <100 kDa, the percentage should be increased.
- When voltage is applied to the gel, proteins migrate at different speeds, and these different speeds result in separation into bands within each lane.

Transfer of Proteins from Gel to Membrane

- Once electrophoresis is complete, the separated proteins are transferred from within the gel onto a membrane made of nitrocellulose, polyvinylidene difluoride, activated paper, or activated nylon. Their thickness is about 100 μm and an average pore size of 0.05–10 μm in diameter.
- Nitrocellulose is the most commonly used membrane. It becomes brittle when dry. The mechanical strength of the membrane has been improved by incorporating a polyester support web. Small proteins tend to move through nitrocellulose membranes and only a small fraction of the total amount actually binds. Using membranes with smaller pores obviates this.
- Electroblotting is the most popular procedure for transferring proteins from the gel to the membrane. This process uses an electric current to pull proteins from the gel onto the membrane. Its main advantages are speed and completeness of transfer. The use of constant voltage provides the best driving force (potential difference) during transfer.

- The efficient transfer of proteins from the gel to membrane also depends on the nature of the gel, the molecular mass of the proteins being transferred, and the membrane used. Transfer is more complete and faster with the use of thinner gels. However, the use of ultrathin gels may cause handling problems and so a 0.4 mm thickness is considered the lower practical limit. Proteins with high molecular weight blot poorly on SDS-PAGE, resulting in low levels of detection on IB assay. However, the efficiency of transfer of such proteins has been facilitated with heat, special buffers, and partial proteolytic digestion of the proteins prior to transfer.

Prevention of Interaction between the Membrane and the Antibody Chosen to Detect the Target Protein

In order to prevent non-specific binding, the membrane is placed in a dilute solution of protein such as bovine serum albumin, 2–5% non/low fat dry milk in 20 mM Tris hydrochloride (HCl) pH 7.5, goat serum or 1% glycine in 0.15 M NaCl and 10 mM Tris HCl pH 7.4, overnight at 4°C. Blocking helps to mask any potential non-specific binding sites on the membrane, thus reducing "background noise", eliminating false positives, and providing a clear result. However, excessive blocking must be avoided as it may produce low signals.

Incubation of Membrane

After blocking, the process is to incubate the membrane with the patient's serum containing the primary auto-antibody, wash and then incubate with secondary antibody, and wash again.

Detection of Antigen/Protein of Interest

The probes that are labeled and bound to the protein of interest have to be detected. For detection, colorimetric, radioactive, and fluorescent methods can be used. Chemiluminescent detection is a sensitive method. The primary antibody binds to the protein of interest and the secondary antibody, linked to horseradish peroxidase or alkaline phosphatase, is used to cleave a chemiluminescent agent. The reaction product produces luminescence, which is related to the amount of protein. The luminescence is detected by photographic film or by a charge-coupled device camera.

Use of fluorescently labeled secondary antibodies instead of chemiluminescence for signal detection, is also done. An advantage is the ability to detect multiple targets by using fluorophores with non-overlapping excitation–emission spectra. However, the relatively poor performance of fluorophores in the visible range is a drawback.

IB assay results in various AIBDs are shown in **Figures 2 to 6.**

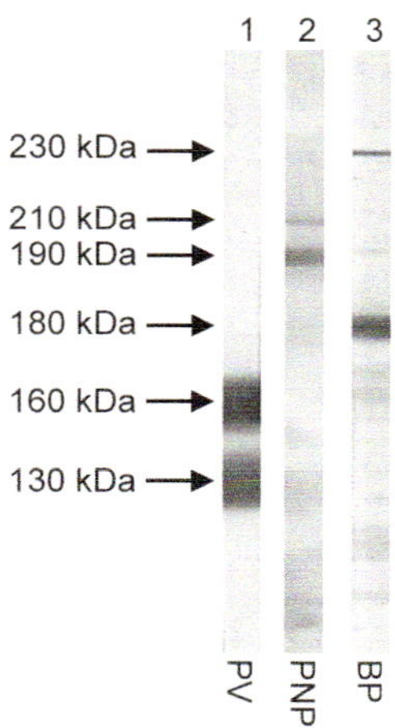

Fig. 2: Immunoblot assay of normal human epidermal extract: Pemphigus vulgaris (PV) serum reacted with the 160 kDa desmoglein 1 (Dsg1) and the 130 kDa Dsg3 (lane 1), paraneoplastic pemphigus (PNP) serum reacted with the 210 kDa envoplakin and the 190 kDa periplakin (lane 2), and bullous pemphigoid (BP) serum reacted with the 230 kDa BP230 and the 180 kDa BP180 (lane 3).

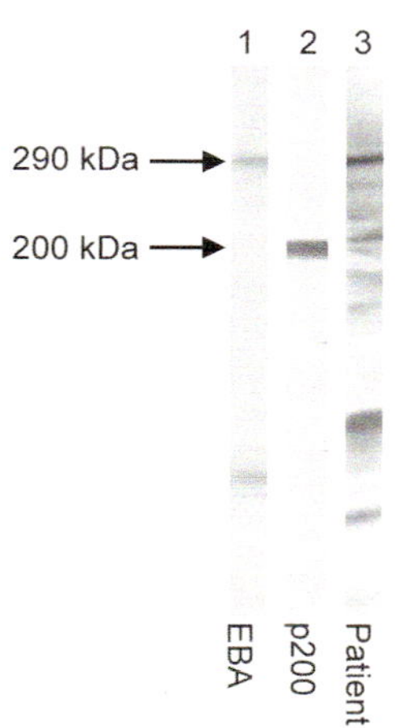

Fig. 3: Immunoblot assay of normal human dermal extract: Epidermolysis bullosa acquisita (EBA) serum reacted with the 290 kDa type VII collagen (EBA antigen) (lane 1), and anti-p200 pemphigoid (p200) serum reacted with the 200 kDa p200 (lane 2).

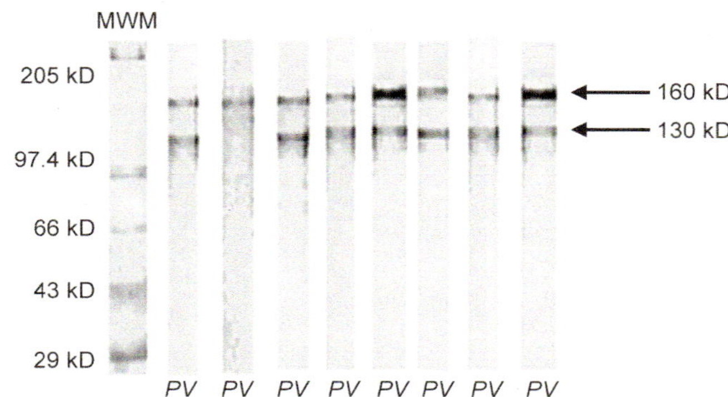

Fig. 4: Immunoblot assay in mucocutaneous pemphigus vulgaris: PV sera reacting with both 130 and 160 kDa antigens.
(MWM: molecular weight marker)

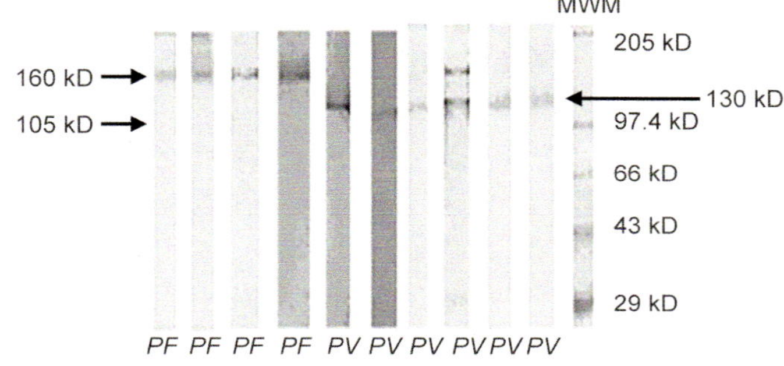

Fig. 5: Immunoblot assay in pure mucosal pemphigus vulgaris (PV) and pemphigus foliaceus (PF): Sera from PF patients reacting with 160 kDa antigen and from PV reacting with 130 kDa antigen.
(MWM: molecular weight marker)

IMMUNOPRECIPITATION

Original IP Steps

1. Substrate for extraction of desired antigens/proteins is taken.
2. The extract is obtained.
3. The extracted epidermal proteins are radiolabeled with ^{125}I, ^{14}C-amino acids, ^{35}S-labeled methionine, or 0.5% Nonidet P-40.
4. Immunoprecipitated proteins/antigens are denatured by boiling for 2 minutes in 100 µl of sample buffer (2% SDS, 10% glycerol, and 0.01% bromophenol blue in 0.0625 M Tris-HCl, pH 6.8).
5. Labeled extracts are sequentially incubated with serum from the patients or controls and protein A—bearing staphylococci
6. Individual immunoprecipitates are resolved by SDS-PAGE electrophoresis.
7. Separated proteins are visualized by autoradiography using enhancing screens.

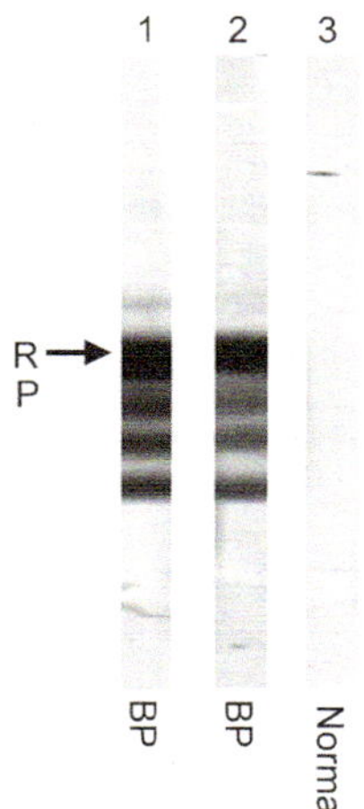

Fig. 6: Immunoblot assay of recombinant protein (RP) of bullous pemphigoid (BP) 180 non-collagenous 16a domain: Two BP sera reacted with this RP (lanes 1 and 2), while normal serum showed negative reactivity (lane 3).

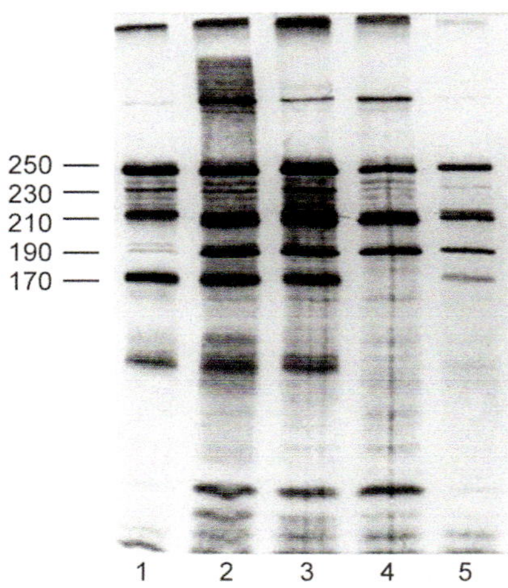

Fig. 7: Immunoprecipitation using the extract of radiolabeled cultured keratinocytes for paraneoplastic pemphigus (PNP) sera: The 5 PNP sera immunoprecipitated the 250 kDa desmoplakin I, 230 kDa bullous pemphigoid (BP) 230, 210 kDa doublet of desmoplakin II and envoplakin, 190 kDa periplakin, and 170 kDa alpha-2 macroglobulin-like protein 1 (α2ML1) in various patterns (lanes 1–5). *Image courtesy*: Grant Anhalt, John Hopkins University, Baltimore, USA.

The result of IP using the extract of radiolabeled cultured keratinocytes for paraneoplastic pemphigus (PNP) sera is depicted in **Figure 7**.

Other Immunoprecipitation Methods

Immunoprecipitation without the use of Radiolabeling

Hashimoto T, *et al* have developed two novel IP assays in which radioisotopes are not used, i.e., IP using silver stain and IP using cell-surface biotinylation. By IP using silver stain to detect immunoprecipitated proteins, PNP sera detected the 250, 210, and 190 kD proteins, while IB showed only 210 and 190 kDa antigens. In addition, three of the four PNP sera specifically reacted with the 130 kDa desmoglein 3 (Dsg3), indicating that PV antigen is involved in PNP.

In addition, IP–IB assay without the use of radioisotope has been recently used **(Fig. 8)** in place of conventional IP with radiolabeling.

SOME OBSERVATIONS IN STUDIES ON AIBDs USING IB AND IP ASSAYS

Table 1 (next page) displays some observations in studies on AIBDs using IB and IP assays.

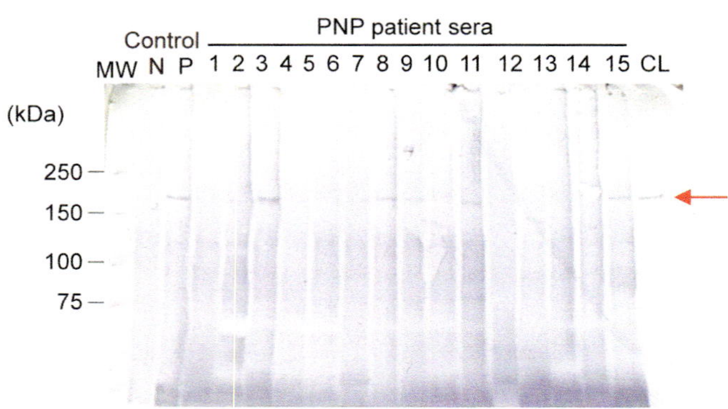

Fig. 8: Immunoprecipitation-immunoblot assay of alpha-2 macroglobulin-like protein 1 (α2ML1) for paraneoplastic pemphigus (PNP) sera: About half of the PNP sera (lanes 1–15) immunoprecipitated the 170 kDa α2ML1 (indicated by a red arrow on the right). *Image courtesy*: Sanae Numata, Kurume University, Kurume, Fukuoka, Japan.

[CL: cell lysate; MW: molecular weight markers (indicated in the left); N: normal control serum; P: positive control PNP serum]

CONCLUSION

IB and IP assays identify specific autoantigens in various AIBDs. They have high specificity, but are expensive, time-consuming and require technical skill. Hence, they are reserved for situations when diagnosis cannot be established by conventional diagnostic modalities.

TAKE HOME MESSAGE

- IB and IP assays in AIBDs identify target antigen(s) to confirm the diagnosis.
- The identification of antigens is done using SDS-PAGE on nitrocellulose membrane.
- Both human and animal substrates, and cultured cell and tumor cell lines are used as substrates to obtain the antigens.
- In IB assay, the antigens/proteins present in a protein extract are first separated according to molecular weight by electrophoresis, then the separated antigens are electrophoretically transferred to an inert membrane filter, and finally the antigen(s) against which the patient's autoantibodies are directed, are visualized.
- In IP, radioisotopes are used to label various substrates. However, IP assays without use of radioisotopes have also been developed including IP using silver stain and IP using cell-surface biotinylation.
- By IB and IP assays, novel antigens targeted by antibodies in both epidermal and subepidermal AIBDs are identified.

TABLE 1: Some observations in studies on AIBDs using IB and IP assays.

Study	Type of assay	Result	Conclusion
Jones, *et al.* 1986	IB assay in PV	The identification of pemphigus antigen by IB assay was considered impossible, probably because most epitopes on Dsg1 (160 kDa antigen) and 3 (130 kDa antigen) are conformational and the antibodies do not react to denatured antigens. This study first detected PV antigen using bovine tongue desmosome preparation as antigen source. Subsequently, detection of PV antigens in normal human epidermal extracts was also shown by using modified extraction procedures	PV and PF antigens can be detected by IB assay using modified extraction procedures
Hashimoto T, *et al.* 1995	IB assay in PV and PF using human epidermal extracts	All PV sera reacted with 130 kDa antigen but not with 160 kDa antigen. By contrast, only half of PF sera reacted with 160 kDa, but none reacted with 130 kDa antigen	The results showed distinct antibody specificity between PV and PF sera. They also suggested that PV sera contain antibodies against linear epitopes present even on the denatured antigen, while some PF sera contain antibodies only against conformational epitopes present on the native antigen
Hashimoto T, *et al.* 1995	IB assay in PV and PF using bovine desmosome preparations	Certain PV sera and an anti-Dsg monoclonal antibody reacted with both 130 kDa and 160 kDa antigens	Affinity purification of PV antibodies suggested that the simultaneous reactivity of the two was produced by two different subsets of antibodies and not by cross-reactivity of single antibodies
Tsuruta D, *et al.* 2013	IB assay in PV and PF	In this study from Chandigarh, in 22 PV and 4 PF patients, DIF and IIF were positive in 95.8% and 56% of patients, respectively. IB assay detected the 130 kDa antigen in 45% and 160 kDa antigen in 4.5% of PV patients. The 190 kDa periplakin was unexpectedly detected in 35% pemphigus patients	The study showed low sensitivity of IB assay in pemphigus
Khandpur S, *et al.* 2010	IB assay in PV and PF on split-skin grafts	In this study from Delhi, sensitivity and specificity of IB assay in PV was 88.9% and 100%, and in PF was 100% and 95.2%, respectively. In PV, 67% cases showed both 130 kDa and 160 kDa antigens, 22% showed only the 130 kDa antigen while 11% showed the 160 kDa antigen. Of 43 mucocutaneous cases, 81% showed both the 130 kDa and 160 kDa bands while 9% showed either the 130 kDa or 160 kDa band. 89% of pure mucosal cases showed only a single band of the 130 kDa antigen, and both pure cutaneous cases demonstrated only the 160 kDa band. All PF cases showed only the 160 kDa band	IB assay can differentiate PV from PF
Jiao D, *et al.* 1997	IB assay in PV and PF	Pemphigus antibodies were detected with equal sensitivity by IIF in patients with PV and PF (i.e., positive in 87% and 86% of sera, respectively). By contrast, IB assay was much less sensitive in PF than in PV (i.e., positive in 45% of PF vs. 83% of PV sera)	IIF better than IB assay in PF, equal in PV
Kricheli D, *et al.* 2000	IB assay on first-degree relatives of PV cases	Circulating PV-IgG was detected in 49% first-degree relatives, and PV-IgG4 in 1.8% relatives by IB assay	Pathogenic antibodies not detected in relatives of PV patients
Cozzani E, *et al.* 1998	IB assay in pemphigus	In 67 pemphigus sera, about one-fourth of patients revealed multiple heterogeneous bands including 13% depicting the 230 kDa band. When challenged with the recombinant protein rBP55, the carboxyl terminal portion of BP major antigen, all 230 kDa-positive-sera proved negative	Caution is recommended in interpreting pemphigus sera with a band migrating to the 230 kDa antigen

Continued

Continued

Study	Type of assay	Result	Conclusion
Cozzani E, *et al.* 1994	IB assay versus IIF in pemphigus	Among 54 sera from pemphigus patients (40 PV and 14 PF), 85% were positive by IIF (46 on monkey esophagus and 41 on rabbit lip) compared with 81.5% by IB assay. IB assay showed positivity in 10% IIF-negative pemphigus cases	IIF and IB assay were equally sensitive in diagnosis of PV while IIF (on rabbit lip) was more sensitive than IB assay in detection of PF autoantibodies
Mohimen A, *et al.* 1995	IB assay in PV by modifications in extraction procedure of the lysate, i.e., by absorption of lysate with normal human serum and by use of an enzygraphic web	Generalized PV cases showed two- to four-fold higher antibody titers by the modified extraction procedure in IB assay than in IIF. All IIF-negative limited PV cases were also IB positive. Moreover, patients in remission and off all therapy for at least 3 years and negative on IIF assay were all positive on IB assay	Sensitivity of IB assay is enhanced over IIF by modifications in epidermal protein extraction procedures
Hashimoto T, *et al.* 1991	IB assay in PV and PF with normal human epidermal extracts and bovine desmosome preparation	All PV sera reacted to the 130 kDa antigen in normal human epidermal extracts and most PV sera reacted to a slightly higher-molecular-weight protein (135 kDa) in bovine desmosome preparation. Sera of one-third PF patients reacted to the 150 kDa protein in human epidermal extracts and in two-thirds of PF sera on bovine desmosomal preparation	There is some variation in antigen profiles in PV and PF in IB assay performed on different substrates
Kawana S, *et al.* 1994	IB assay using normal human epidermal extracts in sera from two PV cases who subsequently developed PF	It was observed that sera during PV reacted exclusively with the 130 kDa antigen and sera during PF reacted exclusively with the 150 kDa antigen	Antigen specificity in PV and PF is maintained even on transformation from PV to PF
Hashimoto K, *et al.* 1994	IB assay on two cases of Hallopeau-type pemphigus vegetans	The cases reacted not only with the PV antigen but also with PF and desmocollin I/II antigens	Multiple antigen reactivity in pemphigus vegetans
Korman NJ, *et al.* 1991	IP on a PF case who later developed BP, utilizing both cultured keratinocytes and suction blister epidermis	The patient had circulating autoantibodies directed against both the PF antigen complex and BP antigen	Co-existence of antibodies against PF and BP antigens in PF later developing BP
Yoshimura K, *et al.* 2014	IB assay in 17 Japanese drug-induced pemphigus patients using normal human epidermal extracts	In addition to positive reactivity with 130 kDa antigen, four patients with no detectable malignancy showed paraneoplastic pemphigus-like reactivity with the 210 kDa envoplakin and the 190 kDa periplakin antigens. Four cases also highlighted 130 kDa antigen without mucosal lesions	Drug-induced pemphigus can show reactivity to few PNP antigens
Korman NJ, *et al.* 1991	IP utilizing extracts of ^{125}I-labeled suction blister epidermis in three patients with drug-induced PF (two due to penicillamine and one due to captopril), and one patient with captopril-induced PV	All three drug-induced PF cases had circulating autoantibodies directed against the PF complex and the one patient with drug-induced PV had circulating autoantibodies directed against the PV antigen complex	The study demonstrated that autoantibodies from drug-induced pemphigus patients have antigenic specificity similar to other pemphigus patients
Joly P, *et al.* 1994	IB assay in PNP using anti-human whole Ig and anti-human IgG subclasses	Using anti-human whole Ig, results were consistent with autoantibody specificities previously described in PNP. On using antihuman IgG subclasses, in two sera, in addition to the anti-desmoplakin I-II, antibodies to 185 kDa, 230 kDa, and 130 kDa antigens were present. In one serum, IgG1 bound to the 250 and 220 kDa bands corresponding to desmoplakin I and II, IgG3 recognized a 185 kDa antigen, and IgG4 bound to the 130 kDa PV antigen	This suggests an overlapping distribution of autoantibody specificities in PNP
Joly P, *et al.* 1999	IB assay on endemic Tunisian pemphigus cases	Most corresponded to PF antigen and additionally showed a high frequency of autoantibodies against a 185 kDa antigen of the desmosomal plaque	Both 160 kDa and 185 kDa antigens detected in endemic Tunisian pemphigus

Continued

Continued

Study	Type of assay	Result	Conclusion
Holtsche MM, *et al.* 2009	IB assay using extracts of human dermis in anti-p200 pemphigoid	IB assay detected 200 KDa antigen	IB assay useful in diagnosis of anti-p200 pemphigoid
Furukita K, *et al.* 2009	IB assay using extract of human dermis in EBA	Type VII collagen-specific autoantibodies mostly directed against the non-collagenous (NC) 1 domain can be detected	IB assay useful in detection of specific antigen in EBA
Sami N, *et al.* 2002	IB assay in 13 recalcitrant BP patients using bovine gingival lysate as substrate	Sera of six patients bound to both the 230 kDa (BP Ag1) and 180 kDa (BP Ag2) protein, while seven sera bound to only a 230 kDa protein. All 13 patients had high levels of antibodies to Dsg3 on ELISA	The authors concluded that in BP patients non-responsive to conventional therapy, presence of two autoimmune diseases or a dual diagnosis should be considered
Paolino G, *et al.* 2017	IB and IP assays in PNP and MMP cases	In PNP, autoantibodies directed against Dsg3, plakins such as BP230, periplakin, envoplakin, desmoplakin 1 and 2, plectin, desmocollins, α-2 macroglobulin-like 1, and epiplakin have been detected. Antibodies against envoplakin and periplakin are most frequent. In MMP, on IIF, autoantibodies can only be detected in 50% of patients. Therefore, IB and IP assays are essential diagnostic tests for MMP (BP180 being target antigen), in which autoantibodies target C-terminal epitopes of BP180 such as LAD-1 and the soluble ectodomain of BP180 using the respective recombinant fragments of the C-terminus of BP180. Both anti-BP180 IgG and IgA are predominant in anti-BP180-type MMP	It is necessary to test for both MMP isotypes

(AIBD: autoimmune bullous disease; BP: bullous pemphigoid; DIF: direct immunofluorescence; Dsg: desmoglein; EBA: epidermolysis bullosa acquisita; IB: immunoblot; IgG: immunoglobulin G; IIF: indirect immunofluorescence; IP: immunoprecipitation; MMP: mucous membrane pemphigoid; PF: pemphigus foliaceus; PNP: paraneoplastic pemphigus; PV: pemphigus vulgaris)

MULTIPLE CHOICE QUESTIONS

1. **In IB assay, transfer of proteins from gel to microporous membrane (blotting) occurs by:**
   (a) Electrophoretic transfer
   (b) Non-electrophoretic transfer
   (c) Both
   (d) None

2. **Which of the following has not been used as a substrate for IB assay?**
   (a) Adult or neonatal foreskin
   (b) HaCaT keratinocyte cell line monolayers
   (c) Hep-2 cell
   (d) Human amniotic membrane

3. **In IB assay, the most popular membrane used to transfer the separated proteins from the gel is?**
   (a) Polyvinyl chloride
   (b) Nitrocellulose
   (c) Polyvinylidene difluoride
   (d) Activated nylon

4. **In IB assay, to obtain epidermal and dermal extracts, the dermo-epidermal separation methods used are:**
   (a) Heat separation
   (b) EDTA separation
   (c) Both (a) and (b)
   (d) Sulfatase separation

5. **In IP, a common radioisotope used to label cultured cells is:**
   (a) Technicium
   (b) Strontium
   (c) Nonidet P-40
   (d) Isotope of glycine

6. **Novel IP assays in which radioisotopes are not used are:**
   (a) IP using silver stain
   (b) IP using cell-surface biotinylation
   (c) IP using method of hydroxylation
   (d) Both (a) and (b)

7. **By IP, which uncommon antigen seems to be involved in paraneoplastic pemphigus?**
   (a) 160 kDa
   (b) 230 kDa
   (c) 260 kDa
   (d) 130 kDa

8. On IB assay, pathogenic antibodies (IgG4) have been detected in relatives of what proportion of PV patients?

(a) 5–10%

(b) <2%

(c) 50%

(d) >75%

9. In drug-induced pemphigus, circulating antibodies can be present against:

(a) 130 kDa antigen

(b) 160 kDa antigen

(c) 45 kDa antigen

(d) Both (a) and (b)

10. On IB assay, in EBA the antibodies are detected against which antigen?

(a) Type VII collagen-specific autoantibodies against the collagenous (NC) 1 domain

(b) Type VII collagen-specific autoantibodies against the non-collagenous (NC) 1 domain

(c) Type XVII collagen-specific autoantibodies against the non-collagenous (NC) 1 domain

(d) Type IV collagen-specific autoantibodies against the collagenous (NC) 1 domain

Answers

1. (c) 2. (c) 3. (b) 4. (c) 5. (c) 6. (d) 7. (d) 8. (b) 9. (d) 10. (b)

SUGGESTED READING

1. Jones JC, Yokoo KM, Goldman RD. Further analysis of pemphigus autoantibodies and their use in studies on the heterogeneity, structure, and function of desmosomes. *J Cell Biol.* 1986;102:1109-17.

2. Otten JV, Hashimoto T, Hertl M, Payne AS, Sitaru C. Molecular diagnosis in autoimmune skin blistering conditions. *Curr Mol Med.* 2014;14:69-95.

3. Jensen EC. The basics of western blotting. *Anat Rec (Hoboken).* 2012;295:369-71.

4. Kurien BT, Scofield RH, Kurien BT, et al. Western blotting: an introduction. *Methods Mol Biol.* 2015;1312:17-30.

5. Hashimoto T, Amagai M, Garrod DR, Nishikawa T. Immuno-fluorescence and immunoblot studies on the reactivity of pemphigus vulgaris and pemphigus foliaceus sera with desmoglein 3 and desmoglein 1. *Epithelial Cell Biol.* 1995;4:63-9.

6. Tsuruta D, Kanwar AJ, Vinay K, Fukuda S, Koga H, Dainichi T, et al. Clinical and immunologic characterization in 26 Indian pemphigus patients. *J Cutan Med Surg.* 2013;17:321-31.

7. Khandpur S, Sharma VK, Sharma A, Pathria G, Satyam A. Comparison of enzyme-linked immunosorbent assay test with immunoblot assay in the diagnosis of pemphigus in Indian patients. *Indian J Dermatol Venereol Leprol.* 2010;76:27-32.

8. Jiao D, Bystryn JC. Sensitivity of indirect immunofluorescence, substrate specificity, and immunoblotting in the diagnosis of pemphigus. *J Am Acad Dermatol.* 1997;37:211-6.

9. Kricheli D, David M, Frusic-Zlotkin M, Goldsmith D, Rabinov M, Sulkes J, et al. The distribution of pemphigus vulgaris-IgG subclasses and their reactivity with desmoglein 3 and 1 in pemphigus patients and their first-degree relatives. *Br J Dermatol.* 2000;143:337-42.

10. Cozzani E, A Parodi A, Rebora A. Prevalence of bands other than 160 and 130 kDa in pemphigus sera (a multicenter immunoblotting study). Gruppo Italiano Studi Epidemiologici in Dermatologia (GISED). *J Eur Acad Dermatol Venereol.* 1998;10:233-6.

11. Cozzani E, Kanitakis J, Nicolas JF, Schmitt D, Thivolet J. Comparative study of indirect immunofluorescence and immunoblotting for the diagnosis of autoimmune pemphigus. *Arch Dermatol Res.* 1994;286:295-9.

12. Mohimen A, Ahmed AR. Comparison of an indirect immuno-fluorescence assay and a modified sensitive immunoblot assay for the study of the autoantibody in pemphigus vulgaris. *Arch Dermatol Res.* 1995;287:202-8.

13. Hashimoto T, Konohana A, Nishikawa T. Immunoblot assay as an aid to the diagnoses of unclassified cases of pemphigus. *Arch Dermatol.* 1991;127:843-7.

14. Kawana S, Hashimoto T, Nishikawa T, Nishiyama S. Shift in clinical features, histologic findings and antigen profiles from pemphigus vulgaris to pemphigus foliaceus-two case studies. *Dermatology.* 1994;189:57-9.

15. Hashimoto K, Hashimoto T, Higashiyama M, Nishikawa T, Garrod DR, Yoshikawa K. Detection of anti-desmocollins I and II autoantibodies in two cases of Hallopeau type pemphigus vegetans by immunoblot analysis. *J Dermatol Sci.* 1994;7:100-6.

16. Korman NJ, Stanley JR, Woodley DT. Coexistence of pemphigus foliaceus and bullous pemphigoid. Demonstration of auto-antibodies that bind to both the pemphigus foliaceus antigen complex and the bullous pemphigoid antigen. *Arch Dermatol.* 1991;127:387-90.

17. Yoshimura K, Ishii N, Hamada T, Abe T, Ono F, Hashikawa K, et al. Clinical and immunological profiles in 17 Japanese patients with drug-induced pemphigus studied at Kurume University. *Br J Dermatol.* 2014;171:544-53.

18. Korman NJ, Eyre RW, Zone J, Stanley JR. Drug-induced pemphigus: autoantibodies directed against the pemphigus antigen complexes are present in penicillamine and captopril-induced pemphigus. *J Invest Dermatol.* 1991;96:273-6.

19. Joly P, Thomine E, Gilbert D, Verdier S, Delpech A, Prost C, et al. Overlapping distribution of autoantibody specificities in paraneoplastic pemphigus and pemphigus vulgaris. *J Invest Dermatol.* 1994;103:65-72.

20. Joly P, Mokhtar I, Gilbert D, Thomine E, Fazza B, Bardi R, et al. Immunoblot and immunoelectronmicroscopic analysis of endemic Tunisian pemphigus. *Br J Dermatol.* 1999;140:44-9.

21. Sami N, Bhol KC, Beutner EH, Plunkett RW, Leiferman KM, Ahmed AR. Diagnostic features of pemphigus vulgaris in patients with bullous pemphigoid. Molecular analysis of autoantibody profile. *Dermatology.* 2002;204:108-17.

22. Holtsche MM, Goletz S, Zillikens D. (Anti-p200 pemphigoid). *Hautarzt.* 2019;70:271-6.

23. Paolino G, Didona D, Magliulo G, Iannella G, Didona B, Mercuri SR, et al. Paraneoplastic Pemphigus: Insight into the Autoimmune Pathogenesis, Clinical Features and Therapy. *Int J Mol Sci.* 2017;18:2532.

24. Sezin T, Avitan-Hersh E, Indelman M, Moscona R, Sabo E, Katz R, et al. Human amnion membrane as a substrate for the detection of autoantibodies in pemphigus vulgaris and bullous pemphigoid. *Isr Med Assoc J.* 2014;16:217-23.

CHAPTER 19

Diagnostic Approach to Autoimmune Bullous Diseases

Anuradha Bishnoi, Shikha Shah, Debajyoti Chatterjee

- Intraepidermal versus subepidermal AIBDs
- Diagnostic approach to pemphigus group of AIBDs
- Diagnostic approach to subepidermal AIBDs

INTRODUCTION

Autoimmune bullous diseases (AIBDs) are broadly categorized into the intraepidermal (pemphigus group) and subepidermal bullous diseases (prototype being bullous pemphigoid) **(Table 1)**.

TABLE 1: Intraepidermal versus subepidermal autoimmune bullous diseases.

	Intraepidermal AIBDs	Subepidermal AIBDs
Autoantibodies	Against intercellular adhesion proteins	Against basement membrane zone proteins
Level of split	Intraepidermal	Subepidermal
Age of presentation	Middle age	Elderly
Clinical presentation	Superficial flaccid blisters and erosions distributed predominantly on trunk with little tendency to heal on their own; mucosal involvement more common	Tense blisters with associated itching/urtication, flexural distribution, healing with dyspigmentation/milia, scarring; mucosal involvement less common
Nature of the blister	Flaccid	Tense, sometimes hemorrhagic
Bedside tests	• Nikolsky positive • *Asboe–Hansen/Lutz test*: Irregular spreading margins • *Tzanck smear*: Acantholytic cells +	• Nikolsky negative (false Nikolsky/Sheklakov sign positive) • *Asboe–Hansen/Lutz test*: Regular extension of bulla • *Tzanck smear*: No acantholytic cells
Classification	• Pemphigus vulgaris (PV) (including pemphigus vegetans) • Pemphigus foliaceus (PF) (including endemic variant, pemphigus erythematosus) • IgA pemphigus • Drug-induced pemphigus • Paraneoplastic pemphigus (PNP)	• Bullous pemphigoid (BP) • Cicatricial pemphigoid (CP) • Mucous membrane pemphigoid (MMP) • Pemphigoid gestationis • Linear IgA disease (LAD), chronic bullous dermatosis of childhood (CBDC) • Epidermolysis bullosa acquisita (EBA) • Bullous systemic lupus erythematosus (BSLE) • Lichen planus pemphigoides • Anti-p200 pemphigoid • Dermatitis herpetiformis (DH) (some experts consider DH not to be classified as subepidermal AIBD since autoantibodies are directed against epidermal components)
Relative therapeutic response and prognosis	Relatively poor	Better

DIAGNOSTIC ALGORITHM

The diagnosis of AIBDs rests on four pillars as depicted in **Figure 1**.

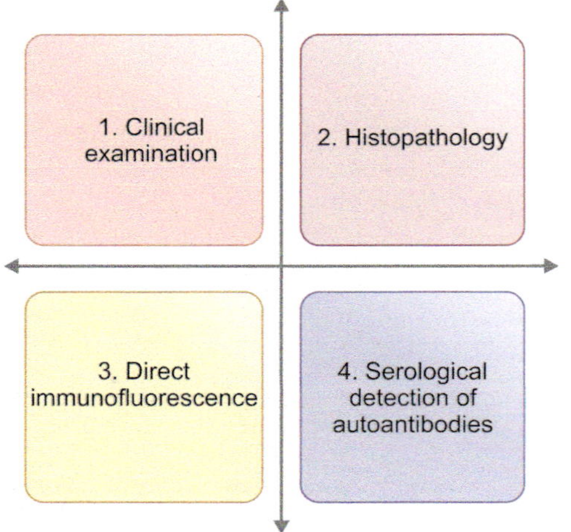

Fig. 1: Four basic diagnostic pillars of autoimmune bullous diseases.

APPROACH TO PEMPHIGUS GROUP OF AUTOIMMUNE BULLOUS DISEASES

For accurate diagnosis of the pemphigus group of disorders, the following steps should be followed:

1. *Clinical examination*: Discerning the lesional morphology, distribution and configuration **(Flowchart 1)**
2. *Bedside investigations*: Tzanck smear
3. Histopathology **(Figs. 2A and B)**
4. Direct immunofluorescence (DIF) **(Figs. 2C and D)**
5. Serology including indirect immunofluorescence (IIF) and enzyme-linked immunosorbent assay (ELISA) **(Table 2)**
6. Antigen detection by immunoblot or immunoprecipitation techniques on epidermal extracts

Investigations

The various findings on investigations in pemphigus group of disorders are mentioned in **Table 2**.

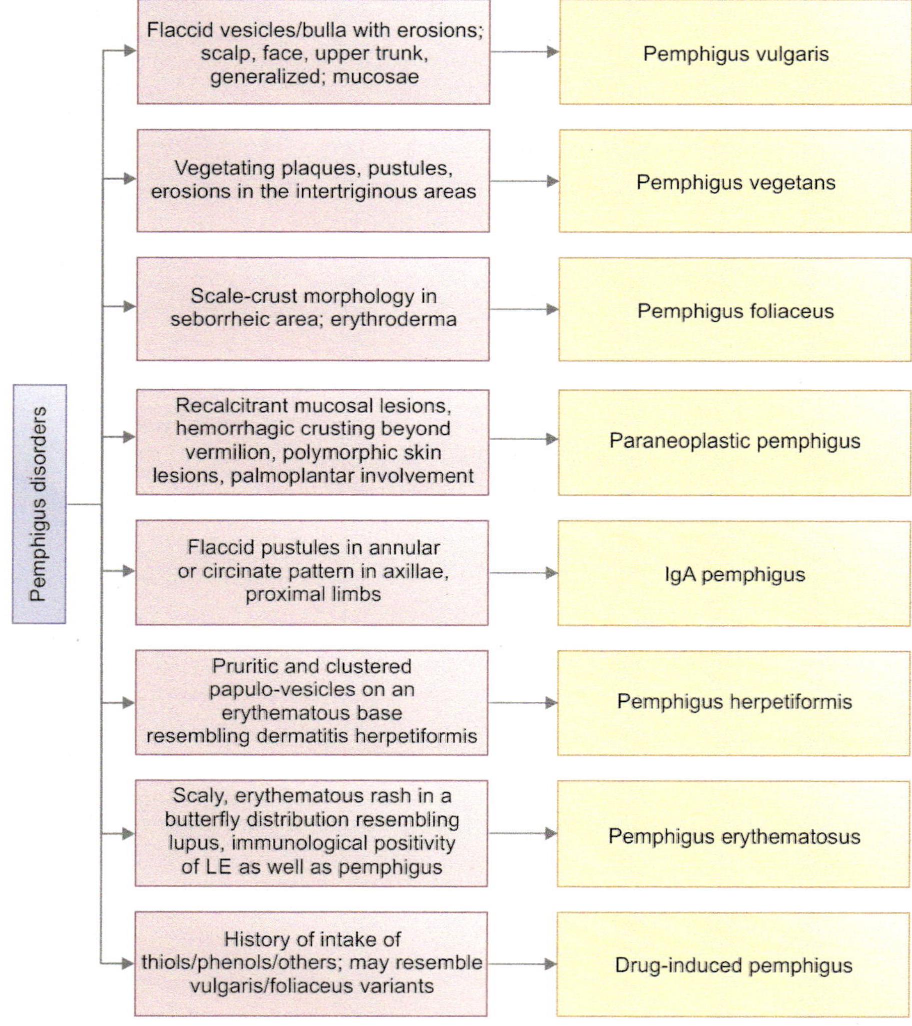

Flowchart 1: Salient clinical features of pemphigus group of disorders.

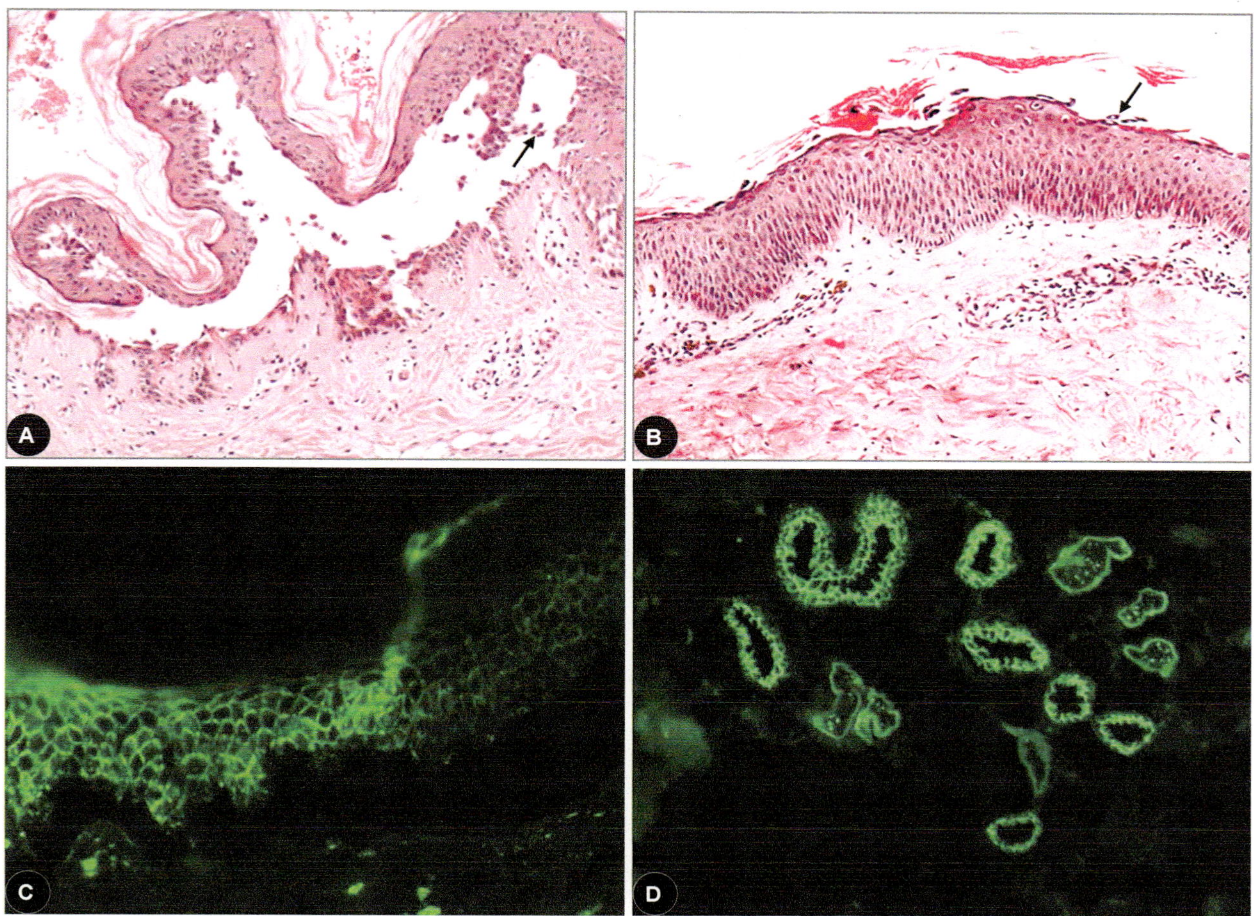

Figs. 2A to D: (A) Pemphigus vulgaris: Histopathology showing a suprabasal split with presence of acantholytic cells (arrow) (H&E, ×200). (B) Pemphigus foliaceus: Histopathology showing subcorneal cleft with few acantholytic cells (arrow) (H&E, ×200). (C) Pemphigus: DIF showing intercellular deposition of IgG in the epidermis in a 'fish-net' pattern (FITC, ×200). (D) Pemphigus vulgaris: DIF showing intercellular deposition of IgG in eccrine ducts (FITC, ×200).

(DIF: direct immunofluorescence; FITC: fluorescein isothiocyanate; IgG: immunoglobulin G)

TABLE 2: Interpretation of investigations in pemphigus group of disorders.

	PV	Pemphigus vegetans	PF	PNP	IgA pemphigus	Pemphigus herpetiformis	PE	Drug-induced pemphigus
Tzanck smear	Acantholytic cells, mourning edges, sertoli rosettes, streptocytes	Similar to PV, inflammatory cells—eosinophils	Acantholytic cells with hyalinized cytoplasm, i.e., dyskeratotic cells	Similar to PV, variable inflammation ± dyskeratosis	Similar to PV, may have neutrophils. Acantholytic cells may be absent	Similar to PV. Acantholytic cells may be absent	Similar to PF	Similar to PV or PF
Histopathology	• Suprabasal split • "Row of tombstone" appearance • Acantholytic cells	• Papillomatosis, acanthosis; pseudoepitheliomatous hyperplasia • Intraepidermal eosinophilic spongiosis or abscess • Suprabasal split, acantholytic cells	• Subcorneal split • Dyskeratotic cells • Acantholytic cells	• Variable split often suprabasal • Erythema multiforme or lichen planus-like patterns of vacuolar and/or lichenoid interface dermatitis	• SCPD or intraepidermal types • Abundant neutrophils, acantholytic cells ±	• Spongiosis with intraepidermal eosinophils or neutrophils or both, and/or intraepidermal split • Acantholysis ±	Resembles PF	• It may resemble PF or PV • More eosinophils

Continued

Continued

	PV	Pemphigus vegetans	PF	PNP	IgA pemphigus	Pemphigus herpetiformis	PE	Drug-induced pemphigus
Immuno-fluore-scence	*IgG, C3*: Intercellular fishnet pattern in the epidermis	*IgG, C3*: Intercellular fishnet pattern in the epidermis	*IgG, C3*: Intercellular fishnet pattern in the epidermis	*IgG*: Intercellular fishnet pattern or linear BMZ pattern; reactivity on rat bladder urothelium on IIF	*IgA*: Intercellular fishnet pattern in the epidermis	*IgG with/without C3*: Intercellular fishnet pattern in the epidermis	*IgG and C3*: Intercellular fishnet pattern in the epidermis + granular IgG and C3 at BMZ	Similar to PF or PV
Serology (ELISA)	Anti-Dsg3 and anti-Dsg1 Ab	Anti-Dsg3 and anti-Dsg1	Anti-Dsg1	Anti-Dsg3, anti-Dsg1, plectin, envoplakin, periplakin, desmoplakin, BPAG1, and A2ML1	Anti-Dsc1, occasionally Dsg1 and 3	Anti-Dsg1/3, occasionally anti-Dsc1/3	Anti-Dsg1 and ANA	Anti-Dsg1/3 in ~70% cases
Immuno-blot assay	Sera reactivity with 130 kDa antigen (Dsg3) and also 160 kDa (Dsg1)	Similar to PV	Sera reactivity with 160 kDa antigen (Dsg1)	Sera reactivity with multiple antigens (130–500 kDa, antigens vide supra)	Sera reactivity with 110 kDa antigen (Dsc1)	Similar to PV	Similar to PF	Similar to PF/PV

(Ab: antibody; A2ML1: alpha-2 macroglobulin-like 1; ANA: antinuclear antibody; BPAG: bullous pemphigoid antigen; BMZ: basement membrane zone; Dsc: desmocollin; Dsg: desmoglein; ELISA: enzyme-linked immunosorbent assay; IIF: indirect immunofluorescence; PE: pemphigus erythematosus; PF: pemphigus foliaceus; PNP: paraneoplastic pemphigus; PV: pemphigus vulgaris; SCPD: subcorneal pustular dermatosis)

APPROACH TO SUBEPIDERMAL AUTOIMMUNE BULLOUS DISEASES

In subepidermal AIBDs, there are two distinct groups: pemphigoid group (where autoantibodies are directed against the structural proteins of the dermo-epidermal junction), and dermatitis herpetiformis (where autoantibodies are directed against epidermal transglutaminase).

In contrast to the pemphigus group, these disorders are complex. They show clinical heterogeneity as well as variable and overlapping immunopathological findings. Since prognosis and treatment responses vary with each subtype, an accurate diagnosis is required in clinical practice.

A step-wise approach to subepidermal AIBDs includes:
1. Clinical examination
2. Histopathology
3. Immunofluorescence—DIF
4. Serology—IIF and ELISA
5. Immunoblot assay and immunoprecipitation on dermal extracts

The clinical approach to subepidermal AIBDs is depicted in **Flowchart 2**.

Investigations

The pemphigoid group of disorders cannot be substantially delineated based on histopathology alone since all these present with a subepidermal split. There are subtle clues on histopathology, especially based on the type of inflammatory cells **(Flowchart 3)**, immunofluorescence (direct and indirect), and whenever available, ELISA test, biochip mosaic, immunoblotting, and immunoprecipitation assays, which help to arrive at the final diagnosis.

DIF is an essential tool for the evaluation of subepidermal AIBDs **(Flowchart 4; Figs. 3 and 4)**. Serration pattern analysis may provide additional information, as pemphigoid group of diseases show an "*n*" serration pattern, while epidermolysis bullosa acquisita (EBA) and bullous systemic lupus erythematosus (BSLE) show a "*u*" serration or a "grass-like" pattern **(Flowchart 5)**. Thus, based on the type of antibody deposition [immunoglobulin G (IgG), IgA, or C3], their pattern of deposition (linear or granular) and the serration pattern (in cases of linear deposits), DIF can help to clinch the diagnosis of subepidermal AIBDs in majority of the cases. For diseases such as EBA and mucous membrane pemphigoid (MMP), the sensitivity of DIF is better than IIF, since circulating antibodies are usually in low titers. However, in some cases, reaching a single accurate diagnosis can be virtually impossible, and an overlap in the clinical and immunological findings of these disorders in certain clinical situations is well-recognized.

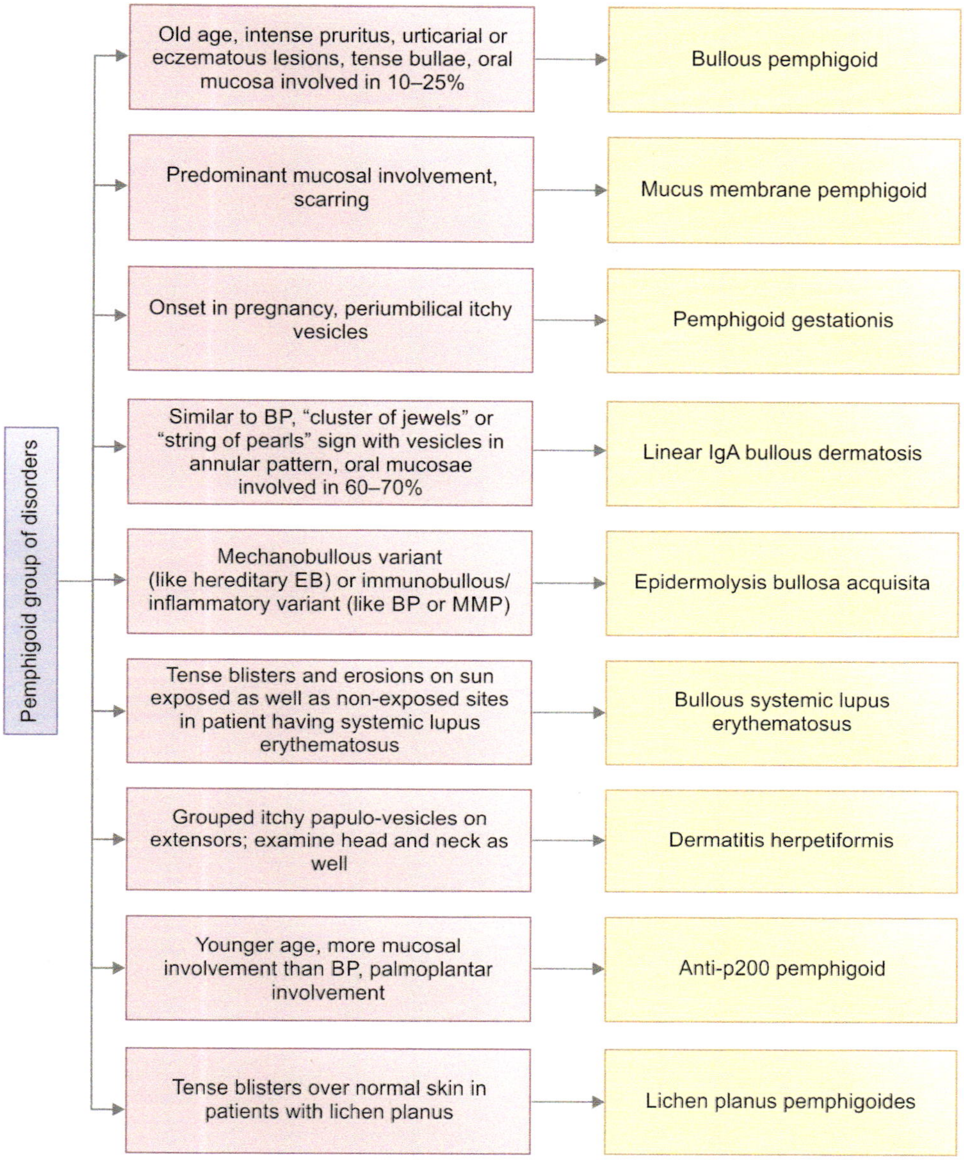

Pemphigoid group of disorders
Old age, intense pruritus, urticarial or eczematous lesions, tense bullae, oral mucosa involved in 10–25%
Bullous pemphigoid
Predominant mucosal involvement, scarring
Mucus membrane pemphigoid
Onset in pregnancy, periumbilical itchy vesicles
Pemphigoid gestationis
Similar to BP, "cluster of jewels" or "string of pearls" sign with vesicles in annular pattern, oral mucosae involved in 60–70%
Linear IgA bullous dermatosis
Mechanobullous variant (like hereditary EB) or immunobullous/ inflammatory variant (like BP or MMP)
Epidermolysis bullosa acquisita
Tense blisters and erosions on sun exposed as well as non-exposed sites in patient having systemic lupus erythematosus
Bullous systemic lupus erythematosus
Grouped itchy papulo-vesicles on extensors; examine head and neck as well
Dermatitis herpetiformis
Younger age, more mucosal involvement than BP, palmoplantar involvement
Anti-p200 pemphigoid
Tense blisters over normal skin in patients with lichen planus
Lichen planus pemphigoides

Flowchart 2: Salient clinical features to diagnose pemphigoid group of disorders.

(BP: bullous pemphigoid; EB: epidermolysis bullosa; MMP: mucous membrane pemphigoid)

Predominant type of cellular infiltration
Neutrophilic
Eosinophilic/Mixed
Non-inflammatory/ Cell-poor
Dermatitis herpetiformis, LABD, CBDC, bullous SLE, inflammatory EBA, anti-p200 pemphigoid
BP, MMP, PG, inflammatory EBA
Mechanobullous EBA Some variants of BP

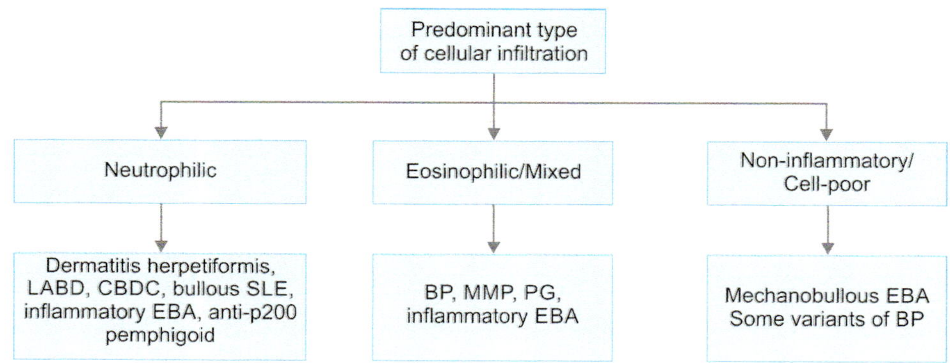

Flowchart 3: Approach to diagnosis of subepidermal autoimmune bullous diseases on histopathology based on type of inflammatory infiltrate.

(BP: bullous pemphigoid; CBDC: chronic bullous dermatosis of childhood; EBA: epidermolysis bullosa acquisita; LABD: linear IgA bullous dermatosis; MMP: mucous membrane pemphigoid; PG: pemphigoid gestationis; SLE: systemic lupus erythematosus)

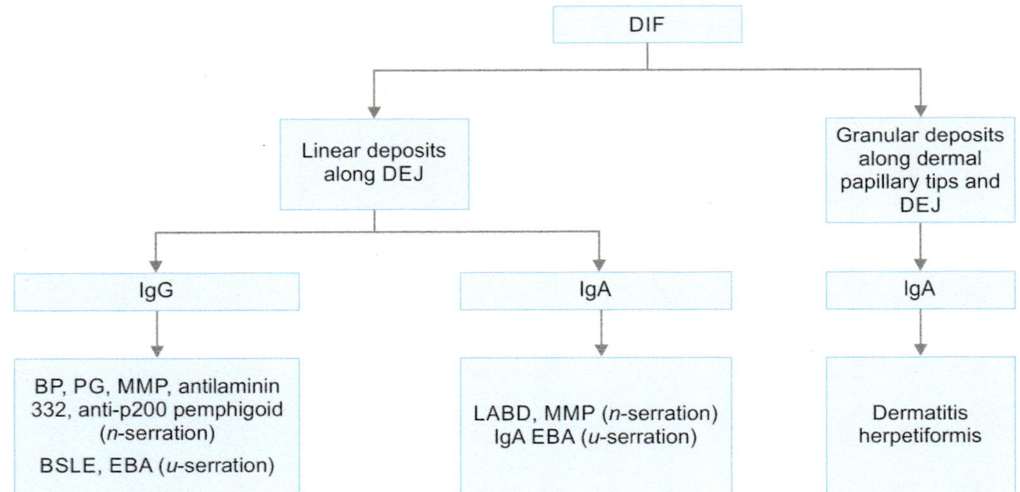

Flowchart 4: Approach to subepidermal autoimmune bullous diseases based on direct immunofluorescence.

(AIBD: autoimmune bullous disease; BP: bullous pemphigoid; BSLE: bullous systemic lupus erythematosus; DEJ: dermo-epidermal junction; DIF: direct immunofluorescence; EBA: epidermolysis bullosa acquisita; IgA: immunoglobulin A; IgG: immunoglobulin G; LABD: linear IgA bullous dermatosis; MMP: mucous membrane pemphigoid; PG: pemphigoid gestationis)

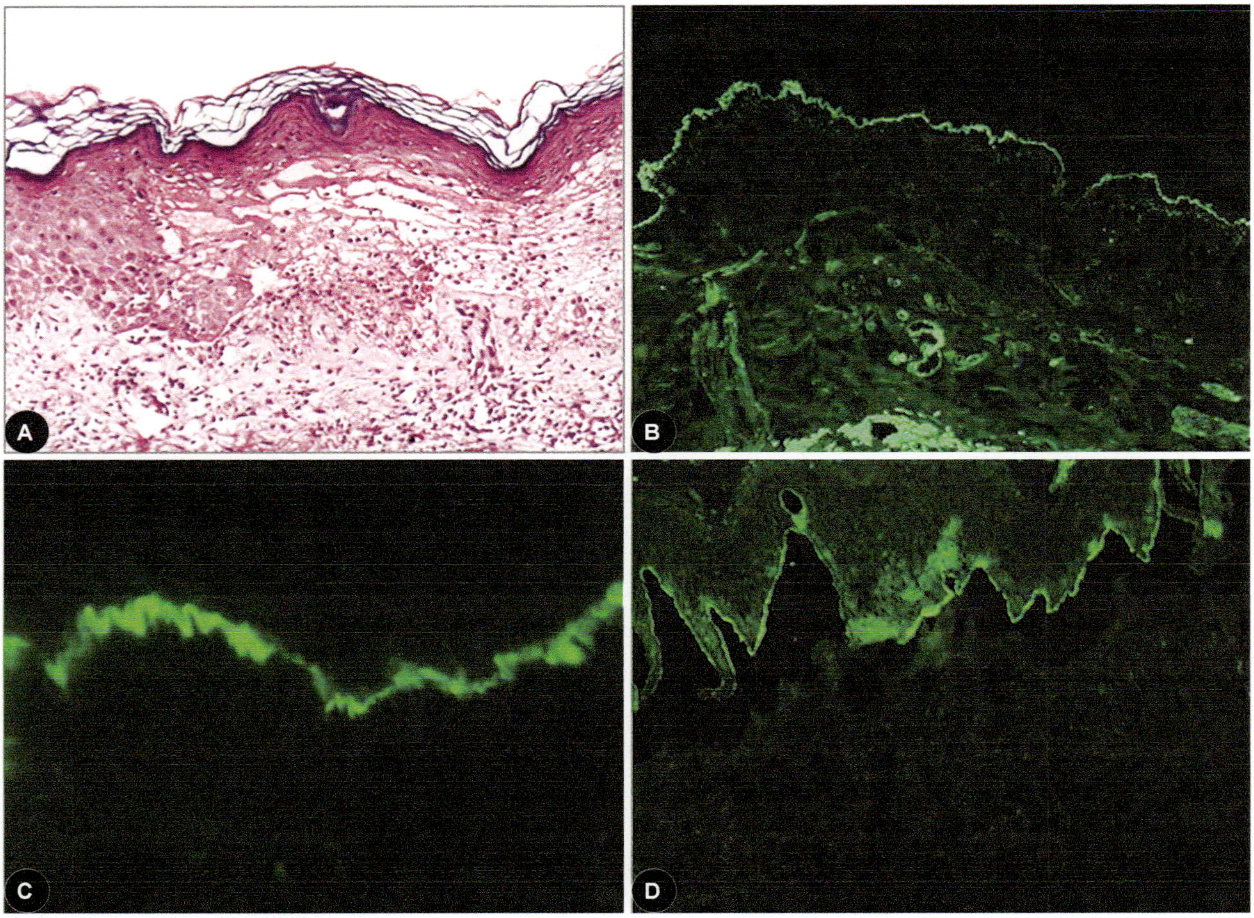

Figs. 3A to D: Bullous pemphigoid. (A) Histopathology showing subepidermal cleft with eosinophils (H&E, ×200). (B) DIF shows linear IgG deposition along dermo-epidermal junction (FITC, ×200). (C) DIF shows "*n*" serration pattern (FITC, ×400). (D) Salt-split IIF shows roof binding of IgG.

(DIF: direct immunofluorescence; FITC: fluorescein isothiocyanate; IgG: immunoglobulin G; IIF: indirect immunofluorescence)

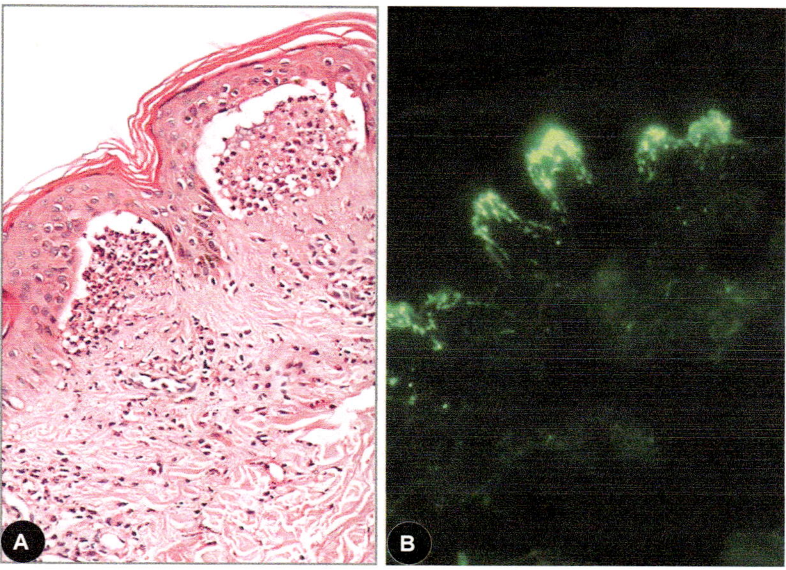

Figs. 4A and B: Dermatitis herpetiformis: (A) Histopathology shows neutrophilic microabscesses along the tips of dermal papillae (H&E, ×400). (B) DIF shows granular IgA deposition at the tips of dermal papillae (FITC, ×200).
(DIF: direct immunofluorescence; FITC: fluorescein isothiocyanate; IgA: immunoglobulin A)

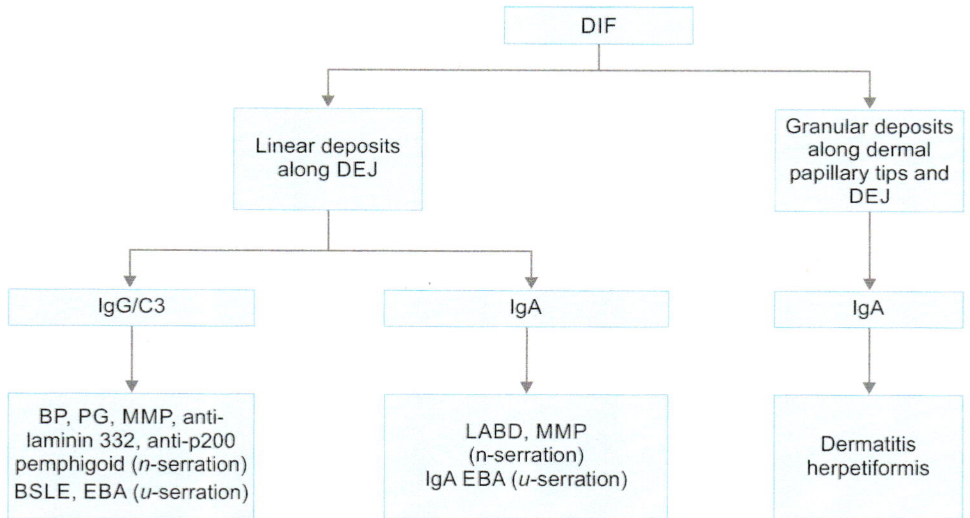

Flowchart 5: Approach to subepidermal autoimmune bullous diseases based on serration pattern analysis on direct immunofluorescence.
(BP: bullous pemphigoid; DEJ: dermo-epidermal junction; EBA: epidermolysis bullosa acquisita; IgG: immunoglobulin G; IgA: immunoglobulin A; LABD: linear IgA bullous dermatosis; MMP: mucous membrane pemphigoid; PG: pemphigoid gestationis)

Additional tests such as salt-split skin technique on IIF **(Flowchart 6)** (to differentiate dermatoses with "roof" from "floor" binding pattern of immunoreactants) and ELISA, for detection of specific antibodies against the common antigens implicated, can further help in delineating the diagnosis.

BIOCHIP mosaic (Euroimmun; **Figs. 5A to D**) is a good screening tool which also helps to differentiate intra-epidermal from subepidermal AIBDs and "roof" from "floor" pattern in many samples (upto 10) at one time .

Immunoblotting and immunoprecipitation identify specific antigens from epidermal or dermal extracts, based on their molecular weight after separation on electrophoresis. Immunoblot requires protein denaturation of substrates and is an easier method. Immunoprecipitation is more taxing to perform since it preserves original conformation of epitopes and requires radioisotopes.

Specific target antigens identified for subepidermal disorders based on these methods are summarized in **Table 3**.

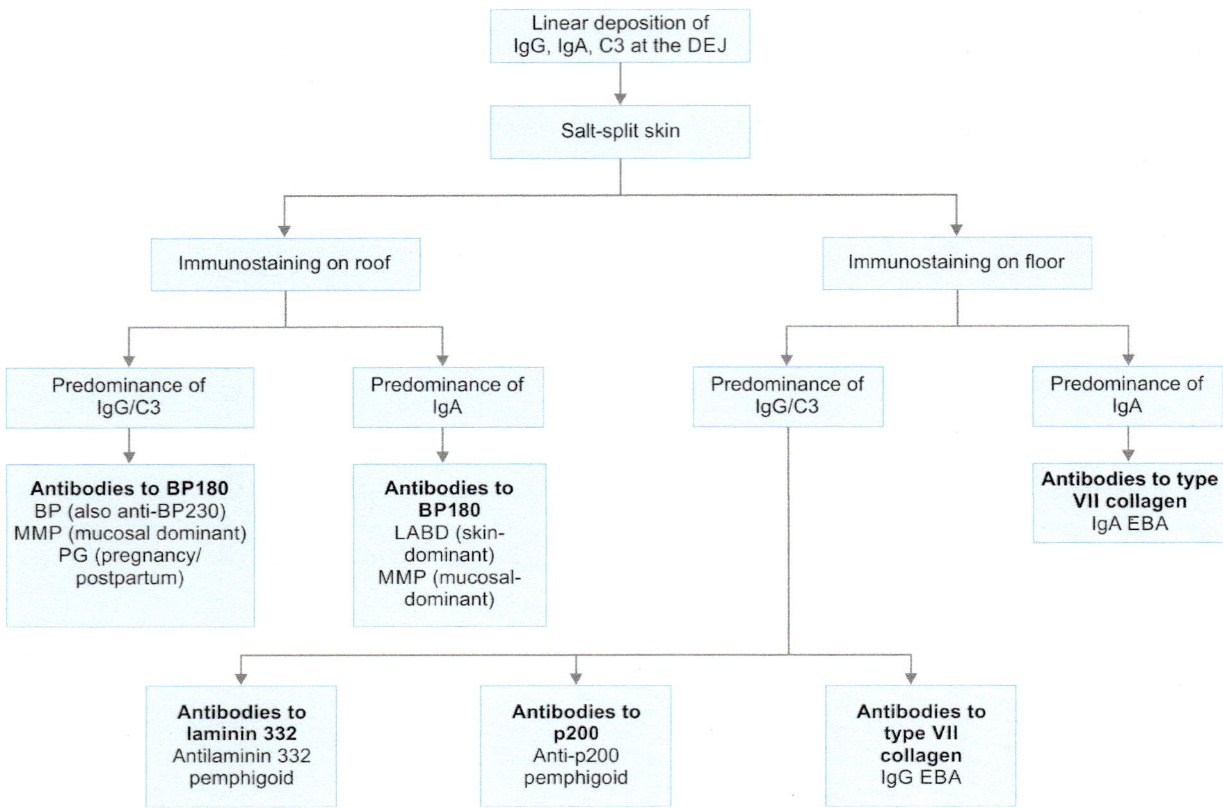

Flowchart 6: Approach to subepidermal autoimmune bullous diseases based on findings on salt-split skin on indirect immunofluorescence. (BP: bullous pemphigoid; DEJ: dermo-epidermal junction; EBA: epidermolysis bullosa acquisita; IgA: immunoglobulin A; IIF: indirect immunofluorescence; LABD: linear IgA bullous dermatosis; MMP: mucous membrane pemphigoid; PG: pemphigoid gestationis)

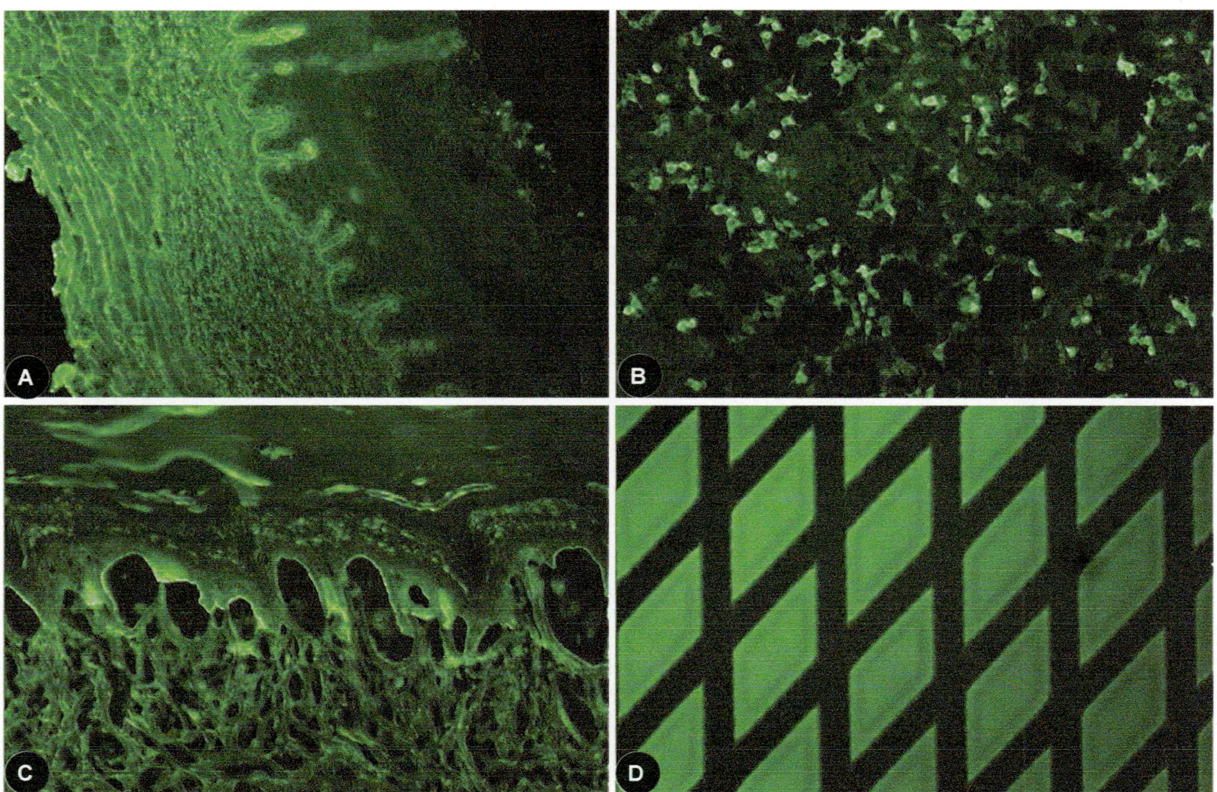

Figs. 5A to D: BIOCHIP mosaic of bullous pemphigoid: (A) Linear IgG deposition along the basement membrane zone (substrate: primate esophagus). (B) Transfected cells showing positivity for BP230. (C) Salt-split skin showing roof binding of immunoreactants, (D) Protein derivative of NC16a domain of BP180 showing positive serum binding.

TABLE 3: Target antigens in various subepidermal autoimmune bullous diseases.

Subepidermal AIBD	Target antigen/s
Bullous pemphigoid	BP180 (NC16 domain), BP230
Mucous membrane pemphigoid	Laminin 332, $\alpha6\beta4$ integrin, BP180 (C-terminal epitopes or NC16 domain), BP230
Pemphigoid gestationis	BP180 (NC16 domain), BP230
Linear IgA bullous dermatosis	BP180 (LABD-97/LAD-1 domain), type VII collagen
Epidermolysis bullosa acquisita	Type VII collagen (290 kDa)
Anti-p200 pemphigoid	Laminin $\gamma1$ (p200)
Lichen planus pemphigoides	BP180 (NC16 domain), BP230
Dermatitis herpetiformis	Epidermal transglutaminase (TG3), tissue transglutaminase (TG2), deamidated gliadin

CONCLUSION

Diagnosis of AIBDs rests on a comprehensive clinical examination, histopathology, and immunofluorescence (both direct and indirect). Newer methods such as ELISA and immunoblot assay complement the other investigations. A very precise classification may sometimes be difficult for certain patients; however, the proposed diagnostic algorithms help to arrive at the best possible diagnosis and henceforth the management plan. It is beneficial for clinicians to revise and update this knowledge from time to time.

TAKE HOME MESSAGE

- Accurate diagnosis of AIBD is crucial to the prognosis as well therapeutic management of the patient.
- Step-wise approach to AIBDs includes clinical evaluation, histopathology, immunofluorescence, and serological tests.
- Broadly, these disorders are intraepidermal and sub-epidermal. The former includes the pemphigus group characterized by flaccid blisters, intercellular fishnet pattern of deposit of immunoreactants by IgG/C3/IgA on DIF and autoantibodies to epidermal adhesion proteins on IIF and ELISA.
- Subepidermal AIBDs include the pemphigoid group characterized by tense blisters, linear deposition of IgG/C3/IgA along the BMZ on DIF, and autoantibodies to structural proteins of the BMZ on IIF and ELISA.
- Serration pattern analysis on DIF can differentiate EBA and bullous LE (*u*-serration) from pemphigoid disorders (*n*-serration).
- Salt-split technique differentiates pemphigoid disorders based on immunostaining on roof versus floor, by inducing a split at the level of lamina lucida.
- Dermatitis herpetiformis is a specific subepidermal AIBD with suprapapillary IgA deposits in picket-fence pattern along with autoantibodies to epidermal transglutaminase.

MULTIPLE CHOICE QUESTIONS

1. **Reactivity to which of the following substrates is a characteristic feature of paraneoplastic pemphigus?**
   - (a) Monkey esophagus
   - (b) Rat bladder
   - (c) Normal human skin substrate
   - (d) Guinea pig esophagus

2. **Intercellular fishnet staining of IgG/C3 in epidermis along with granular staining at basement membrane zone is characteristic of:**
   - (a) Pemphigus foliaceus
   - (b) Pemphigus erythematosus
   - (c) Dermatitis herpetiformis
   - (d) Pemphigus herpetiformis

3. **The level of split induced by 1 M NaCl in salt-split immunofluorescence is:**
   - (a) Lamina lucida
   - (b) Lamina densa
   - (c) Sublamina densa
   - (d) Hemidesmosome

4. **The *n*-serration pattern is found on immunofluorescence in all of the following disorders, *except*:**
   - (a) Epidermolysis bullosa acquisita
   - (b) Bullous pemphigoid
   - (c) Pemphigoid gestationis
   - (d) anti-p200 pemphigoid

5. **"Picket-fence" pattern of IgA deposition is seen in the DIF of which of the following AIBD?**
   - (a) LABD
   - (b) DH
   - (c) IgA EBA
   - (d) IgA MMP

6. **Which of the following AIBD predominantly features neutrophilic infiltration on histopathology?**
   - (a) BP
   - (b) MMP
   - (c) Bullous SLE
   - (d) Classical EBA

7. **What type/s of infiltrates are seen on histopathology of EBA?**
   (a) Neutrophilic
   (b) Eosinophilic
   (c) Cell-poor
   (d) Both (a) and (c)

8. **In salt-split immunofluorescence, anti-p200 pemphigoid would show staining on:**
   (a) Roof
   (b) Floor
   (c) Both (a) and (b)
   (d) None of the above

9. **Which antibody-subtype of MMP has around 30% risk of being associated with underlying malignancies?**
   (a) Laminin 332
   (b) $\alpha6\beta4$ integrin
   (c) BP180
   (d) BP230

10. **BIOCHIP, multiparametric ELISA, and immunoblot are some of the newer assays for accurate diagnosis of AIBDs. Which of the following is/are newer variants of pemphigoid recognized by incorporating such specific assays?**
    (a) anti-p200 pemphigoid
    (b) anti-105 kDa antigen pemphigoid
    (c) anti-type IV collagen pemphigoid
    (d) All of the above

Answers

1. (b) 2. (b) 3. (a) 4. (a) 5. (b) 6. (c) 7. (d) 8. (b) 9. (a) 10. (d)

SUGGESTED READING

1. Witte M, Zillikens D, Schmidt E. Diagnosis of autoimmune blistering diseases. *Front Med (Lausanne)*. 2018;5:296.
2. van Beek N, Zillikens D, Schmidt E. Diagnosis of autoimmune bullous diseases. *J Dtsch Dermatol Ges*. 2018;16:1077-91.
3. Adaszewska A, Woźniak K, Kalińska-Bienias A, Smolarczyk K, Kowalewski C. Diagnostics of autoimmune blistering disorders: an experience of a single tertiary referral centre. *Postepy Dermatol Alergol*. 2022;39:446-53.
4. Beek NV, Zillikens D, Schmidt E. Bullous autoimmune dermatoses: clinical features, diagnostic evaluation, and treatment options. *Dtsch Arztebl Int*. 2021;118:413-20.
5. Saschenbrecker S, Karl I, Komorowski L, Probst C, Dähnrich C, Fechner K, *et al*. Serological diagnosis of autoimmune bullous skin diseases. *Front Immunol*. 2019;10:1974.
6. De D, Khullar G, Handa S, Saikia UN, Radotra BD, Saikia B, *et al*. Clinical, demographic and immunopathological spectrum of subepidermal autoimmune bullous diseases at a tertiary center: A 1-year audit. *Indian J Dermatol Venereol Leprol*. 2016;82:358.
7. Handa S, Dabas G, De D, Mahajan R, Chatterjee D, Saika UN, *et al*. A retrospective study of dermatitis herpetiformis from an immuno-bullous disease clinic in north India. *Int J Dermatol*. 2018;57: 959-64.

Therapeutic Strategies for Pemphigus and other Autoimmune Bullous Diseases

CHAPTER 20

Topical Therapy and Oral Corticosteroids

Sanjeev Handa, Shikha Shah

- Topical therapy
  - Wound management
  - Conventional topical therapies
  - Experimental topical therapies
  - Clinical pearls
- Oral corticosteroids
  - Fundamentals of various corticosteroids
- Dosing regimens
- Therapeutic monitoring
- Adverse events
- Optimization in practice
- Clinical pearls

INTRODUCTION

The mainstay in management of autoimmune bullous diseases (AIBDs) is wound care of the lesions along with specific local and systemic therapies. This chapter aims to highlight the principles and practical aspects of topical therapies and oral corticosteroids in AIBDs.

TOPICAL THERAPY

Principles of topical therapy in AIBDs include:
- *Local site care*: To aid in re-epithelialization of the denuded areas for prevention of infection and for amelioration of pain
- *Topical therapeutic agents*: For control of disease activity in conjunction with systemic agents, as stand-alone therapy in limited disease, for maintenance of clinical remission and/or control of disease flares, and prevention of scarring

The various topical therapies used in AIBDs have been summarized in **Figure 1**.

Wound Management

Local wound management is often the most underrated but pivotal aspect in the management of AIBDs. Cautious and proactive management of raw areas is often rewarding. It is crucial to manage local areas of denudation to prevent disease complications such as sepsis, scarring, and systemic perturbations.

Various aspects of local wound care are discussed in detail in Chapter 27, and include:

Management of Blisters

Blister management depends on their size; larger bullae should undergo sterile puncture and aspiration via large-bore (18 gauge) sterile needle without deroofing, since the intact roof serves as a biological barrier. The blister should

Wound management	Conventional therapies	Experimental therapies
• Managing blisters • Dressings • Cleansing • Mucosal care • Care of infected lesions	• Topical and intralesional corticosteroids • Topical calcineurin inhibitors • Topical cyclosporine* • Topical dapsone* • Topical nicotinamide*	• Pilocarpine eye drops • PGE2 gel • Topical ketamine • Intralesional rituximab • Intralesional platelet-rich plasma • Trichloroacetic acid • Topical mitomycin-C • Amniotic membrane transplant • Topical Bruton tyrosine kinase (BTK) inhibitors • Lights and lasers

*Uncommonly used.

Fig. 1: List of various topical therapies in use for pemphigus and other autoimmune bullous diseases.
(PGE2: prostaglandin E2)

be punctured with the bevel of the needle up, and the site must allow drainage by gravity and prevent refilling. Gentle local cleansing can be accomplished by normal saline and/or topical iodine or silver-based antiseptics after sterile aspiration of bullae, followed by application of bland emollient ointment, e.g., 50% white soft paraffin + 50% liquid paraffin.

Dressings

Dressings must be non-adherent and maintain a moist environment. The suitable options depending upon the extent and type of denudation as well as affordability include non-adherent gauze which may be impregnated with paraffin or silver sulfadiazine, silver-containing dressings, transparent film dressings, hydrogel or hydrocolloid dressings. Newer options include nanocrystalline silver dressings, platelet gel, human recombinant epidermal growth factor, polymeric membrane dressings, and biosynthetic dressings.

A novel and feasible option for non-healing erosions includes use of topical insulin, 0.5–1 mL of 40 IU/mL preparation, sprayed over each erosion twice a day. The mechanism includes promotion of wound healing by increasing angiogenesis and granulation tissue formation by stimulating vascular endothelial growth factor (VEGF), transforming growth factor beta (TGF-β), and Ki-67. Blood sugar levels should be monitored.

Cleansing

Potassium permanganate soaks, 1:10,000 concentration (Condy's solution) can be used for cleansing where there are large areas of denudation and crusting, by dissolving 400 mg of potassium permanganate in 4 L of water. As a rough bedside guide to constituting the required solution from available crystal/powder formulation of potassium permanganate, appropriate dilution to generate a light pink color akin to nail bed, should be advocated.

Mucosal Care

Oral mucosa: The technical difficulty of applying topical agents as well as the salivary dilution of drugs, pose some difficulties in managing oral mucosal lesions. Aspects of mucosal care include maintaining hygiene by employing antiseptic mouth washes, proactive detection and management of superadded candidiasis (by nystatin swishes or clotrimazole paint), dental hygiene management, use of topical lidocaine for pre-meal analgesia, and specific therapies for healing of erosions, besides eating soft, bland food. Oral preparations can be compounded in specific formulations like orabase® to have better efficacy. Oral care has been described in more detail in Chapter 27.

Ocular mucosa: Ocular lubricants should be advocated with timely detection and management of microbial keratitis. An ophthalmology opinion should be sought with a proactive approach to prevent or minimize scarring and its consequences.

Other mucosae: Upper aerodigestive and anogenital mucosae must be cared for with topical steroids and local hygiene to prevent cicatrizing complications, especially in mucous membrane pemphigoid.

Care of Infected Wounds

Wounds that display the telltale signs of inflammation (rubor, calor, dolor, tumor) should be subjected to culture and sensitivity. It is crucial to differentiate between contamination and colonization (which is expected in superficial wounds) versus actual infection that risks delay in wound healing and septicemia, most commonly by staphylococci. Options for dealing with such wounds include the following:

- Cleansing with bleach and water (Dakin's solution)
- Cleansing with bleach, boric acid and water (Eusol solution)
- Use of acetic acid (1 tablespoon vinegar in 1 cup of water)
- *Topical antimicrobials*: Mupirocin or retapamulin (gram positive), metronidazole (anaerobic coverage) after sensitivity reports
- *Iodine or silver-based dressings*: Silver dressings can be used for the initial two weeks to prevent infection, provided that a moist wound environment is maintained (which is quintessential for the release of silver ions that are antimicrobial in nature).

Conventional Topical Therapies

Topical and intralesional corticosteroids (CS) remain the cornerstone of topical therapy in AIBDs. Various guidelines suggest topical corticosteroids to be the first-line of management in localized disease, as well as adjuncts for management of partial remissions or flare.

- *European Academy of Dermatology and Venereology (EADV) updated S2K guidelines*: Class III or IV CS: Limited lesions of "mild pemphigus foliaceus" [BSA <5% and/or Pemphigus Disease Area Index (PDAI) ≤15%]
- *EADV updated S2K guidelines for "mild and moderate bullous pemphigoid" [Bullous Pemphigoid Disease Area Index (BPDAI) <20 and ≥20 and <57, respectively]*: Superpotent topical CS (20–30 g/day) on all lesions except face; for severe cases (BPDAI ≥57), superpotent topical CS (30–40 g/day) are recommended all over the body except the face.
- Guidelines for mucous membrane pemphigoid and epidermolysis bullosa acquisita also suggest use of topical CS (or calcineurin inhibitors) for mild disease, and for pemphigoid gestationis with <10% BSA involvement.

Monitoring for systemic side effects resulting from extensive topical CS use should always be kept in mind. Triamcinolone acetonide can also be injected intra- and peri-lesionally in refractory oral pemphigus lesions as well as in intertriginous plaques of pemphigus vegetans.

Topical calcineurin inhibitors like pimecrolimus 1% cream or tacrolimus 0.1% ointment, have been used as steroid-sparing anti-inflammatory agents that promote re-epithelialization in AIBDs. Topical cyclosporine can be used in oral erosions of AIBDs, and ocular preparation available as 0.05% eyedrops in cases of ocular pemphigoid. Topical dapsone 5% gel has been tried as an adjunct in dermatitis herpetiformis cases. Topical nicotinamide 4% gel has been tried as an adjunctive therapy in refractory pemphigus due to its anti-inflammatory properties, with variable results.

Experimental Topical Therapies

Topical Pilocarpine

Antibodies to acetylcholine receptors have been identified as important mediators of acantholysis and hitherto cholinergic agonism was found to reduce acantholysis and upregulate cadherins. Imbibing this vignette, the readily available topical 2% pilocarpine eyedrops have been advocated in refractory oral lesions of pemphigus as twice daily application on accessible, recalcitrant oral erosions, which have shown good rates of re-epithelialization.

Topical Prostaglandin E2

Prostaglandin analogs like topical PGE2 preparations have been tried in refractory cases of oral pemphigus by virtue of their immunoregulatory and mucoprotective actions.

Topical Ketamine

Topical ketamine has been advocated for its analgesic and anti-inflammatory properties to reduce the pain of severe stomatitis encountered in paraneoplastic pemphigus patients.

Intralesional Rituximab

Intralesional rituximab 10 mg/mL, has been used in oral pemphigus as 5 mg/cm^2 injections on days 1 and 15, adapted from the effectiveness of intralesional rituximab in cutaneous B-cell lymphomas.

Intralesional Platelet-rich Plasma

Autologous platelet-rich plasma (PRP) has been tried in recalcitrant oral erosions of pemphigus by injecting approximately 1 mL of the preparation intralesionally into the base and side of the erosions. Mechanism includes release of various growth factors that promote healing.

Trichloroacetic Acid Application

Topical application of 33% TCA has been tried as a cost-effective modality in refractory buccal erosions of pemphigus by painting the border of the lesions till frost appears as end point. Healing has been reported to occur in 2–6 weeks.

Topical Mitomycin-C

In severe ocular pemphigoid, mitomycin-C delivered by topical or subconjunctival routes, has been tried as an antifibrotic agent.

Amniotic Membrane Transplantation

In cases of persistent ocular epithelial defects in advanced ocular pemphigoid, amniotic membrane transplant has been tried in conjunction with autologous plasma to promote healing.

Bruton Tyrosine Kinase Inhibitors

Pre-clinical trials have shown results with topical Bruton tyrosine kinase (BTK) inhibitors in AIBDs. Akin to its systemic counterparts (oral rilzabrutinib), BTK can exert inhibitory effects on the downstream B-cell signaling, and anti-inflammatory actions.

Lights and Lasers

Low-level light therapy (LLLT) has been shown to accelerate mucosal healing as well as cause analgesia in both oral and cutaneous erosions of pemphigus, by increasing cellular proliferation and collagen synthesis. CO_2 laser irradiated at low power has also been shown to promote healing of mucosal erosions. Photodynamic therapy has paradoxical effects. It can be used in treating refractory ulceration in pemphigus, while having the potential to trigger bullous pemphigoid.

Clinical Pearls

- Local wound care and general measures are rewarding in both inpatient and outpatient care of AIBD patients.
- Aesthesis of topical care and patient dignity should also be borne in mind, especially in the inpatient management of AIBD patients. Adequate privacy must be ensured with simple use of curtain partitions (or burn cages for extensive lesions) in general wards, and the use of insect nets to prevent superinfection by maggots. Use of air beds with frequent change of posture and early mobilization can prevent avoidable complications such as pressure sores or deep vein thrombosis.
- It is advisable to demonstrate dressings as well as preparations of potassium permanganate soaks/compresses to caretakers to ensure correct usage and dilution, while preventing irritation.
- It is equally important to empower the patients to promote self-care by teaching them correct ways to maintain hygiene, and judiciously use topicals agents.
- Conventional corticosteroids remain the mainstay of topical therapy, directed to control the underlying disease.

ORAL CORTICOSTEROIDS

Before the advent of use of systemic CS, AIBDs like pemphigus were considered to be fatal, with reported mortality rates as high as 60–90%. Oral CS remain the main drugs for most AIBDs even till date, warranting detailed knowledge on their practical use.

Fundamentals of Various Corticosteroids

Various corticosteroids are used as systemic therapy in pemphigus and other AIBDs, as summarized in **Table 1**.

Dosing Regimens

Pemphigus foliaceus, Pemphigus vulgaris

EADV updated S2K guidelines:
- *Mild pemphigus foliaceus/vulgaris (BSA <5% and/ or PDAI <15, limited oral lesions not impairing food intake)*: Prednisolone 0.5–1 mg/kg/day monotherapy, or 0.5 mg/kg/day with rituximab, with subsequent rapid decrease and stoppage in 3–4 months
- *Moderate and severe pemphigus foliaceus/vulgaris (BSA >5% and/or PDAI >15 and ≥45 respectively, oral lesions impairing food intake)*: Prednisolone 1–1.5 mg/kg/ day monotherapy and/or with conventional adjuvants; 1 mg/kg/day with rituximab, with subsequent decrease and stoppage in 6 months

Bullous Pemphigoid

EADV updated S2K guidelines:
- *Mild and moderate bullous pemphigoid (BPDAI <20, and ≥20 and <57 respectively)*: Prednisolone 0.5 mg/kg/day for non-localized cases
- *Severe bullous pemphigoid (BPDAI ≥57)*: Prednisolone 0.5 mg/kg/day, increased to 0.75 mg/kg/day if no disease control in 1–3 weeks

For EBA and MMP, oral CS are preferred for moderate and severe disease. MMP lesions are classified as high risk (involvement of ocular, genital, nasopharyngeal, esophageal, laryngeal, or severe involvement of oral mucosa) and low risk, oral CS being the first-line agents along with immunosuppressants, with an aggressive initial treatment to limit scarring.

Therapeutic Monitoring

The various parameters that require monitoring while a patient of AIBD is on oral CS, are summarized in **Figure 2**.

TABLE 1: Various systemic corticosteroids (CS) used in pemphigus and other autoimmune bullous diseases.

Class	Molecule	Equivalent dose	Comments
Short-acting	Hydrocortisone[#]	20 mg	As a switch from intermediate-acting CS on tapering, exogenous Cushing syndrome
	Deflazacort	6 mg	More expensive than prednisolone
Intermediate-acting	Prednisolone/prednisone	5 mg	Most commonly used oral CS preparations, safest oral CS in pregnancy
	Methylprednisolone[$]	4 mg	Lesser mineralocorticoid action, safer CS in hypertension
Long-acting	Dexamethasone[##]	0.75 mg	Long-acting CS, is usually not employed as oral therapy for pemphigus
	Betamethasone	0.6 mg	Crushed betamethasone tablets can be used as mouthwashes in recalcitrant oral erosions

[#]*Intravenous hydrocortisone*: As premedication before rituximab.

[$] *Intravenous methylprednisolone*: As pulse therapy in AIBD; triamcinolone acetonide is another intermediate acting CS used in topical and intralesional preparations in AIBD.

[##] *Intravenous dexamethasone*: As pulse therapy alone (DP) or with cyclophosphamide (DCP).

Baseline workup

- Weight, height, blood pressure, abdominal girth, vaccination history, eye examination
- Fasting glucose or HbA1c, triglycerides, potassium level, screening for hepatitis B, C, HIV, tuberculosis
- Calcium, vitamin D supplementation; proton pump inhibitor if needed

Follow-up monitoring

- Weight, height, blood pressure; eye check-ups 6–12 monthly for cataracts and glaucoma
- At 1 month and repeated once every 2–3 months: Potassium levels, fasting glucose

Special situations

- Bone densitometry (DEXA scan) in suspected osteoporosis (compression fracture, risk assessment by FRAX tool)
- Imaging (MRI) in suspected avascular necrosis (AVN) (antalgic gait, hip pain)
- Fasting cortisol, ACTH in suspected exogenous Cushing syndrome (signs of HPA suppression)

Fig. 2: Monitoring of AIBD patients on oral corticosteroids.
(ACTH: adrenocorticotropic hormone; DEXA: dual-energy X-ray absorptiometry; FRAX: Fracture Risk Assessment; HbA1c: glycated hemoglobin; HIV: human immunodeficiency virus; HPA: hypothalamic–pituitary–adrenal; MRI: magnetic resonance imaging)

Adverse Events

The classical adverse events of oral CS apply to its use in AIBDs as well, which include:

- *Metabolic*: Hyperglycemia, hypertension, hypokalemia, cushingoid habitus, weight gain
- *Gastrointestinal*: Peptic ulcer disease
- *Infectious*: Reactivation of tuberculosis, herpes reactivation, opportunistic infections
- *Bone*: Osteoporosis
- *Psychiatric*: Personality changes, psychosis
- *Muscular*: Myopathy, atrophy
- *Ocular*: Cataract, glaucoma refractive error
- Steroid withdrawal, addisonian crisis

Optimization in Practice

Tapering Guidelines

The consensus is to start tapering CS at the end of consolidation phase, i.e., no new lesions for 2 weeks with almost 80% of existing lesions healed. The conventional teaching to taper oral CS is as follows:

Prednisolone >40 mg/day: Taper by 10 mg/week to 40 mg daily, maintain 40 mg/day for 1 week.

Prednisolone 40 mg/day: Taper by 5 mg/week to 20 mg daily, maintain 20 mg/day for 1 week.

Prednisolone 20 mg/day: Taper by 2.5 mg/week to 5 mg daily, maintain 5 mg/day for 1 week.

Prednisolone 5 mg/day: Taper by 1 mg/week until off prednisolone.

Since 1 mg preparations are not available, practically, 5 mg prednisolone can be tapered as half tablet (2.5 mg) followed by one-fourth tablet (1.25 mg) weekly.

In the era of rituximab use, tapering pattern is rapid with an aim to discontinue CS in 3–6 months depending upon disease activity.

Dealing with Exogenous Cushing's Syndrome

Inappropriate dosing of CS either by quacks or over-the-counter (OTC) use, their abrupt discontinuation/tapering, and erratum in taking oral CS, is not an uncommon clinical encounter. In the setting of a high clinical suspicion of Cushing's syndrome, send a fasting (8 AM) serum cortisol; values <3 µg/dL are diagnostic of exogenous Cushing's syndrome. The subsequent tapering guidelines are summarized in **Table 2**.

Approach to Osteoporosis

The rate of glucocorticoid-induced bone loss is maximum in the initial 3–6 months of therapy, with decreasing risk with its continued use. Initial assessment should include a detailed history on use of oral steroid, additional risk factors for osteoporosis, and any events like fracture. Evidence of spinal tenderness, deformity, and reduced space between the lower ribs and upper pelvis, should be sought.

The Fracture Risk Assessment (FRAX) tool is readily available online which can help clinical assessment

TABLE 2: Tapering schedule of oral corticosteroid in case of exogenous Cushing's syndrome.

Prednisolone dose	Tapering principles
>7.5 mg/day	Decrease by 2.5 mg every third day till 7.5 mg/day dose
5–7.5 mg/day	Decrease by 1 mg every 2–4 weeks till 5 mg/day dose*
5 mg/day	<ul><li>Convert to hydrocortisone equivalent dose: 20 mg/day</li><li>Subsequent hydrocortisone tapering: 2.5 mg/week till 10 mg/day</li><li>Continue hydrocortisone 10 mg/day up to 3 months</li><li>Perform an ACTH stimulation test: continue hydrocortisone if cortisol levels are ≤20 µg/dL; if cortisol >20 µg/dL, discontinue and switch to only stress dosing of hydrocortisone</li></ul>

*Practically tapered by half and one-fourth scoring of 5 mg prednisolone tablet due to non-availability of 1 mg preparation.

(ACTH: adrenocorticotropic hormone)

and predict risk of fractures. It includes the following components: age/sex, weight and height, prior fracture, history of hip fracture in parents, steroid use, current smoking, alcoholism, concurrent rheumatoid arthritis/other disorders associated with secondary osteoporosis, and bone mineral density (BMD) of femur neck (g/cm^2).

Recommendations for management:

- For children and adults <40 years with no clinical features/additional risk factors, only calcium, and vitamin D may be supplemented.
- For patients <40 years but with symptoms/additional risk factors for osteoporosis, and all patients ≥40 years, FRAX assessment with baseline BMD determination is recommended.
- *Low fracture risk*: Treat with calcium (1,000–1,200 mg/day) and vitamin D (600–800 IU/day) along with lifestyle modification (balanced diet, weight reduction, avoidance of smoking/alcohol); BMD testing every 2–3 years.
- *Moderate-to-high fracture risk*: Treat with calcium, vitamin D, and oral bisphosphonates.

Clinical Pearls

- Oral CS were the mainstay of therapy of AIBDs decades back, and are still indispensable even in the era of biologics and small molecules. They stay the "bread and butter" for dermatologists, necessitating in-depth knowledge on their correct use.
- Patients must be educated that appropriate use of CS under adequate monitoring has stood the test of time and remains reasonably safe even till date. The rising "steroid phobia" must be kept in mind while counseling patients.

- Dermatologists must be thorough in evaluation of osteo-porosis and iatrogenic Cushing's syndrome. Liaison with endocrinologist and internist is important in complex cases.

CONCLUSION

Optimization of topical therapies should always be in conjunction with specific management of AIBDs. Practical knowledge on the use of oral corticosteroids is quintessential for residents and practitioners alike.

TAKE HOME MESSAGE

- Topical therapies remain the paradigm in bullous disorders.
- Wound care, dressing, and cleansing of lesions, mucosal care and care of the infected lesions must be advocated with due diligence.
- Oral corticosteroids remain the first-line agents for most AIBDs, and practical aspects of therapeutic monitoring and tapering should be revised and revisited from time to time.

MULTIPLE CHOICE QUESTIONS

1. **The concentration of potassium permanganate in Condy's solution is:**
   - (a) 1:100
   - (b) 1:1,000
   - (c) 1:10,000
   - (d) 1:1,00,000

2. **The upper limit of daily application of topical clobetasol propionate ointment is:**
   - (a) 20 g
   - (b) 30 g
   - (c) 40 g
   - (d) 50 g

3. **Which of the following can be used as topical therapy in refractory oral erosions of pemphigus?**
   - (a) Topical pilocarpine
   - (b) Topical PGE2
   - (c) Trichloroacetic acid application
   - (d) All of the above

4. **Which of the following is an intermediate-acting oral corticosteroid?**
   - (a) Hydrocortisone
   - (b) Dexamethasone
   - (c) Deflazacort
   - (d) Methylprednisolone

5. **Recommended daily dose of calcium and vitamin D supplementation with oral corticosteroids is:**
   - (a) 1,000–1,200 mg, 600–800 IU
   - (b) 500–1,000 mg, 600–800 IU
   - (c) 1,000–1,200 mg, 800–1,000 IU
   - (d) 500–1,000 mg, 800–1,000 IU

Answers

1. (c)   2. (c)   3. (d)   4. (d)   5. (a)

SUGGESTED READING

1. Etesami I, Dadkhahfar S, Kalantari Y. Topical care in pemphigus wounds: a systematic review of the literature. *Dermatol Ther.* 2022;35:e15808.
2. Grada A, Obagi Z, Phillips T. Management of chronic wounds in patients with pemphigus. *Chronic Wound Care Manag Res.* 2019;6:89-98.
3. Zhao W, Wang J, Zhu H, Pan M. Comparison of guidelines for management of pemphigus: a review of systemic corticosteroids, rituximab, and other immunosuppressive therapies. *Clin Rev Allergy Immunol.* 2021;61:351-62.
4. Patel PM, Jones VA, Murray TN, Amber KT. A review comparing international guidelines for the management of bullous pemphigoid, pemphigoid gestationis, mucous membrane pemphigoid, and epidermolysis bullosa acquisita. *Am J Clin Dermatol.* 2020;21: 557-65.
5. Pawar M. Topical insulin in the treatment of nonhealing erosions and ulcers of pemphigus vulgaris. *J Am Acad Dermatol.* 2021;85:e271-2.
6. Vinay K, Kanwar AJ, Mittal A, Dogra S, Minz RW, Hashimoto T. Intralesional rituximab in the treatment of refractory oral pemphigus vulgaris. *JAMA Dermatol.* 2015;151:878-82.
7. De D, Bishnoi A, Shilpa, Kamboj P, Arora AK, Pal A, *et al.* Effectiveness of topical pilocarpine in refractory oral lesions of pemphigus vulgaris: results from an open-label, prospective, pilot study. *Dermatol Ther.* 2022;e15449.
8. Xing Y, Chu KA, Wadhwa J, Chen W, Zhu J, Bradshaw JM, *et al.* Preclinical mechanisms of topical PRN473, a bruton tyrosine kinase inhibitor, in immune-mediated skin disease models. *Immunohorizons.* 2021;5:581-9.
9. John DC, Newell-Price, Richard J. Auchus. The adrenal cortex. In: Melmed S, Koenig R, Rosen C, Auchus R, Goldfine A (Eds). Williams Textbook of Endocrinology, 14th edition. Netherlands: Elsevier; 2019. p. 521.
10. Buckley L, Guyatt G, Fink HA, Cannon M, Grossman J, Hansen KE, *et al.* 2017 American College of Rheumatology guideline for the prevention and treatment of glucocorticoid-induced osteoporosis. *Arthritis Care Res (Hoboken).* 2017;69:1095-110.

Oral Anti-inflammatory and Immunosuppressive Therapies

Chitra Shivanand Nayak, Gayatri Vitthal Gund

- Oral immunosuppressive agents
  - Azathioprine
  - Mycophenolate mofetil
  - Cyclophosphamide
  - Methotrexate
  - Cyclosporine
- Oral anti-inflammatory agents
  - Dapsone
  - Tetracycline
  - Niacinamide
  - Pentoxifylline
  - Sulfasalazine
  - Colchicine
  - Gold
- Immunosuppressants in pregnancy
- Immunosuppressants in children

INTRODUCTION

Autoimmune bullous diseases (AIBDs) produce significant morbidity and mortality, necessitating prompt intervention.

The choice of treatment in AIBDs depends on the severity of the disease, age of the patient, and associated co-morbidities. Hence, treatment must be individualized and chosen carefully based on patient's profile. Besides specific treatment, controlling secondary infection, barrier nursing, nutritional support, and maintenance of fluid and electrolyte balance, are important factors to be taken into consideration. Current treatment options include systemic glucocorticoids, steroid-sparing immunosuppressive agents, anti-inflammatory drugs, and biologics.

Systemic corticosteroids form the backbone of management of AIBDs, but they are associated with gastrointestinal, musculoskeletal, endocrine, vascular, ophthalmic, and hematological side effects. The introduction of steroid-sparing immunosuppressants has allowed use of a lower dose of corticosteroids and tapering of steroids early, thereby decreasing their total cumulative dose (TCD) in order to reduce the adverse effects. The immunosuppressives are not meant for early disease control but to maintain long-term remission and reduce relapse. In a meta-analysis of 10 randomized controlled trials (RCTs), it was shown that adjuvants did not decrease the time to disease control and rate of remission, but decreased relapse rate by 29%. They also reduced the TCD of oral steroids by 25%.

This chapter deals with conventional oral anti-inflammatory and immunosuppressive agents used in AIBDs **(Table 1)**.

TABLE 1: Conventional systemic treatment options in autoimmune bullous diseases.

	Level of evidence in pemphigus	Strength of recommen-dation	Level of evidence in bullous pemphi-goid	Strength of reco-mmen-dation
Systemic corticosteroids				
Oral therapy	1+	B	1+	A
Pulse therapy	4	D (GPP)	–	–
Immunosuppressive agents				
Azathioprine	1+	B	4	D
Mycopheno-late mofetil	1+	B	1–	–
Cyclophospha-mide (oral)	3	D	–	–
Methotrexate	3	D	4	D
Cyclosporine	1–	–	–	–

Continued

Continued

	Level of evidence in pemphigus	Strength of recommendation	Level of evidence in bullous pemphigoid	Strength of recommendation
Anti-inflammatory agents				
Dapsone	1−	−	3	D
Tetracycline/niacinamide	3	−	4	D
Colchicine	−	−	−	−
Sulfasalazine	2−	−	3	−
Pentoxifylline	2−	−	−	−
Gold	3	D	−	−

Level of evidence:

1++ High-quality meta-analyses, systematic reviews of randomized controlled trials (RCTs) or RCTs with a very low risk of bias

1+ Well-conducted meta-analyses, systematic reviews of RCTs or RCTs with a low risk of bias

1− Meta-analyses, systematic reviews of RCTs or RCTs with a high risk of bias

2++ High-quality systematic reviews of case–control or cohort studies. High-quality case–control or cohort studies with a very low risk of confounding, bias, or chance and a high probability that the relationship is causal

2+ Well-conducted case–control or cohort studies with a low risk of confounding, bias, or chance and a moderate probability that the relationship is causal

2− Case–control or cohort studies with a high risk of confounding, bias, or chance and a significant risk that the relationship is not casual

3 Nonanalytical studies (e.g., case reports, case series)

4 Expert opinion, formal consensus

Strength of recommendation:

A At least one meta-analysis, systematic review, or RCT rated as 1++, and directly applicable to the target population or a systematic review of RCTs or a body of evidence consisting principally of studies rated as 1+, directly applicable to the target population and demonstrating overall consistency of results or evidence drawn from a National Institute for Health and Care Excellence (NICE) technology appraisal

B A body of evidence including studies rated as 2++, directly applicable to the target population and demonstrating overall consistency of results or extrapolated evidence from studies rated as 1++ or 1+

C A body of evidence including studies rated as 2+, directly applicable to the target population and demonstrating overall consistency of results or extrapolated evidence from studies rated as 2++

D Evidence level 3 or 4 or extrapolated evidence from studies rated as 2+ or formal consensus

D (GPP) A good practice point (GPP) is a recommendation for the best practice based on the experience of the guideline development group

ORAL IMMUNOSUPPRESSIVE AGENTS

Azathioprine

Azathioprine is a prodrug and its active metabolite 6-thioguanine slowly accumulates in tissues and eventually provides maximal clinical immunosuppression at around 8–12 weeks. Azathioprine carries the advantage of having a better safety profile than cyclophosphamide (which is faster acting) including its safety in patients who have not completed their family. According to the European Dermatology Forum guidelines and British Association of Dermatologists guidelines, it is the first-line adjuvant immunosuppressant in pemphigus. In pulse therapy also, it may be used in place of oral cyclophosphamide [dexamethasone-azathioprine pulse (DAP)].

Mechanism of Action

Azathioprine, a cytotoxic drug, acts during the S phase of the cell cycle and inhibits the formation of adenosine and guanine nucleotides. It affects both T- and B-cell function and has anti-inflammatory properties. It is metabolized by many enzymes including hypoxanthine guanine phosphoribosyltransferase (HGPRT), xanthine oxidase (XO), and thiopurine methyltransferase (TPMT) **(Flowchart 1)**.

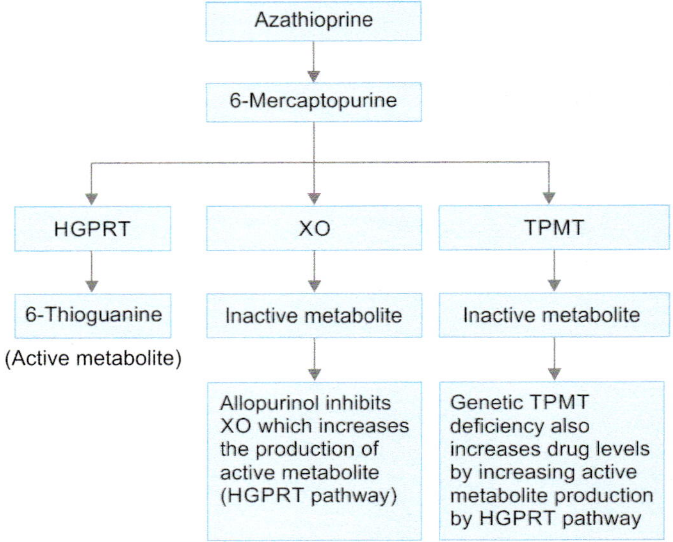

Flowchart 1: Metabolism pathway of azathioprine.

(HGPRT: hypoxanthine guanine phosphoribosyl transferase; TPMT: thiopurine methyltransferase; XO: xanthine oxidase)

TPMT Testing

Certain patients can have low or absent TPMT activity, leading to increased metabolism via the HGPRT pathway, causing higher levels of active metabolite and adverse effects. TPMT testing may be considered in patients with deranged blood counts [complete blood count (CBC)] who are not responding to dose reduction. Dose adjustment is needed in patients with low TPMT activity **(Table 2)**. TPMT testing cannot substitute for CBC monitoring in patients receiving azathioprine.

TABLE 2: Drug dosing by thiopurine methyltransferase (TPMT) level.

TPMT level	Azathioprine dose
High TPMT 15.1–26.4 U/mL	Up to 2–2.5 mg/kg daily
Medium TPMT 6.3–15 U/mL	Up to 1.0 mg/kg daily
Low TPMT < 6.3 U/mL	Do not use azathioprine

Dose

Dose—1–2.5 mg/kg/day. It is available as 25 mg, 50 mg tablet. Injection azathioprine is not available in India.

Contraindications

Azathioprine is contraindicated in patients with hypersensitivity to the drug, and low TPMT activity. Although it is classified as pregnancy category D by Food and Drug Administration (FDA), it is relatively contraindicated in pregnancy and lactation.

Adverse Effects

- Gastrointestinal toxicity—gastritis and pancreatitis
- Hepatic—transaminase elevation and acute cholestatic injury
- Hematological (dose dependent)—leukopenia, agranulocytosis, and pancytopenia
- Dermatological—morbilliform rash, urticaria, erythema nodosum, anagen effluvium, pellagra

Monitoring Guidelines

Baseline CBC, liver function test (LFT) and renal function test (RFT), viral markers, Mantoux test, and chest X-ray should be done. Liver enzymes and CBC should be monitored biweekly for the first 2 months and every 2–3 months thereafter. Azathioprine is generally preferred in patients with renal failure.

Azathioprine is safe in pediatric patients and has a similar side effect profile in children as in adults.

Withhold azathioprine if:
- Total leucocyte count (TLC) < 3,500/cu.mm
- Hemoglobin (Hb) <10 g/dL
- Neutrophils < 2,000/cu.mm
- Platelets <1,00,000/cu.mm
- Aspartate transaminase/alanine aminotransferase (AST/ALT) >two times the upper limit of normal-50% dose reduction is recommended
- Oral ulceration/sore throat
- Unexplained rash or unusual bruising

Mycophenolate Mofetil

Mycophenolate mofetil (MMF) is derived from *Penicillium stoloniferum,* and it is a prodrug of mycophenolic acid. MMF and azathioprine have comparable safety and efficacy in AIBDs, and MMF is non-mutagenic, but its higher cost limits its use in a resource-limited country like India. To induce long-lasting remission, MMF should be administered for > 6 months.

Mechanism of Action

MMF inhibits inosine monophosphate dehydrogenase, the key enzyme in the de-novo pathway of purine (guanine nucleotide) biosynthesis. Both T and B lymphocytes are affected by MMF because these cells lack the salvage pathway and are entirely dependent on de-novo purine synthesis.

Dose

Dose is 2–3 g/day. MMF is available as 250 mg capsule, 500 mg tablet and also as an oral solution. Intravenous preparation of MMF is not available in India. The enteric-coated mycophenolate sodium form of mycophenolic acid is associated with less gastrointestinal side effects.

Contraindications

It is absolutely contraindicated in pregnancy (FDA pregnancy category D) and drug allergy. It is relatively contraindicated in renal, hepatic, and peptic ulcer disease.

Adverse Effects

- Teratogenicity
- Gastrointestinal (dose dependent)—nausea, diarrhea, anorexia, and abdominal pain. MMF should be administered with caution in patients with active serious digestive system disease.
- Hematological (dose dependent and reversible)—neutropenia, anemia, thrombocytopenia, and agranulocytosis
- Neurological—weakness, fatigue, headache, and tinnitus
- Genitourinary—urinary urgency, frequency, and dysuria (does not cause nephrotoxicity)
- Elderly patients are more likely to have reduced hepatic, renal, and cardiac functions, so MMF should be used cautiously in them (FDA, USA).

Monitoring Guidelines

Baseline CBC, LFT, and urinalysis should be done. Repeat CBC every 2–4 weeks following dose escalation, and then every 2–3 months, once the dosage is stable. Urine pregnancy test (within 1 week) before starting treatment should be done. Contraception is advised from 4 weeks before, during, and up to 6 weeks after discontinuing the treatment. During treatment with MMF, use of live attenuated vaccines should be avoided and patients should be informed that vaccinations may be less effective.

MMF has been successfully used in the pediatric population for prevention of renal transplant rejection. Dermatology literature also supports MMF as a safe and effective steroid-sparing adjuvant in pediatric pemphigus.

Cyclophosphamide

Its use in AIBDs has become restricted due to the better safety profile of azathioprine and MMF, although it continues to be prescribed in resource-limited countries as it is inexpensive and has good immunosuppressant action. According to the European Dermatology Forum guideline, it is considered as third-line treatment in recalcitrant pemphigus vulgaris.

Mechanism of Action

It is an alkylating agent, which acts independently of the cell cycle. It has greater effect on B lymphocytes than T lymphocytes.

Dose

Dose is 1–3 mg/kg/day, available as 50 mg tablet and 500 mg injection. In DCP therapy, it is given as four weekly

500 mg IV injection along with daily oral 50 mg tablet. Pulse cyclophosphamide once a month IV infusion (15 mg/kg) along with tapering doses of daily steroids, has also been successfully used.

Contraindications

Cyclophosphamide is contraindicated in pregnancy (FDA pregnancy category D), lactation, drug allergy, prior history of bladder cancer, in men or women who wish to conceive, and depressed bone marrow function. It is relatively contraindicated in hepatic and renal diseases. Live vaccines should be avoided for 2 weeks before and up to 3 months after stopping cyclophosphamide.

Side effects of cyclophosphamide are depicted in **Table 3**. Bladder toxicity and gonadal side effects are dose dependent. Gonadotoxic dose limit of cyclophosphamide for males is <7.5 g/m^2. In female patients, it has age- and dose-dependent effect (cumulative dose limit < 10–15 g/m^2). Hemorrhagic cystitis can occur in 12–41% of patients on cyclophosphamide, and a cumulative dose of >36 g is associated with a greater risk of bladder cancer (incidence of 0.7–7.5%; odds ratio 3.6–100).

Hemorrhagic cystitis is due to the accumulation of metabolite acrolein in the bladder.

Measures to prevent bladder toxicity include:
- Minimizing cumulative dose
- Avoiding night administration and therefore overnight bladder exposure to acrolein
- Forced diuresis with hydration
- Concurrent use of mesna (sodium 2-mercaptoethane sulfonate): If cyclophosphamide is used as IV bolus, IV mesna at 20% of the cyclophosphamide dose is simultaneously administered with cyclophosphamide (w/w) over 15–30 minutes, and the same dose repeated at 4 and 8 hours. Total dose of mesna—60% (w/w) of cyclophosphamide dose.

Mesna binds and inactivates the metabolite acrolein in the bladder and reduces bladder irritation. Monach, *et al* reported low risk of cyclophosphamide-related bladder toxicity among rheumatology patients treated with low-dose cyclophosphamide. As similar dosage of cyclophosphamide (1–2 mg/kg/day) is being used in dermatology patients, concurrent use of mesna is not strongly recommended and can be considered on a case-by-case basis. There are no guidelines regarding use of mesna along with cyclophosphamide in AIBDs. Sheperd, *et al* have reported that good hydration of the patient and mesna have similar efficacy in preventing cyclophosphamide-induced bladder toxicity. Therefore, considering the side effects associated with mesna, hydration can be advised with oral and intravenous cyclophosphamide therapy for prevention of hemorrhagic cystitis.

Cyclophosphamide in special age groups—it should be used cautiously in elderly patients because of decreased renal and hepatic functions. Elderly men are likely to have benign prostatic hyperplasia and urinary retention, which puts them at risk of bladder-related toxicity.

Data from the use of cyclophosphamide in pediatric cancers reports ovarian fibrosis in prepubescent girls, and those with retained ovarian function after completing treatment are at a risk of developing premature menopause. Some degree of testicular atrophy may occur in prepubescent boys treated with cyclophosphamide.

Monitoring Guidelines

Baseline CBC, LFT, RFT, urine analysis, and pregnancy test should be done. CBC and urine analysis should be repeated biweekly for initial 2–3 months and then monthly. Concomitant use of drugs that potentiate myelosuppressive, immunosuppressive, or carcinogenic effects should be avoided.

Methotrexate

Methotrexate is an antimetabolite drug. It may be considered in treatment of AIBD's when the more established first-line drugs cannot be used or have failed.

In bullous pemphigoid, it has been successfully used as an adjuvant. A retrospective analysis has shown methotrexate to be more beneficial in bullous pemphigoid than in pemphigus.

Mechanism of Action

Methotrexate inhibits the enzyme dihydrofolate reductase and decreases formation of tetrahydrofolate, an important co-factor in de-novo purine synthesis. Its immunosuppressive effect occurs because of inhibition of DNA synthesis in immunocompetent cells. It also has anti-inflammatory action and inhibits neutrophil chemotaxis.

Dose

Dose is 0.3–0.4mg/kg/week, available as injection and tablet. Routes of administration are oral, subcutaneous, and

TABLE 3: Adverse effects of cyclophosphamide.

Gastrointestinal	Renal	Hematological	Reproductive	Dermatological
• Anorexia • Stomatitis • Nausea • Vomiting • Diarrhea	• Microscopic hematuria • Hemorrhagic cystitis • Transitional cell carcinoma of bladder	Bone marrow suppression—pancytopenia	• Amenorrhea • Azoospermia • Ovarian failure	• Anagen effluvium • Pigmentation of skin and nails (reversible) • Pigmented band on teeth (irreversible) • Drug rash (Stevens–Johnson syndrome, urticaria)

intramuscular. Usually, low dose is used in elderly patients (5–10 mg/week).

Contraindications

They include pregnancy (FDA pregnancy category X), lactation, alcoholism, alcoholic liver disease, pre-existing blood dyscrasias, and low hemoglobin.

Adverse Effects

- Hepatotoxicity
- Pulmonary toxicity—acute pneumonitis occurs as an idiosyncratic reaction
- Hematological—pancytopenia
- Gastrointestinal—nausea, diarrhea, and vomiting. Supplementation of folic acid decreases gastrointestinal toxicity.
- Reproductive—teratogenicity, abortifacient effect

Monitoring Guidelines

Baseline CBC, LFT, RFT, hepatitis B and C testing, and chest X-ray should be done. A Mantoux test may be done though the evidence for methotrexate reactivating latent tuberculosis is poor. Pregnancy test should be done before initiation of methotrexate. Pregnancy should be avoided if either partner is receiving methotrexate. Contraception should be advised during and for 3 months after stopping treatment with methotrexate in male patients; in women, contraception should continue for at least one menstrual period after the last dose. The drug should be used cautiously in patients with creatinine clearance < 50 mL/min. Though a small test dose (2.5 mg/5 mg) is usually given initially followed by laboratory evaluation before the

second dose, it can be safely omitted in patients with normal renal function. During the escalation period, 1–2 weekly laboratory evaluation is advisable and once the dose is stable, monitoring can be done 1–3 monthly.

Cyclosporine

It is a strong immunosuppressive agent with anti T-cell lymphocyte activity. The British Association of Dermatologists does not recommend cyclosporine as an adjuvant drug in pemphigus and bullous pemphigoid, as there is no additive effect of cyclosporine when combined with a corticosteroid. It can be considered in refractory cases of bullous pemphigoid, but due to renal toxicity, its use is limited in elderly patients.

Cyclosporine has been found to be effective in epidermolysis bullosa acquisita (EBA), but a high dose (>6 mg/kg/day) is required for effective therapy.

Contraindications

These include hypersensitivity to the drug, renal dysfunction, and uncontrolled hypertension.

Monitoring Guidelines

Baseline CBC, LFT, RFT, serum electrolytes, uric acid and fasting lipid profile should be done. Blood pressure and serum creatinine monitoring should be undertaken at regular intervals. The dosage is regulated according to creatinine levels.

A summary of some important studies highlighting the utility of oral immunosuppressive agents in AIBDs is depicted in **Table 4**.

TABLE 4: Summary of studies on utility of various oral immunosuppressive agents in autoimmune bullous diseases.

Authors and year	Study description	Results
Enk AH, *et al.* 1999	• To assess efficacy of mycophenolate mofetil (MMF) in pemphigus vulgaris (PV) with treatment failure to azathioprine and prednisolone (*n* = 12) • Patients had relapsed with azathioprine (1.5–2 mg/kg/day) and prednisolone (2 mg/kg/day) • Combination therapy with MMF (2 g/day) + prednisolone (2 mg/kg/day) administered	• Complete response in 11 cases • No relapse on tapering steroid • During 9- to 12-month follow-up—no relapse
Beissert S, *et al.* 2006	• Prospective multicenter RCT • PV (*n* = 33), PF (*n* = 7) • 2 groups • Methylprednisolone (MP)/azathioprine vs methylprednisolone /MMF	• MMF and azathioprine demonstrated similar efficacy, corticosteroid-sparing effect, and safety profile • *Complete remission*: 　○ MP/azathioprine—72% cases after mean of 74 ± 127 days 　○ MP/MMF—95% cases after mean of 91 ± 113 days (*p* > 0.05) • *Total median cumulative dose of MP*: 　○ MP/azathioprine—8,916 mg 　○ MP/MMF—9,334 mg • *Disease free period*: 　○ MP/azathioprine—258 ± 183 days 　○ MP/MMF—123 ± 103 days (*p* > 0.05) • *Side-effects*: 　○ MP/azathioprine—33% cases 　○ MP/MMF—19% cases (*p* > 0.05)

Continued

Continued

Authors and year	Study description	Results

Chams–Davatchi C, *et al.* 2007	RCT of four regimens in PV (*n* = 120; 30 cases each), follow-up of 1 year:
	1. Prednisolone (P) (2 mg/kg/day) as monotherapy
	2. Prednisolone (2 mg/kg/day) and azathioprine (A) (2.5 mg/kg/day)
	3. Prednisolone (2 mg/kg/day) and intravenous cyclophosphamide pulse (PC) (1 g/month)
	4. Prednisolone (2 mg/kg/day) and MMF (MM) (2 g/day)
		• All adjuvants significantly reduced cumulative steroid dose. The most efficacious cytotoxic drug to do so was azathioprine, followed by pulse cyclophosphamide and MMF
		• Difference between total steroid dose in:
		P vs P/cytotoxic drug—$p = 0.047$
		  – P/A vs P/MM—$p = 0.007$
		  – P/A vs P/PC—$p = 0.971$
		  – P/MM vs P/PC—$p = 0.67$
		• No significant side effects in 4 groups

Olszewska M, *et al.* 2007	Retrospective study
	PV (*n* = 101)
	• Prednisone monotherapy (1.1–1.5 mg/kg/day)
	• Prednisone and cyclophosphamide (1.1–1.5 mg/kg/day)
	• Prednisone and azathioprine (1.1–1.5 mg/kg/day)
	• Prednisone and cyclosporine (2.5–3 mg/kg/day)
		• Prednisone with cyclophosphamide was found to be most effective in terms of time to achieve clinical remission, fastest decrease in circulating pemphigus antibodies, and lowest rate of relapse. All regimens had similar safety profile.
		• *Average time to clinical remission was*:
		  ○ 7.2 ± 13.1 months—prednisone monotherapy
		  ○ 6.8 ± 10.5 months—azathioprine group
		  ○ 8.1 ± 11.8 months—cyclosporine group
		  ○ 4.9 ± 6.9 months—cyclophosphamide group
		• *TCD of prednisone*:
		  ○ 12,058 mg—prednisone monotherapy
		  ○ 8,145 mg—azathioprine group
		  ○ 9,598 mg—cyclosporine group
		  ○ 6,857 mg—cyclophosphamide group

Beissert S, *et al.* 2010	Prospective, randomized, double blind, placebo controlled, parallel group, multicenter, 52-week trial to assess efficacy and safety of adjunct MMF to achieve remission with reduced corticosteroid in active PV: • Group 1—MMF + prednisolone • Group 2—placebo + prednisolone	No significant advantage of MMF on primary endpoint (proportion of patients responding to treatment, i.e., absence of new, persistent oral or cutaneous lesions, and prednisolone dose ≤10 mg/ day)—69% in MMF vs. 64% in steroid only ($p = 0.6$) *Beneficial effect of MMF on secondary endpoints*: • Quicker time to response (6 weeks sooner) ($p = 0.05$) • Quicker time to sustained response (14 weeks sooner) ($p = 0.039$) • Sustained remission of 6 months: 43.1% vs 22.2% ($p = 0.047$) • Longer time to relapse—median 186 days vs 136.5 days • Substantially lower total exposure to corticosteroid over study period (1,000 mg less than in placebo) 7,617.5 mg vs 8,727.5 mg • MMF well tolerated—2 g better than 3 g

Chams–Davatchi C, *et al.* 2013	• RCT. Follow-up for 1 year
	• PV (*n* = 56)
	  ○ Prednisolone (2 mg/kg/day, not exceeding >120 mg daily dose) and azathioprine 50 mg
	  ○ Prednisolone (2 mg/kg/day, not exceeding >120 mg daily dose) and placebo
		Azathioprine was effective and reduced TCD of prednisolone

Sukanjanapong S, *et al.* 2019	• Comparative study—retrospective cohort
	• Pemphigus (*n* = 62) (PV 44, PF 18)
	  ○ Prednisolone (0.53 mg/kg/day) and azathioprine (0.83–1.41 mg/kg/day)
	  ○ Prednisolone (0.48 mg/kg/day) and MMF (910–1,530 mg/day)
		MMF associated with better outcomes in terms of a significantly shorter time to complete remission on and off therapy

Continued

Continued

Authors and year	Study description	Results

Kjellman P, *et al.* 2007	• Retrospective study
	• Methotrexate in bullous pemphigoid ($n = 138$)
	  ○ Methotrexate (2.5–10 mg/week) only
	  ○ Methotrexate plus prednisolone (10–20 mg/day)
	  ○ Prednisolone alone
	  ○ Topical betamethasone gel
		• Methotrexate was safe and effective
		• 2-year remission (percentage of patients with mild disease) was maximum in group 4:
		  ○ Methotrexate only group—43%
		  ○ Methotrexate plus prednisolone—35%
		  ○ Prednisolone alone—0%
		  ○ Topical betamethasone gel—83%
		• Remission occurred after a median treatment time of 11, 20, and 2 months in groups 1, 2, and 4, respectively

Sticherling M, *et al.* 2017	• RCT
	• Bullous pemphigoid ($n = 54$)
	  ○ Oral methylprednisolone (0.5 mg/kg/day) plus azathioprine (1.5–2.5 mg/kg/day)
	  ○ Oral methylprednisolone (0.5 mg/kg/day) plus dapsone (1.5 mg/kg/day)
		Dapsone was as effective and safe as azathioprine, and showed better corticosteroid-sparing effect than azathioprine

(PF: pemphigus foliaceus; PV: pemphigus vulgaris; RCT: randomized controlled trial; TCD: total cumulative dose)

ORAL ANTI-INFLAMMATORY AGENTS IN AIBDs

Dapsone

Dapsone (4,4'-diaminodiphenyl sulfone) is a sulfonamide antibacterial agent. It inhibits neutrophil chemotaxis and formation of neutrophilic respiratory burst. Hence, it has been shown to be effective in AIBDs with abnormal neutrophil accumulation, such as dermatitis herpetiformis (DH), linear IgA bullous dermatosis (LAD), IgA pemphigus, bullous pemphigoid (BP), chronic bullous dermatosis of childhood (CBDC), epidermolysis bullosa acquisita (EBA) and bullous systemic lupus erythematosus (bullous SLE).

- *DH*: A strict gluten-free diet is the treatment of choice as it is able to improve both cutaneous and intestinal manifestations. Dapsone improves cutaneous symptoms but has no effect on intestinal symptoms. During the active phase, a dose of 100–200 mg/day is given. It shows remarkable response in skin lesions in hours to few days. Subsequently, the patient can be maintained on low dose dapsone (0.5–1 mg/kg/day), until benefit of the gluten-free diet is achieved.
- *LAD and CBDC*: It is considered as first-line treatment. In children, dapsone is given as 1–2 mg/kg/day and should not exceed 4 mg/kg/day.
- *Pemphigus*: In IgA pemphigus and pemphigus herpetiformis, it is the first-line agent along with systemic steroid.
  - In mild cases of pemphigus foliaceus, it is given as 50–100 mg/day, along with potent topical steroid. Relapse rate is high with dapsone monotherapy. In an RCT, dapsone failed to demonstrate a corticosteroid-sparing effect in this condition.
  - In pemphigus vulgaris, it can be given during maintenance phase.
- *Bullous pemphigoid* (*BP*): Dapsone is used in mild-to-moderate BP in patients with contraindications to other first-line agents.
- *EBA*: It has been found to be effective in inflammatory EBA when neutrophils are present in the dermal infiltrate.
- *Bullous SLE*: It is given at a dose of 2 mg/kg/day, but has been shown to be effective at even low doses of 25–50 mg/day. Anemia is common in SLE, which can increase the severity of hematological side effect of dapsone, hence, close monitoring of hemoglobin should be done.
- *Mucous membrane pemphigoid*: Dapsone is used in mild-to-moderate disease involving the skin and mucosa. It is administered as 50–200 mg/day, along with cyclophosphamide and systemic corticosteroids.

Adverse Effects

- Gastrointestinal—nausea and vomiting occur in the beginning of treatment and decrease thereafter.
- Woolly headedness—night administration is advised.
- Hematological—hemolytic anemia and methemoglobinemia (dose dependent).
- Dapsone hypersensitivity syndrome
- Hepatotoxicity—cholestatic and hepatocellular hepatitis

Contraindications

These include drug hypersensitivity, low hemoglobin (<8 g%), glucose-6-phosphate-dehydrogenase (G6PD) deficiency (risk of developing severe hemolytic anemia), and blood dyscrasias. It is a pregnancy category C drug.

Monitoring Guidelines

Pretreatment CBC, LFT, RFT and G6PD levels. During the course of treatment, LFT, and CBC should be monitored 1–3 monthly.

Tetracyclines/Niacinamide

Tetracyclines (minocycline, doxycycline, and tetracycline) and niacinamide are used as steroid-sparing agents as they exhibit a variety of anti-inflammatory properties.

Indications

Due to weak steroid-sparing effect of tetracyclines, they are not commonly used in pemphigus. But in bullous pemphigoid, tetracyclines (with or without niacinamide) have shown response, and are well tolerated in elderly patients with co-morbidities. They are recommended in mild-to-moderate cases of bullous pemphigoid. Minocycline is associated with a poorer side effect profile, hence not considered as first choice.

Contraindications

Tetracyclines are FDA pregnancy category D drug. They are contraindicated in pregnancy and pediatric age group (<8 years). They should be avoided in renal disease.

Dosage

Niacinamide is given in doses of 500–2,500 mg/day, tetracycline at 500–2,000 mg/day, doxycycline at 200–300 mg/day, and minocycline at 100–200 mg/day.

Sulfasalazine and Pentoxifylline

They are anti-tumor necrosis factor agents. There are few reports which support the use of sulfasalazine and pentoxifylline as adjuvant therapy in pemphigus. In subepidermal AIBDs, sulfasalazine at a dose of 1–2 g/day can be considered as an alternative in dapsone-responsive patients in whom dapsone is contraindicated.

Colchicine

Colchicine is an antimitotic drug with anti-inflammatory and immunosuppressive action. It has been found useful in LAD, CBDC, and DH patients, who failed to respond to dapsone. It has also been found to be effective in mild forms of EBA and is considered when other immunosuppressants are ineffective. It is initiated at 0.5 mg/day and once the patient tolerates it, dose escalation is done, and a maximum dose of 1.5–3 mg/day can be given. It has gastrointestinal, hematological, and neuromuscular side effects.

Gold

Gold is a historical treatment in pemphigus. It is available as an oral (auranofin) and parenteral formulation (gold sodium thiomalate). Oral formulation is less toxic and preferred. Side effects include renal toxicity, bone marrow suppression, and cutaneous allergic reactions.

Immunosuppressants in Pregnancy

AIBDs in pregnancy should be managed in conjunction with an obstetrician and pediatrician.

Oral glucocorticoids are the mainstay of treatment during pregnancy. Prednisolone is considered safe as it does not cross the placenta. Azathioprine can be used as it is associated with a lower risk of teratogenicity. Dapsone and cyclosporine are also safe in pregnancy but cyclosporine is less effective in treating pemphigus. Methotrexate, cyclophosphamide, and MMF are contraindicated in pregnancy due to their teratogenic effects.

Immunosuppressants in Childhood

Systemic corticosteroids are the cornerstone in the management of pediatric pemphigus. The most commonly recommended steroid-sparing adjuvant in pediatric pemphigus is azathioprine. In active disease, it can be used as 2 mg/kg/day, and during maintenance at a dose of 1 mg/kg/day. Dapsone, methotrexate, cyclosporine, and cyclophosphamide have also been used.

CONCLUSION

Oral anti-inflammatory and immunosuppressive agents are very valuable and economical therapies for pemphigus and other AIBDs. They have been used for many decades for these indications, primarily as steroid-sparing agents.

TAKE HOME MESSAGE

- The decision to initiate immunosuppressive agents depends on disease activity and patient profile.
- A detailed history and physical examination with appropriate investigations should be undertaken before starting immunosuppressants.
- Careful and timely monitoring for adverse effects is necessary, as also clinical and immunological assessment before tapering the dose of immunosuppressants.
- Oral immunosuppressive and anti-inflammatory agents reduce the time to achieve disease remission with lower relapse rates, and also reduce the TCD of oral corticosteroids.

MULTIPLE CHOICE QUESTIONS

1. All of the following immunosuppressants are absolutely contraindicated in pregnancy, *except*:
    - (a) Methotrexate
    - (b) Cyclophosphamide
    - (c) Azathioprine
    - (d) Mycophenolate mofetil

2. Which of the following statement regarding mycophenolate mofetil is incorrect?
    - (a) It is a prodrug
    - (b) MMF inhibits enzyme inosine monophosphate dehydrogenase of pyrimidine biosynthesis

(c) Mycophenolate mofetil is derived from *Penicillium stoloniferum*

(d) It is FDA pregnancy category D drug

3. **All of the following are true regarding cyclophosphamide, *except*:**

(a) Hemorrhagic cystitis is due to accumulation of metabolite acrolein in the bladder

(b) Cyclophosphamide acts mainly by T-cell inhibition

(c) Reproductive side effects of cyclophosphamide are dose dependent

(d) Dose of cyclophosphamide in immunobullous diseases is 1–3 mg/kg/day

4. **All of the following are false, *except*:**

(a) Development of hypertension is a contraindication to continue therapy with cyclosporine

(b) Tetracyclines are pregnancy category C drugs

(c) Cyclosporine is isolated from *Tolypocladium inflatum*

(d) MMF inhibits salvage pathway of purine biosynthesis

5. **How long should contraception be advised in men after stopping methotrexate for immunobullous disorders?**

(a) 1 month

(b) 3 months

(c) 6 months

(d) 1 year

6. **What is the gonadotoxic dose limit of cyclophosphamide in males?**

(a) <2 g/m^2

(b) <5 g/m^2

(c) <7.5 g/m^2

(d) <10 g/m^2

7. **Azathioprine is metabolized to its active form by which enzyme?**

(a) Hypoxanthine-guanine phosphoribosyltransferase (HGPRT)

(b) Thiopurine methyltransferase (TPMT)

(c) Xanthine oxidase

(d) Guanosine monophosphate synthetase

8. **The following is true about azathioprine, *except*:**

(a) It is a prodrug

(b) It is pregnancy category D

(c) Allopurinol decreases active metabolite of azathioprine

(d) Azathioprine should not be used if TPMT activity is <6.3 U/mL

9. **Which is an irreversible side effect of cyclophosphamide?**

(a) Anagen effluvium

(b) Nail pigmentation

(c) Teeth pigmentation

(d) Urticaria and bullous eruption

10. **The following is true about dapsone, *except*:**

(a) In dermatitis herpetiformis, it improves cutaneous symptoms but has no effect on the intestinal symptoms

(b) It is pregnancy category C

(c) It is also known as 4,4'-diaminodiphenyl sulfone

(d) It inhibits synthesis of dihydrofolic acid by competing with para-aminobenzoic acid for the active site of dihydrofolate reductase

Answers

1. (c)   2. (b)   3. (b)   4. (c)   5. (b)   6. (c)   7. (a)   8. (c)   9. (c)   10. (d)

SUGGESTED READING

1. Harman KE, Albert S, Black MM. British association of dermatologists. Guidelines for the management of pemphigus vulgaris. *Br J Dermatol*. 2003;149:926-37.

2. Wolverton SE. Systemic corticosteroids. In: Wolverton SE (Ed). Comprehensive dermatologic drug therapy. Philadelphia: WB Saunders; 2001. pp. 109-38.

3. Kasperkiewicz M, Schmidt E, Zillikens D. Current therapy of the pemphigus group. *Clin Dermatol*. 2012;30:84-94.

4. Gurcan HM, Ahmed AR. Analysis of current data on the use of methotrexate in the treatment of pemphigus and pemphigoid. *Br J Dermatol*. 2009;161:723-31.

5. Harman KE, Brown D, Exton LS, Groves RW, Hampton PJ, Mustapa MFM, *et al*. British association of dermatologist guidelines for the management of pemphigus vulgaris. *Br J Dermatol*. 2017;177: 1170-1201.

6. Venning VA, Taghipour K, MohdMustapa MF, Highet AS, Kirtschig G. British association of dermatologist guidelines for the management of bullous pemphigoid 2012. *Br J Dermatol*. 2012;167:1200-14.

7. De D, Kanwar AJ. Childhood pemphigus. *Indian J Dermatol*. 2006;51:89-95.

8. Monach PA, Arnold LM, Merkel PA. Incidence and prevention of bladder toxicity from cyclophosphamide in the treatment of rheumatic diseases: A data-driven review. *Arthritis Rheum*. 2010;62:9-21.

9. Sheperd JD, Pringle LE, Barnett MJ, Klingemann HG, Reece DE, Philipps GL. Mesna versus hyperhydration for the prevention of cyclophosphamide-induced haemorrhagic cystitis in bone marrow transplantation. *J Clin Oncol*. 1991;9:2016-20.

10. Willsteed E, Lee M, Wong LC, Cooper A. Sulfasalazine and dermatitis herpetiformis. *Australas J Dermatol*. 2005;46:101-3.

CHAPTER 22

Pulse Therapy and its Modifications

Binod K Khaitan, Vishal Gupta, Bhavya Swarnkar

- Dexamethasone cyclophosphamide pulse (DCP) therapy
- Mechanism of action
- Basis and evolution of DCP
- Baseline evaluation and monitoring of patients during pulse therapy
- Efficacy of DCP regimen in pemphigus and other autoimmune bullous diseases (AIBDs)
- Modifications of DCP
- Side effects of DCP
- Criticism of DCP

INTRODUCTION

Systemic corticosteroids have been the mainstay of treatment for autoimmune bullous diseases (AIBDs) since the early sixties. Daily oral corticosteroids, though effective, are limited by the adverse effects of long-term and high-dose therapy, which is required for AIBDs. Pulse therapy with corticosteroids was devised to combat the drawbacks of long-term daily treatment. Pulse treatment involves the administration of a suprapharmacological dose of a drug in an intermittent, cyclical manner to enhance the therapeutic effect and decrease the side effects. Pulsed steroid treatment was first successfully used by Kountz and Cohn for the treatment of renal graft rejection. Subsequently, its use was expanded for the treatment of lupus nephritis, rheumatoid arthritis (RA), and pyoderma gangrenosum. In India, it was first used in Reiter's disease by Pasricha, *et al*, and subsequently in other diseases particularly pemphigus and other AIBDs. Thereafter, it was also used for connective tissue diseases and other inflammatory skin disorders.

Dexamethasone cyclophosphamide pulse (DCP) therapy for pemphigus, pioneered by Pasricha, *et al* in 1982, led to a paradigm shift for patients with AIBDs in general, and pemphigus in particular. Despite the introduction of newer effective treatments like rituximab, DCP still continues to have a place in the therapeutic armamentarium of AIBDs.

DEXAMETHASONE CYCLOPHOSPHAMIDE PULSE THERAPY

The DCP regimen **(Table 1)** was designed by Pasricha, *et al* at the All India Institute of Medical Sciences (AIIMS), Delhi, and has been extensively used for the treatment of pemphigus at various centers. One DCP consists of 100 mg dexamethasone, dissolved in 500 mL of 5% dextrose,

TABLE 1: **Phases of dexamethasone cyclophosphamide pulse (DCP).**

Phase I	DCP every 28 days and daily oral cyclophosphamide till complete healing of all skin and mucosal lesions and discontinuation of daily oral corticosteroid
Phase II	9 additional DCPs with daily oral cyclophosphamide
Phase III	9 months of daily oral cyclophosphamide
Phase IV	Post-treatment surveillance to look for relapse

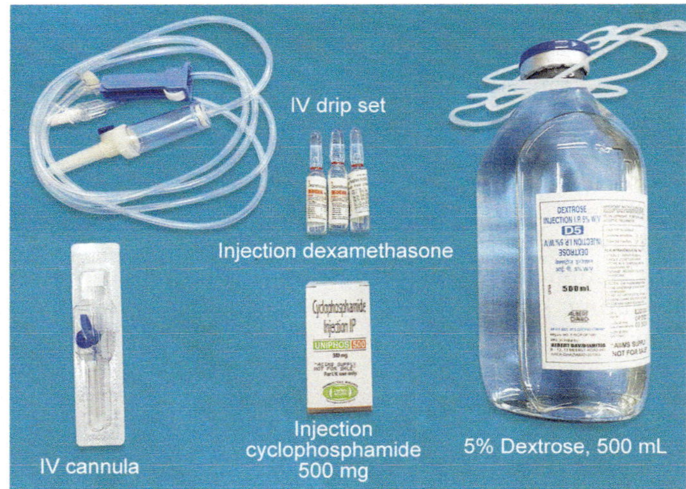

Fig. 1: Medications used in dexamethasone cyclophosphamide pulse (DCP) therapy. *Image courtesy*: Dr Avik Mondal.

given as a slow intravenous infusion over 2–3 hours, on 3 consecutive days. Cyclophosphamide, 500 mg is also given in the same infusion on day 2 **(Fig. 1)**. Such DCPs are repeated at 28 days interval, counted from the first day of the pulse.

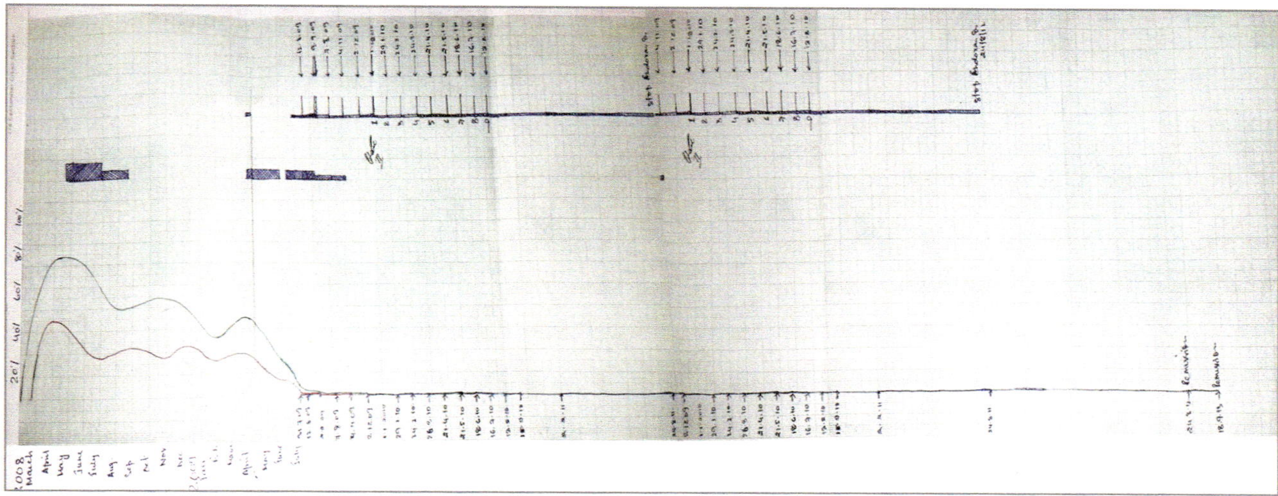

Fig. 2: Image of graph paper depicting charting of the patient on dexamethasone cyclophosphamide pulse (DCP) therapy. The vertical axis shows percentage body surface area (BSA) involved, and the horizontal axis shows the time. The red line corresponds to mucosal involvement and the green line indicates cutaneous involvement. The point at which these two touch the baseline is the point from where phase II begins, meaning clinical remission and also the patient is off daily steroid. The time of each pulse is marked with vertical line along with date, and after the 9th month the pulses are stopped, but the daily cyclophosphamide continues, as seen by the horizontal line.

The different phases of pulse therapy have also been charted on a graph paper **(Fig. 2)**.

MECHANISM OF ACTION

Glucocorticoids have action at both genomic and non-genomic levels. At high doses, the non-genomic effect is predominant and is mediated through interaction with membrane-bound receptors resulting in apoptosis of autoimmune cells and induction of lipomodulin (which inhibits prostaglandins and leukotrienes). At high doses, corticosteroids inhibit nuclear factor kappa B via "transrepression" (direct interaction of glucocorticoid with transcription factors). There are not enough studies to understand the mechanism of action of corticosteroid pulse. However, it has been seen that dexamethasone pulse causes a shift of the T-helper cell (Th) profile toward Th2, and decreases CD3+ and CD4+ T cell phenotypes that recover in 7 days without significant effect on B cells.

Cyclophosphamide is a cytotoxic drug that acts by alkylating the cellular DNA and causing irreversible damage, leading to apoptosis. The use of intermittent high-dose drug probably impairs immune surveillance for a relatively short period of time as compared to a daily dose, thus decreasing adverse effects. At a high dose, it is more toxic to B cells than T cells and natural killer cells, which take 2–4 months to recover.

Therefore, a combination of dexamethasone and cyclophosphamide can target both cellular and humoral aspects of autoimmunity. Monthly pulsed infusions can be effective, while being safer than daily oral administration.

BASIS AND EVOLUTION OF DEXA-METHASONE CYCLOPHOSPHAMIDE PULSE

The selection of drugs and their dosages was completely arbitrary and based upon their availability and convenience. The suprapharmacological dose was conceptually attractive, but the exact dose chosen was intuitive. Using dexamethasone as the steroid of choice was influenced by practical considerations as well as its therapeutic effect. Dexamethasone is easily available and is much cheaper than methylprednisolone, which is more commonly used in the west. A dose of 100 mg was not chosen just arbitrarily, but also based on ease of administration. A 3-day pulse was found to be adequate, convenient, and effective, based on past experience. Dextrose was preferred as the solvent over normal saline because steroids can cause hypernatremia. Similarly, cyclophosphamide dose was kept at 500 mg considering convenience, efficacy, and safety. The daily dose of 50 mg of oral cyclophosphamide was considered safe as it does not produce leukopenia. The interval between pulses was fixed at 4 weeks initially because of convenience, but later it was realized that this schedule needs to be strictly followed to achieve long disease-free remission periods. Those who were irregular on these 4-week schedules showed inferior disease control and/or more relapse. Several patients also showed a trend that new lesions appeared after 3 weeks or more, and therefore they required repeat pulses at regular intervals for proper disease control. Phases II and III were added to prolong the disease-free period, as early relapse was almost universally seen if pulses were stopped after just phase I.

DCP, as we know it today, was not conceptualized in its present form from the very beginning. The regimen has evolved in response to the observations on how patients with pemphigus fared receiving pulse therapy. Initially, only dexamethasone pulses were used. Cyclophosphamide boluses were added because relapses were frequent with dexamethasone pulses alone. Earlier, patients were treated with only monthly steroid pulses; daily oral steroids for the initial few months were added to hasten remission. The current recommendation of 9 months for phases II and III also came up after observing higher relapse rates with other varying durations of these phases of pulse therapy. In the early part of DCP therapy, six DCPs used to be given after remission (phase II) followed by 12 months of oral cyclophosphamide (phase III). Pasricha, *et al* reported a relapse rate of 54% in patients who received incomplete treatment, and 18.2% in those who received pulses irregularly. After increasing the duration of phase II from 6 to 9 months, and shortening phase III from 12 to 9 months, the relapse rate was found to be 19% amongst those who were treated at irregular intervals, and 8% amongst those who took DCPs at 28 days interval. Higher relapse rates were noted in patients who received pulses at variable intervals, leading to the recommendation of pulses being given with regularity every 28 days.

BASELINE EVALUATION AND MONITORING OF PATIENTS DURING PULSE THERAPY

Baseline evaluation includes a complete hemogram, blood sugar, liver and kidney function tests, serum electrolytes, urine microscopy, chest X-ray and electrocardiogram. Before every subsequent pulse, fasting blood sugar and serum electrolytes (Na^+, K^+) should be measured.

Blood pressure and pulse rate is monitored while giving the pulse in both normotensive and hypertensive patients.

EFFICACY OF DCP REGIMEN IN PEMPHIGUS AND OTHER AIBDs

Pemphigus

The advantages of DCP or other pulse protocols include rapid healing of lesions, faster control of disease activity especially in extensive disease, reduction in total cumulative corticosteroid dose (so paradoxically a beneficial steroid-sparing effect), and long-term clinical remission with minimal corticosteroid-induced side effects. On an average, patients achieve significant disease control by 2–3 pulses, and remission in about 6–9 pulses, while the relapse rate has been generally low on long-term observation period (around 10–15% at 5 years and 25% at >20 years of post-treatment follow-up).

Since 1982, more than 2,000 patients of pemphigus have received DCP and followed up over a period of >35 years at AIIMS, Delhi. Of the available recorded data for the initial 500 patients, 435 received pulse therapy; all achieved rapid remission, with relapse occurring in 108 (25%) patients. The relapsed patients were administered a second course of pulse therapy: of the 98 patients who received it, 78 were in remission and 20 relapsed again. The relapses were mild and responded easily to the next course. Overall, 311 (71%) patients enjoyed a disease-free drug-free period for minimum 10 years, the duration of post-treatment follow-up being >20 years for several of these patients. There were 18 deaths during the treatment; eight were due to infections and/or sepsis, two due to malignancies, and the remaining due to unrelated or unknown causes. Some patients having a prolonged phase I received intermediate pulses (called interval pulse) of dexamethasone alone for a single day or daily corticosteroid therapy, in addition to regular DCPs, to hasten regression. Relapses were observed mostly in those patients who had not followed the treatment protocol. The relapses were mild and responded to re-institution of therapy.

Other centers have also shown rapid and prolonged remission with DCP therapy. The reported remission rates with the standard or modified DCP regimen have varied from 55% to 100% in different studies. This wide range may probably be explained by a varying proportion of patients in different phases of pulse therapy regimen at the time of reporting the results; remission rates being close to 100% in patients who had completed phase I.

Unlike phases II and III, the duration of phase I is variable. Phase I is completed when the patients have achieved clinical remission and daily oral steroids have been discontinued. A few studies have shown that phase I duration may be prolonged in patients with more extensive disease. A 10-year retrospective study of 37 patients from Kerala reported that phase I was more likely to exceed 6 months in patients with higher total disease and oral mucosal severity scores, and did not depend on the patient profile or the type of pulse therapy. The type of pemphigus may also influence the time to disease control. A study from Bangalore involving 74 patients reported longer times to achieve disease control in pemphigus foliaceus (PF) ($n = 14$) than pemphigus vulgaris (PV) ($n = 60$) with DCP therapy (10 months for PF vs. 8 months for PV).

A few studies have recently emerged comparing DCP treatment with rituximab, RA protocol, in patients with pemphigus. A retrospective study from Maharashtra involving 14 PV patients (seven patients each treated with rituximab and DCP regimen) found similar efficacy of both treatments, with no statistically significant difference in the mean time to consolidation (5.28 months in DCP arm vs. 3.57 months in rituximab arm). In another retrospective study from Kolkata which included 12 PV patients (six patients each treated with rituximab and DCP regimen), both treatments were seen to significantly reduce disease severity and improve quality of life of the patients. Improvement in skin and mucosal lesions occurred by the first and third month respectively, in both the arms. The daily oral corticosteroids could be stopped in all patients receiving rituximab by 3 months as compared to 6 months in the DCP arm. A study by Khandpur, *et al* from AIIMS, Delhi (under publication) on 37 PV patients (rituximab RA protocol, $n = 15$ or DCP, $n = 22$) showed comparable results, with 93% and 82% patients attaining disease control after median of 2 months, and 93% and 86% attaining remission at 4.5 and 4 months, respectively. Median total cumulative dose of oral steroid with DCP was 2,223 mg as against 2,325 mg in the rituximab group, which was comparable. The change in Th1, 2, and 17 serum cytokine levels were comparable in the two groups at weeks 20 and 52 post-treatment.

Pulse Therapy in Other Autoimmune Bullous Diseases

DCP therapy has been used in patients with other AIBDs as well, such as bullous pemphigoid, cicatricial pemphigoid, and dermatitis herpetiformis, with good results. However, unlike pemphigus, DCP is generally reserved for cases that are refractory to daily oral steroid and conventional immunosuppressive agents, and the available efficacy data is limited.

Modifications of Dexamethasone Cyclophosphamide Pulse

After the reports of successful treatment of pemphigus using DCP regimen at AIIMS, it has been used at several other centers in India and abroad, and a few modifications have been introduced along the way.

A one-day 100 mg dexamethasone pulse ("interval" pulse) may be administered, in addition to the monthly DCPs, in patients whose disease is not getting adequately controlled with the standard regimen, or those with more severe and extensive involvement.

Some dermatologists have used methylprednisolone instead of dexamethasone, while others have used a different dose. Kaur and Kanwar used dexamethasone 136 mg instead of 100 mg as the dose equivalent of methylprednisolone 1,000 mg. However, the dose of methylprednisolone 1,000 mg itself is arbitrary and there is no evidence that 136 mg dexamethasone pulses may be better than the 100 mg pulses. Though comparative trials between dexamethasone and methylprednisolone are lacking in AIBDs, studies done on primary typical optic neuritis and steroid-resistant nephrotic syndrome have reported similar efficacy in both groups.

Some physicians have used oral pulses of dexamethasone or betamethasone in place of intravenous dexamethasone infusions. Oral pulses may be beneficial where patients cannot come to the hospital for 3 days every month.

Other variations include omitting the cyclophosphamide bolus or replacing daily oral cyclophosphamide with another immunosuppressive drug, such as dexamethasone azathioprine pulse (DAP) or dexamethasone methotrexate pulse (DMP). This modification may be used for children, unmarried patients, or those with incomplete families, due to concerns over cyclophosphamide causing gonadal toxicity. In a study by Rao and Lakshmi, DMP was administered to two individuals who failed to finish phase I even after $\geq$12 DCPs/DAPs. Both of them completed phase I within 4–6 months of starting DMP, but scalp/oral lesions relapsed in one of them during phase IV. In a study on 50 pemphigus patients by Hassan, *et al*, three pulse regimes, i.e., DCP, DAP, and DMP were given to different patients (DAP in reproductive age group, DMP in patients with prolonged phase I while on DCP, and DCP in the remaining patients). DCP was found to be the best regimen with the quickest and long-lasting remission, with only 3/30 (10%) patients showing relapse in phase IV. Five of 12 (42%) patients on DAP relapsed in phase III and 4/12 (33%) relapsed in phase IV, while the disease was poorly controlled with DMP.

Another change includes omitting daily oral cyclophosphamide during phases I and II when monthly boluses are being given, and initiating oral cyclophosphamide as the maintenance agent in phase III. This modification is extrapolated from the regimens used in lupus nephritis and systemic sclerosis, where daily cyclophosphamide is not administered along with pulses. Similarly, the choice of maintenance agent during phase III could be another drug such as azathioprine or methotrexate.

One study omitted phase II (nine monthly DCPs) and shifted patients to phase III (daily oral cyclophosphamide × 9 months) directly from phase I, and compared this modified regimen with the standard DCP regimen. Nineteen patients were randomized to phase II ($n = 10$) or phase III ($n = 9$) after remission. The authors found similar relapse rates (one patient each) in both groups in the 9-month post-phase I period. However, the follow-up period was very short to derive any concrete conclusion.

Cyclophosphamide-only pulses have also been tried without the dexamethasone component. Here, cyclophosphamide is administered as an intravenous bolus dose (15 mg/kg) on a single day, along with daily oral corticosteroid in tapering schedule. Cyclophosphamide is dissolved in 200 mL of 5% dextrose or normal saline and infused over 1 hour, followed by hydration with 500 mL 5% dextrose or normal saline, given intravenously over 5–6 hours after the pulse. Mesna (60% of the cyclophosphamide dose) is also added to the cyclophosphamide infusion to avoid risk of bladder toxicity. In addition, patients are advised to increase their daily water intake to $\geq$3 L/day for 3 days, starting 1 day before the cyclophosphamide pulse. Omitting dexamethasone boluses may be preferable in patients with contraindications to high-dose steroids, such as uncontrolled diabetes mellitus, hypertension, or avascular necrosis of bones. In a head-to-head trial, pemphigus patients receiving monthly cyclophosphamide pulses and daily oral steroid ($n = 10$) achieved faster disease control (3.16 vs. 7.33 weeks, $p = 0.02$) and quicker remission (8.4 vs. 13 weeks, $p < 0.001$) compared to those treated with monthly DCPs and daily oral cyclophosphamide ($n = 15$). The relapse rates (40 vs. 33%) and time to relapse (20 weeks in both arms) were largely similar. However, it should be noted that only 40% of the patients in the DCP arm received daily oral steroid as compared to all in the cyclophosphamide pulse arm, and at a lower starting dose (0.5–0.75 mg/kg vs. 1.5 mg/kg).

Another modification of the DCP regimen in diabetics is the addition of 8U of insulin in the infusion to neutralize 5% dextrose as well as to counteract the effect of gluconeogenesis in the liver induced by steroid therapy.

Unlike daily oral corticosteroids, the safety of pulse corticosteroids during pregnancy and lactation is not well studied, therefore their use should generally be avoided. Cyclophosphamide is contraindicated in pregnant and lactating women. Patients with infections such as tuberculosis, human immunodeficiency virus (HIV), hepatitis B or C infection can receive pulse therapy under cover of adequate treatment of the infection and/or once the infection is under control. Such a decision should be based on the risk–benefit ratio of pulse therapy, and in consultation with the infectious disease team on a case-to-case basis.

It should be noted that these modifications of the DCP regimen have been used with variable success in small studies, sometimes with good results in patients who did not respond satisfactorily to the standard regimen. However, good quality clinical trials with adequate sample size and follow-up duration comparing the modified regimens with the standard regimen are largely lacking.

SIDE EFFECTS OF DEXAMETHASONE CYCLOPHOSPHAMIDE PULSE

Serious side effects with DCP are infrequent. Common side effects include a feeling of weakness and tiredness due to corticosteroid withdrawal for 2–3 days after the pulse (can be prevented by prescribing a small tapering dose of oral corticosteroid for 3–5 days post-pulse), bad taste in the mouth (dysgeusia), and diarrhea coinciding with the pulse (usually responds to 7 days of ciprofloxacin or any other appropriate antibiotic). The antibiotic effect probably suggests a change in gut flora that causes diarrhea. Other early side effects include headache, recurrent hiccups, flushing, palpitations, myalgia, and numbness in the feet. The risk of cutaneous bacterial infections, eczema herpeticum, and oral candidiasis is high until the persistence of mucocutaneous erosions of pemphigus. Reactivation of latent tuberculosis, cardiac arrhythmias, and sudden death are rare. The side effects of daily oral corticosteroids including hypertension, diabetes mellitus, peptic ulcer disease, cataract, hirsutism, osteoporosis, and avascular necrosis of bones are not common with pulse therapy unless daily corticosteroid is given concomitantly and for a long period. Hypothalamic–pituitary axis suppression is seen in almost half of the patients, but does not require routine replacement therapy and interestingly, is not related to the duration of therapy.

Side effects due to the cyclophosphamide component are also uncommon. Major side effects include diffuse hair fall and amenorrhea (and azoospermia). Cytopenias and hemorrhagic cystitis are rarely seen. There is a theoretically higher risk of urothelial malignancy, but has not been reported. The main limitation of this regimen is regular visits to the hospital every month for 3 days, though these hospital visits are limited to institution of pulse therapy in convenient day-care settings once the disease is well-controlled.

Other Transient Effects of Dexamethasone Cyclophosphamide Pulse

There is some disturbance in serum electrolyte levels during the 3 days of pulse, however, this disturbance is random, unpredictable, and of little consequence. Once the pulse is stopped, electrolyte levels normalize. Hence, there is no need to do daily monitoring of electrolytes or withhold salt routinely. Minor variations are observed in total leukocyte/platelet count, but they do not require monitoring or treatment. Blood pressure may vary during the 3 days of pulse, but normalizes thereafter. In hypertensives also, pulse therapy is found to be safe, however, recording blood pressure before initiation of the pulse is recommended. Blood sugar rises during pulse therapy in both diabetic and non-diabetic individuals. In non-diabetic individuals, monitoring is not required as the levels normalize later, but in diabetics, 8U of plain insulin is added to neutralize the hyperglycemia caused by the dextrose infusion alone. Blood sugar levels need to be checked on the first day of pulse only.

CRITICISM OF DEXAMETHASONE CYCLOPHOSPHAMIDE PULSE

DCP has its critics too. Some researchers believe that there is not sufficient evidence for DCP to be better than oral corticosteroid and immunosuppressive adjuvant in the treatment of pemphigus for want of good quality randomized controlled trials (RCTs). One randomized double-blind placebo-controlled trial (PEMPULS trial) including 20 PV patients failed to find superiority of oral dexamethasone pulses (300 mg monthly, $n = 11$) over daily oral prednisolone (80 mg/day, $n = 9$). All patients also received daily prednisolone in a tapering protocol, daily azathioprine (3 mg/kg), and were followed up for 1 year. It should be noted that the patients in this study were already receiving high-dose daily prednisolone, i.e., 80 mg/day, which makes administering additional monthly dexamethasone boluses superfluous. It is therefore not surprising that the total cumulative dose of prednisolone in both treatment groups was found to be comparable. The utility of steroid pulses lies in reducing the need of daily steroid, and ideally the study should have used much smaller daily prednisolone doses in the pulse arm (instead of 80 mg/day) to test the utility and comparative efficacy of dexamethasone pulses. Further, demonstrating the beneficial effect of dexamethasone pulses in terms of time to remission and duration of remission would need a larger sample size and a longer follow-up period. All these factors are elaborated upon in detail by Pasricha, *et al* in their published series of 300 patients. Another clinical trial ($n = 123$) comparing methylprednisolone–cyclophosphamide pulse versus oral daily prednisolone (1–2 mg/kg) and azathioprine (1.5 mg/kg), found lesser total cumulative prednisolone dose, hospital stay, and weight gain in the pulse arm. A retrospective case-control study involving patients who did not respond to prednisolone <40 mg/day ($n = 15$), had also shown higher remission rates with or without oral steroid, and lesser duration of daily steroid treatment in the group that was treated with monthly methylprednisolone pulses.

Another concern is about the claimed safety of DCP. It is suggested that the steroid-related adverse effects of DCP therapy may not be majorly due to the daily steroid component, but attributed to the monthly dexamethasone boluses.

Other criticisms include using a fixed dose of drugs irrespective of body weight or disease severity, and dextrose as a solvent in diabetic patients. In the supra-pharmacological dosage schedule, the dose is likely to be high enough in majority of the cases, and hence it need not be adjusted for body weight or disease severity. Dextrose has been chosen as a solvent over normal saline even in diabetics because transient hyperglycemia is less disadvantageous in terms of effects on the body and its management, as compared to hypernatremia.

CONCLUSION

DCP therapy is a safe and effective treatment for the management of AIBDs, producing long-term remission. The regimen can be suitably modified depending on the patient profile. It continues to remain a relevant treatment option even today, in the era of newer treatment options such as anti-CD20 monoclonal antibodies.

TAKE HOME MESSAGE

- Pulse therapy is an effective and inexpensive treatment option for AIBDs especially pemphigus. For more than three decades, this has been the therapeutic regimen of choice in many parts of India for achieving long-term remission
- Its main advantage lies in inducing rapid healing of lesions, faster disease control, and a steroid-sparing effect.
- The regime can be modified and tailored to suit individual patient profile including diabetics, unmarried patients or those with incomplete family, and children.
- Pulse therapy is largely safe, and serious side effects are rare.
- The major limitation is the need to follow the regime strictly every 28 days for optimal disease control, necessitating hospital visits every month.
- Pulse therapy continues to be an important treatment option for AIBDs even after the introduction of newer agents like rituximab, particularly in resource-poor settings.

MULTIPLE CHOICE QUESTIONS

1.   Following are the characteristics of pulse therapy, *except*:
    (a)   Suprapharmacological dose of a drug
    (b)   Intermittent cyclical therapy
    (c)   Decreases the side effect profile of a drug
    (d)   Pharmacological dose of a drug

2.   Which was the first dermatological condition to be treated with pulse therapy in India?
    (a)   Pemphigus vulgaris
    (b)   Psoriatic arthritis
    (c)   Bullous pemphigoid
    (d)   Reactive arthritis

3.   Who introduced DCP therapy in pemphigus vulgaris?
    (a)   Dr Kountz and Cohn
    (b)   Dr Pasricha
    (c)   Dr Niels Finsen
    (d)   Dr VN Sehgal

4.   What are the currently recommended durations of phases II and III of DCP therapy respectively?
    (a)   9, 9 months
    (b)   6, 9 months
    (c)   12, 6 months
    (d)   6, 18 months

5.   Which of the following is an absolute contraindication to dexamethasone pulse (DP) therapy?
    (a)   Pregnancy and lactation
    (b)   Diabetes
    (c)   Hypertension
    (d)   None of the above

6.   What is the ideal interval duration between two dexamethasone cyclophosphamide pulses?
    (a)   31 days
    (b)   15 days
    (c)   28 days
    (d)   30 days

7.   Which phase of DCP includes giving only daily oral cyclophosphamide?
    (a)   Phase I
    (b)   Phase II
    (c)   Phase III
    (d)   Phase IV

8.   Baseline evaluation of a patient planned for DCP includes all of the following, *except*:
    (a)   Chest X-ray
    (b)   Ultrasound abdomen

    (c) Electrocardiography

    (d) Urine microscopy

9. "Interval pulse" includes giving:

    (a) Additional 1 day of 100 mg dexamethasone pulse

    (b) Additional 1 day of 100 mg dexamethasone pulse and 500 mg cyclophosphamide pulse

    (c) Additional 3 days of 100 mg dexamethasone pulse

    (d) Additional 3 days of 100 mg dexamethasone pulse and 500 mg cyclophosphamide pulse on day 2

10. What is the most common side effect of pulse therapy?

    (a) Generalized weakness

    (b) Hiccups

    (c) Giddiness

    (d) Sweating

Answers

1. (d)   2. (d)   3. (b)   4. (a)   5. (d)   6. (c)   7. (c)   8. (b)   9. (a)   10. (a)

SUGGESTED READING

1. Kountz SL, Cohn R. Initial treatment of renal allografts with large intrarenal doses of immunosuppressive drugs. *Lancet.* 1969;1:338-40.

2. Pasricha JS, Seetharam KA. Further experience with dexamethasone pulse therapy in Reiter's disease. *Indian J Dermatol Venereol Leprol.* 1987;53:132.

3. Pasricha JS, Gupta R. Pulse therapy with dexamethasone cyclophosphamide in pemphigus. *Indian J Dermatol Venereol Leprol.* 1984;50:199-203.

4. Pasricha JS, Khaitan BK, Raman RS, Chandra M. Dexamethasone-cyclophosphamide pulse therapy for pemphigus. *Int J Dermatol.* 1995;34:875-82.

5. Pasricha JS, Khaitan BK. Curative treatment for pemphigus. *Arch Dermatol.* 1996;132:1518-9.

6. Ramam M. Dexamethasone pulse therapy in dermatology. *Indian J Dermatol Venereol Leprol.* 2003;69:319-22.

7. Abraham A, Roga G, Job AM. Pulse therapy in pemphigus: ready reckoner. *Indian J Dermatol.* 2016;61:314-7.

8. Hassan I, Sameem F, Masood QM, Majid I, Abdullah Z, Ahmad QM. Non comparative study on various pulse regimens (DCP, DAP and DMP) in pemphigus: our experience. *Indian J Dermatol.* 2014;59:30-4.

9. Mentink LF, Mackenzie MW, Tóth GG, Laseur M, Lambert FP, Veeger NJ, *et al.* Randomized controlled trial of adjuvant oral dexamethasone pulse therapy in pemphigus vulgaris: PEMPULS trial. *Arch Dermatol.* 2006;142:570-6.

10. Kaur S, Kanwar AJ. Dexamethasone-cyclophosphamide pulse therapy in pemphigus. *Int J Dermatol.* 1990;29:371-4.

CHAPTER 23

Rituximab in Pemphigus and other Autoimmune Bullous Diseases

Hitaishi Mehta, Vinay Keshavamurthy

- Pharmacokinetics
- Mechanism of action
- Indications
- Contraindications to rituximab
- Adverse effects and management
- Baseline investigations prior to starting rituximab
- Administration
- Drug interactions
- Use in special groups

INTRODUCTION

Rituximab is a chimeric, murine/human monoclonal antibody that targets the CD20 antigen on B cell surface and triggers B cell depletion. Rituximab was first approved in 1997 for the management of B-cell non-Hodgkin lymphoma (NHL). It subsequently received approval for CD20+ chronic lymphocytic leukemia, granulomatosis with polyangiitis, microscopic polyangiitis, and refractory rheumatoid arthritis (RA). Its first clinical use in dermatology was in paraneoplastic pemphigus (PNP), where rituximab treatment in an NHL patient resulted in improvement of skin and mucosal disease. Subsequently, several reports described successful attainment of remission in pemphigus patients who had failed conventional immunosuppressants. Rituximab received approval for the management of moderate-to-severe pemphigus vulgaris (PV) from Food and Drug Administration (FDA) in 2018 and the European Commission in 2019. Due to favorable efficacy and safety profile, rituximab is now widely regarded as a first-line treatment modality for pemphigus. A recent network meta-analysis comparing first-line steroid-sparing adjuvants in the treatment of PV and pemphigus foliaceus (PF) demonstrated superiority of rituximab over cyclophosphamide and azathioprine in terms of efficacy, safety, and steroid-sparing effect.

PHARMACOKINETICS

The plasma half-life of rituximab on an average is 21 days, but may vary widely depending on the variability in CD20 amount in patients. Serum accumulation of the drug occurs after multiple infusions as B cell depletion reduces the amount of available CD20. Clearance of the drug is primarily through phagocytosis. The patients' age, gender, and weight do not influence pharmacokinetics.

MECHANISM OF ACTION

- Rituximab is a genetically engineered chimeric murine/human monoclonal immunoglobulin G1 (IgG1) kappa antibody that binds to the CD20 antigen on B cell surface.
- CD20 first appears during the early pre-B development and is expressed consistently till before the plasma cell stage. Rituximab targets only the CD20-bearing B cells, which include pre-B, immature B, naïve B and memory B cells, and short-lived plasmablasts. Since plasma cells and the uncommitted precursor stem cells are not affected by rituximab, the effect on pre-existing and new immune function is minimal. Peripheral B cells are renewed to baseline levels by precursor stem cells in majority of the patients within 3–12 months after the therapy.
- After binding to CD20 on B cell surface, rituximab depletes these cells by three major mechanisms: antibody-dependent cell-mediated cytotoxicity, complement-mediated cytotoxicity, and direct cell apoptosis via CD20 signaling (**Fig. 1**). The downregulation of desmoglein 3-specific CD4+ T cells has also been observed in PV patients. Long-term effects include reduction in the number of circulating memory B cells and increase in transitional and naive B cell population.
- Incomplete response and relapse following rituximab infusion may result from inadequate depletion of B cells, appearance of novel lineages of autoreactive B cells,

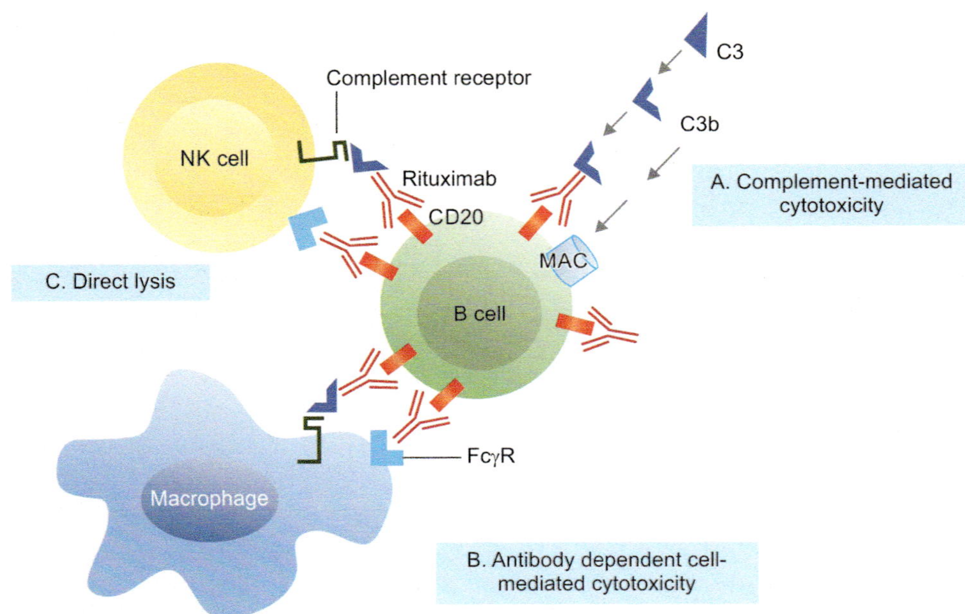

Fig. 1: Mechanism of action of rituximab. Rituximab acts by at least three pathways: A—binding of rituximab to CD20 receptors on B cells resulting in activation of complement pathway, leading to assembly of MAC and culminating in lysis of B cells via complement-mediated cytotoxicity; B—antibody-dependent cell-mediated cytotoxicity is mediated via Fcγ receptor on the surface of granulocytes, macrophages, and NK cells; C—direct lysis of B cells via stimulation of apoptotic pathway.

(CD: cluster of differentiation; FcγR: Fcγ receptor; MAC: membrane attack complex; NK: natural killer)

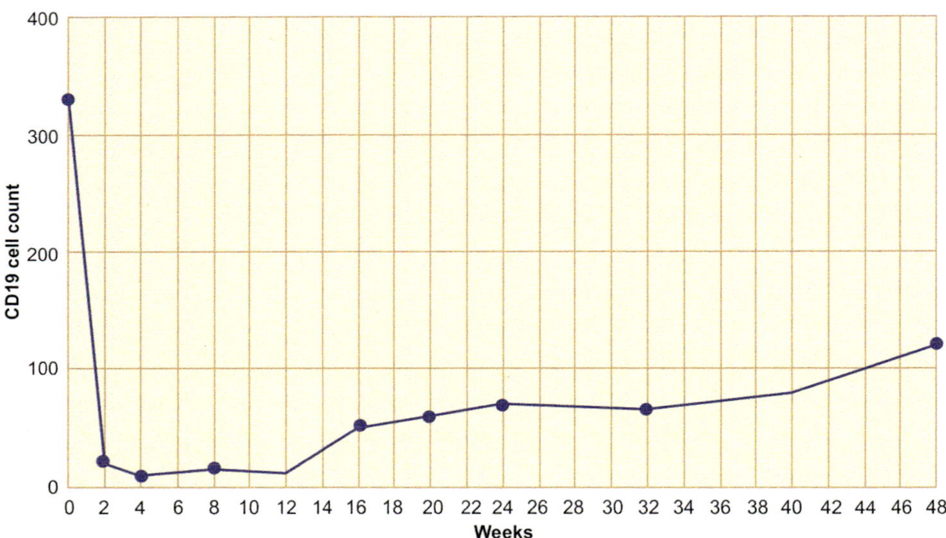

Fig. 2: CD19+ cell count post-rituximab infusion in pemphigus vulgaris patients treated as per rheumatoid arthritis protocol.

Source: Kanwar AJ, *et al*. Clinical and immunological outcomes of high- and low-dose rituximab treatments in patients with pemphigus: a randomized, comparative, observer-blinded study. *Br J Dermatol*. 2014;170:1341-9.

continued release of pathogenic autoantibodies by long-lived plasmablasts, autoreactive CD4+ T helper cells, generation of anti-rituximab antibodies, and biochemical alterations in lipid raft signaling resulting in resistance to rituximab-mediated antibody-dependent cellular cytotoxicity.

Figure 2 represents CD19+ cell count post-rituximab infusion in PV patients treated as per RA protocol.

INDICATIONS

- *PV*: Rituximab is approved for the management of moderate-to-severe PV in adults by FDA and the European Commission. Rituximab (two 1,000 mg intravenous infusions at an interval of 2 weeks) in combination with systemic corticosteroids (oral prednisolone, 0.5–1.5 mg/kg/day) with progressive tapering with the aim of stopping corticosteroids within 6 months, is recommended as first-line treatment in all cases. Patients with relapse, poor response, or intolerance to conventional therapies are also candidates for rituximab therapy. Initiation of treatment with rituximab early in the course of disease may result in more favorable outcomes in terms of response rates and duration of complete remission. Disease remission after one cycle of rituximab persists for an average of 12–15 months. Few patients who fail to achieve complete remission may require additional cycles with or without corticosteroids. Complete remission rates exceeding 90% have been reported with repeat cycles of rituximab. Patients relapsing after a complete remission following the first cycle, are more likely to achieve complete remission with subsequent cycles than patients relapsing after a less favorable outcome, and non-responders.

- *PF*: PF patients treated with rituximab have response rates similar to PV cases. The European guidelines recommend rituximab (two infusions of 1,000 mg 2 weeks apart) as the first-line management option for PF of any severity.
- *PNP*: Multiple case reports have described the efficacious use of rituximab in PNP patients. Most studies have utilized 375 mg/m^2 weekly for 4 weeks, repeated every 6 months. Two infusions of 1 g, 2 weeks apart have also been utilized. The response to rituximab therapy is highly variable. A review of 13 reported PNP cases treated with rituximab found complete response in three patients, all of whom had NHL. One case report of a PNP patient with follicular lymphoma described improvement in mucocutaneous blistering but progression of bronchiolitis obliterans. The limited response to rituximab may be explained on the basis that the drug depletes autoantibodies but has lesser impact on cell-mediated immunity.
- *Bullous pemphigoid (BP)*: Effectiveness of rituximab in BP refractory to conventional therapy has been noted in several retrospective studies. A recent systematic review assessed the efficacy of rituximab (in doses varying from 375 mg/m^2 every 1–4 weeks, to 500 mg weekly for 2 weeks) in BP. Mean duration of therapy was 2.6 months (range: 2 weeks to 13 months). About 85% patients attained complete remission. Most patients had failed to respond to systemic corticosteroids prior to biologic treatment. The recurrence rate was 29% with mean time to recurrence of 10 months.
- *Epidermolysis bullosa acquisita (EBA)*: Several case reports have described successful management with rituximab in refractory disease, in combination with immunosuppressants or immunoadsorption. A literature review assessing 20 cases of recalcitrant EBA found that 56% patients managed with rituximab monotherapy and 75% patients receiving rituximab in combination with immunoadsorption achieved complete remission.

Both the lymphoma and RA protocols were used. The Brazilian Society of Dermatology recommends use of rituximab in either dosage regimens for management of severe EBA refractory to corticosteroids.

- *Mucous membrane pemphigoid (MMP)*: Several small studies have described successful use of rituximab in MMP cases, usually in combination with corticosteroids, with or without other immunosuppressive agents. Both the lymphoma and RA protocols have been used. Complete remission has been obtained in 60–100% of cases, typically occurring in 3–12 months. Rituximab, in combination with corticosteroids, intravenous immunoglobulin (IVIg), or other immunosuppressants can be considered in refractory high-risk disease.

CONTRAINDICATIONS TO RITUXIMAB

The contraindications include:
- Hypersensitivity to either the active drug or any of the components
- Active, serious infection (tuberculosis, sepsis, hepatitis, opportunistic infection)
- Severe immunocompromised state
- Severe cardiac failure or uncontrolled cardiac disease
- Pregnancy
- Caution should be exercised in human immunodeficiency virus (HIV)-infected patients with CD4 count <50/μL

ADVERSE EFFECTS AND MANAGEMENT

Various adverse effects reported with rituximab administration along with their incidence and management have been summarized in **Table 1**.

BASELINE INVESTIGATIONS PRIOR TO STARTING RITUXIMAB

- A clinical history should be obtained regarding active infections, imminent surgical procedures, preceding or current malignancies, cardio-respiratory disease, and pregnancy or lactation
- Complete blood count including differential and platelet count
- *Metabolic panel*: Liver and kidney function tests and serum electrolytes
- *Urine*: Routine and microscopy, stool examination
- Screening for HIV, hepatitis B surface antigen, anti-hepatitis B core antibody, anti-hepatitis C antibody
- Pregnancy testing [serum beta human chorionic gonadotropin (β-hCG) or urine pregnancy test] for women of reproductive potential
- Chest X-ray to screen for active tuberculosis
- Electrocardiogram to screen for cardiac disease
- Serum IgG levels

TABLE 1: Incidence and management of adverse effects following rituximab therapy (incidence rates are derived from product label, unless otherwise specified).

Adverse effect	Description	Incidence	Management
Early			
Infusion reaction	Within 30 minutes to 2 hours of infusion initiation, characterized by fever, chills, headache, nausea, urticarial rash; bronchospasm and hypotension in <10% and anaphylaxis in <5% of cases	12–77% with first infusion, decreases with subsequent infusions	Stop infusion, repeat pre-medication. If reaction subsides → restart at 50% of previous rate. Symptoms such as urticaria, wheeze, and throat tightness are highly suggestive of anaphylaxis and should be specifically sought for. Infusion should be ceased in cases of serious or life-threatening cardiac arrhythmias. Future infusions may be given in case of mild infusion reaction, but therapy should be abandoned in patients who develop serious reactions like anaphylaxis
Cytokine release syndrome	Fever, chills, rigors, nausea, pain, headache not responding to pre-medication or slower infusion rate	Rare, never reported in pemphigus patients. Occurs in cancer patients with high tumor load	Symptomatic treatment with antihistamines, antipyretics, and intravenous fluids in mild cases; intravenous glucocorticoids and interruption of infusion in severe cases
Late			
Late-onset neutropenia	Onset around 3–4 months after infusion, low incidence in pemphigus patients	2.8%	Usually self-limiting, antibiotics or G-CSF may be needed in certain cases
Infections	Reactivation of latent infections, progressive multifocal leukoencephalopathy, *Pneumocystis carinii* pneumonia, sepsis, pyelonephritis, etc.	19–62%, serious infection: 2–11%	Discontinue rituximab and start appropriate anti-microbial treatment
Hypogammaglo-bulinemia	Due to inherent depletion of B cells associated with rituximab infusion, predisposition to serious infections	27–58%	Avoid infusion in patients with low-baseline IgG (<600 mg/dL or below laboratory reference range), replacement Ig should be considered in patients with recurrent infections not prevented by prophylactic antibiotics
Cardiovascular complications	Sinus tachycardia, dysrhythmia, myocardial infarction	5–29%, more common in patients with pre-existing cardiac conditions	Monitoring for cardiac symptoms during and following the infusion, urgent cardiology referral if any cardiac symptoms observed
Immunogenicity	Development of human antichimeric antibodies	56%	May contribute to hypersensitivity and reduced efficacy, exact relevance unclear
Mucocutaneous reactions	Stevens–Johnson syndrome (SJS)/toxic epidermal necrolysis (TEN), maculopapular rash, exfoliative dermatitis, vasculitis, urticaria	Pruritus: ≤17%, skin rash: ≤17%, urticaria: 2–8%, SJS/TEN: rare	Symptomatic treatment for mild reactions; discontinue in patients with severe mucocutaneous reactions
Hepatotoxicity	Elevation in serum aminotransferases, acute liver injury, reactivation of hepatitis B	Hepatobiliary disease: 17%, serum aminotransferase elevation: 13%, acute hepatocellular damage: rare	Screening for HBsAg and Anti-HBc Ab prior to administration, cessation of drug in cases of acute hepatocellular damage, transplantation may be required in fulminant cases
Serum sickness-like reaction	Usually occurs during the first cycle, often with second dose, approximately 7 days after the infusion and presents with fever, arthralgia, and rash	Rare	Oral corticosteroids; slow infusion rates along with pre-treatment and additional glucocorticoid usage during and after infusion may allow for successful re-treatment
Intestinal obstruction and perforation	Presents with abdominal ache and/or recurrent vomiting, mean onset of symptoms in 6 days (range: 1–77 days)	Rare	Urgent referral to gastroenterologist for evaluation of acute abdomen

(G-CSF: granulocyte colony stimulating factor; HBc: hepatitis B core; HBsAg: hepatitis B surface antigen; Ig: immunoglobulin)

ADMINISTRATION

Formulations

- Rituximab is available as 100 mg/mL and 500 mg/50 mL vials for intravenous infusion.
- The original molecule approved by FDA in 1997 was Roche's MabThera/Rituxan.
- Biosimilars are biological products that demonstrate similarity to the original molecule ("innovator") in terms of pharmaceutical quality, biological activity, efficacy, and safety on the basis of a comprehensive clinical and non-clinical study data. They improve patients' access to biologics by substantial reduction of cost. Intended copies refer to biological products which do not meet the stringent criteria for biosimilars and have not been compared adequately with the original molecule analytically or clinically.
- The Indian regulatory bodies do not mandate clinical testing for approval of biosimilars. Several "similar biologics" of rituximab are approved for use in India.

Dosage

- *FDA approved dosage regimen for PV (RA protocol)*: Two, 1 g intravenous infusions 2 weeks apart, along with tapering doses of corticosteroids.
- *Off-label (lymphoma protocol)*: Four infusions of 375 mg/m^2 intravenously at weekly interval.
- *Low-dosage regimens*: A lower dosage regimen (two, 500 mg doses at 2-week interval) has been used successfully for the treatment of pemphigus, with relapses occurring toward the end of second year. An ultra-low dosage regimen (a single 200 mg infusion) was studied in eight pemphigus patients and showed complete and partial remission in five and three patients, respectively. Larger studies to determine the efficacy and advantages of this approach are lacking.
- A systematic review and meta-analysis comparing the various rituximab regimens did not find any difference between the RA and lymphoma protocols in terms of time to complete remission, complete remission and relapse rates. Serious adverse events with the lymphoma protocol (4.8%) were slightly higher than the RA protocol (2.1%). The advantages of the RA protocol over lymphoma protocol include less cost and fewer infusions. High dose rituximab (>2,000 mg) regimens are associated with longer complete remissions as compared to low dose (<1,500 mg) regimens. **Table 2** summarizes findings from a review comparing the efficacy and safety of three rituximab protocols.
- *Intralesional rituximab*: Several case series have described the successful use of intralesional rituximab for refractory mucocutaneous lesions of PV. This mode of administration reduces the total dose of drug required and hence is more economical, particularly in patients with limited disease. Significant decline in peripheral blood CD19+ B-cell count has been documented after intralesional rituximab injection.

How to Administer?

- *Pre-medication*: Antipyretics (paracetamol 650 mg intravenous or 1,000 mg oral), antihistamines (diphenhydramine 50 mg intravenous or pheniramine maleate 22.75 mg intravenous or chlorpheniramine 4 mg oral), and methylprednisolone 100 mg (or hydrocortisone

TABLE 2: Comparison of three rituximab protocols.

Parameters	Lymphoma protocol	Rheumatoid arthritis protocol	Modified rheumatoid arthritis protocol (500 mg)
Number of patients	184	188	21
Dosage	375 mg/m^2 intravenously at weekly interval for 4 weeks	Two 1 g intravenous infusions 2 weeks apart	Two 500 mg infusions 2 weeks apart
Complete remission on therapy	57.6%	46.8%	52%
Complete remission off therapy	27.1%	42%	19%
Follow-up duration (in months)	28.9	21.9	15.5
Incidence of relapse	40.7%	67%	47.6%
Months to relapse	16.9	15.7	15.4
Serious adverse effects	4.8%	2.1%	0%
Comment	Larger total dose and higher cost, higher likelihood of attaining complete remission albeit with slightly higher incidence of adverse effects	Higher incidence of relapse, shorter duration of remission, and lower incidence of serious adverse effects as compared to lymphoma protocol, the difference was, however, not statistically significant	Lower incidence of adverse events, however higher proportion of patients require additional immunosuppression, and rate of relapse may be higher with longer follow-up duration

Source: Adapted from Ahmed AR, *et al*. A comprehensive analysis of treatment outcomes in patients with pemphigus vulgaris treated with rituximab. *Autoimmun Rev*. 2015;14:323-31.

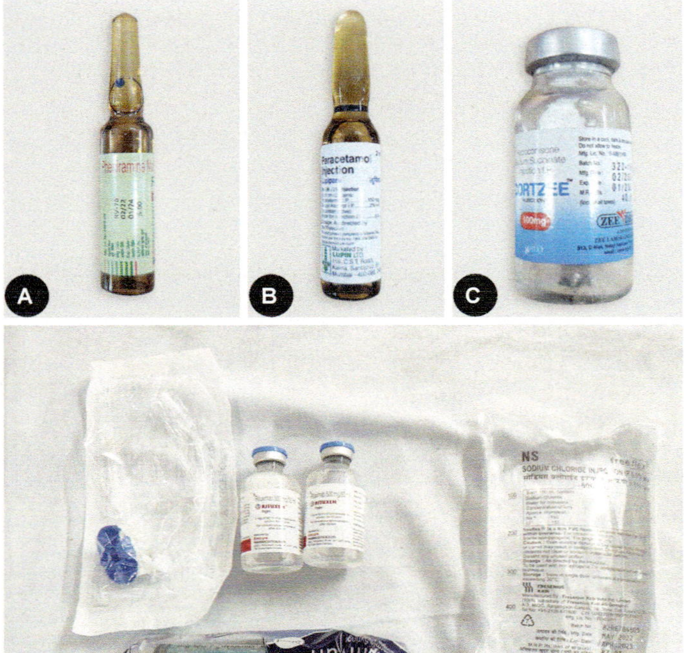

Figs. 3A to D: Administration of rituximab as per rheumatoid arthritis protocol: Pre-medication administered prior to rituximab infusion, includes (A) pheniramine 22.75 mg; (B) paracetamol 650 mg; (C) hydrocortisone 100 mg; (D) two vials of rituximab (500 mg + 500 mg) should be diluted with 400 mL 0.9% normal saline. Use of an infusion pump aids in regulation of rate of administration.

100 mg) intravenous, 30 minutes preceding each rituximab dose **(Figs. 3A to C)**.

- Two vials (50 mL + 50 mL) of rituximab (500 mg + 500 mg) should be diluted in 400 mL, 0.9% sodium chloride solution, to obtain a volume of 500 mL **(Fig. 3D)**. Use of an infusion pump may aid in regulating administration of the drug.
- *Initial infusion*: It is started at 50 mg/h, increased by 50 mg/h every 30 minutes to a maximum of 400 mg/h. Total infusion time is 5–6 hours.
- *Successive infusions*: Started at 100 mg/h; increased by 100 mg/h every 30 minutes to a maximum of 400 mg/h.
- Vitals should be monitored every 15 minutes through the first hour of infusion and every 30 minutes thereafter. It is advisable to keep the patient under observation for a day as infusion reactions may be seen up to 24 hours after administration.

Monitoring

Drug-related Monitoring

- *Physical examination*: Every 1–6 months to assess treatment response and development of infectious or other adverse effects.

- *Complete blood count with differential count*: Repeated 2-weekly during treatment and every 1–3 months thereafter, with special attention to neutrophil count.
- Renal function should be periodically monitored.
- It is advisable to obtain serum Ig levels (total—IgG, IgM, and IgA) before each re-infusion, and in case of occurrence of a serious infectious complication or recurrent infections.

Disease-related Monitoring

- Peripheral blood CD20 levels, and anti-desmoglein 1 and 3 titers are also useful for monitoring response to therapy in pemphigus patients. Serum autoantibodies (anti-desmoglein) should be measured by ELISA at baseline, month 3, and every 3–6 months thereafter.
- Measurement of anti-BP180 IgG by ELISA at days 0, 60 and 150, is recommended for prediction of disease outcome in BP patients.
- ELISA for collagen VII has a low sensitivity for diagnosing EBA. Antibody titers may be utilized to monitor disease activity when positive.

Maintenance Regimen

- Optimum dose, frequency of cycles, and the duration of maintenance therapy with rituximab in pemphigus is yet to be determined.
- An additional cycle of two 1,000 mg infusions 2 weeks apart can be considered in pemphigus patients who do not attain complete remission on or off therapy after 6 months.
- In patients attaining complete remission on or off therapy at 6 months, another 500 mg or 1 g infusion can be considered at month 6 in patients who initially presented with severe disease or had a high titer of anti-desmoglein antibodies at 3 months.
- Additional 500 mg infusions at month 12 and 18 should be considered in patients in complete remission but serum positivity of anti-desmoglein antibodies.
- Infusions after 18 months should be considered in patients who present with reappearance of serum autoantibodies after their initial disappearance.

Predictors of Treatment Response

- The following parameters have been associated with a higher likelihood of relapse following rituximab infusion in pemphigus patients:
  - High baseline pemphigus disease activity index (PDAI >45)
  - Persistent anti-desmoglein 1 antibody enzyme-linked immunosorbent assay (ELISA) level >20 IU/mL and/or anti-desmoglein 3 antibody ELISA level >130 IU/mL, 3 months after rituximab treatment
- Lymphoma protocol, older age, and lower baseline anti-desmoglein-specific antibody titers (<250 IU/mL) have been associated with a higher likelihood of attaining complete remission off therapy.
- Body mass index ≥35 is a negative prognostic factor for complete remission off therapy.

Concomitant Use of Other Immunosuppressants

- *Steroids*: For the management of PV, prednisolone, 0.5–1.5 mg/kg/day should be administered in combination with rituximab for the initial months, with the aim of stopping corticosteroids within 3–4 months for mild disease and 6 months for moderate-to-severe disease.
- *Other immunosuppressants*: Immunosuppressive agents such as azathioprine, cyclophosphamide, and mycophenolate mofetil may increase the risk of infections when combined with rituximab and thus should be used judiciously. However, a combination of methotrexate and rituximab may be considered in view of a long safety record of combination therapy in RA patients.
- Combination therapy with IVIg, intravenous corticosteroid pulses or immunoadsorption can be considered in patients with refractory pemphigus. Concurrent administration of IVIg 2 g/kg every 4 weeks has been shown to aid attainment of complete remission in severe, treatment refractory pemphigus. Two to four cycles of immunoadsorption (consisting of four treatments each) prior to rituximab infusion have been demonstrated to be beneficial in severe, treatment-resistant disease.
- Immunoadsorption-based combination therapy has been observed to result in the fastest disease control.

COST-EFFECTIVENESS OF RITUXIMAB TREATMENT

- Besides having a higher clinical efficacy, rituximab is a more economical management option for pemphigus patients.
- Cost-effectiveness of rituximab has been compared to mycophenolate mofetil in treatment naïve patients with moderate-to-severe pemphigus. Over a period of 24 months, rituximab was observed to be more cost-effective than mycophenolate mofetil, with significantly higher cost reduction and a favorable incremental cost-effectiveness ratio.

DRUG INTERACTIONS

- Immunosuppressive effects may be amplified when used with other immunosuppressants.
- The risk of myelosuppression may be increased when used concomitantly with other myelosuppressive medications.
- Rituximab may attenuate the immunogenicity of vaccines. Immunization with live vaccines should be completed at least 4 weeks prior and with inactive vaccines at least 2 weeks prior to commencing rituximab therapy. Both inactive and live vaccines should be delayed by up to 6–12 months after rituximab infusion.
- There is an increased probability of nephrotoxicity when rituximab is used in conjugation with cisplatin or amphotericin B.

USE IN SPECIAL GROUPS

- No dosage alteration is recommended in individuals with liver or kidney disease.
- Recommendations regarding use of rituximab in children, elderly, pregnant, and nursing women are summarized in **Table 3**.

TABLE 3: Recommendations on use of rituximab in special groups.

Special group	Recommendations
Pediatric	• Off-label use in dermatology, dose—375 mg/m^2 weekly for 4 weeks • Vaccination should be brought up-to-date, preferably with killed or subunit vaccines as per the current immunization guideline recommendations • Immunization with live vaccines should be completed at least 4 weeks prior and with inactive vaccines at least 2 weeks prior to commencing rituximab therapy • Both inactive and live vaccines should be delayed by up to 6–12 months after rituximab infusion
Elderly	No dosage adjustment recommended
Pregnancy	• Rituximab passes through the placental barrier and has been found in newborn serum. Lowest risk of exposure is during the stage of organogenesis • May interfere with neonatal B cell development, resulting in increased risk of infections; premature births have also been reported • Food and Drug Administration (FDA) category C • Women of reproductive age group should utilize effective contraceptive methods during therapy and for a minimum of 1 year following infusion
Lactation	• According to the manufacturer, breastfeeding is not recommended during rituximab administration and for ≥6 months after the last infusion • American College of Rheumatology (ACR) strongly recommends rituximab as compatible with breastfeeding in patients with rheumatic and musculoskeletal disease; unlikely to be absorbed via infant gastrointestinal tract
Latent tuberculosis infection	• No increase in risk of tuberculosis reactivation after rituximab infusion; literature does not support treatment for latent tuberculosis infection prior to rituximab treatment • ACR guidelines do not recommend screening for latent tuberculosis prior to commencement of rituximab therapy • European guidelines recommend chest X-ray and tuberculin skin test or quantiferon test in case of elevated risk of tuberculosis

CONCLUSION

Rituximab has emerged as a promising treatment option for patients with AIBDs, specifically pemphigus vulgaris. It has also shown good response in patients of pemphigus foliaceus, bullous pemphigoid, and mucous membrane pemphigoid. Clinical trials have shown that rituximab is effective in inducing remission and reducing disease activity in these conditions, including patients who are refractory to conventional therapies. Its mechanism of action, which involves depletion of B cells, makes it a promising alternative to traditional immunosuppressive therapies that target a broad range of immune cells. In addition, rituximab has a favorable safety profile with a low incidence of serious adverse events.

Despite these promising results, there are still some areas that require further research, such as optimal dosing regimen and duration of treatment. The use of rituximab in pregnant and lactating women, as well as in children, also needs to be further studied.

TAKE HOME MESSAGE

- Rituximab is an IgG1, chimeric, monoclonal antibody that binds to the B cell surface antigen CD20, triggering depletion of B cells.
- Initially utilized as a management option for pemphigus refractory to conventional immunosuppressants, rituximab is now widely regarded as first-line treatment for this disease.
- Other autoimmune bullous diseases where rituximab has shown promise include BP, EBA, and MMP.
- Prior to commencement of therapy, patient should be screened for active infections, cardiopulmonary disease, pregnancy, prior or current malignancy. Vaccinations should be brought up-to-date.
- The depletion of B cells by rituximab is sustained for an average of 6 months and peripheral blood B cell levels return to baseline within 1 year of treatment, hence majority of patients require maintenance therapy with periodic re-infusions.

MULTIPLE CHOICE QUESTIONS

1. **All of these are well-known complications of rituximab, *except*:**
   (a) Infusion reaction
   (b) Late-onset neutropenia
   (c) Candidiasis
   (d) Hypogammaglobulinemia

2. **A 56-year-old lady presents to emergency department with complaints of fever and dizziness. She had been recently discharged from dermatology ward after rituximab infusion for pemphigus vulgaris. On examination, she has a blood pressure of 90/60, heart rate of 120 bpm, and cutaneous erosions particularly in axilla and back have a purulent discharge. You suspect that she has developed sepsis. All of the following pre-treatment investigations are essential to prevent infectious complications, *except*:**
   (a) Complete blood count
   (b) Human immunodeficiency virus antibodies
   (c) Hepatitis B core antibody
   (d) Peripheral blood CD20 counts

3. **A patient diagnosed with pemphigus vulgaris presents to you inquiring about rituximab treatment. He is particularly curious about the durability of treatment response. Which of the subsequent statements is/are correct with respect to disease remission after treatment with rituximab?**
   (a) Nearly complete depletion of plasma cells is observed 2–3 weeks after infusion

   (b) Weight of the patient has significant impact on pharmacokinetics and duration of action of rituximab
   (c) Majority of patients attain complete remission off therapy within few months and do not require maintenance therapy
   (d) Anti-desmoglein antibodies are useful in predicting disease relapse after rituximab infusion

4. **While administering rituximab infusion to a pemphigus patient, you notice development of urticarial rash over the skin. The patient also complains of throat tightness. An expiratory wheeze is evident on auscultation and blood pressure of 90/60 mm Hg. All of the following are correct regarding further management, *except*:**
   (a) Immediate cessation of rituximab infusion
   (b) Establishment of airway and intramuscular epinephrine injection
   (c) Rapid bolus of normal saline
   (d) Resumption of infusion at a lower rate after repeating pre-medication

5. **A 17-year-old boy presents to dermatology outpatient department with pemphigus vulgaris of moderate severity. He has previously received oral corticosteroids along with azathioprine and mycophenolate mofetil with minimal response. You decide to commence rituximab therapy according to lymphoma protocol. Which of the following statements regarding protocols of rituximab infusion is true?**
   (a) Lymphoma protocol employs weight-based dosing and hence is preferable in children and adolescents

(b) Lymphoma protocol has the advantage of fewer infusions

(c) Duration of remission is similar in both lymphoma protocol and rheumatoid arthritis protocol

(d) Low-dose rheumatoid arthritis protocol is associated with more relapse and lesser remission rate

6. The most common adverse effect associated with rituximab infusion is:

(a) Infusion reaction

(b) Injection site reaction

(c) Mild-to-moderate transaminitis

(d) Sinus tachycardia

7. As per the FDA labeling, which pregnancy category does rituximab belong to?

(a) Category A

(b) Category B

(c) Category C

(d) Category D

8. All of the following are cutaneous adverse effects of rituximab, *except*:

(a) Urticaria

(b) Night sweats

(c) Pruritus

(d) Drug rash with eosinophilia and systemic symptoms

9. Minimum period of effective contraception following rituximab infusion should be:

(a) 6 months

(b) 9 months

(c) 12 months

(d) 18 months

10. Which of the following parameters requires careful monitoring in weeks following rituximab infusion?

(a) Hemoglobin

(b) Total leukocyte count

(c) Absolute neutrophil count

(d) Absolute eosinophil count

Answers

1. (c)   2. (d)   3. (d)   4. (d)   5. (d)   6. (a)   7. (c)   8. (d)   9. (c)   10. (c)

SUGGESTED READING

1. Huang A, Madan RK, Levitt J. Future therapies for pemphigus vulgaris: Rituximab and beyond. *J Am Acad Dermatol*. 2016;74: 746-53.

2. Joly P, Horwath B, Patsatsi A, Uzun S, Bech R, Beissert S, *et al*. Updated s2k guidelines on the management of pemphigus vulgaris and foliaceus initiated by the European Academy of Dermatology and Venereology (EADV). *J Eur Acad Dermatol Venereol*. 2020;34:1900-13.

3. Joly P, Maho-Vaillant M, Prost-Squarcioni C, Hebert V, Houivet E, Calbo S, *et al*; French study group on autoimmune bullous skin diseases. First-line rituximab combined with short-term prednisone versus prednisone alone for the treatment of pemphigus (RITUX 3): A prospective, multicentre, parallel-group, open-label randomised trial. *Lancet*. 2017;389:2031-40.

4. Wang HH, Liu CW, Li YC, Huang YC. Efficacy of rituximab for pemphigus: A systematic review and meta-analysis of different regimens. *Acta Derm Venereol*. 2015;95:928-32.

5. Vinay K, Kanwar AJ, Sawatkar GU, Dogra S, Ishii N, Hashimoto T. Successful use of rituximab in the treatment of childhood and juvenile pemphigus. *J Am Acad Dermatol*. 2014;71:669-75.

6. Kremer N, Snast I, Cohen ES, Hodak E, Mimouni D, Lapidoth M, *et al*. Rituximab and omalizumab for the treatment of bullous pemphigoid: A systematic review of the literature. *Am J Clin Dermatol*. 2019;20:209-16.

Other Therapeutic Interventions for Pemphigus and other Autoimmune Bullous Diseases

Intravenous Immunoglobulin, Omalizumab, Newer Therapeutic Interventions including Emerging Therapies

Rajat Choudhary, Vishal Gupta

- Intravenous immunoglobulin
- Omalizumab
- Emerging therapies in pemphigus
    - Anti-CD20 molecules other than rituximab
    - FcRn antagonists
- Bruton tyrosine kinase inhibitors
- Cholinomimetic drugs
- Stem cell therapy
- Chimeric autoantibody receptor (CAAR)-T cell therapy

INTRODUCTION

Systemic corticosteroids and other conventional immuno-suppressive agents have been the mainstay of treatment of autoimmune bullous diseases (AIBDs) for a long time. Due to their broad immunosuppressive effect, adverse effect profile, and the need for long-term administration of medications, search for more effective and safer drugs is ongoing. Rituximab, an anti-CD20 monoclonal antibody, is now viewed as the first-line agent for the treatment of pemphigus vulgaris (PV), and has been recently approved by Food and Drug Administration (FDA) for moderate-to-severe disease.

In this chapter, we will discuss a few other therapeutic options for AIBDs, namely, intravenous immunoglobulin (IVIg) and omalizumab, as well as some of the promising emerging therapies.

INTRAVENOUS IMMUNOGLOBULIN (IVIg)

IVIg is a concentrate of human immunoglobulin G (IgG) in supraphysiological doses along with trace amounts of other immunoglobulins which are derived from the plasma of multiple human donors. It was initially developed for the treatment and prevention of viral infections, and for treatment of primary immunodeficiency syndromes. Since the late 1980s, its use has been expanded for the treatment of autoimmune and inflammatory disorders as well.

Mechanism of Action

The exact mechanism of IVIg is not known, but many have been postulated for its action in a variety of disorders, ranging from providing passive immunity in immunodeficiency disorders to neutralizing toxins in infections, and immunomodulation in various autoimmune and inflammatory disorders.

The following mechanisms have been put forward to explain the efficacy of IVIg in autoimmune diseases:
- "Anti-idiotypic" antibodies bind and neutralize pathogenic antibodies.
- Suppression of antibody production by IgG binding via its Fc fragment to the corresponding surface receptors on B lymphocytes leading to the downregulation of pathogenic autoantibody production.
- *Accelerated antibody catabolism*: IgG is taken up by non-specific pinocytosis into the endosomes. At low pH (approximately pH 6), IgG binds to FcRn (a neonatal Fc receptor) in the wall of the endosomes, after which the IgG–FcRn complexes are recycled to the cell surface, where IgG is released because of higher pH. IgG not bound to FcRn is delivered to lysosomes and degraded. High-dose IVIg in AIBDs causes saturation of FcRn, resulting in a smaller proportion of the endocytosed IgG rescued by FcRn from degradation in the lysosomes, leading to increased catabolism of IgG including that of autoantibodies.
- IVIg binds to C3 and C5 convertase, blocks complement activation at an early stage, and interferes with the formation of the terminal membrane-attack-complex.
- IVIg binds to Fc receptors on macrophages and causes saturation and downregulation of these receptors; this leads to the inhibition of autoantibody-mediated cellular activation.
- Anti-Fas receptor antibodies block keratinocyte apoptosis.

- IVIg downregulates the expression of co-stimulatory molecules, like lymphocyte function-associated antigen-1 (LFA-1) on activated T cells, leading to interference with T-cell activation.
- It increases glucocorticoid receptor sensitivity and synergizes suppression of lymphocyte activation with steroids.

Pre-treatment Investigations

There is no absolute test required before infusion of IVIg. The role of baseline testing for serum IgA levels is controversial. Although patients with low or absent serum IgA are at risk of developing IgG antibody against IgA, majority of such patients tolerate IVIg. Further, currently available IVIg preparations have very low IgA content. On the other hand, patients without IgA deficiency or anti-IgA antibodies can also develop anaphylaxis. Hence, screening for IgA deficiency and anti-IgA antibodies may lead to an unnecessary delay and even needlessly restrict its use in some patients. Pre-treatment testing of viral infections such as hepatitis B and C should be done, since after IVIg infusion the source of pathological antibodies cannot be determined.

Contraindications

- Hypersensitivity to human Ig products
- History of anaphylaxis to IVIg
- IgA deficiency and presence of anti-IgA antibodies is considered a relative contraindication by some authors.

Boxed Warning

- Caution should be observed in the presence of risk factors for thrombosis (advanced age, prolonged immobilization, hypercoagulable conditions, history of venous or arterial thrombosis, use of estrogens, indwelling central vascular catheters, hyperviscosity,

and cardiovascular risk factors). Such patients should be given slow infusion with adequate pre-infusion hydration.
- Renal dysfunction, acute renal failure, osmotic nephrosis, and death may occur with the IVIg products in predisposed patients (pre-existing renal insufficiency, diabetes mellitus, age >65 years, volume depletion, sepsis, paraproteinemia, or patients receiving known nephrotoxic drugs).

Pregnancy Status

Traditional FDA category C; new rating: compatible.

Adverse Effects

Adverse reactions to IVIg occur in about 5–15% of IVIg infusions. Infusion reactions are the most common; more than half of them occur immediately or within few hours of infusion, and mostly occur with first infusion or with the change in product. Most infusion reactions are mild and transient. Potentially serious reactions have been reported in 2–6% of patients. Anaphylactic reactions (prevalence: 1 in 20,000 to 1 in 50,000) and transfusion-related acute lung injury are serious but are rare side effects. **Table 1** summarizes the acute and delayed adverse effects of IVIg.

Use in Autoimmune Bullous Diseases

Pemphigus Vulgaris (Level of Evidence: 1b)

Currently systemic corticosteroids and rituximab are the mainstay of treatment for moderate-to-severe PV. As both these agents are immunosuppressives, they are not suitable when the patient has concomitant systemic infection. Further, rituximab takes about 4–6 weeks to control the disease, and is therefore not useful for managing acute flares. IVIg is rapidly acting, and can be used in patients with concurrent infections.

TABLE 1: Adverse effects of intravenous immunoglobulin (IVIg) and its management.

Adverse effect	Manifestation	Management
Infusion reaction (around 6–30% patients)	• Flushing, nausea, fatigue, fever, chills, malaise, lethargy • Occurs within the first hour of infusion	Slow infusion rate, antihistamine, and paracetamol
Dermatological adverse effects (around 6%)	Urticaria and pompholyx can occur till 2 weeks of infusion	Conservative and symptomatic management
Arrhythmia and hypotension (rare)	• Supraventricular tachycardia, bradycardia in patients with heart disease • Anaphylaxis-like reaction	Stopping of infusion, restart infusion at slow rate if reaction is non-life threatening
Transfusion-related acute lung injury (few reports)	Acute respiratory distress and bilateral pulmonary edema without any other cause	• Corticosteroids • Might require ventilatory support
Thrombotic events (1–17%)	Thrombosis of arteries, veins, and intracranial sinuses, arterial thrombotic events (such as stroke, myocardial infarction, pulmonary embolism)	• Pre-infusion hydration and slow infusion • Consider anticoagulation in high-risk patients
Neurological disorders	Headache, aseptic meningitis (0.5–1%), posterior reversible encephalopathy syndrome (PRES), seizure and abducens nerve palsy	Conservative management in consultation with neurologist
Hematologic disorders	Hemolytic anemia and neutropenia (asymptomatic, around 1.5%)	Self-resolving

Various IVIg protocols have been used in pemphigus:

- *Sequential therapy*: Mostly IVIg is used as rescue therapy in pemphigus for rapid control of disease, and in patients with contraindications to immunosuppressives. After rapid control of disease activity or treatment of underlying infections, conventional immunosuppressives or rituximab are used for sustained remission. In a randomized controlled trial including 61 patients with steroid-dependent pemphigus, a single cycle of IVIg led to a significantly faster clinical improvement and fall in circulating autoantibody levels as compared to placebo.

- *IVIg as a sole adjuvant to systemic corticosteroids*: Ahmed and Dahl proposed it as the sole adjuvant in PV. They proposed its use at a dose of 2 g/kg over 3–5 days every 4 weeks until control of disease activity off systemic steroids is achieved, and then increasing the infusion interval by 2 weeks till a 16-week interval is achieved, followed by stopping IVIg. This regimen was used in 15 patients with moderate-to-severe steroid-dependent PV. Steroids could be tapered over a mean period of 4 months, and five (30%) patients had 1–3 relapses in the 6-year follow-up period which were managed by increasing the frequency of IVIg infusions. This protocol has not been widely used due to its high cost, repeated five-day long infusions, and adverse effects of repeated IVIg infusions.

- *Combination therapy*: In the combination protocol, IVIg is given along with other immunosuppressive agents. When using IVIg with other immunosuppressive agents, its efficacy increases from 56% to around 90%. Combination of cytotoxic therapy with IVIg leads to faster clearance of pathogenic autoantibodies.

Ahmed, *et al* have proposed a new treatment protocol for management of pemphigus, in which multiple cycles of rituximab are given along with IVIg. In phase 1 (B cell depletion phase), initially IVIg 2 g/kg (monthly) is given along with weekly rituximab (375 mg/m^2) for 8 consecutive weeks, followed by monthly infusions for 4 months. Phase 2 (B cell re-population phase) is of flexible duration and ends till CD19-positive cells reach 15% re-population. In this phase, patients receive monthly cycles of IVIg. In phase 3 (immune restoration phase), patients receive additional six cycles of IVIg at 6, 8, 10, 12, and 14 weeks. Apart from the synergistic effect of this combination, the other proposed advantage of this protocol is the immunoprophylaxis offered by IVIg against rituximab-induced risk of infections. Ahmed, *et al* have used this protocol in various AIBDs such as PV (21 patients), bullous pemphigoid (BP) (12 patients), mucous membrane pemphigoid (MMP) (6 patients), and epidermolysis bullosa acquisita (EBA) (5 patients). In a follow-up period (after stopping all immunosuppressive drugs) of 11 years in PV, 6 years in BP, and 9.8 years in MMP, no patient developed relapse, any significant infection, hospitalization or malignancy. Although this treatment protocol is longer and costly, it provides significantly longer remissions.

Bullous Pemphigoid (Level of Evidence: 4)

Various case reports and case series have published the use of IVIg in BP. Majority of the reports have used IVIg at a dose of monthly 2 mg/kg, either as monotherapy or in combination with other immunosuppressives, and >80% patients had significant improvement by 3 months. Few case reports have also demonstrated good efficacy of IVIg in infantile BP after one or two cycles of relatively low doses (~1.5 g/kg).

Mucous Membrane Pemphigoid/Cicatricial Pemphigoid (Level of Evidence: 4)

More than 70 MMP patients treated with IVIg have been reported in the literature. Of these 70 patients, 65 responded completely, two had partial improvement, and three patients had no improvement (two out of three discontinued IVIg therapy). Most of the patients had control of conjunctival inflammation and halt in progression of their disease for up to 12 months. In view of serious mucosal complications, the authors have generally used IVIg every 2 weeks along with other immunosuppressives. Leverkus, *et al* reported improvement in 90% (*n* = 9/10) of their patients at 6 months with this regimen. At five-year follow-up, 8 of 10 patients maintained clinical remission. In a retrospective study of 12 patients of ocular MMP, six patients who received a combination of IVIg and rituximab did not have progression of disease, whereas six patients who received other aggressive therapies experienced disease progression and became blind in both eyes by 55-week follow-up period.

Other Autoimmune Bullous Diseases (Level of Evidence: 4)

There are a few reports of the use of IVIg in pemphigoid gestationis, EBA, and linear IgA disease. Most of them have used IVIg at a dose of 1–2 g/kg/cycle, repeated at 4 weeks interval, and have demonstrated significant improvement in most patients at 3–4 months.

OMALIZUMAB

Omalizumab is an anti-IgE monoclonal antibody which was first approved for asthma in early 2000. Later, its use was extended to dermatological diseases, primarily chronic urticaria. Recently, it has also been tried in AIBDs mainly in BP.

Some studies have shown a positive correlation between the severity of BP and circulating levels of anti-BP 180 IgE antibodies as well as linear IgE deposition at the dermo-epidermal junction. A meta-analysis reported a positive correlation between the severity of BP and serum IgE levels. Therefore, omalizumab may be effective in BP by decreasing the pathogenic IgE levels.

Dose: 150 mg/300 mg subcutaneously every 4 weeks.

Adverse Effects and Contraindications

Anaphylaxis is the most severe adverse drug reaction, and has been reported in 0.1 to 0.2% patients. This reaction can be delayed in onset; hence patients should be observed for 2 hours after the first three doses, and for 30 minutes in subsequent doses. Anaphylactic reactions have been reported even after 1 year of regular omalizumab dosing. Hence, it should always be given under appropriate medical supervision. Other adverse effects such as injection site reaction, headache, and urticaria are minor and self-limiting.

Use in Autoimmune Bullous Diseases

Bullous Pemphigoid (Level of Evidence: 4)

A recent systematic review reported that 68% patients (36 out of 53 patients) had complete remission after omalizumab treatment, which was similar to rituximab (70% of 122 patients) in BP. However, recurrences were lesser (29% vs. 80%), and remissions were longer (10.4 vs. 3.4 months) in the rituximab group as compared to omalizumab arm.

The updated S2K guidelines for the management of BP also recommend that omalizumab should be considered for patients having urticarial plaques, high serum IgE levels, and associated neoplasia. However, a recent systematic review of 56 patients, found no difference in baseline serum IgE level (2,486.52 IU/mL vs. 4,222 IU/mL; p value = 0.84) and eosinophil count (2,631 cells/μL vs. 1,446 cells/μL; p value = 0.79) among the responders (n = 31) and partial or non-responders (n = 25).

Omalizumab appears to be a promising drug for BP without causing significant immunosuppression. It can be an option in corticosteroid-dependent and relapsing BP cases in whom other immunosuppressives are contraindicated. However, well-designed comparative trials are needed to ascertain its therapeutic status in BP.

EMERGING THERAPIES IN PEMPHIGUS

Rituximab has brought a paradigm shift in the management of AIBDs, particularly pemphigus. However, there is still a need for treatment options that have a more targeted immunosuppression with better safety profile, and that produce faster and longer remissions including a potential to cure.

The following upcoming therapies seem promising for the treatment of pemphigus (**Table 2**).

TABLE 2: Emerging therapies for the treatment of pemphigus.

Class of drug	Proposed mechanism of action	Drugs	Available evidence
Anti-CD20 antibodies (other than rituximab)	Antibody-dependent and complement-dependent lysis of B cells	Ofatumumab veltuzumab, ocrelizumab, tositumomab, obinutuzumab	Level 4
FcRn antagonist	Block the binding of IgG to FcRn, thereby accelerating their breakdown and inducing a reduction in overall plasma IgG levels	Efgartigimod	• Level 4 • Phase 3 trial undergoing
Bruton tyrosine kinase (BTK) inhibitors	BTK inhibition leading to reduced antibody production and thereby inflammatory cytokines	• Rilzabrutinib • Ibrutinib	• Level 4 • Phase 3 trial discontinued due to insignificant effect from treatment
Cholinomimetic drugs	Increase expression of desmosomes by reducing its phosphorylation	• Pilocarpine (topical) • Pyridostigmine (oral)	• Level 2b • Level 4
Stem cell therapy	Depletion of autoreactive cells and repopulation of self-tolerant cells		Level 4
CAAR-T (chimeric autoantibody receptor-T cell) therapy	CAAR-T therapy selectively targets pathological B cells and memory cells	Desmoglein 3 (Dsg3)–CAAR-T	Phase 1 clinical trial undergoing
Other potential therapies			
Phosphatidylinositol-3 kinase (PI3K)	PI3K inhibition leading to reduced activation and survival of B cells	• Paraclisib • Duvelisib	Phase 2 trial in pemphigus was discontinued due to lack of interest from participants
B-cell activating factor (BAFF) inhibitor	BAFF inhibition leading to elimination of autoreactive B cells and reduced longevity of plasma cells	• Ianalumab • VAY736	Phase 2 trial in pemphigus vulgaris was prematurely terminated
Interleukin-4 (IL-4) inhibitor	Reducing T helper 2 cytokine response leading to reduced production of anti-Dsg antibody	Dupilumab	Level 4
Polyclonal regulatory T cells (PolyTregs)	Restore the lost immune tolerance against Dsg		Phase 1 trial undergoing in pemphigus vulgaris and pemphigus foliaceus
Monoclonal antibodies targeting CD19 positive cells	Killing of long-lived plasmablasts producing anti-Dsg IgG autoantibodies	Inebilizumab	Not yet used in pemphigus

(Dsg: desmoglein)

Anti-CD20 Antibodies other than Rituximab

Anti-CD20 antibodies can be divided into two types based on the mechanism of action and site of binding. Type 1 monoclonal antibodies (rituximab, ofatumumab, veltuzumab, and ocrelizumab) mainly cause complement-dependent cytotoxic effect, whereas type 2 antibodies (tositumomab or obinutuzumab) cause direct cell death and antibody-mediated cytotoxicity, with minimal effects due to complement activation **(Table 3)**. Recently, a new mechanism, "trogocytosis" has been proposed for the action of type 1 monoclonal antibodies in which macrophages remove monoclonal antibody-CD20 complexes by transferring plasma membrane, which in turn leads to triggering of cell death. In contrast to rituximab which is chimeric, these newer anti-CD20 molecules are humanized antibodies and therefore less immunogenic, which may translate into a lesser risk of infusion reactions and potentially better long-term patient outcomes.

Among the newer anti-CD20 antibodies, veltuzumab, obinutuzumab, and ofatumumab have been tried in pemphigus. Veltuzumab and ofatumumab have been used in isolated cases of rituximab-resistant PV with excellent response and without significant adverse effects. A phase 3 clinical trial was also started for ofatumumab in PV, but it was discontinued without disclosing results due to change in sponsor of drug. Similarly, obinutuzumab has been used in a patient of follicular lymphoma with paraneoplastic pemphigus (PNP), with excellent improvement in both lymphoma and PNP. It will be interesting to compare the efficacy and safety of these newer anti-CD20 monoclonal antibodies with rituximab in larger studies.

TABLE 3: Type 1 and 2 anti-CD20 monoclonal antibodies.

	Type 1 monoclonal antibody	Type 2 monoclonal antibody
Modulation of CD20 antigen and its redistribution to lipid raft	Yes	No
Complement-dependent cytotoxicity	High	Minimal
Antibody-dependent cytotoxicity	High	High
Apoptosis induction	Caspase-dependent	Lysosome-mediated
Homotypic adhesion	Weak	Strong
Example	Rituximab, ofatumumab, veltuzumab, and ocrelizumab	Tositumomab, obinutuzumab

FcRn Antagonists

FcRn is a neonatal Fc receptor, which provides short-term humoral immunity to neonates by recycling IgG antibodies transferred from the mother. In adults, FcRn is expressed in muscles, vascular endothelial cells, and skin. FcRn-bound IgG is pinocytosed in acidic lysosomes and is released back into the circulation after recycling. This recycling process is responsible for the long half-life of IgG antibodies, and its recycling rate is around 40% higher than new IgG production. Thus, FcRn plays an important role in maintaining serum IgG levels. Anti-FcRn monoclonal antibodies like efgartigimod (recently approved for myasthenia gravis), and syntimmune bind to FcRn receptors and cause reduction in the level of circulating IgG antibodies in serum, without affecting other classes of immunoglobulins. A decrease in circulating autoantibodies can also reduce downstream inflammatory cytokines. Apart from these effects, these monoclonal antibodies also prevent FcRn-mediated presentation of antigen to IgG, which may result in inhibition of activation of T and B lymphocytes. As these drugs are acting at the downstream pathway to antibody production from B cells (unlike rituximab and steroids which mainly act at B cell level), they will hopefully be faster-acting and might require less cumulative dose of corticosteroids. However, they share the disadvantages of current therapies such as non-specific immunosuppression, parenteral route of administration, risk of infections, and short-lasting effect. As compared to IVIg, which also acts mainly at the antibody level, the anti-FcRn monoclonal antibodies do not provide multipronged immunomodulatory effects. Hence, these drugs may not be used in patients with concurrent infections. Although a rapid drop in the levels of pathogenic antibodies appears promising, its effect on other aspects of autoimmunity (such as T and B cells, plasma cells, inflammatory cytokines), as well as other parameters, such as the duration of remission, adverse effects, and development of anti-drug antibodies might decide its future in the treatment of pemphigus.

A multicenter phase 2 open-label feasibility trial of efgartigimod was conducted in 34 patients with mild-to-moderate PV or PF. About 90% of patients had early disease control after a median of 17 days with efgartigimod alone or in combination with steroids, and 64% patients reached prednisolone dose <0.5 mg/kg/day at median time of 13 weeks. IgG and anti-desmoglein antibody levels decreased and correlated with improvement in the pemphigus disease area index (PDAI) scores. Minor adverse effects were seen in 84% and 87% patients with 10 mg/kg and 25 mg/kg dose of efgartigimod, respectively, and two patients had serious adverse effects (pneumonia and tibia fracture) at 10 mg/kg dose which were probably unrelated to the drug. A phase 3 multicenter trial is currently underway which will provide better insights into its efficacy and safety profile.

Bruton Tyrosine Kinase Inhibitors

Bruton tyrosine kinase (BTK) is one of the many known signaling molecules which leads to B cell activation. BTK inhibitors act by reducing antibody production and subsequently reducing the inflammatory cytokines. Ibrutinib, a BTK inhibitor, has been approved for treatment for graft-versus-host disease, and has shown promising results in pre-clinical trials of rheumatoid arthritis.

Rilzabrutinib, an oral, reversible, covalent BTK inhibitor, has been tried in 27 PV patients (9 newly diagnosed and 18 relapsing; 11 with moderate disease and 16 with moderate-to-severe disease) in a single-arm multicenter phase 2 trial. In this trial, 52% patients achieved disease control on zero-to low-dose steroids, at 4 weeks. Common adverse effects included nausea, vomiting, and throat discomfort and only one patient developed a grade 3 adverse effect (cellulitis). Following this, a phase 3 clinical trial (PEGASUS) was conducted but showed disappointing results, with similar remission rates in the drug and placebo arms. Currently, it appears that this class of drugs may not create significant impact in the management of PV in the foreseeable future.

Cholinomimetic Drugs

Desmosomes and adherence junctions play a critical role in cell-to-cell adhesion of keratinocytes, and acetylcholine (ACh) axis increases their expression on the cell surface. Due to antibody formation against ACh (anti-ACh) receptors in pemphigus, this axis is not maintained, leading to phosphorylation of the desmosomes and weakening of intercellular adhesions. Although anti-ACh antibodies are not the primary culprit antibodies in pemphigus, they augment the effects of anti-desmosomal antibodies by reducing desmosomal expression on cell surface. Some pre-clinical studies have suggested that cholinergic drugs can prevent acantholysis in subjects without anti-ACh receptor antibodies by producing a positive effect in the ACh axis and increasing the expression of desmosomes.

Subsequently, cholinomimetic drugs such as oral pyridostigmine and topical pilocarpine have been tried in pemphigus patients. In a small, open-label study, eight patients (six PV, one PF, and one PNP) were given oral pyridostigmine alone or with low-dose corticosteroids. Complete remission was observed in one patient, partial remission in one patient and improvement in two patients, with no improvement observed in four patients. In a double-blind placebo-controlled trial, 64 cutaneous lesions in three PV patients were treated with either pilocarpine 4% gel or placebo gel. After 15 days, the epithelization index of lesions treated with topical pilocarpine was significantly better than placebo (mean 40.3 vs. 24.4, $p < 0.001$). In an open-label study, 20 PV patients having resistant oral erosions were given topical pilocarpine 2% drops, twice daily for 180 days along with continuation of systemic immunosuppression at

the same dose throughout the study. After 180 days, there was significant reduction in the mean area of erosions. Pre- and post-treatment levels of anti-desmoglein 1 and 3, and anti-ACh receptor antibodies, however, in both the serum and saliva were similar.

These preliminary studies suggest a potential adjuvant effect of cholinomimetic drugs, however this needs to be confirmed in larger studies.

Stem Cell Therapy

Stem cells are undifferentiated cells in various tissues with properties of self-renewal, differentiation, and plasticity. These cells reside in stem cell niche and help in homeostasis and tissue repair. Based on the source of these cells, they can be divided into embryonic, somatic, and induced pluripotent cells. In autoimmune diseases, hematopoietic stem cells have been used which cause the depletion of autoreactive cells and re-population of self-tolerant cells. Hematopoietic cells can be taken from self-donor (autologous) or human leukocyte antigen (HLA)-matched donor (allogenic). Stem cell therapy has been reported in recalcitrant pemphigus with both autologous and allogenic stem cell transplantation from various centers (including a series of 11 patients from Ahmedabad, India). Among all reported patients, 90–100% patients achieved clinical remission on tapering the dose of steroids at 6 months, and around 75–100% patients had drug-free remission at 5 years in various series. Most common adverse effects were infection including sepsis, and one patient died among the 24 reported cases. Major disadvantages of this treatment are high cost, risk of infection, and complications of stem cell treatment such as graft-versus-host disease and Epstein–Barr virus-associated lymphoproliferative disorders. As safer and cheaper alternatives such as rituximab have become available, stem cell therapy has not gained much popularity in the management of pemphigus. Stem cell therapy has also been discussed in Chapter 25.

Chimeric Autoantibody Receptor-T Cell Therapy

Chimeric antigen receptor (CAR) technology is a promising emerging treatment for cancers and autoimmune diseases. CAR is an antigen receptor which directs T cells towards the cells expressing target antigens in a major histocompatibility complex (MHC)-independent manner. In this therapy, engineered CAR is inserted into isolated and activated T cells of the host via viral or non-viral technology. These CAR-T cells are infused back into the patients after multiplication and this leads to the selective destruction of target cells.

In AIBDs, T cells expressing chimeric autoantibody receptor T (CAAR-T cells) targeting pathogenic B cells is the latest treatment model. In pre-clinical studies, CAAR-T cells created by combining desmoglein 3 to the various signaling domains were able to eliminate autoreactive B cells with minimal toxicity. If effective in clinical setting, it will not only act as a specific immunosuppressant, but might also lead to long remissions or even cure of pemphigus by depleting the memory B cells. Due to the small number of target cells, adverse effects such as cytokine release and tumor lysis syndrome are also theoretically less expected as compared to in cancers.

The major postulated limitation of this therapy is the presence of multiple pathogenic antibodies in pemphigus besides desmoglein 3, hence targeting single type of such T cells might not provide an expected clinical remission or cure. Another limitation might be the high cost associated with this treatment. FDA has approved tisagenlecleucel, a CD19-targeted CAAR-T for the treatment of hematological malignancy. For mucosal pemphigus, desmoglein 3–CAAR-T is under phase 1 trial, which is expected to be completed in 2026.

CONCLUSION

Systemic corticosteroids and rituximab have brought a paradigm shift in the management of AIBDs, but search for more effective and safer treatments continues. In this chapter, we have discussed a few other therapeutic interventions including some emerging treatments. The newer treatment options appear promising, but large-scale trials are needed to confirm their therapeutic status in the management of AIBDs.

TAKE HOME MESSAGE

- IVIg is a fast-acting immunomodulatory drug which is mainly used for rapid control of the disease ("crisis") and in patients with concomitant infections. Various dosing schedules and combinations with other immuno-suppressive drugs have been tried.
- Omalizumab has shown promising results as an immunomodulatory adjuvant in bullous pemphigoid. However, its exact therapeutic status in the management of bullous pemphigoid, and factors predicting good response to omalizumab remain to be identified.
- Some of the newer promising therapies for pemphigus include newer anti-CD20 antibodies, FcRn antagonists, BTK inhibitors, cholinomimetic drugs, stem cell therapy, and CAAR-T therapy.
- These newer targeted therapies have been proposed largely based on the experience in other immunological diseases, and large-scale controlled clinical trials are needed to ascertain their utility in AIBDs.

MULTIPLE CHOICE QUESTIONS

1. **Which of the following anti-CD20 monoclonal antibody acts by direct cell death and antibody-mediated cytotoxicity, without activation of complements?**
    (a) Ofatumumab
    (b) Veltuzumab
    (c) Rituximab
    (d) Obinutuzumab

2. **Which of the following statements regarding omalizumab is correct?**
    (a) Omalizumab is a chimeric monoclonal antibody
    (b) Omalizumab is first-line drug for treatment of bullous pemphigoid
    (c) Remission rates achieved in bullous pemphigoid by omalizumab and rituximab are comparable
    (d) Relapse rates in bullous pemphigoid by omalizumab and rituximab are comparable

3. **Which of the following drugs acts by reducing IgG levels by inhibiting recycling of circulating IgG?**
    (a) Veltuzumab
    (b) Rilzabrutinib
    (c) Efgartigimod
    (d) Paraclisib

4. **Which of the following statements about CAAR-T therapy is true?**
    (a) It has been first proposed and developed exclusively for pemphigus
    (b) It is an FDA approved drug for pemphigus vulgaris
    (c) It has been approved for treatment of diffuse large B cell lymphoma and follicular lymphoma
    (d) It acts primarily by inhibiting formation of pathological T cells

5. **Which of the following drugs is NOT likely to be helpful in management of pemphigus vulgaris?**
    (a) Tropicamide
    (b) Pilocarpine
    (c) Pyridostigmine
    (d) Edrophonium

6. **Which of the following are absolute contraindications for IVIg?**
    i.   IgA deficiency
    ii. Anti-IgA antibodies
    iii. Sepsis
    iv. History of anaphylaxis in IgA deficient patients

Choose combination of correct answers:

(a) i, ii, iii

(b) iii only

(c) i, ii, iv

(d) iv only

7. **Phase 2 in Ahmed protocol for treatment of autoimmune bullous diseases is:**

(a) Immune depletion phase

(b) B cell re-population phase

(c) Clinical remission phase

(d) Immune restoration phase

8. **CAAR-T therapy for pemphigus vulgaris is in which phase of clinical trial?**

(a) Pre-clinical phase

(b) Phase 1

(c) Phase 2

(d) Phase 3

9. **CAAR-T therapy is reminiscent of which organism?**

(a) Leopard

(b) Zebra

(c) Angler fish

(d) Crocodile

10. **Which of the following drugs is available in oral formulation?**

(a) Rilzabrutinib

(b) Veltuzumab

(c) Efgartigimod

(d) Omalizumab

Answers

1. (d) 2. (c) 3. (c) 4. (c) 5. (a) 6. (d) 7. (b) 8. (b) 9 (c) 10 (a)

SUGGESTED READING

1. Ahmed AR, Dahl MV. Consensus statement on the use of intravenous immunoglobulin therapy in the treatment of autoimmune mucocutaneous blistering diseases. *Arch Dermatol.* 2003;139:1051-9.

2. Ahmed AR, Spigelman Z, Cavacini LA, Posner MR. Treatment of pemphigus vulgaris with rituximab and intravenous immune globulin. *N Engl J Med.* 2006;355:1772-9.

3. Czernik A, Toosi S, Bystryn JC, Grando SA. Intravenous immuno-globulin in the treatment of autoimmune bullous dermatoses: an update. *Autoimmunity.* 2012;45:111-8.

4. Cao P, Xu W, Zhang L. Rituximab, omalizumab, and dupilumab treatment outcomes in bullous pemphigoid: a systematic review. *Front Immunol.* 2022;13:928621.

5. Borradori L, Beek N van, Feliciani C, Tedbirt B, Antiga E, Bergman R, *et al.* Updated S2 K guidelines for the management of bullous pemphigoid initiated by the European Academy of Dermatology and Venereology (EADV). *J Eur Acad Dermatol Venereol.* 2022;36: 1689-704.

6. Goebeler M, Bata-Csörgő Z, de Simone C, Didona B, Remenyik E, Reznichenko N, *et al.* Treatment of pemphigus vulgaris and foliaceus with efgartigimod, a neonatal Fc receptor inhibitor: a phase II multicentre, open-label feasibility trial. *Br J Dermatol.* 2022;186:429-39.

7. D'Aguanno K, Gabrielli S, Ouchene L, Muntyanu A, Ben-Shoshan M, Zhang X, *et al.* Omalizumab for the treatment of bullous pemphigoid: a systematic review of efficacy and safety. *J Cutan Med Surg.* 2022;26:404-13.

8. Didona D, Maglie R, Eming R, Hertl M. Pemphigus: current and future therapeutic strategies. *Front Immunol.* 2019;10:1418.

CHAPTER 25

Miscellaneous Therapies

Krina Bharat Patel, Pooja Desai

- Plasmapheresis
- Immunoadsorption
- Extracorporeal photopheresis
- Stem cell therapy

INTRODUCTION

Autoimmune bullous diseases (AIBDs) cause significant morbidity and mortality requiring prompt intervention. Several therapeutic modalities are available such as systemic corticosteroids, oral immunosuppressive and anti-inflammatory agents, and biologics, with majority of the patients responding to these agents. In recalcitrant cases, interventions such as plasmapheresis, immunoadsorption, stem cell therapy and other miscellaneous, and experimental treatments, either used alone or in combination with conventional agents, may be helpful.

PLASMAPHERESIS

Plasmapheresis was first successfully used in the autoimmune disease Goodpasture's syndrome in 1975. It was first applied in the treatment of pemphigus vulgaris (PV) after 3 years. Since then, many case reports and series demonstrating its effectiveness in inducing partial or complete remission in recalcitrant AIBDs have been published.

Principle of the Procedure

Plasmapheresis is an extracorporeal blood purification procedure in which plasma proteins are non-selectively removed from the circulation. In this process, patient's blood is continuously driven from the body and separated in to plasma and cellular components by a plasma separator. The cellular components are then returned to the patient's circulation, whereas plasma is replaced with plasma substitutes such as albumin or fresh frozen plasma **(Fig. 1)**.

There is no standardized protocol for plasmapheresis in AIBDs. Many experts suggest 4–5 plasma exchanges, each consisting of around 1–1.5 plasma exchanges, over a period of 7–10 days, while others suggest one or two plasma exchanges. Plasmapheresis can be done using the conventional blood centrifuge device, but recently double-

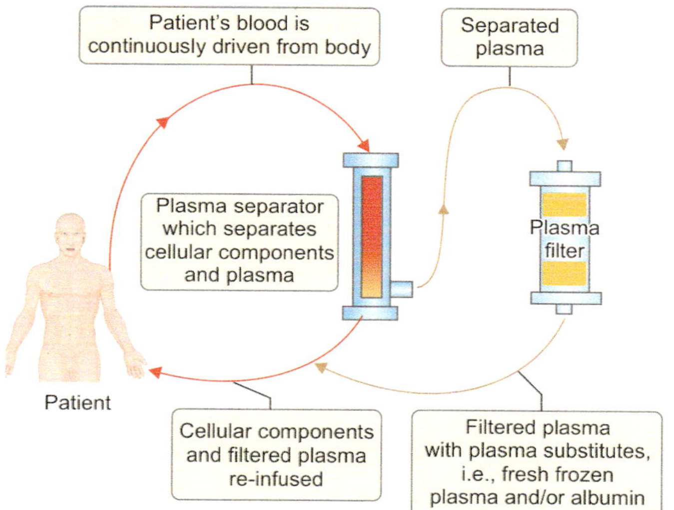

Fig. 1: Schematic diagram showing the procedure of plasmapheresis.

plasmapheresis is being used to selectively remove the immunoglobulins and reduce albumin loss.

Rationale in AIBDs

The rationale behind the procedure is that disease severity correlates with the titers of circulating pathogenic antibodies. However, plasmapheresis only removes the antibodies but does not halt their production, as after their removal there is a negative feedback to the effector B-cells leading to rebound production of these antibodies. Antibody titers have been shown to increase as early as within 3 hours of the procedure and reach pre-treatment levels or even higher within 7–14 days after plasmapheresis. This rebound increase can be prevented by giving concomitant immuno-suppressive therapy which halts antibody production by destroying the active B-cells, thereby providing long-lasting effect of plasmapheresis.

Safety Profile

It is a relatively safe procedure. In patients with compromised cardiac function or problems of fluid overload, it can cause hypertension, pulmonary edema, and severe problems of homeostasis. Adverse events reported post-plasmapheresis include thrombocytopenia, hypogammaglobulinemia, hypoproteinemia, anemia, leukopenia, hypocalcemia, and risk of infection (due to concomitant use of immuno-suppressive agents).

IMMUNOADSORPTION

Immunoadsorption (immunopheresis) of plasma with protein A cellulose columns was first developed in the 1970s to selectively remove immunoglobulin G (IgG) antibodies from plasma. It is also an extracorporeal blood purification procedure that leads to the removal of disease-specific antibodies such as anti-desmoglein 1 (Dsg1) and 3 antibodies in PV and other disease-specific antibodies in other AIBDs.

Rationale in AIBDs

Immunoadsorption is more safe and efficient than plasmapheresis as it selectively removes disease-specific immunoglobulins and immune complexes. Other blood components such as hormones, albumin and clotting factors are not affected, thereby mitigating the need for plasma substitutes.

Principle of the Procedure

Immunoadsorption is done by removing blood from the patient's body and then separating it into plasma and cellular components. Plasma is passed through columns with specific ligands to remove specific immunoglobulins. The absorbed plasma is then re-infused into the patient's circulation along with cellular components **(Fig. 2)**.

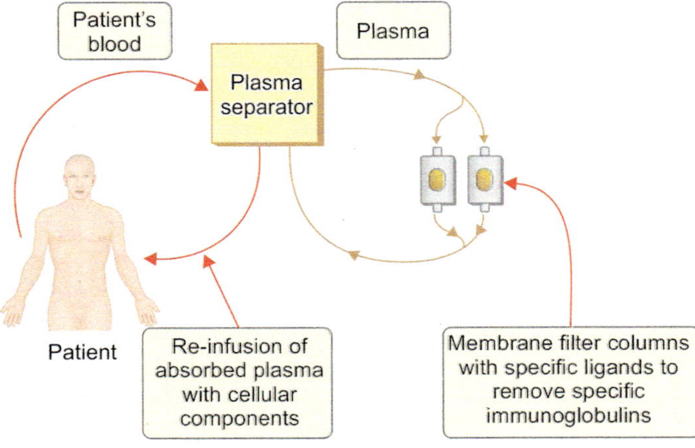

Fig. 2: Schematic diagram showing steps of immunoadsorption.

It was claimed that after a single cycle of immuno-adsorption and immunoadsorption sessions on 3 consecutive days, IgG concentration against Dsg1 and 3 could be reduced by 75% and 95%, respectively. The recommended sessions include four treatments on 4 consecutive days (usually 2.5-fold plasma volume/day). The procedure is repeated after 4 weeks, if required. The efficacy of immunoadsorption is enhanced by concomitant treatment with immunosuppressive agents to reduce rebound production of antibodies.

Safety Profile

It is usually well tolerated. It is superior to plasmapheresis in terms of safety and efficacy. Less common adverse effects include hypotension, anaphylaxis, bradycardia, deep vein thrombosis, and herpes zoster infection.

Contraindications to immunoadsorption are cardio-vascular diseases, sepsis, treatment with angiotensin-converting enzyme inhibitors, bleeding diathesis, and hypersensitivity to components of the immunoadsorption column.

EXTRACORPOREAL PHOTOPHERESIS

Extracorporeal photopheresis (ECP) was introduced in the early 1980s for the palliative treatment of erythrodermic cutaneous T-cell lymphoma and it is FDA approved for the same. ECP is also advocated for other chronic skin conditions such as chronic graft-versus-host disease, PV, atopic dermatitis, systemic sclerosis, and systemic lupus erythematosus.

ECP is based on the principle that infusion of autologous haptenated cells in which apoptosis is induced by 8-methoxypsoralen/ultraviolet A (8-MOP/UVA), produces immunological tolerance. This immunological tolerance is due to the induction of regulatory T cells (Tregs), which may be the reason behind the beneficial effect of ECP in a wide range of inflammatory diseases, and with no generalized immunosuppression after ECP therapy.

Principle of the Procedure

The process involves the passage of blood from an arm vein through a photopheresis machine and then back into the patient's circulation. Discontinuous flow cell separator in the machine harvests peripheral blood mononuclear cells (PBMC) within the buffy coat collection. The red cell component is returned to the patient without any further treatment. In the PBMC fraction, 8-MOP solution is directly added. This is then exposed to 2 J/cm^2 of UVA light and re-infused into the patient's circulation **(Fig. 3)**. The procedure is usually undertaken on 2 successive days and repeated after 2–4 weeks interval.

Multiple case reports have shown efficacy of ECP in drug-resistant PV, pemphigus foliaceus, and epidermolysis bullosa acquisita.

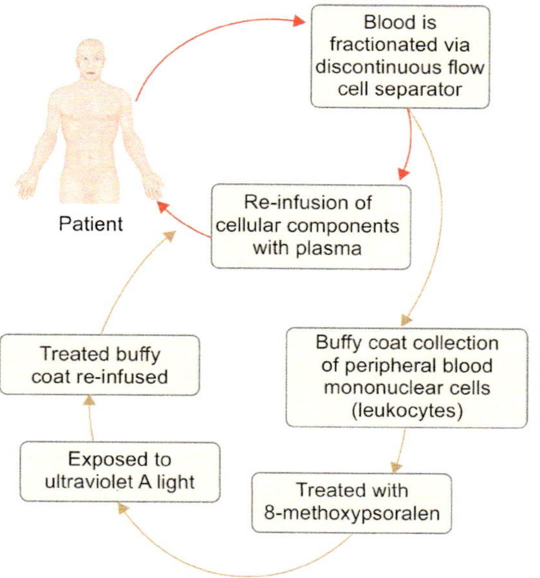

Fig. 3: Schematic diagram showing steps of extracorporeal photopheresis.

Safety Profile

ECP is a safe modality and adverse effects are generally uncommon. Hypotension, dizziness, temporary itching, low-grade fever and vasovagal reflex due to volume shifts during treatment, have been reported.

STEM CELL THERAPY

Stem cells are those which have the ability to differentiate into different types of cells, and are present in many tissues. Stem cells have three characteristics—(1) self-renewal (2) differentiation, and (3) plasticity. On the basis of their differentiation capacity, they are classified as totipotent, pluripotent, multipotent, oligopotent, and unipotent **(Fig. 4)**. Based on their source, they may be embryonic, somatic (adult) and induced pluripotent stem cells.

Stem cell transplantation (SCT) is a procedure in which a patient (recipient) receives healthy stem cells to replace damaged or diseased cells. SCT is of two types, autologous (patient's own cells), and allogeneic (stem cells from donor).

In refractory cases of PV, hematopoietic stem cell transplantation (HSCT) using different mobilization and conditioning regimens, has been used with success. The onset of response is as early as 24 hours postHSCT, with remissions occurring at 2–9 months and disease-free period varying from 5 months to 8 years.

Hematopoietic stem cells (HSCs) work by repopulating the immune system, which leads to decline in autoreactive immune cells and this helps in restoring the balance in the immune system. Allogeneic HSCs have also been transplanted into the thymus, bone marrow, and periphery for treatment of refractory pemphigus.

Safety Profile

Infection is the most common adverse event. Culture-negative neutropenic fever, nausea, anorexia, arthralgia, arthritis, headache, transaminitis, sepsis, and occasionally death, have been reported with this therapy.

CONCLUSION

The above therapies provide an impetus to the treatment of recalcitrant AIBDs. However, their lack of easy accessibility and expertise in many centers is a limiting factor in exploring their utility optimally.

TAKE HOME MESSAGE

- In patients who are resistant or intolerant to conventional modalities, miscellaneous therapies such as plasmapheresis, immunoadsorption, ECP, and stem cell therapy may provide a ray of hope.

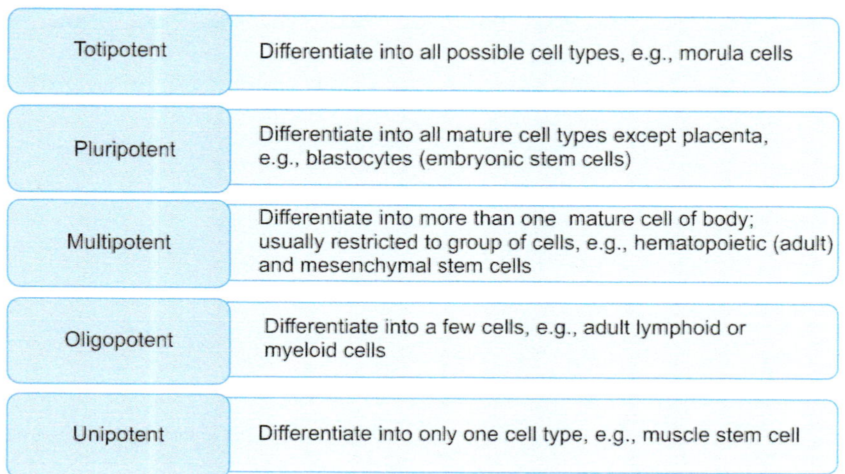

Fig. 4: Classification of stem cells based on their differentiation capacity.

- Plasmapheresis and immunoadsorption are extracorporeal blood purification procedures, of which immunoadsorption is superior as it selectively removes pathogenic IgG antibodies.
- ECP is based on the principle that infusion of autologous haptenated cells in which apoptosis is induced by 8-MOP/UVA, produces immunological tolerance, thereby producing benefit in inflammatory diseases including AIBDs, without causing generalized immunosuppression.
- Both autologous hematopoietic stem cell therapy and allogeneic stem cell transplant have shown benefit in recalcitrant pemphigus.

MULTIPLE CHOICE QUESTIONS

1. **Plasmapheresis is an extracorporeal blood purification procedure in which plasma proteins are _______________ removed from the circulation.**
   - (a) Selectively
   - (b) Non-selectively
   - (c) All of the above
   - (d) None of the above

2. **Extracorporeal photopheresis is FDA approved for:**
   - (a) Pemphigus vulgaris
   - (b) Bullous pemphigoid
   - (c) Erythrodermic cutaneous T-cell lymphoma
   - (d) Graft-versus-host disease (GvHD)

3. **In extracorporeal photopheresis, which solution is added to the cellular component?**
   - (a) 8-methoxypsoralen (8-MOP)
   - (b) 4, 5, 8 trimethylpsoralen (trimop)
   - (c) 5-methoxypsoralen (5-MOP)
   - (d) 6-methoxypsoralen (6-MOP)

4. **All are correct in the classification of stem cells according to differential capacity, *except*:**
   - (a) Totipotent.
   - (b) Multipotent
   - (c) Embryonic
   - (d) Pluripotent

5. **The rebound increase in antibody titers after plasmapheresis can be prevented by:**
   - (a) Giving immunosuppressant therapy in combination with plasmapheresis
   - (b) Giving frequent plasmapheresis
   - (c) Giving immunosuppressant before plasmapheresis
   - (d) Giving immunosuppressant one month after plasmapheresis

6. **How much decrease in plasma titer of antibodies occurs after single session of immunoadsorption?**
   - (a) 75%
   - (b) 80%
   - (c) 95%
   - (d) 85%

7. **Stem cells are not transplanted into:**
   - (a) Bone marrow
   - (b) Thymus
   - (c) Periphery
   - (d) Skin

8. **Which light rays are used for extracorporeal photopheresis?**
   - (a) UVB
   - (b) UVA
   - (c) Infrared
   - (d) Visible light

9. **How much plasma volume exchange is done in one day session of immunoadsorption?**
   - (a) 1 fold of plasma volume
   - (b) 1.5 fold of plasma volume
   - (c) 2 fold of plasma volume
   - (d) 2.5 fold of plasma volume

10. **Plasmapheresis is a more efficient modality than immunoadsorption in treatment of refractory cases of pemphigus:**
    - (a) True
    - (b) False

Answers

1. (b)   2. (c)   3. (a)   4. (c)   5. (a)   6. (a)   7. (d)   8. (b)   9. (d)   10. (b)

SUGGESTED READING

1. Ranugha P, Kumari R, Kartha LB, Parameswaran S, Thappa DM. Therapeutic plasma exchange as a crisis option in severe pemphigus vulgaris. *Indian J Dermatol Venereol Leprol*. 2012; 78:508-10.

2. Knobler R, Arenberger P, Arun A, Assaf C, Bagot M, Berlin G, *et al*. European dermatology forum: Updated guidelines on the use of extracorporeal photopheresis 2020—Part 2. *J Eur Acad Dermatol Venereol*. 2021;35:27-49.

3. Mazzi G, Raineri A, Zanolli FA, Da Ponte C, De Roia D, Santarossa L, *et al*. Plasmapheresis therapy in pemphigus vulgaris and bullous pemphigoid. *Transfus Apher Sci*. 2003;28:13-8.

4. Eming R, Hertl M. Immunoadsorption in pemphigus. *Auto-immunity*. 2006;39:609-16.

5. Sen S, Rudra O, Gayen T. Extracorporeal therapy in dermatology. *Indian J Dermatol*. 2021;66:386-92.

6. Khandpur S, Gupta S, Gunaabalaji DR. Stem cell therapy in dermatology. *Indian J Dermatol Venereol Leprol*. 2021;87:753-67.

CHAPTER 26

Treatment Guidelines, Consensus Statements, Appraisal of Evidence for Pemphigus and other Autoimmune Bullous Diseases, Management in COVID Era

Dipankar De, Hitaishi Mehta, Rahul Mahajan

- Treatment guidelines for:
  - Pemphigus vulgaris
  - Bullous pemphigoid
  - Mucous membrane pemphigoid
  - Epidermolysis bullosa acquisita
  - Dermatitis herpetiformis
- Management of autoimmune bullous diseases in the COVID era

INTRODUCTION

Autoimmune bullous diseases (AIBDs) are a group of potentially life-threatening disorders. Management guidelines have been proposed for AIBDs from various regions of the globe. However, a universal standard of care is lacking. Most guidelines are consensus-based and cater to the prevalent healthcare system. Some recommendations made in these guidelines may not be feasible or applicable to the Indian scenario. This chapter summarizes the guidelines by various expert groups in order to provide a collective assessment of management recommendations. Special considerations in the management of AIBDs during the coronavirus disease 2019 (COVID-19) era are also enumerated. Since the evidence for management of these diseases is evolving, so are the guidelines. The readers are expected to update themselves with the evolving management strategies.

PEMPHIGUS VULGARIS

Corticosteroids are recommended as first-line therapy in all the pemphigus guidelines. The European and British guidelines recommend oral prednisolone in combination with adjuvants. British guidelines recommend intravenous pulsed corticosteroids as first-line therapy in patients with severe disease. If the disease is not controlled with the recommended dose of systemic corticosteroids alone for baseline, the dose may be increased and an adjuvant should be considered. If the patient is already receiving an adjuvant, switching to an alternative adjuvant may be considered.

Rituximab is now recommended as the first-line treatment option for management of moderate-to-severe pemphigus vulgaris (PV), alone (in mild disease) or in combination with corticosteroids. The European guidelines recommend rituximab as first-line therapy in mild pemphigus as well. Rituximab-treated patients with relapse should be managed with an additional infusion cycle. Other adjuvants are not usually combined with rituximab due to the potential of severe immunosuppression. Mycophenolate mofetil (MMF) and azathioprine, as adjuvants to systemic corticosteroids, are favored over other immunosuppressants in most guidelines. The European and British guidelines do not recommend cyclosporine for the management of pemphigus. Methotrexate is recommended as a third-line treatment option in the British and Brazilian guidelines. European guidelines do not recommend methotrexate for the treatment of pemphigus. **Table 1** compares the European, Brazilian, and British guidelines for the management of PV.

Critical Appraisal of Current Guidelines

- Steroid-tapering schemes have not been clearly delineated, particularly when corticosteroids are used in combination with adjuvants.
- Pneumocystis pneumonia (PCP) is a potentially life-threatening complication of immunosuppression. In rheumatology patients, prophylaxis against PCP is recommended in patients receiving >20 mg of prednisolone per day in combination with a second immunosuppressive agent. PCP prophylaxis may be considered in pemphigus patients, particularly in those receiving rituximab infusions. Real-world studies from pemphigus patients not receiving routine PCP prophylaxis have observed the incidence of PCP to be low.
- European Academy of Dermatology and Venereology (EADV) guidelines recommend determination of serum levels of anti-desmoglein 1 (Dsg1) and/or Dsg3 by enzyme-linked immunosorbent assay (ELISA) at baseline, after 3 months and thereafter every 3–6 months. In patients attaining clinical remission with rituximab treatment, maintenance infusion (rituximab

TABLE 1: Comparison of guidelines for the management of pemphigus vulgaris.

	European Academy of Dermatology and Venereology	Brazilian Society of Dermatology	British Association of Dermatologists
Year of publication	2020	2019	2017
First-line	• Rituximab, alone or with systemic corticosteroids • Prednisolone with or without azathioprine or MMF	• *Mild*: Oral corticosteroids • *Moderate*: Prednisone + azathioprine • *Severe*: Prednisone or methylprednisolone + azathioprine	Systemic corticosteroids + azathioprine or MMF or rituximab
Second-line	Higher dose of systemic corticosteroids; add immunosuppressants in patients treated with prednisolone alone	• *Mild*: Dapsone, MMF or azathioprine • *Moderate*: Rituximab • *Severe*: IVIg and/or rituximab	Switch to alternate immunosuppressive agent
Third-line	Cyclophosphamide	Cyclophosphamide, methotrexate, cyclosporine, immunoadsorption	Cyclophosphamide, methotrexate, immunoadsorption, plasma exchange, IVIg
Refractory cases	IVIg, immunoadsorption, intravenous corticosteroid pulse		IVIg, immunoadsorption, plasma exchange

(IVIg: intravenous immunoglobulin; MMF: mycophenolate mofetil)

500 mg or 1 g) is recommended in patients who initially presented with severe disease or had high anti-Dsg antibody titers at month 3. Maintenance treatment with rituximab 500 mg is recommended at months 12 and 18, particularly in patients with persistent anti-Dsg antibodies. However, it is difficult for the management to be guided based on immunological parameters instead of clinical parameters in resource-constrained settings.

BULLOUS PEMPHIGOID

The current European guidelines recommend diagnosis of bullous pemphigoid (BP) based on the following criteria:

- *Three out of four clinical characteristics*: Age >70 years, absence of atrophic scarring, absence of mucosal involvement, absence of predominant bullous lesions on the head and neck
- Positive direct immunofluorescence (DIF)
- Presence of IgG antibodies binding to the epidermal side on salt-split skin on indirect immunofluorescence (IIF) and/or raised anti-BP180 or anti-BP230 by ELISA.

The EADV guidelines recommend use of superpotent topical corticosteroid (clobetasol propionate, 0.05% cream), 20–30 g/day in mild-to-moderate disease [mild disease— Bullous Pemphigoid Disease Activity Index (BPDAI) score <20 and moderate disease—BPDAI score ≥20 and <57] and 30–40 g/day in extensive disease (BPDAI score ≥57), initially administered once or twice daily, over the entire body including both normal and diseased skin (except the face), until control of disease activity is achieved (till new lesions cease to form and existing lesions begin to heal). Once control is attained, progressive tapering over the next 4–12 months is recommended.

An initial prednisolone dose of 0.5 mg/kg/day is recommended in patients with mild/moderate and severe BP. The dose is gradually tapered to 0.1 mg/kg/day within 6 months of treatment initiation. In patients with

corticosteroid-dependent, relapsing or recalcitrant BP, immunosuppressive agents such as azathioprine, MMF, and methotrexate are recommended. In patients with poor general condition or in those with contraindications to immunosuppressives, dapsone, omalizumab, and doxycycline may be considered. **Table 2** compares the European, Japanese, Brazilian, British, Italian, and German guidelines for the management of BP.

Critical Appraisal of the Guidelines

- As average life expectancy in India is 70 years, the clinical diagnostic criteria of age >70 years may not be applicable to Indian scenario.
- IIF and ELISA to confirm the diagnosis of BP may not be feasible due to scarce availability and affordability issues with these investigations. However, serration pattern analysis on DIF can be adopted and is helpful in reaching a diagnosis in an appropriate clinical setting with reasonable accuracy.
- Cost of topical steroid therapy may be prohibitive in their use as first-line treatment modality in BP patients.
- As patients are generally cared for by relatives or by themselves, topical application of topical corticosteroids twice a day may be a difficult proposition. It is also often considered messy to be applied on eroded skin.
- The current European guidelines mention the importance of a thorough drug history in BP patients, particularly for gliptins and immune checkpoint inhibitors. However, the effect of cessation of the triggering drug on disease prognosis is unclear and the guidelines suggest that switch to an alternative agent may be considered.
- The clinician should be aware of the various co-morbidities associated with BP such as neurological and cardiovascular diseases, thrombo-embolism, osteoporosis and autoimmune diseases, and related history and examination findings should be sought.

TABLE 2: Comparison of treatment guidelines for the management of bullous pemphigoid.

Treatment recommen- dation	European Academy of Dermatology and Venereology	Japanese Dermatological Association	Brazilian Society of Dermatology	British Association of Dermatologists	Italian guidelines	German guidelines
Year	2022	2019	2018	2012	2018	2021
First-line	Superpotent TCS for localized disease, oral corticosteroids for non-localized disease	• *Mild*: TCS + adjuvants • *Moderate/severe*: Oral corticosteroids + TCS ± tetracycline/minocycline + nicotinamide, dapsone	• *Localized*: TCS • *Extensive*: Oral corticosteroids + TCS	• *Mild*: TCS, oral corticosteroids ± TCS, anti-inflammatory antibiotics ± nicotinamide • *Moderate/severe*: Oral corticosteroids ± TCS, TCS, anti-inflammatory antibiotics ± nicotinamide	• *Localized disease with mild activity*: TCS (localized disease—lesions only, mild disease—whole body except face) • *Generalized*: TCS on whole body except face, oral corticosteroids	• *Mild*: TCS • *Moderate*: TCS ± oral corticosteroids or adjuvants • *Severe*: TCS + oral corticosteroids or adjuvants
Second-line	Doxycycline, dapsone	• *Mild*: manage as severe • *Moderate/severe*: Addition of adjuvants	• *Extensive*: Adjuvants • *Mucosal*: Dapsone	Consider switching to or the addition of adjuvants	• *Localized disease with mild activity*: Adjuvants, topical tacrolimus, oral corticosteroids • *Generalized*: Adjuvants	-
Adjuvants	Methotrexate, MMF/MPA, azathioprine	• *Mild*: Tetracycline/minocycline + nicotinamide, dapsone, oral corticosteroids • *Moderate/severe*: Azathioprine, cyclosporine, mizoribine, oral cyclophosphamide, dapsone, MMF, MPA, methotrexate, intravenous cyclophosphamide pulse, IVIg	Oxytetracycline, doxycycline ± nicotinamide, azathioprine, MMF, methotrexate, dapsone, chlorambucil	Oral corticosteroids ± TCS, anti-inflammatory antibiotics ± nicotinamide, azathioprine, methotrexate, dapsone, chlorambucil, MMF	• *Mild disease*: Tetracycline + nicotinamide, dapsone, sulfonamide • *Generalized*: Tetracycline + nicotinamide, azathioprine, MMF, methotrexate, chlorambucil	Dapsone, doxycycline ± nicotinamide, azathioprine, MMF, methotrexate
Refractory cases	Rituximab, omalizumab, dupilumab, IVIg, immunoadsorption	Intravenous cyclophosphamide pulse, plasma exchange, rituximab	Rituximab, omalizumab, IVIg, plasma exchange, oral cyclophosphamide	IVIg, cyclophosphamide, plasma exchange	Rituximab, omalizumab, IVIg, immunoadsorption, plasma exchange, cyclophosphamide	Rituximab, omalizumab, IVIg, immunoadsorption, cyclophosphamide

(IVIg: intravenous immunoglobulin; MMF: mycophenolate mofetil; MPA: mycophenolic acid; TCS: topical corticosteroids)

European guidelines also recommend relevant workup, including mental status examination, osteodensitometry, echocardiography, and an age-appropriate malignancy screening.

MUCOUS MEMBRANE PEMPHIGOID

The European S3 guidelines of mucous membrane pemphigoid (MMP) defines mild/moderate MMP as a disease involving the oral mucosa, with or without skin involvement. Severe MMP involves the following extraoral mucosae: ocular, genital, nasopharyngeal, laryngeal, and/or esophageal mucosa. The diagnosis is based on clinical findings along with the detection of anti-BMZ antibodies by DIF, IIF, ELISA, or immunoblotting. Nearly 50% patients with ocular MMP do not meet the immunopathological criteria for the diagnosis of MMP. In such patients, diagnosis of ocular MMP should be made when compatible clinical features are present and other cicatricial conjunctival diseases have been excluded.

Management strategy depends on whether only oral mucosa or other mucosae are also involved. Since extraoral involvement may be associated with the potential for significant morbidity, these patients need to be managed with more aggression.

For the management of mild-to-moderate disease, first-line management options include dapsone, methotrexate, tetracycline, and/or topical corticosteroids. In patients with treatment failure, contraindications or intolerance to first-line therapies, the second-line treatment options include dapsone in combination with tetracyclines, topical corticosteroids, oral corticosteroids or MMF; azathioprine or methotrexate with oral corticosteroids. In patients with severe MMP, first-line treatment is dapsone in combination with oral or intravenous cyclophosphamide, with or without oral corticosteroids. In patients with therapeutic failure, contraindications, or intolerance, dapsone in combination with rituximab is recommended. Addition of intravenous immunoglobulin (IVIg) and tumor necrosis factor alpha (TNF-α) inhibitor may be considered as third- and fourth-line therapies, respectively. **Table 3** compares the management guidelines for MMP recommended by the European, Japanese, Brazilian, and International consensus guidelines.

Critical Appraisal of the Guidelines

- The diagnosis of MMP is hampered by low-serum autoantibody titers and unavailability of standardized assays for the detection of autoantibodies against the diverse target antigens.
- As per the European S3 guidelines, determination of positivity for anti-laminin 332 antibodies is warranted. If these are detected, a malignancy screen is warranted. Larger prospective studies are however required to determine the extent of association between anti-laminin 332 MMP and internal organ malignancy.
- All guidelines recommend the use of oral corticosteroids along with an immunosuppressant in patients with severe disease. Intravenous pulsed cyclophosphamide and corticosteroids are recommended for rapidly progressive severe disease. Most guidelines are based on uncontrolled studies and expert opinion due to lack of randomized controlled trial (RCT) data in MMP patients.
- A growing body of evidence suggests that rituximab is effective in MMP.

TABLE 3: Comparison of guidelines for the management of mucous membrane pemphigoid.

Treatment recommendation	European Academy of Dermatology and Venereology	Japanese Dermatological Association	Brazilian Society of Dermatology	International Consensus
Year	2021	2019	2018	2002
First-line	• *Mild/moderate*: Dapsone, methotrexate, tetracycline and/or topical corticosteroids • *Severe*: Dapsone in combination with oral or intravenous cyclophosphamide, with or without oral corticosteroids	• *Mild/moderate*: Topical corticosteroids + tetracycline/minocycline, nicotinamide, dapsone • *Severe*: Oral corticosteroids with azathioprine or cyclophosphamide	• *Mild/moderate*: Topical corticosteroids, intralesional corticosteroids, adjuvants • *Severe*: Oral corticosteroids, azathioprine, cyclophosphamide, MMF	• *Mild/moderate*: Topical corticosteroids • *Severe*: Dapsone (50–200 mg/day) for 3 months. If response not satisfactory, oral corticosteroids + cyclophosphamide (oral/intravenous) or azathioprine
Second-line	• *Mild/moderate*: Dapsone + tetracyclines/topical corticosteroids/oral corticosteroids/MMF/azathioprine, or methotrexate with oral corticosteroids • *Severe*: Dapsone + rituximab	• *Mild/moderate*: Treat as severe disease • *Severe*: Oral corticosteroids with MMF, methotrexate, IV corticosteroid pulse, IVIg or plasma exchange	• *Mild/moderate*: Dapsone, oral corticosteroids, anti-inflammatory antibiotics • *Severe*: Oral corticosteroids + IV cyclophosphamide, IVIg, rituximab	• *Mild/moderate*: Tetracyclines + nicotinamide • *Severe*: Oral corticosteroids + cyclophosphamide (oral/intravenous)
Refractory disease	Add IVIg, TNF-α inhibitor	IV cyclophosphamide, rituximab	TNF-α inhibitors (etanercept, infliximab)	IVIg

(IV: intravenous; IVIg: intravenous immunoglobulin; MMF: mycophenolate mofetil; TNF-α: tumor necrosis factor alpha)

EPIDERMOLYSIS BULLOSA ACQUISITA

The Brazilian and French guidelines define severe disease as EBA involving the ocular, laryngeal, and esophageal mucosa or EBA with widespread skin involvement. The BPDAI is recommended as the standard tool for assessing disease severity in EBA patients. The first-line management options include topical corticosteroids, colchicine, and dapsone. Severe EBA can be treated with oral or intravenous corticosteroids, IVIg or other immunosuppressants. **Table 4** presents a comparison of the management guidelines for EBA recommended by the Japanese, Brazilian, and French dermatology societies.

Critical Appraisal of the Guidelines

- Treatment of EBA is difficult and often unsatisfactory. Evidence is largely based on anecdotal case reports.
- Treatment has been reported to be particularly challenging in cases with mechanobullous EBA, with poor response to immunosuppressants. The guidelines do not recommend differentiation of treatment among the inflammatory and mechanobullous subtypes.
- Nearly 20 cases of EBA with hematological malignancies have been reported, however, unlike anti-laminin 332 MMP, paraneoplastic screening is not recommended in EBA patients.

DERMATITIS HERPETIFORMIS

As per the European guidelines, diagnosis of dermatitis herpetiformis (DH) should be made if both the major criteria are fulfilled: clinical picture compatible with DH and a positive DIF on microscopy. If the clinical picture is incompatible, diagnosis cannot be made. If DIF is repeatedly negative, diagnosis can be made by the combination of minor criteria: histopathology compatible with DH, a positive serology (antibodies against transglutaminase 2, transglutaminase 3, endomysial antigen), a duodenal biopsy showing features of celiac disease, human leukocyte antigen (HLA) testing compatible with DH, a positive iodine patch test, rapid response to dapsone, and response to gluten-free diet over the long term. The Brazilian guidelines also consider DIF as the gold standard diagnostic test for DH.

Both the European and Brazilian guidelines recommend gluten-free diet (GFD) as the mainstay of management of DH. Wheat, barley, and rye should be excluded from the diet, and oats may be consumed if cross-contamination with wheat can be ruled out. Nutritional supplementation (iron, folate, calcium, vitamin D, vitamin B12) are recommended when their deficiencies are confirmed.

Dapsone is regarded as the drug of choice in both the guidelines. As cutaneous lesions have a slow response to GFD, dapsone is required for initial disease control. Serum glucose-6-phosphate dehydrogenase (G6PDH) deficiency should be ruled out prior to initiation of therapy. The Brazilian guidelines recommend a uniform starting dose of 50 mg/day in all cases, with a gradual increase to 200 mg/day as per tolerance and therapeutic response. The European guidelines recommend tailoring the initial dose as per disease severity. Patients with milder disease may be commenced on 25–50 mg/day of dapsone. A higher initial dose of 100–150 mg/day should be considered in patients with severe skin involvement and extreme pruritus. Both guidelines recommend a maximum dose of 200 mg/day and a maintenance dose of 0.5–1 mg/kg/day.

Alternative treatments recommended in patients with contraindications, intolerance and non-response to dapsone include sulfapyridine, sulfasalazine, sulfamethoxypyridazine, tetracycline, and nicotinamide. Topical steroids may be useful in the short term. The Brazilian guidelines recommend methotrexate, azathioprine, and MMF in refractory cases. Both the European and Brazilian guidelines recommend against use of systemic corticosteroids in DH due to inefficacy.

TABLE 4: Comparison of guidelines for the management of epidermolysis bullosa acquisita.

	Japanese Dermatological Association	Brazilian Society of Dermatology	French Society of Dermatology
Year	2019	2018	2011
First-line	• *Mild*: Topical corticosteroids ± colchicine/dapsone/oral corticosteroids • *Moderate/severe/resistant*: Topical corticosteroids + oral corticosteroid ± dapsone/colchicine/azathioprine/cyclophosphamide/cyclosporine/MMF/methotrexate/intravenous corticosteroids/plasma exchange/rituximab	• *Non-severe*: Colchicine or dapsone • *Severe*: IVIg + oral corticosteroids or intravenous corticosteroid pulse	• *Non-severe*: Topical corticosteroids • *Diffuse form*: Colchicine, dapsone, sulfasalazine, topical corticosteroids • *Severe*: Cyclosporine or IVIg
Second-line	• *Mild*: Manage as moderate/severe/ resistant • *Moderate/severe/resistant*: IVIg	• *Non-severe with partial response*: Systemic corticosteroids • *Severe*: Add MMF, cyclosporine or azathioprine to systemic corticosteroid	• *Non-severe*: Cyclosporine or MMF • *Severe*: Rituximab or extracorporeal photopheresis
Third-line	IVIg	• *Non-severe*: Systemic corticosteroids • *Severe*: Rituximab	*Non-severe*: IVIg, rituximab, extracorporeal photopheresis

(IVIg: intravenous immunoglobulin; MMF: mycophenolate mofetil)

Critical Appraisal of the Guidelines

Adherence to a GFD is difficult in the Indian scenario, and food items lack "gluten-free" labeling. Grains such as rice, bajra, maize, and ragi can be incorporated in meals instead of wheat, barley, and rye. The few available gluten-free cereals are expensive. Exacerbation of DH due to aerosolized wheat in an Indian farmer has been documented. As most beers are made of grains and other additives that contain gluten, they should be avoided.

A high incidence of anemia in the Indian population presents a relative contraindication to dapsone therapy. Further, dapsone is only available as a 100 mg tablet, making dose titration quite difficult. Sulfapyridine is not available in the Indian market.

MANAGEMENT OF AUTOIMMUNE BULLOUS DISEASES IN THE COVID ERA

As social distancing is among the most effective strategies in the prevention of COVID-19 infection, patients with mild disease should be followed up using teledermatology. Choice of therapy should be individualized based on disease severity, age, co-morbidities, and infection risk. Oral corticosteroids and immunosuppressants should be prescribed in a minimum necessary dose to induce and maintain remission. Immunosuppressive treatment should not be halted as interruption may lead to cytokine dysregulation, disease exacerbation, and an increased risk of viral infection and mortality. Immunosuppressants such as rituximab, MMF, and azathioprine have been associated with an increased risk of COVID-19 infection and COVID-19 related hospitalization. Dexamethasone cyclophosphamide pulse therapy may not be suitable due to requirement of hospital admission and an increased risk of exposure to COVID-19. Patients on immunosuppressants represent a susceptible population who should be monitored closely for infectious complications and should observe strict precautions in the context of the ongoing pandemic. Patients should preferably be managed via teledermatology instead of physical visits wherever possible in order to minimize risk of exposure.

New-onset AIBD and disease exacerbation after COVID-19 vaccination have been documented in literature; controlled studies to determine causality are lacking. Most exacerbations can be controlled with adjustments in immunosuppressant dosages. However, such reports should not discourage physicians from promoting vaccination among AIBD patients. Every AIBD patient without contraindications to vaccination should be administered the COVID-19 vaccine. Since the risk of COVID-19 infection and COVID-19-related hospitalization is higher in patients on immunosuppression than the broader vaccinated population, vaccination should preferably be performed while the patient is in remission or prior to initiation of the immunosuppressant. Immunosuppression should, however, not be decreased during the vaccination period due to the risk of disease exacerbation. In case of rituximab, the entire vaccination series should be completed 4 or more weeks prior to infusion, or be given 12–20 weeks after the administration of an infusion cycle.

CONCLUSION

The treatment guidelines and consensus statements for pemphigus and other AIBDs provide a valuable framework for clinicians to manage these complex and potentially life-threatening conditions. The COVID-19 pandemic has posed unique challenges for the management of AIBDs, with the need to balance disease control with the potential risks of immunosuppressive therapy and infection. The available evidence suggests that most patients with AIBDs can continue their treatment regimens during the pandemic, with appropriate precautions.

TAKE HOME MESSAGE

- Various expert groups have published guidelines and consensus statements on the management of AIBDs.
- These guidelines highlight several gaps in research, including lack of high-quality evidence from RCTs, owing to the rarity of these disorders.
- The guidelines differ in their choice of therapeutic modalities for several disorders, and integration of these would provide a physician with a wider range of suggestions regarding the optimal management of their patients.
- As there is underrepresentation of guidelines from India, some special considerations pertinent to the Indian scenario have been highlighted.
- The management of pemphigus during COVID-19 requires special considerations which may take precedence over the guidelines.

MULTIPLE CHOICE QUESTIONS

1. Which of the following is not recommended as a steroid-sparing adjuvant in pemphigus?
   - (a) Azathioprine
   - (b) Mycophenolate mofetil
   - (c) Cyclosporine
   - (d) Rituximab

2. As per the recommendations by EADV, the entire COVID-19 vaccine schedule should be completed how many weeks prior to initiation of rituximab therapy?
   - (a) 2 weeks
   - (b) 4 weeks
   - (c) 6 weeks
   - (d) 8 weeks

3. **According to the updated S2k guidelines for the management of pemphigus vulgaris, what is the recommended target dose range of prednisolone for induction therapy for severe disease?**
   (a) 0.5–1 mg/kg/day
   (b) 1–1.5 mg/kg/day
   (c) 1.5–2 mg/kg/day
   (d) 2–2.5 mg/kg/day

4. **As per the EADV guidelines, what is the recommended daily dose of topical superpotent corticosteroids in patients with extensive bullous pemphigoid?**
   (a) 10–20 g
   (b) 20–30 g
   (c) 30–40 g
   (d) 40–50 g

5. **All of the following are considered high-risk types of mucous membrane pemphigoid, *except*:**
   (a) Ocular mucous membrane pemphigoid
   (b) Nasal mucous membrane pemphigoid
   (c) Genital mucous membrane pemphigoid
   (d) Oral mucous membrane pemphigoid

6. **Detection of which of the following warrants malignancy screening in patients with mucous membrane pemphigoid?**
   (a) Anti-BP180
   (b) Anti-laminin 332
   (c) Anti α6β4 integrin
   (d) Any of the above

7. **Treatment of choice for the management of dermatitis herpetiformis is:**
   (a) Dapsone
   (b) Oral corticosteroids
   (c) Topical corticosteroids
   (d) Gluten-free diet

8. **A person on gluten-free diet may consume all of the following, *except*:**
   (a) Rice
   (b) Maize
   (c) Oats
   (d) Rye

9. **Which of the following criteria is not recommended by the current European guidelines for the diagnosis of bullous pemphigoid (BP)?**
   (a) Age > 70 years, absence of atrophic scarring, absence of mucosal involvement, absence of predominant bullous lesions on the head and neck
   (b) Positive direct immunofluorescence (DIF)
   (c) Presence of IgG antibodies binding to the epidermal side on salt-split skin on indirect immunofluorescence (IIF)
   (d) Subepidermal bullae with eosinophilic infiltrate on histopathology

10. **All of the following are accepted first-line management options for epidermolysis bullosa acquisita, *except*:**
    (a) Dapsone
    (b) Colchicine
    (c) Rituximab
    (d) Topical corticosteroids

Answers

1. (c) 2. (b) 3. (b) 4. (c) 5. (d) 6. (b) 7. (d) 8. (d) 9. (d) 10. (c)

SUGGESTED READING

1. Joly P, Horvath B, Patsatsi A, Uzun S, Bech R, Beissert S, *et al.* Updated S2K guidelines on the management of pemphigus vulgaris and foliaceus initiated by the European Academy of Dermatology and Venereology (EADV). *J Eur Acad Dermatol Venereol.* 2020;34:1900-13.

2. Borradori L, Van Beek N, Feliciani C, Tedbirt B, Antiga E, Bergman R, *et al.* Updated S2 K guidelines for the management of bullous pemphigoid initiated by the European Academy of Dermatology and Venereology (EADV). *J Eur Acad Dermatol Venereol.* 2022;36:1689-704.

3. Schmidt E, Rashid H, Marzano AV, Lamberts A, Di Zenzo G, Diercks GFH, *et al.* European Guidelines (S3) on diagnosis and management of mucous membrane pemphigoid, initiated by the European Academy of Dermatology and Venereology - Part II. *J Eur Acad Dermatol Venereol.* 2021;35:1926-48.

4. Ujiie H, Iwata H, Yamagami J, Nakama T, Aoyama Y, Ikeda S, *et al.* Committee for Guidelines for the Management of Pemphigoid Diseases (Including Epidermolysis Bullosa Acquisita). Japanese guidelines for the management of pemphigoid (including epidermolysis bullosa acquisita). *J Dermatol.* 2019;46:1102-35.

5. Santi CG, Gripp AC, Roselino AM, Mello DS, Gordilho JO, Marsillac PF, *et al.* Consensus on the treatment of autoimmune bullous dermatoses: Bullous pemphigoid, mucous membrane pemphigoid and epidermolysis bullosa acquisita - Brazilian Society of Dermatology. *An Bras Dermatol.* 2019;94:33-47.

6. Görög A, Antiga E, Caproni M, Cianchini G, De D, Dmochowski M, *et al.* S2k guidelines (consensus statement) for diagnosis and therapy of dermatitis herpetiformis initiated by the European Academy of Dermatology and Venereology (EADV). *J Eur Acad Dermatol Venereol.* 2021;35:1251-77.

7. Vale ECSD, Dimatos OC, Porro AM, Santi CG. Consensus on the treatment of autoimmune bullous dermatoses: dermatitis herpetiformis and linear IgA bullous dermatosis - Brazilian Society of Dermatology. *An Bras Dermatol.* 2019;94:48-55.

8. Kasperkiewicz M, Schmidt E, Amagai M, Fairley JA, Joly P, Murrell DF, *et al.* Updated international expert recommendations for the management of autoimmune bullous diseases during the COVID-19 pandemic. *J Eur Acad Dermatol Venereol.* 2021;35: e412-4.

Nursing Care in Autoimmune Bullous Diseases

Rochelle C Monteiro, Amitha Ramesh, Ramesh Bhat M

- Nursing care, compresses, and dressings
  - Goals of wound management
  - Maintenance of barrier function
  - Management of moist/exudative erosions
  - Dressings
- Management of extensive skin involvement and acute skin failure
- Care of the mucosae
- Periodontal therapy

INTRODUCTION

Current advances in therapeutics have made the management of disorders with high mortality easier to accomplish. However, in dermatologic disorders, especially in autoimmune bullous diseases (AIBDs), primary skin care with optimum aseptic barrier maintenance, is the most important step in the management. A well-trained nursing team with adequate support from other specialties, especially critical care units, general physicians, otolaryngologists, ophthalmologists, dentists, etc., is pertinent for care of these patients. Healing of skin erosions depends on barrier care, methods of dressing/soaks used, and prevention of infection.

In this chapter, we will enumerate all these supportive modalities, which although labeled supportive, form the backbone of management of these disorders. We will also discuss the management of acute skin failure, a serious complication of this group of disorders.

NURSING CARE, COMPRESSES, AND DRESSINGS

An active case of AIBD especially of the pemphigus group, produces extensive cutaneous erosions due to skin fragility. Therefore, careful handling of cutaneous surfaces is of paramount importance. Educating the doctors, dermatology nurses, and family members is necessary. It is equally essential to pay attention to fluid and electrolyte balance, thermoregulation, prevention of secondary infection due to breach in barrier function, prevention of further skin trauma, management of pain, and nutritional and psychological support.

Goals of Wound Management

The goals of wound management include:
- Protection of wound
- Prevent secondary infection
- Maintain a moist environment
- Minimize scarring

Maintenance of Barrier Function

Maintaining the barrier function in patients with AIBDs is necessary to reduce transcutaneous water loss and encourage skin re-epithelialization. A bland emollient containing equal amounts of soft white paraffin and liquid paraffin is preferred. It is applied to the whole skin including the erosions. Emollients can be applied directly on the skin or over the primary dressings. The principle of using dressings is to provide moisture in dry wounds and absorb excess exudate in weepy lesions. Aerosolized preparations of emollients are preferred if available, as they prevent shearing off of the skin during application. Emollients containing irritants and sensitizers should be avoided.

Management of Moist/Exudative Erosions

Soaks are helpful in patients with moist, oozy, and crusted erosions. Potassium permanganate ($KMnO_4$) soaks as 1:10,000 solution (Condy's compress/soak) can be used, which is prepared by adding a 400 mg tablet in 4 L of water, to form a light pink-colored solution that matches the pink color of the nail bed **(Fig. 1)**. $KMnO_4$ crystals can also be dissolved in water to prepare the soaks. During preparation of the soaks, metallic containers should be avoided and caution should be exercised that no crystals

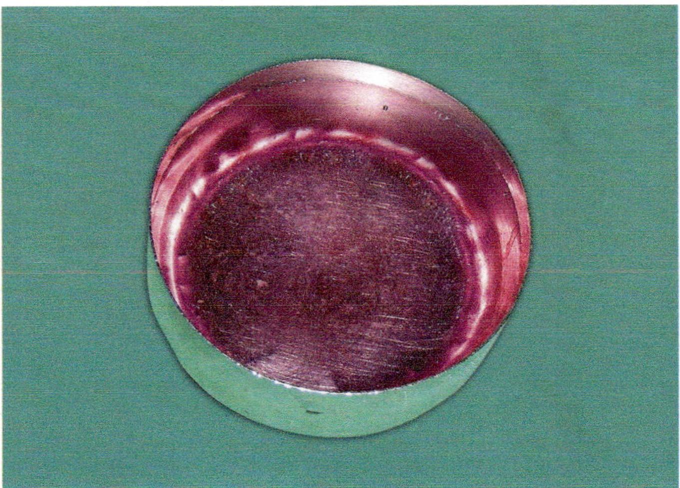

Fig. 1: Condy's solution: Potassium permanganate diluted 1:10,000 to light pink color for use as soaks to remove crusts.

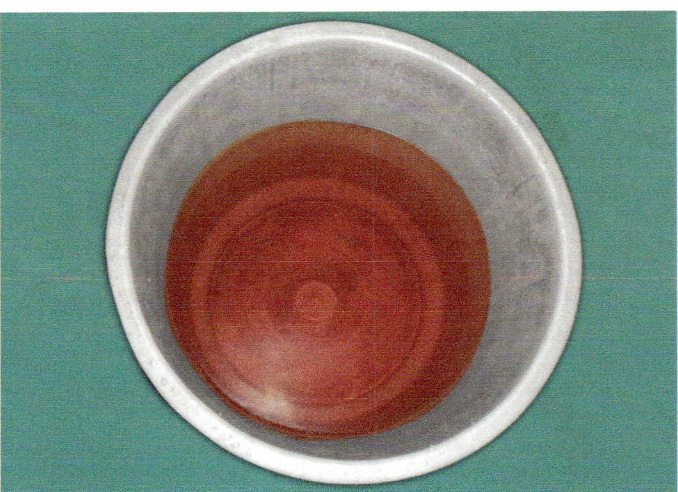

Fig. 2: Condy's bath: Potassium permanganate solution prepared in a bucket for taking bath by patients with extensive erosions and crusting.

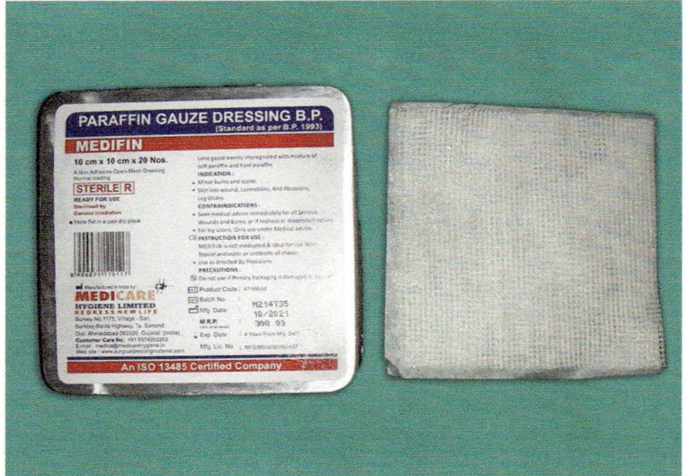

Fig. 3: Paraffin gauze: It is used as a primary dressing over the erosions.

Fig. 4: Gauze pad: It is used as a secondary dressing over the primary dressing to absorb exudate.

remain undissolved at the bottom of the container. Soaks are applied for a maximum of 15 minutes, after which they become ineffective due to oxidation of the product. For treating large areas, baths (Condy's bath) are more practical **(Fig. 2)**. Patient counseling is essential when using this modality as the discoloration produced may cause distress to some patients. They should be explained about the temporary nature of discoloration. To prevent discoloration of the nails, they may be covered with soft white paraffin before soaking in Condy's solution.

Other applications such as paraffin gauze **(Fig. 3)** or dressing pads **(Fig. 4)** can be directly applied on the crusted erosions.

Dressings

The role of dressings is to reduce fluid loss, prevent secondary infection, and decrease pain. The selection of an appropriate dressing must take into account the wound characteristics and specific features of the dressings, such as hydrating quality, absorptive capacity, adhesive quality, and comfortability.

There is no clear consensus on the superiority of any dressing, however, non-adherent dressings are preferred. Prevention of fluid loss is accomplished by using moisture-retentive dressings, either occlusive or semi-occlusive.

Types of Dressings

Dressings can be of the following types **(Fig. 5 and Table 1)**:
- ***Sterile paraffin gauze***: It maintains a humid environment, prevents drying of the erosions, and is non-adherent **(Fig. 3)**. In addition, it promotes pain reduction, provides more mobility and comfort to the patient, and improves sleeping patterns. It should be changed every day and the erosions cleaned with normal saline (NS).
- ***Films***: These are thin, elastic, see-through dressings, available in various shapes and sizes conforming to the wound dimensions. They are mainly composed of polyurethane. They can be used on erosions and superficial ulcers. Non-adherent films should be used.

Advantages: They provide an excellent barrier to bacterial invasion and are waterproof, but provide a one-way exit for excess moisture and CO_2.

Disadvantages: They are non-absorbent, thus their use is limited to minimally exudative and superficial erosions.

- **Hydrogel dressings:** They are available in two forms: sheets and amorphous form. They are composed mainly of water (97%) and polyethylene. They are non-adherent, so may require a secondary dressing such as a xeroform gauze or film for stabilization and moisture retention.

Advantages: Due to high moisture content, they are particularly useful in dry wounds and have a soothing and cooling effect on the skin.

Disadvantages: They cannot be used on infected or heavily exudative wounds as they are non-absorbent.

- **Polymeric membrane dressings (PMDs):** They are multi-functional dressings composed of a hydrophilic polyurethane membrane matrix backed by a continuous semipermeable polyurethane film. They are used in superficial erosions.

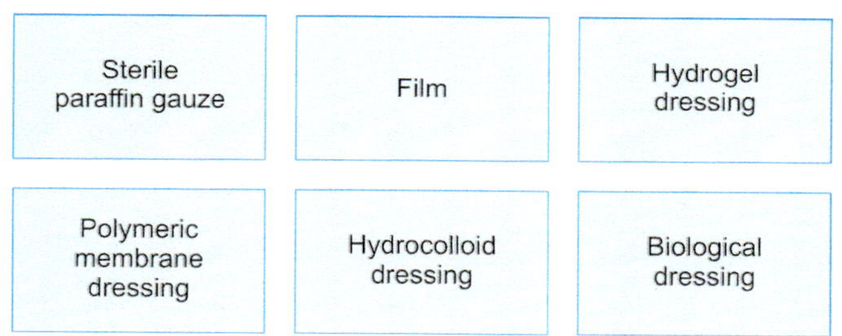

Fig. 5: Types of dressings used in autoimmune bullous diseases.

Advantages: They contain ingredients that work together to promote debridement and wound healing.

- **Hydrocolloid dressings:** They are available as sheets and in gel form, the main composition of which is carboxymethyl cellulose, gelatin, and pectin (**Figs. 6 and 7**). The sheet hydrocolloid dressing has two layers, an internal layer and an external semipermeable layer.

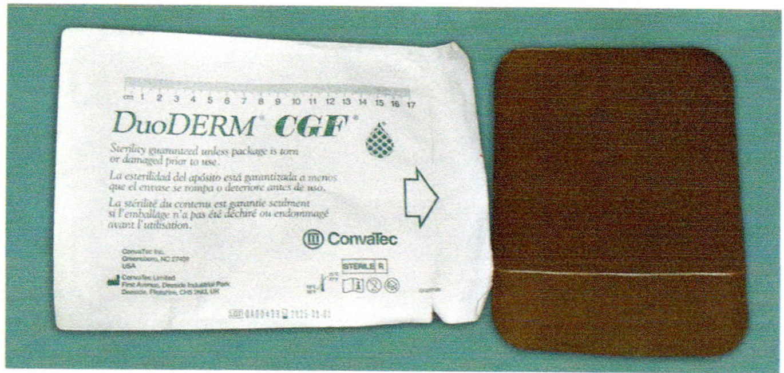

Fig. 6: Hydrocolloid dressing, adhesive side up: It is a waterproof, absorptive dressing for exudative wounds.

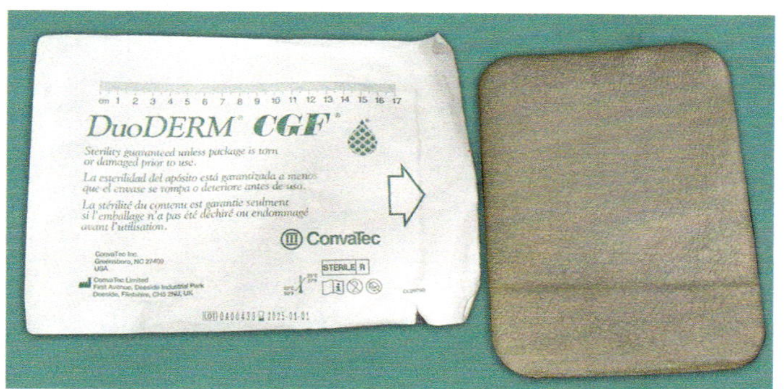

Fig. 7: Hydrocolloid dressing, absorptive side up: It is a waterproof, absorptive dressing for exudative wounds.

TABLE 1: Types of dressings used in autoimmune bullous diseases.

Type of dressing	Advantages	Disadvantages	Some available brands	Price in INR (size)
Sterile vaseline/ paraffin gauze	• Non-adherent • Prevents dryness • Reduces pain	Has to be changed every day	• JELONET™-10 no. • Medrop™ • Medifin™-20 no.	• 744 (10 × 10 cm) • 399 (10 × 10 cm) • 640 (10 × 10 cm)
Film	• Excellent barrier • Waterproof • Allows inspection of wound	• Non-absorbent • Use is limited to minimally exudative, superficial wounds	• Tegaderm™ HP + Pad film (8582IN)™ • Velflix™-TPad (5510)™	• 145 • 266 (10 × 30 cm)
Hydrogel dressing	Useful in dry wounds due to high moisture content	Non-absorbent hence cannot be used in infected/exudative wounds	McKesson™	307 (4 × 4 inch)—available online
Polymeric membrane dressing	Promotes debridement and wound healing	Expensive	• PolyMem™ • DuoDERM™	• 7,663 (4 × 4 inch), 15 no. • 8,714 (4 × 4 inch), 10 no.
Hydrocolloid dressing	• Waterproof • Absorptive • Painless debridement	• Skin shearing due to the adhesive • Contact dermatitis	• Smith & Nephew™ • Convatec DuoDERM™	• 9,528 (1.5 × 2.5 inch), 30 no. • 1,430 (10 × 10 cm), 10 no.
Biological dressing	Cheap, easy to procure; collagen-based ones have limited availability and are expensive	• Non-absorbent • Has to be changed frequently	Kollagen™	1625 (15 x 30 cm) per unit

Advantages: They are absorptive, help in painless debridement, need not be changed for several days and so are cost-effective.

Disadvantages: They have the potential to cause contact dermatitis, and the adhesive content in them causes the skin to shear off. Caution: They produce a malodorous yellow gel on the inside which can be confused for infection.

- ***Biological dressings:*** Sterile banana leaves **(Fig. 8)**, potato peels and amnion are the various biological dressings available. Collagen-based skin substitutes have limited availability and are expensive **(Figs. 9A and B)**.
- ***Others:*** Plastic sheets coated with unsaturated fatty acid, which is well absorbed by the body, inhibits free radicals that prevent healing, has potent antioxidant action, and protects the skin DNA.

Method of Doing Dressing in Eroded Skin

For the primary dressing, a soft silicone mesh dressing is preferred, which is coated with an emollient such as a 50:50 mix of soft white paraffin and liquid paraffin, or in some cases, a topical antimicrobial. The secondary dressing should be an absorbent, e.g., soft silicon foam or foam dressing. A knitted tube dressing may aid in optimal securing of the dressing. In resource-poor settings, sterile paraffin gauze can be used as the primary dressing over erosions **(Fig. 10)**, and an absorbent gauze pad **(Fig. 4)** as the secondary dressing.

Fixed guidelines that dictate the frequency of change of dressings do not exist. Factors that should be considered while deciding this include, the stage of wound healing, presence of infection, and the appearance of strikethrough (a breach in barrier of the dressing such that bacteria go

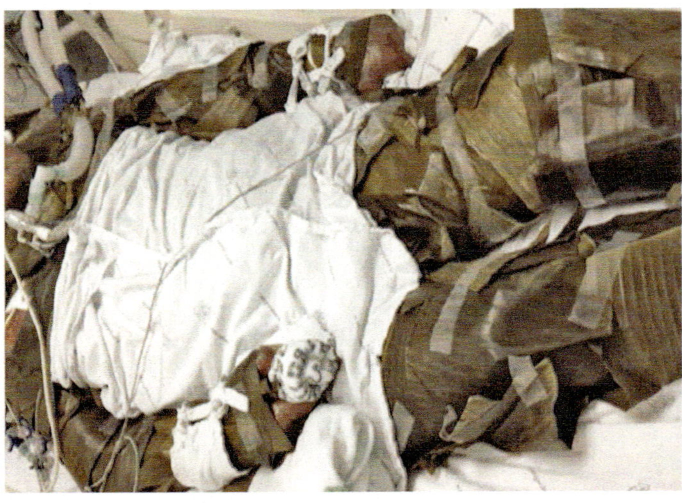

Fig. 8: Banana leaf dressing: Indigenously prepared biological dressing to promote re-epithelialization of wounds, often used over extensive skin erosions.

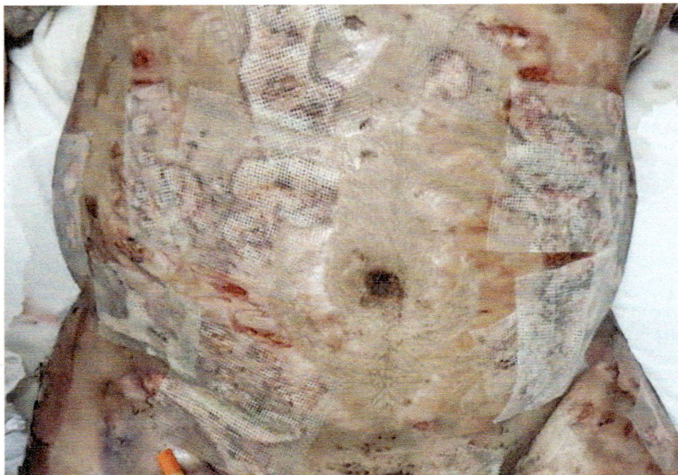

Fig. 10: Paraffin gauze dressing (primary dressing) applied over erosions in pemphigus vulgaris.

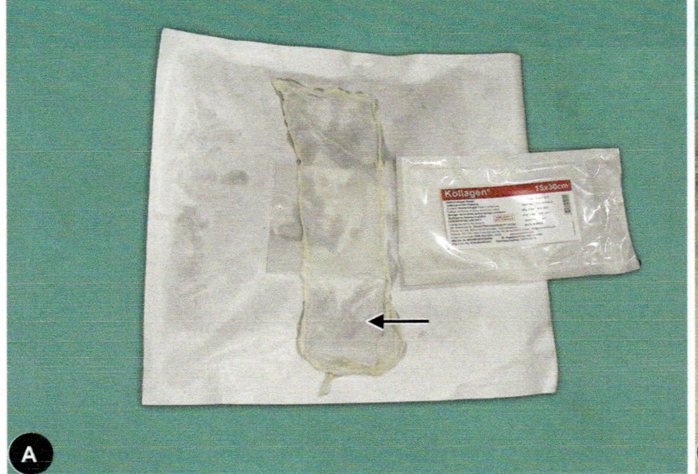

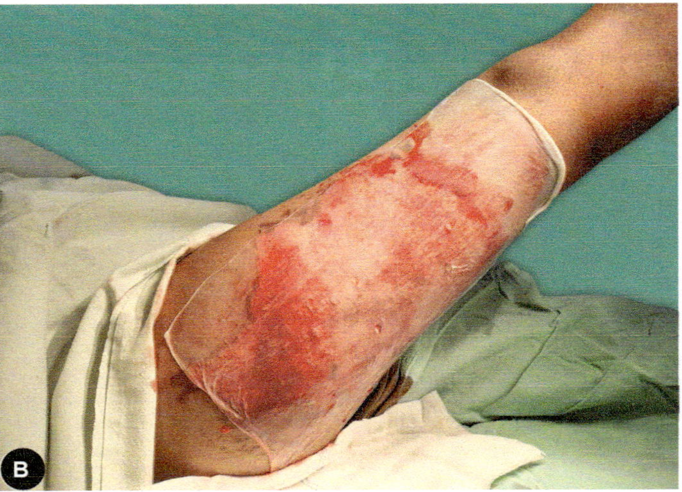

Figs. 9A and B: Collagen dressing: (A) A biological dressing (arrow) used on erosions and wounds. (B) Collagen dressing applied on extensive erosion on the limb.

down the dressing to the wound bed) over the secondary dressing. Thus, in the acute stage, daily change of dressing may be warranted. Toward the later stages of healing, it may be advised to change only the secondary dressing while leaving the primary dressing in place so that erosions may heal undisturbed. If further topical applications are required, they can be applied over the primary dressing.

Crusts must be removed to facilitate healing. The removal of dressings is as critical as the application process. If the dressing has dried and adheres to the skin surface, it should be soaked in saline and gently removed to prevent further shearing.

Pain control is an essential part of wound care and should not be trivialized; taking help from a pain management team is advisable.

Care of the Dressing

Dressings should be changed using aseptic precautions. In patients with extensive erosions, barrier nursing methods must be employed. It is vital to look for signs of infection as it can lead to sepsis causing significant morbidity and even mortality. Infection also increases the risk of scarring. If the patient is sick, a swab must be sent for bacterial and viral cultures, supplemented with blood culture. It is important to clean the dressing daily with an antimicrobial solution like povidone-iodine, but use of topical antimicrobials should be limited to short periods. Systemic antibiotics should be started whenever clinically deemed necessary, i.e., at the earliest sign of local or systemic infection.

Management of Blisters

Intact bullae should not be de-roofed as they can compromise barrier function of the epidermis. The recommendation is to decompress the bulla by piercing it, with the roof left intact, which serves as a biological dressing. Prior analgesia can be offered to patients sensitive to pain as the procedure may cause discomfort. Maintaining a daily blister chart is recommended to monitor disease progression in the acute phase.

The steps for decompressing a bulla are as follows:
- Gently sterilize the area over and around the bulla with an antimicrobial solution, ensuring it does not rupture.
- Using a sterile needle with the bevel facing upward, pierce the bulla at the base, at a site that will ensure fluid drainage by gravity. In case of a large bulla, using a wide-bore needle and multiple piercings may be necessary.
- Sterile gauze swabs can be used to compress the bulla and ensure drainage and absorption of the fluid.
- It is vital to ensure that the bulla is not de-roofed.
- After draining the contents of the bulla, it is gently cleaned with an antimicrobial solution such as povidone-iodine.
- Application of a non-adherent dressing like sterile paraffin gauze may be necessary after draining the contents of the bulla.

MANAGEMENT OF EXTENSIVE SKIN INVOLVEMENT AND ACUTE SKIN FAILURE

The management of extensive skin involvement and acute skin failure is a complex task and involves certain principles **(Flowchart 1)**.

Establishing a skin intensive care unit (ICU), or at least a high dependency unit (HDU) or an isolation room for barrier nursing is important, since in severe disease with extensive skin involvement, acute skin failure can occur. This produces complications such as hypothermia, electrolyte imbalance, hypovolemia, renal insufficiency, and sepsis.

Risk factors for developing skin failure are:
- Increasing age
- Increased body surface area (BSA) of involvement
- Patients with bowel or bladder incontinence
- Immunocompromised patients, or patients with multiple co-morbidities

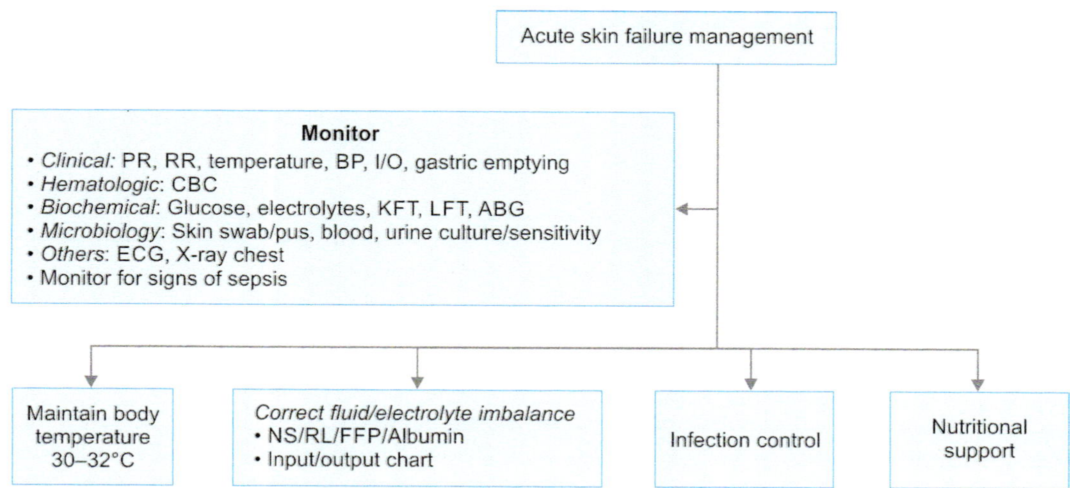

Flowchart 1: Management of extensive skin involvement and acute skin failure in autoimmune bullous diseases.
(ABG: arterial blood gas; BP: blood pressure; CBC: complete blood count; ECG: electrocardiogram; FFP: fresh frozen plasma; I/O: fluid input/output; KFT: kidney function test; LFT: liver function test; NS: normal saline; PR: pulse rate; RL: Ringer's lactate; RR: respiratory rate)

The principles of management of acute skin failure in extensive AIBDs include:

- **Initial assessment of the extent and severity of skin and mucosal involvement:** This helps in the overall management.
- **Periodic monitoring of the patient:** The important parameters that must be monitored regularly are as follows:
  - *Clinical:* Pulse and respiratory rate, body temperature, blood pressure, urine output, gastric emptying
  - *Hematological:* Total and differential count, platelet count
  - *Biochemical:* Blood glucose, serum electrolytes, liver and renal function tests, serum proteins, arterial blood gas
  - *Microbiological:* Culture/sensitivity of skin lesions, blood and urine culture
  - *Others:* X-ray chest, electrocardiogram
  - *Monitoring for signs of sepsis:* Change in mental status or decreasing consciousness, decrease in urine output, sudden hypothermia with hypotension and tachycardia, fever or rigors after the fourth day in a euthermic patient, reduced respiratory rate or gastric emptying.
- **Maintenance of body temperature:** To prevent hypothermia, an ideal room temperature of 30–32°C should be maintained. This can be achieved by using an infrared lamp, steamer, or a burn cage (**Figs. 11 and 12**).
- **Management of fluid and electrolyte imbalance:** In patients with ≥50% BSA involvement, fluid loss can be ≥4–5 L/day. It is therefore pertinent to quickly replenish intravascular fluid loss. A daily input–output charting and body weight monitoring should be performed. An intravenous (IV) line should be inserted in all cases at admission, and urinary catheter in required cases.
- **Prevention and treatment of wound infection:** Patients with extensive erosions bear a threat of superimposed infection due to breakdown of skin barrier, or treatment-associated immune suppression. *Staphylococcus aureus* skin infection is the most frequent cause of septicemia and death in these patients. Secondary bacterial infection impairs wound healing and increases recovery time, resulting in refractoriness to therapy. Therefore, prevention of wound infection is critical for recovery. Patients should be educated about the warning signs of early infection and instructed not to open or drain blisters.

Signs of wound infection include erythema, raised local temperature, tenderness, edema, and increased wound discharge, which may be purulent and malodorous. If a wound infection is suspected, culture and sensitivity profile of skin swab or pus should be performed. Quantitative swabs are helpful, and culturing of 1×10^6 organisms/g of tissue indicates infection. It is a reliable method for quantifying the number of viable bacteria. In open wounds, the swab bacterial count correlates well with the bacterial count obtained from a tissue biopsy. These swabs are inoculated into blood agar. The results are reported as 1+, 2+, 3+ or 4+, or as trace, few, moderate or abundant. However, it is also important to recognize that presence of bacteria in the wound does not always mean infection. It may be attributed to (1) contamination: bacteria are present on the surface without clinical disease; (2) colonization: bacteria multiply on the surface without signs and symptoms of infection; (3) infection: bacterial proliferation with local host reaction, delay in healing and tissue damage.

Blood and urine cultures are also sent in addition to skin swab cultures.

Topical antiseptics that may be used to cleanse infected lesions are eusol solution (Edinburgh University solution—1.25 g boric acid, 1.25 g bleaching powder, 100 mL sterile water), acetic acid (1–5%), and Dakin's solution (a mixture of sodium hypochlorite 0.4–0.5%,

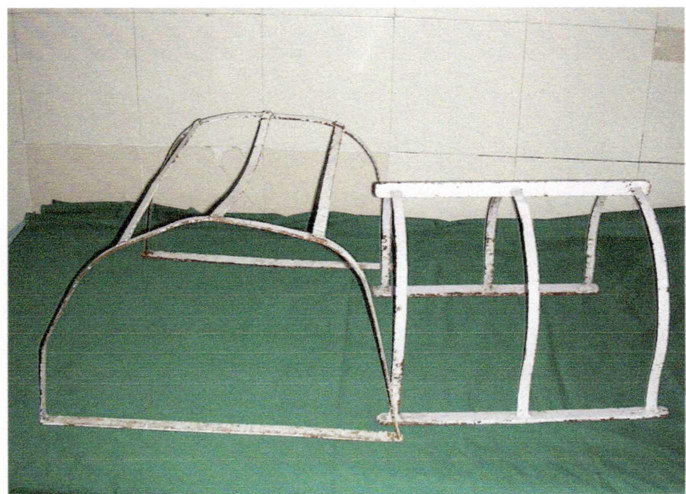

Fig. 11: Burn cage.

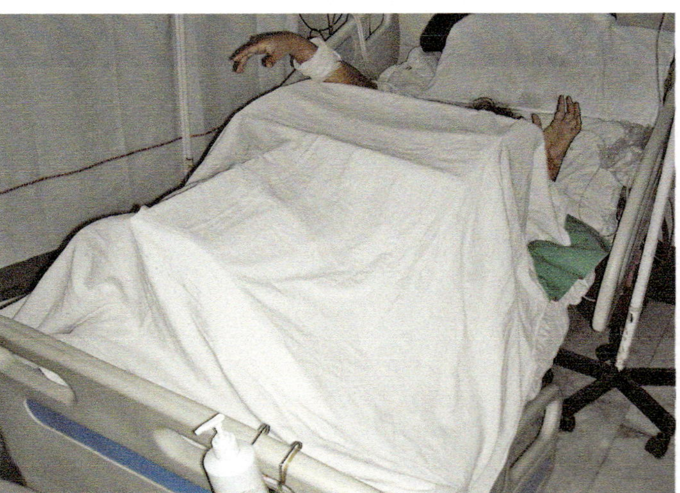

Fig. 12: Burn cage: A patient of severe pemphigus vulgaris being covered with it for thermoregulation and to prevent erosions from sticking to the sheets.

boric acid 4%, diluted in water). Among the topical antimicrobials, both mupirocin and retapamulin are effective against gram-positive organisms, and topical metronidazole is effective against anaerobic organisms. These agents are applied directly to the wound bed.

Iodine and silver-based dressings **(Figs. 13A and B)** are non-cytotoxic, and preferred for infected wounds. Cadexomer iodine dressing (Iodoflex) is bactericidal against both gram-positive and gram-negative bacteria and fungi, and hastens wounds healing. In addition, it provides a moist environment for healing. Silver is a broad-spectrum, microbicidal agent. Their antimicrobial action is due to release of silver ions, for which a moist environment is essential. Traditional silver dressings were found to be cytotoxic. Hence, newer dressings such as PMD with silver (sterizone dressing; Ferris Polymem silver) are preferred nowadays.

Local treatment can be undertaken for 2 weeks followed by re-evaluation of the wound, and an appropriate decision regarding continuation of local treatment, or switching to more aggressive broad-spectrum, systemic antibiotic therapy (covering gram-positive and gram-negative organisms) especially if sepsis is setting in.

In addition, daily cleansing and removal of crusts from the oral, nasal, genital, and ocular mucosa are important.

- **Fluid Replacement:**
  Calculation of fluid replacement: Parkland's formula used in the setting of acute burns, can be used to calculate fluid requirement.

Fluid requirement in first 24 hours = 4 mL × total body weight × %BSA involved

About half to three quarters of the estimated requirement is given as there is overestimation of fluid requirement with this formula, and overcorrection of hypovolemia can result in pulmonary edema. Half of this is given in the first 8 hours and the remaining half over the next 16 hours.

In the initial 24 hours, the preferred fluids are normal saline (NS) 0.7 mL/kg, Ringer's lactate, or human albumin (diluted in NS, 40 g/L) 1 mL/kg body weight per %BSA (if the involved BSA is >40%).

- *Maintenance fluids*: Thereafter, the choice of fluid is governed by the previous day's output. The fluids should be gradually decreased. NS is the fluid of choice for maintenance.

The total requirement of maintenance fluid is calculated to maintain an ideal urine output of 1 mL/kg/h (approximately 1,500 mL/day).

The formula for maintenance fluid: Input of previous day (oral feeds + IV fluids) + 1,500 mL – urine output of previous day.

In case of electrolyte imbalance, potassium phosphate is supplemented in the initial 24 hours. In patients with hypokalemia, injection potassium chloride, 40 mmol/L in 5% dextrose saline or 5% dextrose/NS is administered. NS 500 mL/day, is also used to manage hypokalemia.

- **Nutritional support:**
  Nasogastric feeding: In cases where it is indicated, initially 1,500–2,000 mL in the first 24 hours is given, which provides 1,500–2,000 kcal. Thereafter it can be progressively increased by 500 kcal/day up to 3,000–4,000 kcal/day.

The caloric requirement is calculated based on the formula: 25 kcal/kg + 40 kcal per %BSA involved, to be given daily. Protein supplementation is calculated as: 1 g/kg + 3 g per %BSA involved, given daily. In general, the caloric requirements are 30–35 kcal/kg/day, and protein requirement is 1.5 g/kg/day.

Hot, cold, and acidic foods are preferably avoided, and soft, bland meals are preferred. Locally available foods such as mashed banana/rice/potato, dal, soft-boiled vegetables, and porridge provide adequate nutrition and are easily palatable. The addition of ghee and jaggery increases palatability, the oil coats the gastric mucosa and also aids in the absorption of fat-soluble vitamins.

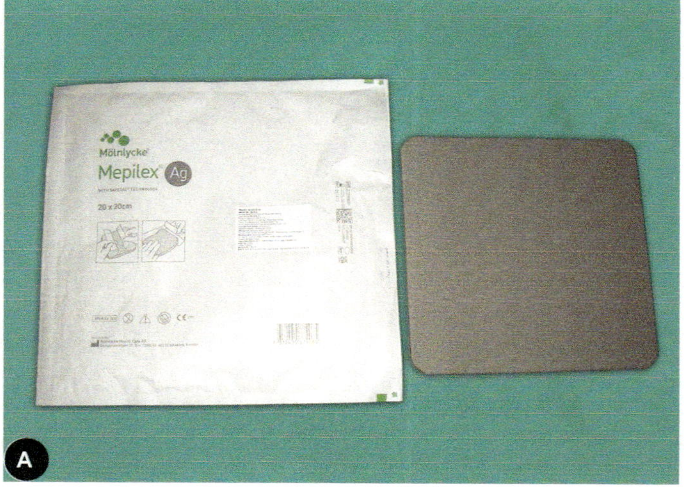
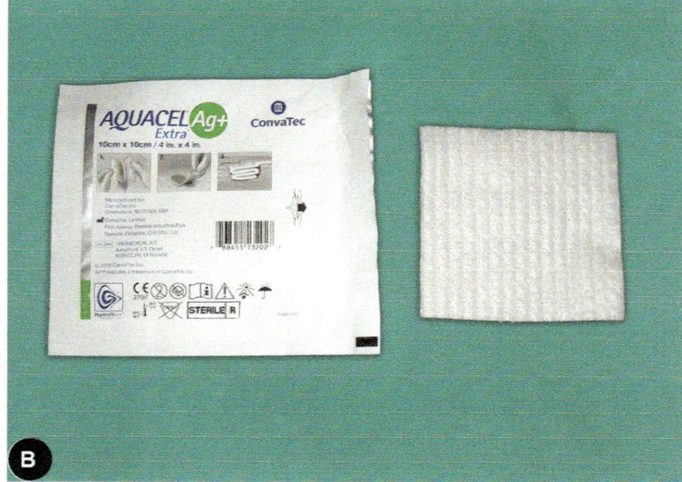

Figs. 13A and B: Silver dressing: It is used on infected wounds.

In hypokalemia, milk, fruit juice, coconut water, honey, and potassium chloride syrup can be supplemented. Optimum supplementation of essential fatty acids and micronutrients should be done.

CARE OF THE MUCOSAE

- *Care of the eyes*: Eyelids should be cleaned with saline wipes from one end to the other. Regular lubrication of the ocular surface with ointments and artificial tears is essential to prevent synechiae. A glass rod or cellulose sponge spear is used to sweep the fornices under local anesthesia, especially in ocular pemphigoid if adhesions form.
- *Nasal and respiratory mucosa*: Use of NS nasal drops aids in softening and loosening of the nasal crusts; pooling of saliva and secretions in the throat can potentially cause aspiration, hence they should be cleared regularly, sometimes with a suction apparatus.
- *Genital mucosa*: Regular examination of the genital mucosa is advocated. Application of white soft paraffin to both the mucosal surfaces in females can prevent synechiae. Urethral catheterization prevents formation of urethral strictures.
- *Oral mucosa*: Oral cavity hygiene must be maintained.
  - Brush with a pediatric toothbrush and fluorinated toothpaste twice daily.
  - Rinsing the mouth with diluted chlorhexidine 0.12% mouthwash **(Fig. 14)** or 2% povidone-iodine mouthwash/gargle **(Fig. 15)**, is recommended.
  - Mouthwashes containing non-steroidal anti-inflammatory drugs (NSAIDs) like benzydamine hydrochloride (e.g., maxtra gargle, mucobenz) are preferred for pain relief.
  - Alternately, rinsing the mouth with 5 mL of betamethasone elixir and/or triamcinolone suspension can be done.
  - Triamcinolone acetonide, 0.1% paste/gel in orabase, may be applied locally on the erosions, with avoidance of food or water for about 2 hours after application.
  - The efficacy of topical tacrolimus ointment has been found to be comparable to topical steroid.
  - Cyclosporin mouthwash/oral suspension (100 mg/mL), 5 mL used three times per day, is effective
  - Topical prostaglandin E2 (PGE2) has been used successfully in some cases of oral pemphigus
  - Whenever lips are involved, saline compresses help to remove crusts, followed by application of white soft paraffin
  - Prophylactic use of 1% w/v clotrimazole mouth paint is recommended to prevent oral candidiasis

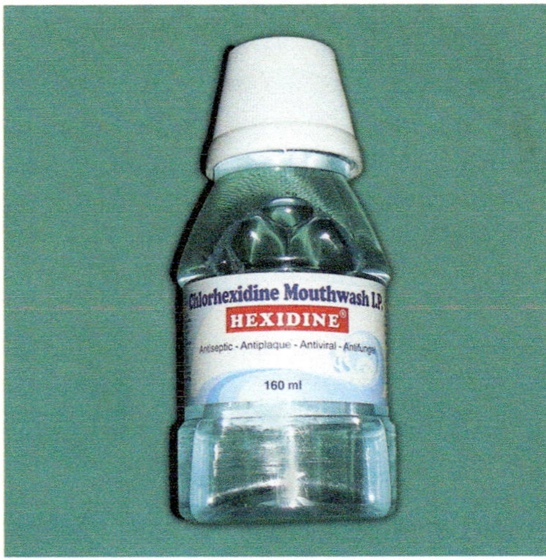

Fig. 14: Chlorhexidine mouthwash: To rinse oral cavity in patients with oral erosions.

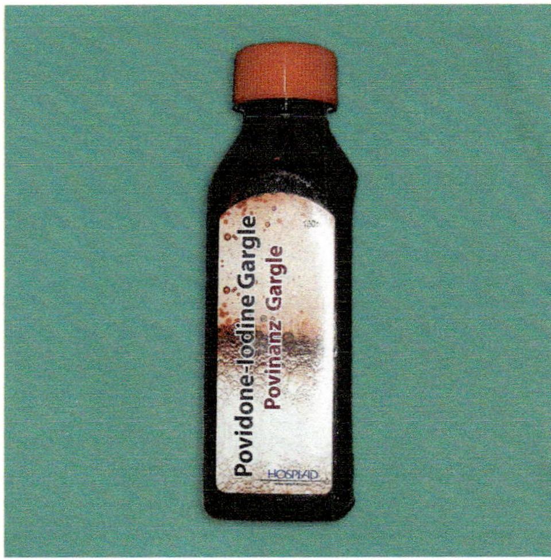

Fig. 15: Povidone-iodine mouthwash: To rinse oral cavity and do gargles in patients with oral erosions.

PERIODONTAL THERAPY

In conjunction with medical therapy, elimination of trauma and infection is beneficial for patients with oral manifestations; in this context, non-surgical periodontal therapy consisting of scaling and root planning, and effective bacterial plaque control is important.

AIBDs cause pain and blister formation in the oral cavity. These patients tend not to remove plaques adequately in painful areas or in those sites where blisters appear more easily. This causes gingival inflammation with further plaque deposits and increase in pain. Therefore, these patients must undergo professional oral hygiene appointments every 3–4 months to avoid these issues.

Carious/jagged teeth should also be promptly extracted.

CONCLUSION

Along with specific drug therapy, barrier nursing, management of mucosae, fluid replacement, prevention of secondary infection and astute management of acute skin failure form the cornerstone in the management of AIBDs. Optimum selection of the type of dressing is paramount in early recovery. A multidisciplinary team comprising various specialties will aid in early recovery and reduce morbidity and mortality for the patient.

TAKE HOME MESSAGE

- In patients with extensive skin loss secondary to bullous disorders, the goals of therapy are to restore barrier function, prevent secondary infection, and maintain adequate nutrition and electrolyte balance.
- Soaks and dressings form the main supportive skin therapy; soaks help to remove crusts and absorb excessive fluid in oozy lesions, while dressings help to maintain adequate skin hydration, prevent skin infection, and reduce pain.
- The choice of dressing depends on wound characteristics, and specific features of the dressing.
- Acute skin failure is a dermatologic emergency and should be managed in an ICU or burns unit, or if unavailable, at least an HDU or an isolation room for barrier nursing.
- Adequate care of the mucosae is very important.
- In addition to nursing and supportive care, pain management and counseling of the patients and their family members is vital.

MULTIPLE CHOICE QUESTIONS

1. **The following statement about emollients is true, *except*:**
   (a) Emollients should be applied over normal and eroded skin
   (b) A bland preparation is preferred
   (c) Creams are preferred to aerosols
   (d) Emollients containing irritants and sensitizers should be avoided

2. **A non-absorbent type of dressing preferred in superficial erosions is:**
   (a) Films
   (b) Hydrocolloid dressing
   (c) Hydrogel dressing
   (d) Polymeric membrane dressing

3. **The following is bactericidal against gram-positive and negative organisms and fungi:**
   (a) Mupirocin
   (b) Retapamulin
   (c) Cadexomer iodine
   (d) Metronidazole

4. **All of the following are signs of sepsis, *except*:**
   (a) Tachycardia
   (b) Reduced urine output
   (c) Increase in respiratory rate
   (d) Hypotension

5. **The following topical agents are used in the management of oral lesions in pemphigus:**
   (a) Benzydamine hydrochloride
   (b) Diluted chlorhexidine 0.12% mouthwash
   (c) Clotrimazole
   (d) All of the above

6. **Dakin's solution contains all, *except*:**
   (a) Sodium hypochlorite 0.4–0.5%
   (b) Boric acid 4%
   (c) Water
   (d) Bleaching powder

7. **EUSOL has the following constituents, *except*:**
   (a) 1.25 g boric acid
   (b) 1.25 g bleaching powder
   (c) Sterile water
   (d) Sodium hypochlorite, 0.5%

8. **The caloric and protein requirement in a patient with extensive skin disease are:**
   (a) 10 kcal/kg/day and 0.5 g/kg/day
   (b) 30–35 kcal/kg/day and 1.5 g/kg/day
   (c) 60–70 kcal/kg/day and 3 mg/kg/day
   (d) 100 kcal/kg/day and 1 mg/kg/day

9. **In the initial 24 hours of fluid management in a patient with extensive skin erosions, the preferred fluids are:**
   (a) Dextrose, dextrose saline or Ringer's lactate
   (b) Ringer's lactate, dextrose or normal saline
   (c) Normal saline, Ringer's lactate or human albumin
   (d) Dextrose, human albumin or normal saline

10. **Which formula is used in the setting of acute burns to calculate the fluid requirement?**
    (a) Parkland
    (b) Saraswat
    (c) Eular
    (d) Fitzpatrick

Answers

1. (c) 2. (a) 3. (c) 4. (c) 5. (d) 6. (d) 7. (d) 8. (b) 9. (c) 10. (a)

SUGGESTED READING

1. Harman KE, Brown D, Exton LS, Groves RW, Hampton PJ, Md Mustapa MF, *et al*. British Association of Dermatologists' guidelines for the management of pemphigus vulgaris 2017. *Br J Dermatol*. 2017;177:1170-201.

2. Norman RA, Coatney G. Acute skin failure: concept, causes, consequences, and care. In: Wolf R, Davidovici B, Parish J, Parish L (Eds). Emergency Dermatology. Cambridge, England: Cambridge University Press; 2011. pp. 62-5.

3. Valeyrie-Allanore L, Oro S, Roujeau JC. Acute skin failure. In: Revuz J, Roujeau JC, Kerdel FA, Valeyrie-Allanore L (Eds). Life-threatening Dermatoses and Emergencies in Dermatology. Berlin: Springer; 2009. pp. 45-56.

4. George NM, Potlapati A, Shivanna R. Fluid and diet management in acute skin failure. *Clin Dermatol Rev*. 2022;6:1-5.

5. Inamadar AC, Palit A. Acute skin failure: concept, causes, consequences and care. *Indian J Dermatol Venereol Leprol*. 2005;71:379-85.

6. Vaishampayan SS, Senger SS, Lachhiramani RR, Gupta A. Acute skin failure. In: Vasudevan B, Verma R (Eds). Dermatological Emergencies, 1st edition. Boca Raton: CRC press; 2019. pp. 9-20.

7. Grada A, Obagi Z, Phillips T. Management of chronic wounds in patients with pemphigus. *Chronic Wound Care Manag Res*. 2019;6:89-98.

Index

Page numbers followed by *f* refer to figure, *fc* refer to flowchart, and *t* refer to table.

I